Contemporary Sleep Medicine
For Physicians

Editor

Octavian C. Ioachimescu

Guest Editor

Teofilo Lee-Chiong

Motto: *Nullius in verba. Per ardua ad astra.*

eBooks End User License Agreement

DEDICATION

With great gratitude for what they have done for me, for their unconditional trust and love, to my parents,

Victoria and Gheorghe Ioachimescu

Motto: *Nullius in verba. Per ardua ad astra.*

CONTENTS

Part IV: SLEEP AND SPECIFIC CONDITIONS

Guest Editor's Foreword

A Two-Thirds World

Needless to say, conventional medicine was, at least until recently, a two-thirds science, and clinicians and medical researchers had limited their practice and queries, respectively, to a 2/3 patient and the world. Human physiology and pathologic processes were examined only in awake people and mostly during the day; changes in these systems brought about by circadian rhythms and sleep were often ignored and considered unimportant.

Several factors could explain this penchant or, worse, prejudice, for disregarding the influence of sleep on the health, or lack thereof, of individuals and of society as a whole. Firstly, there was a lack of resources to conduct research at night. Unlike clinical medicine that had to meet the needs of the ill patients twenty-four hours a day, medical researchers never fully embraced the idea of shift work in their research career. Even among clinicians, the end of the typical "working" day is greeted with the time-honored *sign-out* as patient care is handed over to the doleful nocturnist (i.e., a physician working only at night) who responds begrudgingly to nighttime calls from patients, pharmacies or the hospital staff. Nighttime for the medical clinician and researcher is, similar to most other professions, a time for uninterrupted repose and rest.

Secondly, there was a lack of resources to conduct research on the sleeping person. How is he/she to be evaluated: by observation alone (relatively inexpensive but admittedly poorly sensitive and specific) or using polysomnography? Is he/she to be awakened as biologic processes (e.g., airflow or intraocular pressure) are measured, or left undisturbed? Often, these are dictated not by the specific physiologic parameters being monitored, but simply by the tools available to study them.

Finally, and most importantly, there was a lack of appreciation that humans are not an 18-hour species. Almost every biologic system affects, and is affected, by sleep. In addition, circadian rhythms alter physiologic processes to such an extent that measurements obtained in the daytime are commonly significantly different from nighttime results (e.g., hormones and inflammatory markers). The incidence of pathologic disorders wax and wane throughout the course of a 24-hour day as, for example, sudden cardiac death, asthma and sleep-related seizures tend to occur more often during the night and early morning. Finally, medical disorders and interventions used to treat them are affected as well by sleep (e.g., effects of the timing of hemodialysis on the prevalence and severity of sleep disordered breathing in patients with end-stage renal failure).

Medicine is increasingly becoming "holistic" but unless it addresses the totality of a person's health-related physical, psychological, spiritual and social needs including the often-overlooked eight-hour period from "lights-out" to "lights-on", can it truly and honestly claim to be so?

Teofilo Lee-Chiong, MD
Guest Editor
Professor of Medicine, School of Medicine - University of Colorado Denver
Chief, Division of Sleep Medicine, Department of Medicine - National Jewish Health
Denver, Colorado

Editor's Preface

We live in an interesting world. We are fueled every day by strong curiosity and desire to know, understand and fix problems, illnesses and abnormal conditions, and that's probably the main reason why we are all in this noble profession of medicine. Healing power is, as we all know, daughter of the mother Knowledge. Day in and day out, we take care of patients using our skills and profound of knowledge, learning new facts, embracing new technologies and applying new methodologies, all subdued to the purpose of curing diseases, taking care of patients, understanding the human body and mind, preventing future illnesses and epidemics.

I have been privileged to get trained in multiple fields, starting with Internal Medicine and followed by Pulmonary, Critical Care and last, but not least, Sleep Medicine. Among all medical fields, Sleep Medicine is a very young subspecialty and it seems to me that it lives golden age of childhood in a ravishing, very fast-transforming world. Sleep Medicine is not only an offspring of an era, but also a significant and active participant in this amazing cognitive journey. Let me state upfront my strong conviction that understanding why and how we sleep and how various sleep disturbances influence our life is not a minor task or duty. We owe this to us, to our patients, to the society, to previous and future generations.

Typically, our biological sciences' cognitive travels start in the lab, or at the bench side, with various simplified animal models which are put in place in order to answer simple or more complex questions; the results may show some "significance", especially if we are "lucky". They are generally followed by necessary confirmatory, small-scale, human studies, which may reproduce the previous research findings, again, if we are "lucky". Ultimately, in the quest of more statistical power and strength of significance, we end-up designing and conducting more complex, expensive and sometimes multi-decade long epidemiological studies. The problem is that, once completed, these studies are either negative (and then we stimulate our sharp analytical activity to explain why) or show some type of connection or "association". In this latter scenario, we discover what we already knew, i.e., that the epidemiological studies do not establish causality, or we start refining the analyses by correcting for multiple confounders (some of which not completely independent from each other) and, in the end, we dilute most of the findings towards neutrality. Curious beings, the human researchers have the natural tendency to go back to the laboratory and design other experiments, which start other quests for proof. Isn't this the abbreviated and at the same time the short journey of medical knowledge? How many times didn't we reverse written-in-stone axioms? How many times didn't we flip positions? How many times didn't we accept to be shattered in our strongest beliefs? The time may have come to change our research paradigms.

There are many ways we can improve our knowledge grasp, learning efficiency and the application of what we find in daily life. One of them is to revamp and reform the research methodologies and study designs. But equally important, especially for our learning of where we are in our journey, is that we need better localization methodologies (like GPS technology?), better collaborative models and better integrative approaches to research and information. At the same time, our information and data repositories need to become more interactive, up-to-date and more available.

Stemming from these convictions, and in order to improve our knowledge gaps and inherent lags, we created this electronic textbook called "Contemporary Sleep Medicine". We acknowledge that this is just a modest beginning at the feet of a new era, that of online open-source data and information and of a body of knowledge that has only upward potential of development, from design, content, delivery, accessibility or any other attribute. We designed this publication for a very wide audience, from patients, or "red" section readers, to physicians and other healthcare providers, who can navigate between the "green belt" or summary level, to "blue belt" or intermediate level, all the way to Research Outlook, or "black belt", of those readers who have an advanced level of knowledge and want to be up-to-date with the latest developments and directions in research in that particular field or condition without a need to read extensive, frequently outdated and often redundant materials. My task, the illustrious chapter authors' and that of the Guest Editor's has not been negligible at all, I can assure you. But with great vision, persistence and excellent skills of all the people involved, this publication comes to light to give us a glimpse of what we know and an even more flickery view of what we would like to find out in the future.

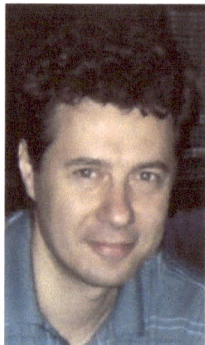

Octavian Ioachimescu, MD, PhD
Editor
Assistant Professor of Medicine, Emory University
Adjunct Clinical Assistant Professor of Medicine
Morehouse University
Medical Director, Sleep Disorders Center
Atlanta VA Medical Center
Atlanta, Georgia
USA

List of Contributors

Allam, J. Shirine, M.D.

Assistant Professor of Medicine - Emory University; Adjunct Clinical Assistant Professor of Medicine – Morehouse School of Medicine, Division of Pulmonary, Critical Care and Sleep Medicine, Emory University School of Medicine, Atlanta Veterans Affairs Medical Center, Atlanta, GA 30033, USA

Babayeuski, Alexander, M.D.

Atlanta Medical Center 303 Parkway Dr NE, Atlanta, GA, USA

Carney, Paul R., M.D., M.S.

Wilder Professor and Chief, Division of Pediatric Neurology, Departments of Pediatrics, Neurology and Neuroscience, J Crayton Pruitt Department of Biomedical Engineering, University of Florida Mc Knight Brain Institute, Gainesville, Florida, USA

Cohen, Dan, M.D.

Instructor in Neurology, Harvard Medical School - Beth Israel Deaconess Medical Center; Associate Physician, Brigham and Women's Hospital, Boston, MA, USA

Dubrovsky, Boris, M.D.

Center for Sleep Medicine, Department of Neurology, New York Presbyterian Hospital, Weill Cornell Medical College, New York, NY, USA

Endeshaw, Yohannes, M.D., M.P.H.

Associate Professor, Department of Aging and Geriatric Research, College of Medicine, University of Florida, Gainesville, FL, USA

Fine, Lina, M.D.

Cognitive Neuroscience Doctoral Program, Department of Psychology, The City College of New York, City University of New York, New York, NY, USA

Foldvary-Schaefer, Nancy, D.O., M.S.

Associate Professor of Medicine, Cleveland Clinic Lerner College of Medicine of Case Western Reserve University; Director, Cleveland Clinic Sleep Disorders Center, Cleveland Clinic Neurological Institute, 9500 Euclid Avenue, FA20, Cleveland, Ohio 44195, USA

Geyer, James D., M.D.

Director, Sleep Program, Associate Professor of Neurology and Sleep Medicine, Alabama Neurology and Sleep Medicine, Tuscaloosa, Alabama, USA

Guilleminault, Christian, M.D.

Professor of Medicine, Department of Psychiatry and Behavioral Sciences, Stanford University, Stanford, CA, USA

Harrington, John, M.D.

National Jewish Health, 1400 Jackson Street, Denver, CO 80213, USA

Ioachimescu, Octavian C., M.D., Ph.D.

Assistant Professor of Medicine - Emory University; Adjunct Clinical Assistant Professor of Medicine – Morehouse School of Medicine; Medical Director, Atlanta Veterans' Affairs Sleep Disorders Center, Division of Pulmonary, Critical Care and Sleep Medicine Emory University School of Medicine, Atlanta Veterans Affairs Medical Center, Atlanta, GA 30033, USA

Kakkar, Rahul, M.D.

North Florida South Georgia VA Health System, St. Augustine, FL, USA

Kanathur, Naveen, M.D.

National Jewish Health, 1400 Jackson Street, Denver, CO 80213, USA

Koo, Brian, M.D.

Assistant Professor of Neurology, Case Western Reserve School of Medicine, 11100 Euclid Avenue, Cleveland OH 44106, USA

Kotha, Kavitha S., M.D.

Senior Fellow, Division of Pulmonary, Allergy, Critical Care and Sleep Medicine, Department of Medicine, Emory University School of Medicine, USA

Kryger, Meir H., M.D.

Clinical Professor of Medicine, University of Connecticut School of Medicine and Director of Research and Education,Gaylord Sleep Medicine, 400 Gaylord Farm Road, Wallingford CT 06492, USA

Lee-Chiong, Teofilo, M.D.

National Jewish Health, 1400 Jackson Street, Denver, CO 80213, USA

Littleton, Stephen W., M.D.

Attending Physician, John H. Stroger Jr. Hospital of Cook County; Assistant Professor, Rush University Medical Center, 1900 W. Polk St. Room 1416 Chicago, IL 60612, USA

Malik, Vipin, M.D.

National Jewish Health, 1400 Jackson Street, Denver, CO 80213, USA

Mignot, Emmanuel, M.D., Ph.D.

Professor of Medicine, Department of Psychiatry and Behavioral Sciences, Stanford University, Stanford University Center for Narcolepsy, 701b Welch Rd Room 145, Palo Alto, CA, USA

Mokhlesi, Babak, M.D., M.Sc.

Associate Professor of Medicine, Section of Pulmonary and Critical Care Medicine; Director, Sleep Disorders Center and Sleep Medicine Fellowship Program, University of Chicago Pritzker School of Medicine, 5841 S. Maryland Ave, MC0999, Room L11B, Chicago, IL 60637, USA

Neme-Mercante, Silvia, M.D.

Associate Staff, Cleveland Clinic Sleep Disorders Center, 9500 Euclid Avenue, FA20 Cleveland, Ohio 44195, USA

Olson, Eric J., M.D.

Associate Professor of Medicine, Mayo College of Medicine; Consultant, Division of Pulmonary and Critical Care Medicine; Co-Director, Center for Sleep Medicine, Mayo Clinic, Rochester, MN, USA

Qamar, Arman, M.D.

University of Delhi, Delhi, India

Ramar, Kannan, M.B.B.S., M.D.

Assistant Professor of Medicine, Mayo College of Medicine; Consultant, Division of Pulmonary and Critical Care Medicine, Mayo Clinic, Rochester, MN, USA

Roux, Francoise, M.D., Ph.D.

Assistant Professor of Medicine, Section of Pulmonary and Critical Care Medicine, Yale University School of Medicine, 333 Cedar Street, Post Office Box 208057, New Haven, CT 06520-8057, USA

Roy, Asim, M.D.

Assistant Clinical Professor of Neurology, University of Pittsburgh Medical Center, Pittsburgh, PA, USA

Budur, Kumar S., M.D., M.P.H.

Associate Medical Director: Clinical Science – Neuroscience, Takeda Global Research and Development Inc., 675 North Field Drive, Lake Forest, IL 60045, USA

Schulman, David A., M.D.

Assistant Professor of Medicine - Emory University, 615 Michael Street, Suite 205, Atlanta, GA 30322, USA

Singh, Randip, Ph.D.

Overlake Sleep Disorders Center, Bellevue, WA, USA

Spielman, Arthur J., Ph.D.

Cognitive Neuroscience Doctoral Program, Department of Psychology, The City College of New York, City University of New York, New York, NY, USA

Talathi, Sachin S., Ph.D.

Division of Pediatric Neurology, Department of Pediatrics, University of Florida, Gainesville, Florida, USA

Teodorescu, Mihai, M.D.

University of Wisconsin, William S. Middleton VA Medical Center, Madison, WI, USA

Venkateshiah, Saiprakash, M.D.

Assistant Professor of Medicine - Emory University; Adjunct Clinical Assistant Professor of Medicine – Morehouse School of Medicine , Division of Pulmonary, Critical Care and Sleep Medicine, Emory University School of Medicine, Atlanta Veterans Affairs Medical Center, Atlanta, GA 30033, USA

Yaggi, Henry K., M.D. M.P.H.

Associate Professor of Medicine, Yale University School of Medicine, Section of Pulmonary and Critical Care Medicine, Medical Director, VA CT Center for Sleep Medicine, Clinical Epidemiology Research Center, 950 Campbell Ave, Building 35 Annex, West Haven, CT 06516, USA

Famous Quotes about Sleep

'Sunt geminae Somni portae, quarum altera fertur

Cornea, qua veris facilis datur exitus umbris,

Altera candenti perfecta nitens elephanto,

Sed falsa ad caelum mittunt insomnia Manes.'

There are two gates of Sleep, one of which it is held is made of horn and by it easy egress is given to real ghosts; the other, shining, fashioned of gleaming white ivory, but the shades send deceptive visions that way to the light.'

Publius Vergilius Maro (Virgil, 70-19 BC), Aeneid bk. 6, l. 893

'And the Lord God caused a deep sleep to fall upon Adam, and he slept; and he took one of his ribs, and closed up the flesh instead thereof; And the rib, which the Lord God had taken from man, made he a woman.'

The Bible (authorized version, 1611; transl. by William Tyndale), Old Testament: Genesis, ch. 2, v. 21

'To be or not to be: that is the question:

Whether 'tis nobler in the mind to suffer

The slings and arrows of outrageous fortune,

Or to take arms against a sea of troubles,

And by opposing end them? To die: to sleep;

No more; and, by a sleep to say we end

The heart-ache and the thousand natural shocks

That flesh is heir to, 'tis a consummation

Devoutly to be wished. To die, to sleep;

To sleep: perchance to dream: ay, there's the rub;

For in that sleep of death what dreams may come

When we have shuffled off this mortal coil,

Must give us pause.'

William Shakespeare (1564-1616), 'Hamlet', 1601, act 3, sc. 1, l. 56

'Why let the stricken deer go weep,

The hart ungallèd play;

For some must watch, while some must sleep:

So runs the world away.'

William Shakespeare (1564-1616), 'Hamlet', 1601, act 3, sc. 2, l. 287

'Not poppy, nor mandragora,

Nor all the drowsy syrups of the world,

Shall ever medicine thee to that sweet sleep

Which thou owedst yesterday.'

William Shakespeare (1564-1616), 'Othello', 1602-1604, act 3, sc. 3, l. 331

'Bien haya el que inventó el sueño, capa que cubre todos los humanos pensamientos, manjar que quita la hambre, agua que ahuyenta la sed, fuego que calienta el frío, frío que templa el ardor, y, finalmente, moneda general con que todas las cosas se compran, balanza y peso que iguala al pastor con el rey y al simple con el discreto.'

'Blessings on him who invented sleep, the mantle that covers all human thoughts, the food that satisfies hunger, the drink that slakes thirst, the fire that warms cold, the cold that moderates heat, and, lastly, the common currency that buys all things, the balance and weight that equalizes the shepherd and the king, the simpleton and the sage.'

Miguel de Cervantes Saavedra (1547-1616), 'Don Quixote', 1605, pt. 2, ch. 74

'You lack the season of all natures, sleep.'

William Shakespeare (1564-1616), 'Macbeth', 1606, act 3, sc 4, l.141

'Our revels now are ended. These our actors,

As I foretold you, were all spirits and

Are melted into air, into thin air;

And, like the baseless fabric of this vision,

The cloud-capped towers, the gorgeous palaces,

The solemn temples, the great globe itself,

Yea, all which it inherit, shall dissolve

And, like this insubstantial pageant faded,

Leave not a rack behind. We are such stuff

As dreams are made on, and our little life

Is rounded with sleep.'

William Shakespeare (1564-1616), 'The Tempest', 1611, act 4, sc 1, l.148

'We term sleep a death, and yet it is waking that kills us, and destroys those spirits which are the house of life.'

Sir Thomas Browne (1605-1682), Religio Medici, 1643, pt. 2, sect. 12

'One hour's sleep before midnight is worth two after'. (mid-17th century proverb)

'The winds come to me from the fields of sleep.'

William Wordsworth (1770-1850), 'Ode. Intimations of Immortality', 1807, st. 3

'Our birth is but a sleep and a forgetting...'

William Wordsworth (1770-1850), 'Ode. Intimations of Immortality', 1807, st. 5

'I shall sleep, and move with the moving ships,

Change as the winds change, veer in the tide'.

Algernon Charles Swinburne (1837-1909), 'The triumph of time', 1866.

'I have come to the borders of sleep,

The unfathomable deep

Forest where all must lose

Their way.'

Edward Thomas (1878-1917), 'Lights out', 1917

CHAPTER 1

Why Do We Sleep? Human Sleep: Neurobiology and Function

J. Shirine Allam, M.D.[1,*] and Christian Guilleminault, M.D.[2]

[1]*Assistant Professor of Medicine, Division of Pulmonary, Critical Care and Sleep Medicine, Emory University School of Medicine, Atlanta Veterans Affairs Medical Center, Atlanta, GA, USA and* [2]*Professor of Medicine, Department of Psychiatry and Behavioral Sciences, Stanford University, Stanford, CA, USA*

Abstract: Sleep is defined as a reversible state of reduced responsiveness to environmental stimuli. It roughly occupies one third of a human life. The science of sleep has greatly evolved over the past century. From a state of passive inactivity, sleep has come to be regarded as a complex physiologic state, with characteristic brain activity.

The neurobiology of sleep is complex. Transection studies have led to the description of the ascending reticular activating system as responsible for the awake state, with the main neurotransmitters involved being acetylcholine, norepinephrine, glutamate, serotonin, dopamine, histamine and orexin. Similarly, specific brain regions have been involved in the active generation of sleep. Non rapid eye movement (NREM) sleep is generated in the basal forebrain and anterior hypothalamus, containing the neurotransmitters gamma amino butyric acid (GABA) and galanin. These areas send inhibitory signaling to the excitatory regions of the brain. Rapid eye movement sleep (REM) is generated in the caudal pons and rostral mesencephalon area. It consists of several features, divided into tonic and phasic phases. Each of these is produced by a specific group of neurons. Acetylcholine is one of the major neurotransmitters in REM sleep.

Sleep has been described in the developing human fetus as early as 28 weeks of gestation. At birth, the human infant sleeps up to 16-18 hours a day and spends half of that time in REM sleep. This high fraction of sleep in the human infant has led to the hypothesis that REM is important in brain maturation.

TOPIC DISCUSSION (CLINICAL OUTLOOK)

Definitions of Sleep

Sleep roughly occupies a third of the human life and has always fascinated human beings. Scientific interest in sleep has emerged and greatly developed over the past century. In its simplest definition, sleep is a reversible state of reduced responsiveness to environmental stimuli. Historically, sleep was indeed thought to represent a passive state of all physiological and intellectual functions of the organism. It was not until the early 20th century that electrical activity recordings of the human brain demonstrated clear differences between the awake and asleep brain activity [1]. This was followed in the 1950's by the description by Kleitman and Aserinski of periods of rapid-eye movements (REM) occurring during sleep, which were associated with vivid dream recollections when subjects were awakened during their presence [2]. The REM periods were found to occur in a cyclical pattern throughout the night by Dement and Kleitman, who further described a cyclical variation of associated EEG patterns that is present during sleep [3]. Michel Jouvet added that the sleep associated with the rapid eye movements was a very different type of sleep that he called "paradoxical" and was a "state" in itself [4]. This suggested that sleep was not simply a passive inactivity of the brain, but rather represented a complex physiologic state, separate from the waking state.

The current behavioral definition of sleep is a state of behavioral quiescence in a species specific posture, that is characterized by a high arousal threshold, is reversible upon stimulation and displays a rebound after deprivation [5].

Neurobiology of Sleep

Neuroanatomy of Wakefulness

In the early 1900's several researchers set out to elucidate the mechanisms for sleep and wakefulness in the brain. A well known set of early experiments include those performed by Bremer who carried out several transection experiments on cats [6] One such preparation, called *cerveau isolé* consisted of transecting the brainstem just below the level of the oculomotor nerve, therefore isolating the brain from all sensory input except the optic and olfactory

---

*Address correspondence to J. Shirine Allam: Assistant Professor of Medicine, Division of Pulmonary, Critical Care and Sleep Medicine, Emory University School of Medicine, Atlanta Veterans Affairs Medical Center, Atlanta, GA, USA; E-mail: shirine.allam@emory.com

ones. The resulting brain electroencephalographic recording showed a state of constant sleep. Bremer thus hypothesized that the absence of the wake state was due to interruption of the sensory input to the brain.

Magoun and Moruzzi later challenged this explanation in 1949. They suggested that it was not the sensory interruption but rather the interruption of signals from the brainstem reticular formation that resulted in a sleep state. They showed that stimulation of the reticular formation in the brainstem resulted in the generation of fast EEG activity in the cortex that is characteristic of wakefulness. On the other hand, lesions in that same region resulted in loss of this fast activity and its replacement with cortical slow waves with a resulting behavioral state of inactivity [7]. This region was called the *ascending reticular activating system* (ARAS).

We now know that there are several clearly defined cell groups that make up the ARAS and contribute to arousal. They are located in the brainstem, hypothalamus, thalamus and basal forebrain and each has its specific neurotransmitter. The ARAS consists of two main pathways: a direct pathway, the ventral tegmental pathway that bypasses the thalamus and sends excitatory signals directly to the hypothalamus and cortex; and an indirect pathway, the dorsal tegmental pathway, that activates the thalamus, which in turn, through thalamocortical projections, induces the high frequency cortical EEG pattern seen during wakefulness [8]. The ventral tegmental pathway comprises the following nuclei and neurotransmitters: the *locus coeruleus* (LC, norepinephrine), the *dorsal raphe* nuclei (DR, serotonin), the *substantia nigra* and ventral tegmental area (SN & VT, dopamine), the tuberomamillary nuclei (TMN, histamine) and the basal forebrain (BF, acetylcholine). The dorsal tegmental pathway is formed by the cholinergic pedunculopontine tegmental (PPT) and the laterodorsal tegmental nuclei (LDT) (Fig. **1**).

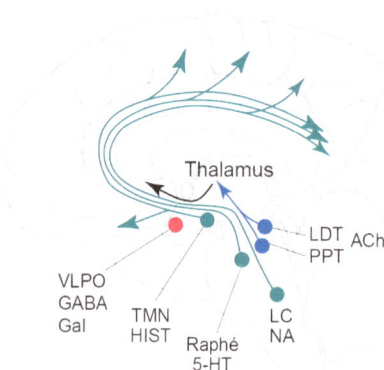

Figure 1: The ascending arousal system send projections from the brainstem and posterior hypothalamus throughout the forebrain. Neurons of the laterodorsal tegmental nuclei and pedunculopontine tegmental nuclei (LDT and PPT) (blue circles) send cholinergic fibers (Ach) to many forebrain targets, including the thalamus, which then regulate cortical activity. Aminergic nuclei (green circles) diffusely project throughout much of the forebrain, regulating the activity of cortical and hypothalamic targets directly. Neurons of the tuberomamillary nucleus (TMN) contain histamine (HIST), neurons of the raphé nuclei contain 5-HT and neurons of the locus coeruleus (LC) contain noradrenaline (NA). Sleep- promoting neurons of the ventrolateral preoptic nucleus (VLPO,red circle) contain GABA and galanin (Gal). (Reproduced with permission from: Saper CB, Chou TC, Scammel TE. The sleep switch: hypothalamic control of sleep and wakefulness. Trends Neurosci 2001; 24(12): 726-731).

Neurotransmitters in Sleep and Wakefulness

Acetylcholine is highly implicated in the regulation of sleep and wake behaviors. During wakefulness, the cholinergic neurons in the PPT and LDT nuclei as well as those in the basal forebrain fire rapidly. Their rate drops at the onset of NREM sleep, especially during slow wave sleep. Their rate accelerates again during REM sleep [9]. A pharmacological correlate of acetylcholine's role in the generation of wakefulness is seen in the activating effect of cholinergic agonists and the impaired cognition seen with the administration of anticholinergic drugs.

Histaminergic neurons of the tuberomamillary nuclei, **noradrenergic** neurons in the locus coeruleus, **serotonergic** neurons in the raphe nuclei and **hypocretin** neurons of the hypothalamus all have an important role in maintaining wakefulness. They have been shown to have a high firing rate during wakefulness; their rate decreases during NREM and they become nearly silent during REM sleep. These neurons have been shown to increase wakefulness when activated [10-12]. They receive direct inhibitory innervations from **GABA**ergic sleep active neurons [10].

The neurotransmitter **glutamate** is a major excitatory neurotransmitter and is located diffusely throughout the cortex.

NREM Sleep Generation

Normal human sleep is entered through NREM sleep and is associated with decreased responsiveness to external stimuli resulting from altered neurotransmission at the level of the thalamus. It was long believed that sleep resulted from the simple interruption of stimuli from the ARAS. However, we now know that specific brain regions exist that actively control NREM and REM sleep.

NREM sleep is generated by neurons in the anterior hypothalamus and basal forebrain. Stimulation of these regions will induce sleep and lesions in this area will greatly reduce sleep. The first clues about this date from the early 20th century, when von-Economo studied cases of encephalitis lethargica and concluded from examination of autopsy materials that lesions to the anterior hypothalamus produced insomnia and lesions to the posterior hypothalamus caused excessive sleepiness [13, 14]. More recent studies have clearly shown the existence of GABAergic "sleep active" neurons in the preoptic area of the anterior hypothalamus and in the basal forebrain [15-17]. The neurons on the preoptic area also contain the inhibitory neurotransmitters GABA and galanin. These "sleep active" neurons project to the wake promoting regions of the brainstem (TMN, LC, DR and LDT/PPT) and coordinate their inhibition, therefore producing sleep [8] (Fig. **2**). Benzodiazepines and barbiturates bind to GABA receptors and induce sleep by enhancing these pathways.

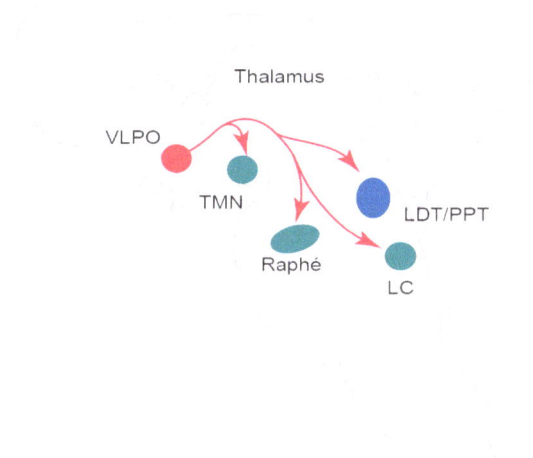

Figure 2: The projections from the ventrolateral preoptic nucleus (VLPO) to the main components of the ascending arousal system. Axons from the VLPO directly innervate the cell bodies of the proximal dendrites of neurons in the major monoamine arousal groups. Within the major cholinergic groups, axons from the VLPO mainly innervate interneurons, rather than the principal cholinergic cells. Abbreviations: LC, locus coeruleus; LDT, laterodorsal tegmental nuclei; PPT, pedunculopontine tegmental nuclei; TMN, tuberomammillary nucleus; VLPO, ventrolateral preoptic nucleus. (Reproduced with permission from: Saper CB, Chou TC, Scammel TE. The sleep switch: hypothalamic control of sleep and wakefulness. Trends Neurosci 2001; 24(12): 726-731).

The neurons of the preoptic area of the hypothalamus and the basal forebrain are also thought to contribute to sleep homeostasis by responding to various substances that accumulate during wakefulness, including adenosine and prostaglandin D2 [10, 18].

Two characteristic waveforms of N2 stage of NREM sleep are sleep spindles, produced by reticular thalamic nuclei and K-complexes, which represent cortical depolarization.

REM Sleep Generation

REM sleep has been termed "paradoxical sleep", "activated sleep" or "active sleep" because of the high level of cerebral activity that characterizes it, with increases in cerebral blood flow, oxygen and glucose consumption.

Features of REM sleep are divided into "tonic" features, present throughout the REM period and "phasic" features that occur episodically. The tonic features consist of a low voltage, mixed frequency EEG recording and muscle atonia. The phasic features are the rapid, conjugate eye movements, brief, fine twitches of the peripheral and middle ear muscles and ponto-geniculo-occipital (PGO) waves. The PGO waves are high voltage bursts that have been recorded in the geniculate nucleus in animals and in humans [19], and that, as their name indicates, originate in the pons and can be detected in the occipital lobe after an additional delay. They occur around 30 seconds prior to the onset of REM sleep, usually shortly followed by rapid eye movements.

Transection studies have demonstrated that the region of the rostral pons and caudal mesencephalon is crucial for the generation of REM sleep [20]. Within this region, groups of neurons that are maximally active during REM sleep ("REM-on" cells) have been identified. They contain the neurotransmitters GABA, glutamate, glycine and, most importantly, acetylcholine. The REM-on cells are involved in the generation of REM sleep and include the nucleus reticularis pontis oralis (RPO), the nucleus sub-coeruleus (SubC) and the PPT-LDT nuclei. These areas also contains "REM-off" cells that are minimally active during REM and contain norepinephrine, epinephrine, serotonin, histamine and GABA [10, 20].

Each of the manifestations of REM sleep is generated by a specific subgroup of REM-on cells. The PPT/LDT nuclei are rapidly firing during REM sleep and release acetylcholine in the thalamus, activating it and producing the typical REM sleep cortical desynchrony [8]. The PGO waves described above are generated in the nucleus sub-coeruleus (SubC).

Muscle atonia is produced by a polysynaptic pathway starting in the pontine inhibitory area (sub-coeruleus region, SubC), which activates the nucleus reticularis gigantocellularis and the nucleus magnocellularis in the medulla, through the lateral tegmento-reticular tract. In turn, these nuclei will directly inhibit (hyperpolarize) ventral horn motor neurons by releasing GABA and glycine through the ventrolateral reticulospinal tract. Atonia is also produced by a loss of excitation, which consists of a decrease in the brainstem noradrenergic and serotonergic excitatory release on spinal motor neurons [10, 21]. The latter mechanism explains the loss of REM atonia that is seen in individuals who are taking selective serotonin re-uptake inhibitors (SSRIs), which results from continued excitation of the motor neurons.

Table 1 summarizes the neuroanatomy of NREM and REM sleep.

Table 1: Neurobiology of sleep

Sleep stage/phenomenon	Brain area	Neurotransmitter
NREM sleep	Anterior hypothalamus (VLPO) Basal Forebrain	GABA and Galanin
REM sleep: PGO waves	Pons → lateral geniculate nucleus→occipital lobe	
Low voltage, mixed frequency EEG	PPT/LDT nuclei activating the thalamus	Acetylcholine
Muscle atonia	Pons (Sub-coeruleus area) →lateral tegmento-reticular tract →medulla (nucleus magnocellularis and gigantocellularis) →ventrolateral reticulospinal tract →ventral horn motor neurons	GABA and Glycine

NREM: Non Rapid Eye Movement Sleep; VLPO: ventro-lateral preoptic nucleus; GABA: gamma amino-butyric acid; PGO: ponto-geniculo-occipital; EEG: electroencephalogram; PPT/LDT: pedunculo-pontine tegmental/laterodorsal tegmental

Ontogeny of Sleep in Humans

The generation of sleep clearly involves complex neurological pathways. Its development in fetuses is therefore linked to the maturation of the central nervous system.

As in adult humans, sleep occurs in two different states in infants and fetuses: "active sleep" (AS, REM equivalent) and "quiet sleep" (NREM equivalent). The human fetus exhibits a wide range of movements as early as 8-12 weeks of gestational age (GA) [22]. These movements are episodic, with periods of activity alternating with periods of quiescence. The cycles become longer with advancing gestational age [23]. The emergence of sleep states has been described at about 28 weeks of GA. However, clearly defined periods of REM sleep or active sleep, with correlation of heart rate variability, fetal movements and rapid eye movement are not seen before 30-32 weeks of GA [24, 25].

At birth, newborns spend 16 to 18 hours per day sleeping. Fifty to sixty percent of their sleep is composed of active sleep. Over the first 3-5 months of life the fraction of active sleep drops to 40%. Between 6 and 24 months of age, total sleep time will decrease to 13 hours per day and will consist of 25-30% REM sleep. The percentage of REM sleep will reach the adult levels of 20% by the age of 3-5 years.

The large amount of time spent in AS by fetuses and infants has led to the hypothesis that AS induces CNS development. Prior experiments in cats have shown that deprivation of newborn kittens from normal visual experience leads to a permanent alteration of the brain response to visual stimuli. Active sleep is therefore thought to provide early sensory CNS stimulation prior to birth to allow adequate brain development [26-28].

Electroencephalographic (EEG) Characterization of Sleep

Normal human sleep is composed of two main stages: Rapid eye movement sleep (REM) and non rapid eye movement sleep (NREM). The latter is divided into 3 stages N1 though N3.

Stage N1 is characterized by a low voltage, mixed frequency EEG pattern in the range of 4-7 Hz, frequently accompanied by slow rolling eye movements. Vertex sharp waves can be seen during stage N1 (Fig. **3**) [29].

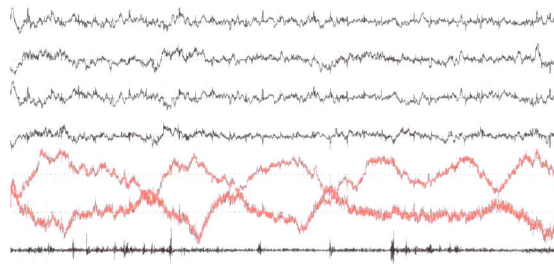

Figure 3: Thirty second epoch representing stage N1 with low voltage, mixed frequency EEG in the range of 2-7Hz, as well as slow rolling eye movements. Each horizontal line represents one second. The first four leads are EEG leads, followed by two eye leads (in red) and a chin EMG lead.

Stage N2 is characterized by the presence of K-complexes and/or sleep spindles. K-complexes are high voltage waves that consist of a sharp negative deflection followed by a slower positive deflection, lasting at least 0.5 seconds, usually best seen using frontal EEG derivations. Sleep spindles are high frequency (11-16Hz, but most commonly 12-14 Hz) waves, shaped in a crescendo-decrescendo pattern, that last at least 0.5 seconds and are best seen using central EEG derivations (Fig. **4**) [29].

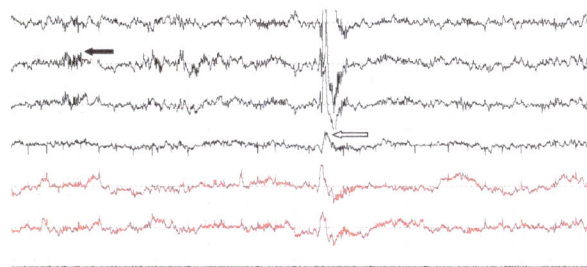

Figure 4: Thirty second epoch representing stage N2 which is characterized by K complexes (white arrow) and spindles (black arrow). Each horizontal line represents one second. The first four leads are EEG leads, followed by two eye leads (in red) and a chin EMG lead.

Stage N3 is comprised of more than 20% slow wave activity, with a frequency range of 0.5 to 2 Hz and a peak to peak amplitude of at least 75 µV measured over the frontal regions (Fig. **5**) [29].

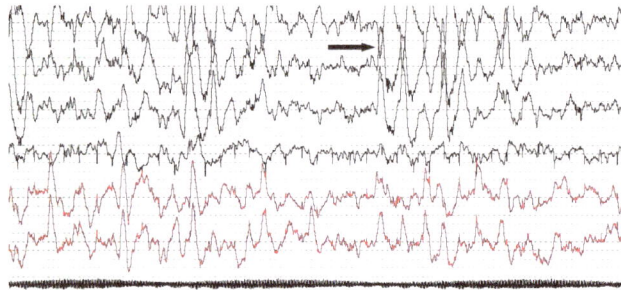

Figure 5: Thirty second epoch representing stage N3 which is characterized by more than 20% delta waves (arrow). Delta waves are low frequency waves (0.5 to 2Hz) with an amplitude exceeding 75µV. Each horizontal line represents one second. The first four leads are EEG leads, followed by two eye leads (in red) and a chin EMG lead.

Stage REM necessitates the presence of 3 factors: a low voltage, mixed frequency EEG pattern, resembling the awake EEG; the lowest chin EMG amplitude reached during the entire recording, as well as conjugate rapid eye movements. The initial deflection of rapid eye movements usually lasts less than 500 msec (Fig. **6**). Sawtooth waves are sharply contoured triangular waves of 2-6 Hz frequencies, often seen at the beginning of a REM period, just preceding a burst of rapid eye movement (Fig. **7**) [29].

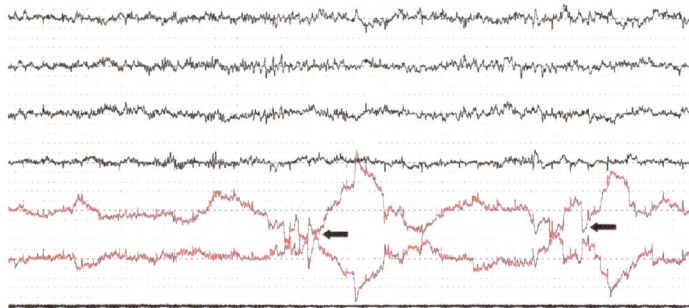

Figure 6: Thirty second epoch representing stage REM. The EEG has a typical low voltage mixed frequency pattern, rapid conjugate eye movements are seen (arrows) and the chin EMG has a very low amplitude. Each horizontal line represents one second. The first four leads are EEG leads, followed by two eye leads (in red) and a chin EMG lead.

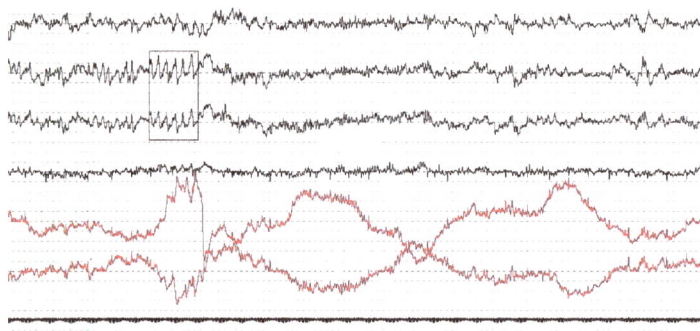

Figure 7: Sawtooth waves (boxed) can be seen during REM sleep, usually preceding a rapid eye movement. They are best seen in central EEG leads.

In a healthy young adult, sleep is composed of 2-5% stage N1, 45-55% Stage N2, 13-23% Stage N3, and 20-25% REM sleep. The normal sleep architecture in the young healthy adult is shown in Fig. **3**. Sleep is usually entered through NREM sleep, usually stage N1.

RESEARCH OUTLOOK

The question of "why do we sleep?" has been occupying scientists and clinicians alike for many years. Despite great advances in our knowledge about the science of sleep, this question remains a matter of great debate. Sleep is highly conserved throughout evolution, despite it seeming a rather maladaptive feature. Sleep is also homeostatically controlled and its deprivation leads to serious physiologic consequences, at times ending in death. These observations may lead one to believe that sleep must have a necessary function for the organism. Several hypotheses have been put forth. One theory claims that sleep is merely a way to keep the organism safe during periods when it is likely to encounter predators or injury. Another theory holds that sleep allows the brain to regenerate energy, in the form of ATP and glycogen, consumed during wakefulness. Newer experiments have lent support to this theory but shown that the overall process is more complex then the mere glycogen and adenosine pathways.

Another role of sleep is memory and learning consolidation. REM sleep has been mainly involved in the consolidation of motor tasks and NREM sleep in that of declarative memory. Functional neuroimaging studies have revealed the fascinating neuroplasticity processes, which occur during sleep, leading to the generation of new neuronal circuitry after learning a new task. Finally, microarray studies have shown that synthesis of macromolecules might be upregulated during sleep.

What do we know:

Several observations testify to the importance of sleep in the animal kingdom and lead us to believe that it must have a functional importance for the human body:

1. Sleep has been conserved throughout evolution: it is ubiquitous among the higher orders of the animal kingdom, namely mammals, birds and reptiles [30]. Although not meeting the electrophysiological criteria for sleep in the higher orders, sleep may also present in simpler forms of life such as arthropods, as evidenced by studies in the fruit fly [31, 32]. This evolutionary conservation of a feature that may seem maladaptive points to an important role for sleep.

2. Sleep deprivation experiments in rats lead to serious physiologic consequences ending in death after 2-3 weeks of total sleep deprivation and 5 weeks after selective REM sleep deprivation [33, 34]. Human experiments show a near-linear increase in neurobehavioral deficits with accumulating sleep deprivation after a critical time of wakefulness of about 15.84 hours [35].

Sleep is homeostatically regulated. Sleep deprivation usually leads to rebound sleep, with an architecture different from normal sleep. In acute sleep deprivation, rebound human sleep will have a higher density of slow wave sleep (SWS) [36]. In chronic sleep deprivation, SWS is conserved at the expense of other NREM stages and REM sleep [37, 38].

Many theories have emerged about the function of sleep and a lot of data has been generated, however no one theory has yet gained acceptance as the central role for sleep. Some regard sleep as an evolutionary mistake without a specific purpose [39]. However most sleep scientist believe that sleep has a central function. It is likely that sleep has not one but many roles in the organism. We will review below the main hypotheses about the roles of sleep and the evidence behind each of them.

Environmental Adaptation Theory

The environmental adaptation theory holds that sleep has evolved as a state of adaptive inactivity, that is rapidly reversible and that enables the animal to remain out of harm's way when the risk of injury and predation is high. One important validation for this theory is that sleep duration and intensity in different animals, can often be explained by an environmental variable. For example, large herbivores need to stay awake to consume a large amount of (low caloric) food to meet their energy requirements, which explains their short sleep duration. In addition, their size would put them at higher risk for predation during sleep and minimizing sleep time would be highly adaptive in their case. By contrast, one of the longest sleeping mammals is the brown bat, which sleeps 20 hours and feeds on mosquitoes and moths. It is typically awake during dusk hours, when its prey is maximally active. This adaptation allows it to make the most out of its wake time, and to be sheltered at other times when its food source is not available and it would be exposed to predators with better vision and flight abilities [40]. What the environmental adaptation theory fails to explain is why does the body need sleep *per se* and not restful immobility, which would achieve the same environmental benefits.

The Energy Theory

Bennington and Heller first proposed the energy theory in 1995. They suggested that wakefulness resulted in depletion of glycogen storage in the brain and the accumulation of adenosine in the basal forebrain as a result of ATP and AMP degradation. The effects of adenosine accumulation on neurons would produce the EEG manifestations of increased sleep need [41]. A considerable amount of work was done since then to test this theory. Adenosine has been indeed found to accumulate during wakefulness in certain areas of the brain, namely the basal forebrain and the cortex [42, 43]. Increasing the levels of extracellular adenosine in the basal forebrain leads to a decrease in wake, and an increase in slow wave sleep during NREM sleep, similar to the response to sleep deprivation [43, 44].

Brain glycogen content has also been extensively studied. It was found to be depleted after time spent awake, and repleted after brief sleep. However, if wakefulness continues, glycogen stores are repleted again, at times to levels above resting. This led to the hypothesis that glycogen repletion, not depletion is the stimulus for sleep [45].

Although new work had made clear that the control of brain energy utilization is more complex than what is reflected by ATP and glycogen variations alone, the energy theory has largely been validated. Several energy pathways are altered with sleep, wake and sleep deprivation. They include antioxidant enzymes, the electron transport system, the unfolded protein response and more. A comprehensive review of the subject can be found in Scharf *et al* 2008 [45].

Learning and Memory Theory and Neuroplasticity

The observation that sleep enhances memory has been supported by strong evidence over the past few years (Stickgold, 2005). On one hand, sleep after learning has been shown to stabilize newly encoded information making it more resistant to interfering inputs. On the other hand, delayed retrieval of memory was improved when learning was followed by a period of sleep [46-51].

Memory is divided into two main types: *declarative memory*, which refers to the retention of facts (semantic, e.g., the number of eggs in a dozen) or events (episodic, e.g., what you had for breakfast), and *non-declarative memory*, which is used without conscious recollection. One subtype of non-declarative memory is procedural memory, e.g., riding a bicycle [46, 52].

The different types of memory are thought to be stored in different formats and in different brain regions and have therefore been studied separately. The evidence gathered thus far seems to point to NREM sleep benefiting mostly, but not exclusively, declarative memory and REM sleep benefiting mostly, but not exclusively, non-declarative memory, namely procedural and emotional enhancement [46]. More recently, some doubt has been shed on the involvement of REM sleep in procedural learning, when the introduction of REM suppressing medications did not impair, but rather improved the consolidation of motor tasks [53].

Learning seems to have an effect on sleep architecture as well. Indeed, increases in REM sleep duration and REM density have been observed after the acquisition of a procedural task [54]. An increase in stage 2 (non-REM2, N2) sleep duration and spindle density has been described with consolidation of procedural and declarative memory [55-57]. Neuroimaging studies have demonstrated the reappearance during REM sleep of a pattern of brain activity present during motor task learning [58]. Such changes during sleep may be indicative of a modification of synaptic circuitry in specific brain areas that leads to the refining of the motor task. Functional MRI studies have shown the presence of this neuroplasticity after learning a motor task by documenting changes in brain activation during the performance of a task after an intervening period of sleep. The documented changes involved an increased activation of motor control areas of the brain and decreased activation of the areas involved in conscious spatial monitoring and emotions [59].

Macromolecule Biosynthesis

The advent of microarray studies gave scientists an opportunity to study the gene expression characteristics of sleep as compared to wakefulness. One such study focused on the cortex and hypothalamus of mice and found significant changes in gene expression during sleep. In particular, the largest group of genes found to have increased expression during sleep were those involved in biosynthesis and transport. The authors concluded that one of the functions of sleep consists of the rebuilding of cellular components that have been depleted during wakefulness [60].

What we don't know:

Our knowledge about sleep has greatly increased over the past century; nevertheless, the important question of the function of sleep has continued to spark heated debates. While each of the above-described functions of sleep plays a significant role for the organism, a search for one primordial function is still ongoing and would explain why a seemingly maladaptive feature has been so highly conserved in evolution.

Other questions remain to be answered:

- What are all the factors that control sleep homeostasis?
- How to accurately predict the need for sleep, or the duration of sleep?
- What are the mechanisms involved in neuroplasticity during sleep?
- Which stages of sleep are responsible for memory consolidation and what are the exact mechanisms underlying that?
- What is the specific role of REM (R) sleep?

There is still much to learn in the domain of Sleep Medicine. It has been clear from prior research and observation that sleep is necessary for health. Future research, aiming at elucidating some of these questions hold great promise for the improvement of both physical and mental health.

REFERENCES

[1]   Berger H. Ueber das Elektroenkephaligramm des Menschen. J Psycholo Neurol 1930; 40: 160-179.
[2]   Aserinski E, Kleitman N. Regular occurring periods of eye motility, and concomitant phenomena, during sleep. Science 1953; 118: 273-274.
[3]   Dement W, Kleitman N. Cyclic variations in EEG during sleep and their relation to eye movements, body motility and dreaming. Electroencephalog Clin Neurophysiol 1957; 9: 673-690.
[4]   Jouvet M, Michel F, Courion J. On a stage of rapid cerebral electrical activity in the course of physiological sleep. (French). C R Seances Soc Biol Fil 1959; 153: 1024-1028.
[5]   Vassalli A, Dijk DJ. Sleep function: current questions and new approaches. Eur J Neurosci 2009; 29: 1830-41.
[6]   Bremer F. Cerveau "isolé" et physiologie du sommeil. C R Soc Biol 1935; 118:1235-1241.
[7]   Moruzzi G, Magoun H. Brainstem reticular formation and activation of the EEG. Electroencephalog Clin Neurophysiol 1949; 1: 455.
[8]   Espana RA, Scammell TE. Sleep neurobiology for the clinician. Sleep 2004; 27: 811-20.
[9]   Lee MG, Manns ID, Alonso A, Jones BE. Sleep-wake related discharge properties of basal forebrain neurons recorded with micropipettes in head-fixed rats. J Neurophysiol 2004; 92: 1182-98.
[10]   Siegel JM. The neurobiology of sleep. Semin Neurol 2009; 29: 277-96.
[11]   Ramesh V, Thakkar MM, Strecker RE *et al.* Wakefulness-inducing effects of histamine in the basal forebrain of freely moving rats. Behav Brain Res 2004; 152: 271-8.
[12]   John J, Wu MF, Boehmer LN, Siegel JM. Cataplexy-active neurons in the hypothalamus: implications for the role of histamine in sleep and waking behavior. Neuron 2004; 42: 619-34.
[13]   von-Economo C. Encephalitis Lethargica. Wiener Klinische Wochenschrift. 1917; 30: 581–585
[14]   von-Economo C. Sleep as a problem of localization. J Nerv Ment Dis 1930; 71: 29-259.
[15]   Suntsova N, Szymusiak R, Alam MN *et al.* Sleep-waking discharge patterns of median preoptic nucleus neurons in rats. J Physiol 2002; 543: 665-77.

[16]   Szymusiak R, Gvilia I, McGinty D. Hypothalamic control of sleep. Sleep Med 2007; 8: 291-301.

[17]   Torterolo P, Benedetto L, Lagos P *et al.* State-dependent pattern of Fos protein expression in regionally-specific sites within the preoptic area of the cat. Brain Res 2009; 1267: 44-56.

[18]   Szymusiak R, McGinty D. Hypothalamic regulation of sleep and arousal. Ann N Y Acad Sci 2008; 1129: 275-86.

[19]   Fernandez-Mendoza J, Lozano B, Seijo F *et al.* Evidence of subthalamic PGO-like waves during REM sleep in humans: a deep brain polysomnographic study. Sleep 2009; 32: 1117-26.

[20]   Boissard R, Gervasoni D, Schmidt M. The rat ponto-medullary network responsible for paradoxical sleep onset and maintenance: a combined microinjection and functional neuroanatomy study. Eur J Neurosci 2002; 16: 1959-1973.

[21]   Mileykovskiy BY, Kiyashchenko LI, Siegel JM. Cessation of activity in red nucleus neurons during stimulation of the medial medulla in decerebrate rats. J Physiol 2002; 545: 997-1006.

[22]   de Vries JI, Visser GH, Prechtl HF. The emergence of fetal behaviour. I. Qualitative aspects. Early Hum Dev 1982; 7: 301-22.

[23]   Dierker LJ, Jr., Pillay SK, Sorokin Y, Rosen MG. Active and quiet periods in the preterm and term fetus. Obstet Gynecol 1982; 60: 65-70.

[24]   Okai T, Kozuma S, Shinozuka N *et al.* A study on the development of sleep-wakefulness cycle in the human fetus. Early Hum Dev 1992; 29: 391-6.

[25]   Visser GH, Poelmann-Weesjes G, Cohen TM, Bekedam DJ. Fetal behavior at 30 to 32 weeks of gestation. Pediatr Res 1987; 22: 655-8.

[26]   Roffwarg HP, Muzio JN, Dement WC. Ontogenetic Development of the Human Sleep-Dream Cycle. Science 1966; 152: 604-619.

[27]   Wiesel TN, Hubel DH. Single-Cell Responses in Striate Cortex of Kittens Deprived of Vision in One Eye. J Neurophysiol 1963; 26: 1003-17.

[28]   Peirano P, Algarin C, Uauy R. Sleep-Wake states ad their regulatory mechanisms throughout early human development J Pediatr 2003; 143: S70-S79.

[29]   Iber C, Ancoli-Israel S, Chesson A, Quan S. The AASM Manual for the Scoring of Sleep and Associated Events: Rules, Terminology and Technical Specifications. In: 2007.

[30]   Rechtschaffen A. Current perspectives on the function of sleep. Perspect Biol Med 1998; 41: 359-90.

[31]   Shaw P. Awakening to the behavioral analysis of sleep in Drosophila. J Biol Rhythms 2003; 18: 4-11.

[32]   Hendricks JC, Finn SM, Panckeri KA *et al.* Rest in Drosophila is a sleep-like state. Neuron 2000; 25: 129-38.

[33]   Everson CA, Bergmann BM, Rechtschaffen A. Sleep deprivation in the rat: III. Total sleep deprivation. Sleep 1989; 12: 13-21.

[34]   Kushida CA, Bergmann BM, Rechtschaffen A. Sleep deprivation in the rat: IV. Paradoxical sleep deprivation. Sleep 1989; 12: 22-30.

[35]   Van Dongen HP, Maislin G, Mullington JM, Dinges DF. The cumulative cost of additional wakefulness: dose-response effects on neurobehavioral functions and sleep physiology from chronic sleep restriction and total sleep deprivation. Sleep 2003; 26: 117-26.

[36]   Dement W, Greenberg S. Changes in total amount of stage four sleep as a function of partial sleep deprivation. Electroencephalogr Clin Neurophysiol 1966; 20: 523-6.

[37]   Guilleminault C, Powell NB, Martinez S *et al.* Preliminary observations on the effects of sleep time in a sleep restriction paradigm. Sleep Med 2003; 4: 177-84.

[38]   Brunner DP, Dijk DJ, Borbely AA. Repeated partial sleep deprivation progressively changes in EEG during sleep and wakefulness. Sleep 1993; 16: 100-13.

[39]   Rial RV, Nicolau MC, Gamundi A *et al.* The trivial function of sleep. Sleep Med Rev 2007; 11: 311-25.

[40]   Siegel JM. Sleep viewed as a state of adaptive inactivity. Nat Rev Neurosci 2009; 10: 747-53.

[41]   Benington J, Heller H. Restoration of brain energy metabolism as the function of sleep. Prog Neurobiol 1995; 45: 347-360.

[42]   Porkka-Heiskanen T, Strecker RE, McCarley RW. Brain site-specificity of extracellular adenosine concentration changes during sleep deprivation and spontaneous sleep: an *in vivo* microdialysis study. Neuroscience 2000; 99: 507-17.

[43]   Methippara MM, Kumar S, Alam MN *et al.* Effects on sleep of microdialysis of adenosine A1 and A2a receptor analogs into the lateral preoptic area of rats. Am J Physiol Regul Integr Comp Physiol 2005; 289: R1715-23.

[44]   Porkka-Heiskanen T, Strecker RE, Thakkar M *et al.* Adenosine: a mediator of the sleep-inducing effects of prolonged wakefulness. Science 1997; 276: 1265-8.

[45]   Scharf MT, Naidoo N, Zimmerman JE, Pack AI. The energy hypothesis of sleep revisited. Prog Neurobiol 2008; 86: 264-80.

[46]   Marshall L, Born J. The contribution of sleep to hippocampus-dependent memory consolidation. Trends Cogn Sci 2007; 11: 442-50.

[47]   Ellenbogen JM, Hulbert JC, Stickgold R *et al.* Interfering with theories of sleep and memory: sleep, declarative memory, and associative interference. Curr Biol 2006; 16: 1290-4.

[48]   Korman M, Doyon J, Doljansky J *et al.* Daytime sleep condenses the time course of motor memory consolidation. Nat Neurosci 2007; 10: 1206-13.

[49]   Fischer S, Hallschmid M, Elsner AL, Born J. Sleep forms memory for finger skills. Proc Natl Acad Sci U S A 2002; 99: 11987-91.

[50]   Gais S, Plihal W, Wagner U, Born J. Early sleep triggers memory for early visual discrimination skills. Nat Neurosci 2000; 3: 1335-9.

[51]   Stickgold R, James L, Hobson JA. Visual discrimination learning requires sleep after training. Nat Neurosci 2000; 3: 1237-8.

[52]   Stickgold R. Sleep-dependent memory consolidation. Nature 2005; 437: 1272-8.

[53]   Rasch B, Pommer J, Diekelmann S, Born J. Pharmacological REM sleep suppression paradoxically improves rather than impairs skill memory. Nat Neurosci 2009; 12: 396-7.

[54]   Smith CT, Nixon MR, Nader RS. Posttraining increases in REM sleep intensity implicate REM sleep in memory processing and provide a biological marker of learning potential. Learn Mem 2004; 11: 714-9.

[55]   Gais S, Molle M, Helms K, Born J. Learning-dependent increases in sleep spindle density. J Neurosci 2002; 22: 6830-4.

[56]   Huber R, Ghilardi MF, Massimini M, Tononi G. Local sleep and learning. Nature 2004; 430: 78-81.

[57]   Aeschbach D, Cutler AJ, Ronda JM. A role for non-rapid-eye-movement sleep homeostasis in perceptual learning. J Neurosci 2008; 28: 2766-72.

[58]   Peigneux P, Laureys S, Fuchs S *et al.* Learned material content and acquisition level modulate cerebral reactivation during posttraining rapid-eye-movements sleep. Neuroimage 2003; 20: 125-34.

[59]   Stickgold R, Walker MP. Sleep-dependent memory consolidation and reconsolidation. Sleep Med 2007; 8: 331-43.

[60]   Mackiewicz M, Shockley KR, Romer MA *et al.* Macromolecule biosynthesis: a key function of sleep. Physiol Genomics 2007; 31: 441-57.

CHAPTER 2

Epidemiology of Sleep Disorders

Mihai Teodorescu, M.D.[1,*] **and Rahul Kakkar, M.D.**[2]

[1]*Assistant Professor, University of Wisconsin, William S. Middleton VA Medical Center, Madison, WI, USA and* [2]*Assistant Professor, North Florida South Georgia VA Health System, St. Augustine, FL, USA*

Abstract: Obstructive sleep apnea (OSA) is estimated to affect about 24% of adult males and 9% of adult females. The prevalence rate of OSA with excessive daytime sleepiness was reported to be 5-7 % in adult males and 3-4 % in adult females. Since these publications, the incidence and prevalence of obesity, a major risk factor for OSA, has increased significantly.

Central sleep apnea (CSA)m is a conglomerate of different conditions, including: primary CSA, Cheyne-Stokes breathing-CSA (CSB-CSA) pattern, high-altitude periodic breathing, CSA due to medical conditions not Cheyne-Stokes, and CSA due to drugs or substances. Another newly recognized CSA syndrome is complex sleep apnea, which is seen during treatment of OSA, generally before the obstructive events are completely abolished by positive airway pressure (PAP). Primary CSA is uncommon in adults and is seen in less than 10% of patients presenting polysomnography (PSG). The prevalence of primary CSA, high-altitude periodic breathing, and CSA due to medical conditions in the general population are unknown. The obesity-hypoventilation syndrome (OHS) is also known as obesity-associated hypoventilation or Pickwickian syndrome. Criteria for OHS includes a BMI ≥ 30 kg/m^2 and chronic alveolar hypoventilation leading to daytime hypercapnia, in the absence of pulmonary or neuromuscular disease.

Epidemiological data on insomnia has been confounded by multiple definitions; most of the studies account for three insomnia symptoms: difficulty falling asleep, difficulty maintaining sleep and early morning awakenings. Insomnia symptoms were reported to be present in about one-third of the general population. Non-restorative sleep, which is also part of the insomnia definition (ICSD-2), is rarely explored. When daytime consequences of insomnia are taken into account, the prevalence is estimated to be around 10%. Overall, daytime consequences may be as prevalent as 2/3 of insomnia subjects.

Narcolepsy is classically defined by sleepiness and abnormal rapid eye movement (REM) sleep-related symptoms (cataplexy, hypnagogic hallucinations, and sleep paralysis). In one study, the prevalence of narcolepsy with or without cataplexy has been reported as 30.6 per 100,000 people (18 years or older), narcolepsy with cataplexy as 21.8/ 100,000 people and narcolepsy with HLA-DQB1*0602 as 15.3/ 100,000 people. In 18,980 randomly selected subjects, representative of a target population of 205 million European inhabitants, excessive daytime sleepiness was reported by 15% of the sample, napping two times or more in the same day was reported by 1.6% of the sample, while cataplexy (episodes of loss of muscle function related to a strong emotion) was found in 1.6% of the sample. A narcolepsy diagnosis was reported in 47/100,000 people, severe for 26/100,000 and moderate in 21/100,000. Multiple sleep-onset REM periods and short mean sleep latencies (of less than 8 minutes) were reported in about 4% of the general population.

EPIDEMIOLOGY OF SLEEP RELATED BREATHING DISORDERS

Obstructive Sleep Apnea

Obstructive sleep apnea (OSA) is estimated to currently affect about 24% of adult males and about 9% of adult females [1]. Studies from different countries have consistently shown a prevalence rate of OSA *and excessive daytime sleepiness* of about 5-7 % in adult males and 3-4 % in adult females. Since these publications, the incidence and prevalence of obesity, a major risk factor for OSA, has increased. In United States, between 1980 and 2004 the prevalence of obesity increased from 15% to 33% among adults and the prevalence of excessive weight in children increased from approximately 6% to 19% [2]. African Americans and Hispanics have prevalence rates of obesity of 31% and 23%, respectively.

---

*Address correspondence to Mihai Teodorescu: Assistant Professor, University of Wisconsin, William S. Middleton VA Medical Center, Madison, WI, USA; E-mail: mct@medicine.wisc.edu

RISK FACTORS

The prevalence of OSA increases with increasing body mass index (BMI), neck circumference, age, certain disease states, family history of OSA, craniofacial abnormalities and certain races. While OSA is most commonly seen in adults between the ages of 30 to 60, particularly obese men, many sleep apneics do not belong to this group.

Body Weight

Obesity is the most important epidemiologic risk factor for development of OSA. Studies have consistently shown a graded increase in the risk of OSA with increase in body weight [1-4]. In the Wisconsin Sleep Cohort, an increase in BMI by one standard deviation was associated with a 4-fold increase in disease prevalence. A 10% increase in weight over a period of 4 years resulted in a 32% worsening of apnea hypopnea index (AHI), while the risk of having moderate to severe sleep apnea increased six-fold; a 10% weight loss was associated with 26% decrease in AHI. In the Sleep Heart Health Study a 10 kg weight gain in men was associated with 5.2-fold the odds of increase in the AHI by more than 15 events per hour.

For *women*, the same amount of weight gain was associated with 2.5-fold the odds of a similar increase in their AHI. The effect of weight and age on AHI appears non linear over time, obese older men being at the highest risk of an increase in OSA severity[5]. Reported values of BMI of *Asians* with OSA are lower than in their Caucasian counterparts; however, population-based studies have demonstrated that obesity is still the major risk factor for OSA in Asians.

Weight loss is associated with a decrease in the severity of OSA, but residual OSA may persist after bariatric surgery[6]. Data from ten studies showed that an overall decrease in BMI from 55 to 38kg/m2 resulted in a decrease in the AHI by 38.2 events/hour. However, more than 62% patients had residual OSA at least moderate in severity with only 25% of individuals achieving an AHI < 5 events/hour and less than half (44%) achieving an AHI < 10 events/hour.

Gender

Differences in the relative proportion of male to female in clinic-based populations (5-8:1) and epidemiological studies (2-3:1) [7] have been explained by: (a) OSA is less severe in women, being milder during non-rapid eye movement (NREM) sleep; (b) women have a greater clustering of respiratory events during rapid eye movement (REM) sleep than men do; (c) REM OSA is disproportionately more common in women than in men; and (d) supine OSA is disproportionately more common in men than in women [8]. Women with AHI > 10 per hour were found to have lower levels of 17-OH progesterone, progesterone, and estradiol than women with AHI of < 10 per hour [9]. In contrast, excess endogenous or exogenous testosterone increases the predisposition to OSA in women.

Age

OSA becomes most prevalent in midlife, with the largest age-related increase occurring before the age of 65, with some excess prevalence in women after menopause. Studies have additionally found a higher prevalence of OSA in individuals older than 65, although the estimates have ranged widely. OSA in the elderly may have a different clinical presentation. Obesity seems to have a weaker association with OSA in elderly patients than in the middle-age patients [10, 11].

Ethnicity

Despite a lower prevalence of obesity in Asia, the prevalence of OSA is similar to that in the West. For a given age, gender, and BMI, the disease severity in Asians seem to be greater than that of the Caucasians. The increased predisposition in Asians may partly be explained by differences in craniofacial morphology; however, other factors, possibly genetic, may play a role. Middle-age African-Americans have a similar prevalence of OSA as Caucasians. BMI appears to be more strongly associated with OSA in Caucasians than in African Americans or Polynesians.

Genetics

There appears to be a substantial familial aggregation of OSA[12]. First degree relatives of OSA patients have a higher risk of developing the disease than individuals without a first degree relative with OSA. One study of elderly twins found the heritability of both the respiratory disturbance index (RDI) and the oxygen desaturation index (ODI) to be nearly 40% [13]. Study of non-obese OSA patients revealed a strong genetic risk. Linkage scans of OSA from Cleveland Family Study have reported heritability of OSA in both Caucasians and African Americans to be ~ 33%, and heritability of obesity to be more than 50% [14, 15]. Heritability of OSA persisted after controlling for BMI, indicating that about half of genetic variation of OSA is obesity-related and about half is independent of OSA. Other factors known to be important in the pathogenesis of OSA, like cephalometric variables, lateral pharyngeal wall fat distribution and ventilatory control have certain heritability [16].

Craniofacial Abnormalities

Craniofacial abnormalities associated with tonsillar hypertrophy, macroglossia or increased size of soft palate, inferiorly positioned hyoid bone, maxillary and mandibular retroposition, and decreased posterior airway space increase the risk of OSA [17]. In Caucasians, certain craniofacial features may predict the risk of developing OSA [18]. Mandibular length, mandibular nasion angle, mandibular triangular area and anterior neck space area are smaller, while mandibular width-length angle and face width-midface depth angle are larger in OSA compared with controls [18]. Mandibular body length appears to be, among cephalometric measurements, the strongest predictor of OSA [19].

Exogenous Factors

OSA is more common in smokers [20]. Current smoking, in contrast to past smoking, is associated with increased risk of developing OSA, presumably due to increased inflammation and swelling of the upper airway. Alcohol ingestion prior to bedtime can induce OSA in otherwise asymptomatic patients and can worsen the severity and oxygen desaturation in established OSA. Recreational drug use was associated with increased risk of developing OSA in truck drivers. Patient on long-term opiates are also known to have a high prevalence of OSA (39%) and combined OSA and CSA (8%).

Endocrine Conditions

Polycystic ovary syndrome (PCOS), hypothyroidism, type II diabetes mellitus, pregnancy and acromegaly are associated with high prevalence of OSA. Strong correlation between diabetes mellitus type II and OSA led the International Diabetes Federation Task Force on Epidemiology and Prevention to recommend screening diabetes patients for OSA, and, conversely, screening OSA patients for hyperlipidemia, hypertension and type II DM [21]. Approximately 40% adults diagnosed with OSA will have diabetes mellitus type II [22, 23].

In patients with known diabetes, the prevalence of OSA has been reported to be 23-77% [24, 25]. In a large longitudinal study of 1,233 Veterans, presence of sleep apnea was a significant risk factor (HR 1.43; CI 1.1-1.86) for the development of diabetes and adherence to CPAP treatment seemed to attenuate this risk [26].

Hypertension

About 30% of patients with hypertension have OSA [27, 28]. In patients with refractory hypertension, the prevalence of OSA is estimated to be more than 80% [29].

Coronary Artery Disease

The prevalence of OSA in patients with coronary artery disease (CAD) is estimated to be two times that in the reference population [30, 31].

Arrhythmias

The European Multicenter Polysomnographic study showed a high prevalence of OSA in patients who had pacemakers implanted (59%) [32]. A high prevalence of OSA (50%) in patients admitted to hospital with atrial fibrillation (AF) has been reported as compared to a prevalence of 30% in patients admitted to a general cardiology floor [33].

Heart Failure

Prevalence of OSA in patients with heart failure ranges from 11% to 37%[34-36]. Heart failure patients with obesity and snoring are at an increased risk of having OSA. Patients with diastolic dysfunction are more likely to have OSA than patients with systolic dysfunction [37]. In men, the likelihood of OSA is related to BMI whereas in women it is more closely linked to age [38].

Stroke

The studies on the prevalence of OSA in patients with stroke have yielded conflicting results. Since stroke may cause sleep disordered breathing, Bassetti and Aldrich examined the prevalence of OSA in patients with transient ischemic attacks (TIA) and compared it to the prevalence in normal subjects and those with stroke [39, 40]. They found a high prevalence of OSA in patients with TIA (62%) and stroke (65%) compared with normal individuals (12%). However, a larger case control study found that patients with TIA did not have increased prevalence of OSA (50%) compared with controls (60%). High prevalence of OSA in controls could be due to selection bias in this study since many individuals declined participation in study as controls and it is possible that more symptomatic individuals agreed to participate as controls [41].

Asthma

Asthma patients have been reported to have an increased risk for OSA. In the European Community Health Respiratory Survey, the prevalence of self-reported habitual snoring and apnea were higher in asthmatics as compared to normal subjects (14.7% vs. 9.2% and 3.8% vs. 1.2%, respectively) [42], independent of BMI, age, gender and smoking[42]. Symptomatic asthma almost doubles the risk of snoring (OR = 1.8), independent of upper respiratory tract symptoms (*e.g.*, rhinitis), cigarette smoking and race. In a prospective study from Australia spanning 14 years, asthma was found to be an independent risk factor for development of habitual snoring (RR=2.8), even after adjusting for BMI at baseline and BMI change [43]. A clinic-based study [44] revealed a high prevalence of self-reported snoring with any frequency (86%), habitual snoring (38%) and witnessed apnea (31%), with 44% of subjects having a high OSA risk on a validated scale [45]. Lastly, two studies using nocturnal polysomnography (PSG) found a high prevalence of OSA in more severe asthmatics. Twenty one out of 22 (95.5%) difficult-to-control asthma patients had OSA on PSG [46]. OSA was also found to be more prevalent among those with severe (88%) versus moderate asthma (58%), and more prevalent in moderate or severe asthma patients versus controls (12%) [47]; these rates were higher than the expected incidence for the degree of excess body weight observed. No correlation was found between OSA severity and BMI or neck circumference [46].

COPD

The combination of COPD and obstructive sleep apnea is referred as *overlap syndrome*. Individuals with COPD have a higher prevalence of sleep-related symptoms including snoring (OR 1.34), apneas, (OR 1.46) and excessive daytime sleepiness (OR=2.04), compared to non-COPD patients [48]. Based on prevalence estimates of COPD prevalence of 10% and SDB of 5 to 10% in the general population, the prevalence of overlap syndrome is approximately 0.5-1% of the population over the age of 40 [49, 50]. The prevalence of cor pulmonale in patients with overlap syndrome is close to 80%, with 5 year survival of about 30% [51].

RESEARCH OUTLOOOK

What do we know:

OSA is an under-recognized disease with profound effects on cardiovascular and neurocognitive function. Many of these effects are preventable and reversible with proper treatment of OSA. However, high suspicion and proper recognition of OSA remain key to outcomes success.

What we don't know:

Although obesity and male sex are strong risk factors, there are many patients who lack the conventional characteristics of OSA phenotype. A high index of suspicion in patients with cardiovascular disease, diabetes, hypothyroidism and certain ethnicities could help identify those patients early and may impact the outcomes.

Central Sleep Apnea

Central sleep apnea (CSA), unlike obstructive sleep apnea, is not one entity, it is a conglomerate of different conditions. These disorders are further divided into primary forms: those for which the exact etiology is unknown and those due to a known cause.

The vast majority of patients with CSA have concomitant obstructive sleep apnea. Furthermore, treatment of obstructive sleep apnea results in the emergence of central sleep apnea and vice versa, indicating the commonality of pathogenesis between the 2 seemingly distinct, but probably overlapping, breathing disorders during the sleep state [52, 53]. The *International Classification of Sleep Disorders, Second Edition* (*ICSD-2*) describes several different entities grouped under central sleep apnea with varying signs, symptoms, and clinical and polysomnographic features. The CSA syndromes afflicting adults include *primary CSA, Cheyne-Stokes breathing-CSA (CSB-CSA) pattern, high-altitude periodic breathing, CSA due to medical conditions not Cheyne-Stokes,* and *CSA due to drugs or substances.* Another newly recognized CSA syndrome is *complex sleep apnea*, which is seen during treatment of obstructive sleep apnea, generally before the obstructive events are completely abolished by positive airway pressure (PAP).

Primary CSA is uncommon in adults and is seen in less than 10% of patients presenting for PSG. The prevalence of primary central apnea, high-altitude periodic breathing, and CSA due to medical conditions in the general population is unknown.

Cheyne Stokes Breathing (CSB-CSA)

Cheyne Stokes breathing is a cyclical variation in the amplitude of respiration characterized by hypopneic or apneic periods alternating with hyperpnea. Common causes are: congestive heart failure (most common condition associated with CSB-CSA), stroke and high altitude. The prevalence of CSA-CSB can be as high as 60% of patients with CHF, suggesting a special link between this breathing disorder and CHF [54, 55]. In a prospective study of 100 patients with systolic heart failure (LVEF < 45%), the prevalence of CSA-CSB was found to be 37%[56]. Poorer functional classification, atrial fibrillation, P_aCO_2 < 36 mm Hg, LVEF < 20%, and nocturnal ventricular arrhythmias predicted a higher prevalence of CSA-CSB. Patients with CSA are commonly thin and most do not snore. In a French cohort of 316 patients, the prevalence of CSA was 30 % and was associated with more severe heart failure and a more elevated AHI than an obstructive pattern [57]. Patients with CHF and CSR-CSA tend to have higher brain natriuretic peptide (BNP) levels than those without CSR-CSA [58].

CSA-CSB has been reported in both chronic and acute left ventricular dysfunction. In stable heart failure patients, the prevalence of CSA-CSB was reported as high as 15% [59]. In a study of 50 patients admitted with acute coronary syndrome (ACS), 6 patients had CSB-CSA [60]. Patients with acute myocardial infarction with impaired LV function were more likely to exhibit CSA-CSB [60]. Repeat polysomnography performed 6 months after the ACS demonstrated that CSA-CSB had largely resolved, while OSA persisted. No large scale studies are available on prevalence of CSA-CSB in patients with diastolic dysfunction. The presence of CSR or CSA in a patient with heart failure is associated with increased morbidity and mortality and impaired quality of life [61].

CSA-CSB has also been observed in patients with stroke. In a small study of 31 patients, Hermann et al observed CSA in 10% of patients [62]. It partially resolved within weeks.

Central Sleep Apnea Due to Drug or Substance

In a study of 98 patients on chronic opiate therapy, 24% had central sleep apnea and 21 % had mixed central and obstructive sleep apnea [63]. Walker et al found a dose response relationship between opiates and prevalence of central sleep apnea and ataxic breathing. 92% of patients taking a morphine dose equivalent of 200 mg or more showed ataxic breathing compared with 61% of the patients taking a morphine dose equivalent of < 200 mg a day [64].

Central Sleep Apnea due to Medical Conditions not Cheyne Stokes

In a study of 119 patients undergoing dialysis, Tada et al found that 12% of patients had CSA [65]. However, since they initially screened patients with overnight oximetry and only 46 patients underwent polysomnography, the true prevalence could be in fact, higher. PaO_2, $PaCO_2$ and cardio-thoracic ratio were predictors of CSA. Chiari malformation is associated with increased risk of both CSA and OSA. In a study of 26 adults, central sleep apnea was found to be prevalent in about 15% patients with Chiari malformation. Predictors for presence of central sleep apnea were age, type II Chiari malformation and vocal cord paralysis [66]. Traumatic brain injury is also associated with a high prevalence of central sleep apnea [67]. One study found a high prevalence of CSA after lung transplantation. In that study the prevalence of central sleep apnea after lung transplant was 25% and use of cyclosporine was associated with a higher risk of developing CSA [68]. Whether the incidence of CSA is high after other organ transplantation is unknown.

Complex Sleep Apnea (CxSA)

Central sleep apnea is occasionally seen during positive airway pressure (PAP) titration for treatment of OSA. Sometimes it is severe and can cause disruption in sleep and oxygen desaturations. Incidence of CxSA (central sleep apnea index or CAI > 5) has been reported to be between 5-15% [69]. In a large retrospective study of 1,286 patients undergoing CPAP titration for OSA, Javaheri et al found the incidence of CxSA to be 6.5 %. Half of these patients returned for a second titration study and CxSA was eliminated in 78.6% patients with 8 week therapy with CPAP. Persistence of CxSA on CPAP was associated with higher CAI, severity of OSA at baseline and with opioid use and was estimated to be about 1.5% [70].

RESEARCH OUTLOOK

What do we know:

Central sleep apnea is a heterogeneous group of disorders with different causes and manifestation. Central sleep apnea is associated with heart failure, stroke and high altitude. Cheyne Stokes breathing portends a poor prognostic value.

What we don't know:

The epidemiology of many types of central sleep apnea is not clear yet. New types of central sleep apnea and conditions associated with CSA are being identified.

Sleep-Related Hypoventilation

The obesity-hypoventilation syndrome (OHS) is also known as obesity-associated hypoventilation or Pickwickian syndrome. Criteria for OHS include a BMI $\geqslant$30 kg/m^2 and chronic alveolar hypoventilation leading to daytime hypercapnia, in the absence of pulmonary or neuromuscular disease. These patients frequently have hypoxemia with an arterial partial pressure of oxygen (PaO$_2$) less than 70 mm Hg. Sleep-induced hypoventilation is characterized by elevated levels of PaCO$_2$ while asleep, defined as a level > 45 mm Hg or a rise in PaCO$_2$ during sleep by 10 mm Hg or more above wakefulness [71]. Sleep-related hypoxemia is defined by the International Classification of Sleep Disorders-2 as "SaO$_2$ (oxyhemoglobin saturation) during sleep of less than 90% for more than five minutes, with a nadir of at least 85%" or ">30% of total sleep time with an SaO$_2$< 90%".

Risk Factors

Obesity

Obesity is one of the diagnostic criteria for OHS. The prevalence of morbid obesity (BMI > 40 kg/m^2) quadrupled between 1986 and 2000 from 0.5 to 2% of the adult population and that of BMI > 50 kg/m^2 increased five times. Morbid obesity appears to be an important contributor to OHS: the prevalence of OSA has been demonstrated to be close to 70% and OHS in the range of upper 20%, as opposed to 60% for OSA and 10% for OHS in non-morbidly obese [72].

Obstructive Sleep Apnea

The prevalence of OHS among patients with OSA is estimated between 10-20%, higher in the subgroup of patients with extreme obesity [71]. While the majority (90%) of patients with OHS have OSA, the remaining 10% of patients do not [71].

Daytime Hypercapnia

Sleep hypoventilation is present in 70% of hypercapnic subjects. The prevalence of daytime hypercapnia is related to the severity of obesity and obesity-related impairment in lung function, and reaches >20% in massive obesity [73]. This could be mediated by obstructive OSA, probable through an alteration of the ventilatory drive. In 1,141 patients with chronic respiratory insufficiency due to OSA needing CPAP therapy, the prevalence of daytime hypercapnia (PaCO$_2$ > 45 mm Hg) was 11% [73]. The prevalence of daytime hypercapnia was approximately 7% in the non-obese, 10% in moderate obesity (BMI 30-40), and 24% in morbidly obese (BMI >40). P$_a$CO$_2$ level was positively associated with age, BMI, neck circumference, waist circumference, AHI, TST$_{SaO2<90\%}$ and negatively correlated with forced expiratory volume in one second as % of predicted value (FEV$_1$%), FVC%, and PaO$_2$ [72]. Other contributors include mean apnea duration and decreased functional reserve capacity (FRC) [74]. Awake hypercapnia appears also to correlate with the maximum voluntary ventilation (MVV) [75], with the prevalence of OHS much less in normal compared to low MVV (5% vs. 25%, respectively).

Bariatric and Hospitalized Populations

Bariatric surgery and hospitalized patients are at increased risk for OHS. In 3,451 bariatric surgery patients, the overall OHS prevalence was 3.3%, higher in the Medicare group (10%) [76], while the general OSA prevalence was 30%. Male patients had an OHS prevalence of approximately 10% and an OSA prevalence of 57%. In 77 patients referred for bariatric surgery, an AHI >10 was detected in 40% of patients and AHI above 15 in 22% [77]. Hypoxemia (PaO$_2$ < 80 mmHg) was observed in 27% and hypercapnia (PaCO$_2$> 45 mm Hg) in 8% patients. In 4,332 patients admitted to the hospital, 31% of severely obese (BMI > 35 kg/m^2) patients had hypercapnia unexplained by other disorders [78].

RESEARCH OUTLOOK

What do we know:

Obesity-hypoventilation syndrome is under-recognized, but increasingly prevalent condition associated with significant adverse morbidity and mortality.

Prevalence of obesity-hypoventilation syndrome parallels the emergence and spread of the obesity epidemic.

OHS is frequently associated with OSA, but can occur also in its absence, depending on the predominant mechanism (obstructive versus central).

What we don't know:

If OHS is the end of a continuous spectrum of evolution of SDB severity, *i.e.*, if a patient with OHS progresses in time from primary snoring, to severe OSA and then to OHS.

EPIDEMIOLOGY OF INSOMNIA

Due to the evolving view of insomnia from symptom to a distinct disorder, epidemiological data has been dependent (and confounded) by multiple definitions: insomnia symptoms, insomnia symptoms with daytime consequences and insomnia diagnoses [79]. Most of the studies account for three insomnia symptoms: difficulties falling asleep, difficulties maintaining sleep and early morning awakenings. Insomnia symptoms were reported to be present in about one-third of a general population [79]. Non-restorative sleep, which is also part of the insomnia definition (ICSD-2), is rarely explored. Daytime consequences of insomnia have also been absent in many of the early studies. When daytime consequences of insomnia (*e.g.* excessive sleepiness, irritability, depressive or anxious mood) are taken into account, the prevalence has been estimated to be around 10%. However, daytime consequences may be as prevalent as 2/3 of insomnia subjects [79]. The last definition, corresponding to a decision-making diagnosis, has been estimated at a prevalence at 6% [79].

Risk Factors

Most data comes from cross-sectional studies correlating insomnia to coincident demographic traits, health status, occupation, or social functioning. In the case of most acquired characteristics found to predict insomnia, such studies imply possible risk but do not confirm it.

Gender

Women/men ratio for insomnia symptoms is about 1.5 [80]. In a sample of 5469 young adults (ages 20-39) part of the 3rd National Health and Nutritional Examination Survey (NHANES-III), women were more likely to report insomnia symptoms than men (16.7% vs. 9.2%), correlating with a higher prevalence of affective disorders among women [81]. Unemployment, lower socio-economic status, alcohol consumption, regular medication use and psychiatric disturbances were associated with higher risks of insomnia in both genders [82]. Lower education level and being retired were reported to be associated with a higher risk of insomnia in males; being a housewife, divorced/widowed, and complaining of a nocturnal noisy environment were associated with a higher risk of insomnia in females [82]. Menopausal women appear to have an increased prevalence of insomnia as compared with pre-menopausal women [83].

Age

Increasing age is associated with increased prevalence of insomnia symptoms, reaching almost 50% in subjects older than 65 years of age. However, there appears that there is no increase in prevalence in healthy older adults, which seem to sleep as well as younger adults. Prevalence of insomnia with daytime consequences is less clear, with studies demonstrating stable rates versus increased prevalence with aging [79].

Marital Status

There appears to be a higher prevalence of insomnia in divorced or widowed subjects, with a stronger association noted in women [84].

Occupational Status

Insomnia symptoms are reported more often by non-working subjects compared with working individuals. The highest risk was noted in retirees and homemakers [85].

Comorbidities

Approximately half of all insomnia subjects have been reported to have long-term medical problems [86]. The preferred term for insomnia that co-exists with health conditions that may disturb sleep is *co-morbid* insomnia; differentiating if the accompanying condition plays a causal role in the insomnia, is the consequence of insomnia or is incidental to insomnia can be challenging for the provider.

Mental Health Conditions

Mental health conditions are often associated with complaints of difficulties with sleep. Sleep disruption is, in fact, a part of the diagnostic criteria for many psychiatric disorders. To be an independent diagnosis, insomnia has to be distinct of the complaints and more prominent than usually present in mental disorders [87].

Depressive and Bipolar Disorders

Insomnia in the primary care setting shows a stronger association to depression than any other medical disorder [88]. Approximately three quarters of depressed adults and older adults complain of difficulty falling or staying asleep, or being tired during the day [89, 90]. These subjective sleep complaints may persist beyond the resolution of depressive symptoms [91]. Prevalence of symptoms is comparable between genders [92]. Insomnia was shown to be a strong risk factor for future depression [93]. Insomnia at baseline and one year later increased 8 times the risk of development of depression [94]. Insomnia can precede manic episodes as a first symptom in as many as 77% of cases [95]. Furthermore, sleep loss may trigger manic episodes, emphasizing a need to clinically monitor sleep changes, and address sleep disrupting factors in an attempt to decrease such exacerbations [95].

Bereavement and Grief

In a cross-sectional study of 170 women at 4-60 months (average 26 months) from the loss event, insomnia was reported by 13% of subjects [96]. Baseline complicated grief scores of recently widowed individuals were significantly associated with sleep difficulties at 18-month follow-up [97]. Higher grief tended to be associated with less time spent asleep and reduced alertness at 8 pm [98].

Anxiety Disorder

Generalized anxiety disorder, a condition of generalized hyperarousal, is the most prevalent condition of subjects complaining of insomnia who have a mental health diagnosis in the adult population [99]. Sleep disturbance is endorsed in about 2/3 of patients with this diagnosis [100]. Objective findings include: more awakenings, longer time to fall asleep, decreased sleep efficiency and time, with less consistent findings of more stage N2, and decreased slow wave sleep (SWS) [101, 102].

Panic Disorder

Panic disorder is associated with difficulty falling sleep, disturbed and restless sleep, as well as nocturnal panic attacks. Nearly a quarter of patients with panic disorder report either short sleep duration ($\leq$ 5h) or long sleep duration ($\geq$9h) [103]. Nocturnal panic attacks are similar to daytime panic attacks, occur at least weekly in 18-45% of panic disorder patients [100, 104], usually in the first few hours of sleep, in transition from stage N2 to slow wave sleep (SWS) [105]. People with nocturnal panic attacks have higher rates of insomnia and depression than people with panic disorder without nighttime episodes [106, 107].

Post-Traumatic Stress Disorder (PTSD)

Difficulties initiating and maintaining sleep are *DSM-IV* criteria and prominent symptoms of PTSD. Insomnia seems to be common early after trauma leading to PTSD [108]. Nightmares that are similar to trauma memories seem to be relatively specific to developing PTSD. More recent studies do not indicate that sleep initiation and maintenance is markedly more impaired among those developing PTSD, pathogenesis appears to rather implicate shorter continuous periods of REM sleep before stage shifts or arousals and increased sympathetic nervous system activity during REM sleep [109].

Medical Conditions and Sleep

Pain

Pain is a common contributor to insomnia. In a population of adults aged 55-84, 19% reported that pain disrupted their sleep at least a few nights per week and 12% reported almost nightly sleep fragmentation due to pain [110]. In referral populations of patients with chronic pain, prevalence rates of insomnia can range between 50-70% [111]. Painful conditions are frequently associated with reduced total sleep time, reduced REM sleep, frequent brief arousals and increased wakefulness after sleep onset [112, 113].

Arthritis

Insomnia has been described in 30-80% of patients with osteoarthritis [114]. Adults over age 65 with knee arthritis have been observed to have problems initiating sleep (31%), maintaining sleep (81%), and a tendency to awaken early in the morning (51%) [115]. The prevalence of insomnia complaints in patients with rheumatoid arthritis (RA) is greater than 50%. Although these complaints may involve problems with sleep onset, the most significant differences between patients with RA and healthy controls appear to be in sleep maintenance, sleep quality, and restorative sleep [116]. Insomnia is also highly prevalent (>75%) in fibromyalgia patients [116].

Gastroesophageal Reflux Disease (GERD)

In population surveys, between 50-70% of individuals with GERD report nighttime symptoms and reduced sleep quality [117]. In a sample of 11,685 survey respondents with GERD, 89% experienced nighttime symptoms, 68% sleep difficulties, 49% difficulty initiating asleep and 58% difficulty maintaining sleep. Subjects with nighttime GERD symptoms were more likely to experience sleep difficulties (odds ratio, 1.53) and difficulties with initiation of sleep (odds ratio, 1.43) and maintenance of sleep (odds ratio, 1.56) [118].

Hypertension and Heart Disease

In 432 patients with hypertension, 48% were identified as having insomnia, more frequent in women (61%) and coronary artery disease (CAD) patients [119]. In stable CAD patients, women had a higher prevalence of "too little sleep" (42%) compared with men (24%) [120]. Among 3,309 adults presenting with acute coronary syndrome (ACS), 26% of the individuals were awakened from sleep [121]. In 223 patients with CHF (New York Heart Association class II–IV), consistent difficulties maintaining sleep were reported by approximately 20% of sample, while 25% of the subjects were awake up to 3 hours/night [122]. In another sample of 106 CHF patients, 31%

reported symptoms suggestive of chronic insomnia; paroxysmal nocturnal dyspnea (PND) had an odds ratio (OR) of 3.5 for a complaint of insomnia [123].

Chronic Obstructive Lung Disease

Chronic lung disease increases sleep stage changes, decreases total sleep time and increases number of arousals [124]. Mechanisms include: nocturnal cough, wheezing, and shortness of breath due to worsening of pulmonary mechanics and gas exchange during sleep. Hypoxemia, which is common in COPD during rapid eye movement (REM) sleep, correlates with an increase in arousal and excessive daytime sleepiness.

Nocturnal Asthma

Nocturnal asthma symptoms resulting in nighttime awakenings may occur in over 70% of persons with asthma. A survey of 7,729 asthmatics reported that 74% awoke at least once per week with asthma symptoms, while 64% reported nocturnal symptoms at least 3 times per week and 39% experienced symptoms nightly [125]. In a study of 3,129 asthmatic patients who maintained a record of 1,631 acute asthma episodes, asthma was approximately 70-fold more frequent between 4:00-5:00 am than between 2:00-3:00 pm [126]. As the number of nocturnal breathing problems increase, there appears to be an increase of difficulty in initiating sleep, maintaining sleep and nocturnal wakefulness [127, 128]. Asthma control and $FEV_1\%$ correlate with global Pittsburgh Sleep Quality Index (PSQI) [129] and quality of sleep [130]. Circadian peak expiratory flow (PEF) variation was found to be the strongest factor influencing PSG-documented time spent awake at night in nocturnal asthmatics [131]. However, asthmatics have increased prevalence of sleep symptoms even with optimal asthma control [130].

Menopause

Peri-menopause, approximately 40-50% of women report sleep difficulties following cessation of menstruation. While some of this is transient during the years of hormonal changes ("hot flashes"), symptoms may continue years later. Hormone replacement therapy (HRT) has been shown to improve subjective but not objective sleep measures [132].

Urologic and Chronic Renal Diseases

The incidence and severity of nocturia increase with age. Nocturia was listed as a self-perceived cause of disrupted nocturnal sleep "every night or almost every night" by 53% of a sample of 1,424 subjects (ages 55-84), which was over four times as frequently as the next most often cited cause of poor sleep, pain (12%) [133]. Nocturia was an independent predictor both of self-reports of insomnia (75% increased risk) and reduced sleep quality (71% increased risk).

In a Danish population of 2,799 men and women aged 60–80 years, prevalence of nocturia (≥ 1 void) was 75% in women and 78% in men. While urinary incontinence, recurrent cystitis and diabetes mellitus were found to be strongest risk factors for nocturia [134], other factors include polyuria, low bladder capacity, sleep apnea, intake of excessive fluid before bedtime, alcohol, caffeine, diuretics, medical disorders such as hypertension, congestive heart failure and prostatic disease, as well as nocturnal polyuria syndrome, characterized by normal or only moderately increased 24-hr urine output but inappropriate nocturnal urine output, often an undetectable nocturnal plasma ADH, and increased thirst, particularly at night [135].

Fifty-seven percent of patients with end-stage renal disease report sleep maintenance problems, and 55% report early morning awakening [136]. Prevalence of insomnia in hemodialysis (HD) patients may be as high as 80% [137]. Quality of sleep was associated with hemoglobin level, serum albumin and depression [138]. Conversely, the treatment of anemia with erythropoietin improved sleep quality [139].

Cancer

Patients with cancer may have sleep effects from the disease itself, its treatment or the psychological response to the diagnosis [140]. Large epidemiological studies reported sleep problems being present in 55-87% of patients [140, 141]; approximately ½ of patients reported onset within six months pre-diagnosis to 18 months post-diagnosis [142]. In a study of 867 patients newly diagnosed with breast, colorectal, lung, or prostate cancer, insomnia remained present in 23% of patients at 1 year from their diagnosis. A high attrition rate may have influenced the observed lessening of insomnia over time [143].

Neurologic Disorders

Different neurologic disorders, including Parkinson's disease (PD) and Alzheimer's disease (AD), are associated with a high prevalence of insomnia. In PD, insomnia may be the result of motor symptoms, psychiatric symptoms, and/or treatment with dopaminergic agents [144]. Difficulty in maintaining sleep is particularly burdensome in patients with AD, and both insomnia and nocturnal agitation/sleep schedule disruption (*e.g.*, "sundowning") being present in as many as a quarter of patient and often leading to institutionalization [145].

RESEARCH OUTLOOK

What do we know:

Insomnia is a common chronic condition and may have a spectrum of severity and co-morbidities.

There appears to be an increased prevalence related to gender (women are more affected than men) and also with advancing age.

What we don't know:

There is little data in regard to what makes a person more prone to develop insomnia as well as what daytime consequences are to be expected from insomnia and to what degree.

EPIDEMIOLOGY OF HYPERSOMNIA SYNDROMES

Narcolepsy

Narcolepsy is clasically defined by sleepiness and abnormal rapid eye movement (REM) sleep-related symptoms (cataplexy, hypnagogic hallucinations, and sleep paralysis). In a study of narcolepsy in King County, state of Washington, USA, prevalence of narcolepsy with or without cataplexy has been reported as 30.6 per 100,000 people (18 years or older), narcolepsy with cataplexy as 21.8/ 100,000 people and narcolepsy with HLA-DQB1*0602 as 15.3/ 100,000 people [146]. The median age of onset was 14 years. Estimated prevalence was higher in African-Americans than other racial groups. Prevalence of narcolepsy in the Finnish Twin Cohort population of over 11,000 individuals was 26/100,000 [147]. In 18,980 randomly selected subjects (age 15-100, 51% women), representative of a target population of 205 million European inhabitants, excessive daytime sleepiness was reported by 15% of the sample, while napping two times or more in the same day was reported by 1.6% of the sample [148]. Cataplexy (episodes of loss of muscle function related to a strong emotion) was found in 1.6% of the sample. A narcolepsy diagnosis was reported in 47/100,000 people, severe for 26/100,000 and moderate in 21/100,000. With the exception of cataplexy, other narcolepsy symptoms (sleep paralysis, hypnagogic hallucinations) are not necessarily specific of narcolepsy and some are highly prevalent in the general population: 6.2% for sleep paralysis and 24.1% for hypnagogic hallucinations[148]. Multiple sleep-onset REM periods (SOREMPs) and short mean sleep latencies (MSL ≤ 8 mins) were reported in about 4% of the general population [149].

Risk Factors

Hypocretin

Impairement of hypocretin neurotransmission is thought to be a major mechanism in narcolepsy. Hypocretin-1 levels below 110 pg/mL are considered diagnostic for narcolepsy, while values above 200 pg/mL are considered normal. In a study of cerebrospinal fluid (CSF) hypocretin level in 9 people with narcolepsy (all HLA-DR2/DQB1*0602 positive), hypocretin-1 concentrations were below the detection limit of the assay (<40 pg/mL) in 7 patients, while it was detectable in all controls [150]. In another study of 38 successive narcolepsy-cataplexy cases [36 HLA-DQB1*0602-positive and 34 matched controls], hypocretin-1 was decreased (<100 pg/mL) in 32 of 38 patients (all HLA-positive) [151]. Low CSF hypocretin-1 levels appears to be specific for HLA DR2-positive narcolepsy, and the deficiency is thought to be established at the early stage of the disease [152].

Genetics

Most cases do not appear genetically linked; however, genetic factors have been suggested by twin and family studies. Narcolepsy appears to be associated with HLA-DR2 phenotype, HLA-DQB1*0602 being the main susceptibility allele, particularly for narcolepsy with cataplexy. Among narcoleptic patients with cataplexy, 61% were positive for HLA-DQB1*0602, and among the ones who were positive for HLA-DQB1*0602, 82% had cataplexy [146]. HLA-DQB1*0602 positivity is lower in narcolepsy without cataplexy (56%), and idiopathic hypersomnia (52%) [153]. DQB1*0602 is also present in controls, with numbers as high as 38% of controls[153] and as low as 6.8% (reported in Israel), suggesting a wide variation in genetic susceptibility to develop narcolepsy depending on population [154].

In a study of 12 Hong Kong Chinese narcoleptic subjects, 34 first-degree relatives, and 30 healthy controls, the frequency of narcolepsy in first degree relatives was 2.9% [149]. Nearly 30% of the relatives fulfilled the criteria of narcolepsy spectrum disorder (shortened mean sleep latency and/or the presence of sleep onset REM periods). The odds ratio of narcolepsy spectrum disorder in first-degree relatives was 5.8 compared to healthy controls. There were 6 families in which all 10 relatives were found with narcolepsy spectrum disorders and were positive for HLA DQB1*0602.

Obesity

In a cross-sectional, case-control study of 138 patients with narcolepsy compared with a population of 10,696 people, the prevalence of obesity was 33% in narcoleptics vs. 12.5% in controls [155]. Excess body fat, as reflected in waist circumference, was more common in patients with narcolepsy [155].

Race

In a population-based case control study of narcolepsy with cataplexy from King County, Washington, USA, being African American was associated with an odds ratio of 7.6 [156].

Gender

Some studies suggest that narcolepsy is more common in men than women [154]. For narcolepsy with cataplexy, the relative risk was estimated at 1.2:1, and prevalence ratio was 1.4:1. For all patients with narcolepsy, the relative risk was 1.6:1, and prevalence ratio was 1.8:1, suggesting that the gender difference is greater in those without cataplexy [154].

Immunological Factors

Comparing 9 cases and 9 controls, auto-antibodies enhancing postganglionic cholinergic neurotransmission were found in immunoglobulin G fraction of patients with narcolepsy, but not in controls [157]. Comparing 20 narcoleptic patients with 20 controls, narcoleptics had immunoglobulin G in their CSF that reacted to a rat hypothalamic protein extract containing hypocretin-secreting cells [154]. In a population-based case control study of narcolepsy with cataplexy investigating a wide range of exposures in early life, a history of physician diagnosed strep throat before age 21 was associated with a 5-fold increase [156].

Secondary Narcolepsy

Sporadic cases of narcolepsy associated with head trauma, encephalitis, and Guillain-Barré syndrome, autosomal dominant cerebellar ataxia, vascular and tumoral hypothalamic lesions, Prader-Willi syndrome, myxedema coma secondary to Hashimoto thyroiditis [153].

RESEARCH OUTLOOK

What do we know:

Hypocretin-1 is a major neurotransmitter involved in the complex regulation of wake-sleep cycle

What we don't know:

In regard to narcolepsy geographic differences in prevalence, we don't know if a low prevalence in some countries is due to methodological differences, genetic susceptibility pool, exposure to etiologic risk factors, etc.

Evidence to support an immune mechanism is emerging, but the etiologic or initiating events have not been identified yet.

Idiopathic Hypersomnia

Idiopathic hypersomnia (IH) is characterized by chronic, daily excessive daytime sleepiness, despite normal sleep. Naps are typically long and unrefreshing. Patients may also report prolonged difficulty waking, presenting automatic behavior, confusion, and repeated returns to sleep, *i.e.*, "sleep drunkenness" or "sleep inertia". Idiopathic hypersomnia is now divided in hypersomnia with or without long sleep time. Available series and the expert clinical opinions suggest that IH is a rare disease with a ratio of 8:10 to 1:10 compared with patients having narcolepsy; the current prevalence is estimated at 5/100,000 people [158].

Topic Discussion (Clinical Outlook)

Genetics

The HLA DQB1*0602 genotype was found equally in IH (24.2%) and controls (19.2%)[158].

Obesity

Idiopathic hypersomnia subjects were not reported to be overweight, suggesting a major difference from narcolepsy [158]. Patients with long sleep time ($\geq$ 10 hours) appear to have a lower BMI versus than those without long sleep time [158].

Hypocretin-1

IH cases were reported to have normal hypocretin-1 CSF levels [159]. Objectively, these cases can be differentiated from narcolepsy without cataplexy by MSLT; IH patients tend to have < 2 SOREMPS during MSLT [159].

RESEARCH OUTLOOK

What do we know:

Idiopathic hypersomnia is a distinct entity, thought to be rarer than narcolepsy, with a specific clinic picture. Most cases of excessive daytime sleepiness have other causes than idiopathic hypersomnia.

What we don't know:

There are only a few series of patients described in literature with little data in regard to epidemiological aspects, such as general population prevalence and factors increasing the risk for this disorder.

EPIDEMIOLOGY OF PARASOMNIAS

NREM Parasomnias

NREM parasomnias tend to arise from slow wave sleep (SWS) (stage N3 of NREM sleep) and, thus, typically occur during the first 1 to 2 hours of sleep. Confusional arousals typically are brief, simple motor behaviors that occur without significant affective expression or responsiveness to the environment. They are associated with mental confusion on arousal or awakening.

In an European study of 13,057 subjects, confusional arousals were reported by 2.9% of the sample [160]. About 1% of the sample also admitted memory deficits (54%), disorientation in time and/or space (71%), or slow mentation and speech (54%); the rest reported confusional arousals without associated features. Younger subjects (< 35 years) and shift or night workers were at higher risk of reporting confusional arousals. These arousals were associated with the presence of a mental disorder (especially bipolar and anxiety disorders) with odds ratios ranging from 2.4 to 13.5 as well as with obstructive sleep apnea [160].

REM Sleep Behavior Disorder

REM sleep behavior disorder (RBD) is characterized by loss of normal skeletal muscle atonia during rapid eye movement (REM) sleep, associated with vivid dreaming and complex motor activity during sleep, even violent behavior during sleep. RBD may be idiopathic in approximately 60% cases.

Little is known about the prevalence of this condition in the general population. In a sample of 2,078 men and 2,894 women between the ages of 15 to 100 years, 2% of respondents of a telephone interview reported experiencing violent behavior during sleep [161].

Neurodegenerative Disorders

RBD may occur during or precede a neurodegenerative disease, most often alpha-synucleinopathies, such as Parkinson's disease (PD), dementia with Lewy bodies, multiple system atrophy *etc.* Prevalence of probable RBD (based on a sleep questionnaire) in a community-based cohort of PD patients has been reported to be 15%, with about 20% of subjects developing new RBD at 4 years follow-up [162]. Prevalence of RBD was found to be 12% in Huntington disease[163]. Other neurologic conditions involving the brainstem, such as cerebrovascular disease, tumors and demyelinating lesions may result in RBD.

Medications

RBD has been associated with use or withdrawal of barbiturates, bisoprolol, caffeine, and alcohol [164]. Selective serotonin re-uptake inhibitors (SSRI's), such as fluoxetine, paroxetine and venlafaxine, were also associated with RBD [165]. Overall, it has been estimated that this is an uncommon side effect, particularly when taking into account the number of individuals receiving these medications [164].

Age

In a population of patients with RBD presenting to a regional sleep laboratory, more than one-third of patients were <50 years of age at the time of diagnosis [165]. Idiopathic cases accounted for more than half of cases, and the secondary form of the disorder was responsible for 49% of cases in patients younger than 50 years of age and 36.5% of cases in the older group. RBD occurring in patients under 50 years of age was associated with narcolepsy in 38% of patients, while in those over 50 years old RBD was associated with a synucleinopathy in 29% of cases [165].

In another study, younger patients had significantly more psychiatric diagnoses (85% vs. 46% and 85% vs. 36%, for past and present diagnoses) and antidepressant use (80% vs. 46%) compared to the late-onset group [164].

Gender

RBD has been consistently reported to occur in males more frequently than females with a M:F proportion smaller (M:F=1.4:1) in subjects younger than 50 years of age compared a ratio M:F=3:1 observed in subjects older than 50 [165].

RESEARCH OUTLOOK

What do we know:

The incidence of parasomnias varies by category, with disorders of arousal being the most common. Simple sleep talking (somniloquy) is common and is often part of normal phenomenons of sleep. One the the hand, REM sleep behavior disorder has been associated with certain medication use or neurological, especially neurodegenerative, disorders. RBD occurs most common in middle-aged and older men.

What we don't know:

The mechanisms behind parasomnias remain poorly understood. Why RBD is primarily a male disorder remains unknown.

EPIDEMIOLOGY OF RESTLESS LEGS AND PERIODIC LEG MOVEMENTS OF SLEEP

Restless Legs Syndrome

RLS is generally diagnosed from a patient's report of specific symptoms. However, no single diagnostic test has been shown to detect the presence or absence of the disease. Self-defined, non-standard definitions of RLS characterized earlier studies, until the International Restless Legs Syndrome Study Group released four "minimal diagnostic criteria" in 1995, leading to development of a standardized questionnaire then implemented in epidemiologic studies[166]. The prevalence of RLS has been reported to be between 6% and 12% [166]. The highest prevalence has been found in northern European and North American populations (5–10%), and the lowest among individuals from Asia and the Middle East (0.1–2%) [167].

In a European study of 18,980 subjects representative of 205,890,882 inhabitants, unpleasant feelings in the legs at bedtime occurred daily for 0.9% of the sample, at least one night per week for 6.4% of the sample and several times per month in 3.1% of the sample [168]. Subjects meeting minimal criteria for RLS represented 5.5% of the sample. In a survey of 23,000 patients from primary care physician practices, the prevalence rate was 11.1% for any degree of symptoms, while 9.6% of patients reported weekly RLS symptoms. The prevalence rate of clinically significant RLS was 2.7% in this primary care population [169]. In a general population of >15,000 subjects, symptoms of any frequency occurred in 7.2% of the population. 5% had at least weekly symptoms, and 2.7% had symptoms at least twice weekly that were moderately or severely distressing [167].

Risk Factors

Genetic Factors

There have been described two separate phenotypes of RLS, one with a high degree of familial penetrance and symptoms starting early (before age 45), and another one with a much lower degree of familial penetrance and symptoms starting later (after age 45) [170]. The risk to first-degree relatives of the affected patient has been reported as high as approximately 25-50%, in some cases suggestive of an autosomal dominant genetic disorder with nearly 100% penetrance [170]. While gene identification studies using these and similar families have been generally unsuccessful, a significant linkage on chromosome 12q has been reported occurring in some RLS families [170].

Age

RLS prevalence increases 2- to 3-fold from young age (20–29 years) to older age (60–69 years)[166]. In the above noted large European sample, prevalence of symptoms was 2.5 times higher in subjects 50 years or older as compared to those under 40 years [168].

Gender

Higher prevalence of RLS in women than in men has been described repeatedly, in many studies. Women are affected approximately twice as often as men [166]. For example, in a community-based epidemiological study of 714 participants drawn from a roster of 61,730 adult individuals aged 65 years and older, while the RLS prevalence was 8.3%, women had an almost two-fold higher prevalence (10.2%) than men (5.7%) [171]. The increased prevalence in women has been proposed to be linked to transitory hormonal changes, such as those occurring during pregnancy, or alternatively, as well as depletion of iron stores triggering the disorder in predisposed women[166]. As such, females have been reported to have lower levels of ferritin (average 44 ng/mL) compared with males (91 ng/mL) [172].

Pregnancy

In a sample of 271 pregnant women admitted to the hospital for delivery, 30% satisfied diagnostic criteria of RLS [173]. Family history of RLS (OR 8.43), history of RLS in prior pregnancy (OR 53.74), history of RLS in past even when non-pregnant (OR: 12.91) and hemoglobin of 11 g/dL or less (OR 2.05) were found to be independent predictors of RLS during pregnancy. Family history of RLS (OR 3.06) and anemia (OR 1.89) were associated with de novo RLS, and family history of RLS (OR 12.39) and multiparity (OR 6.84) were predictors of pre-existing RLS. In another large sample of 16,528 pregnant women living in Japan, the prevalence of RLS was found to be 19.9%, increasing in the later stages of pregnancy [174].

Iron Metabolism

Conditions that compromise iron availability appear to increase the risk of RLS [175]; as such, some patients with RLS with marginal CNS iron status can become insufficient when normal access to adequate peripheral iron is limited or may become insufficient even with normal access to adequate peripheral iron supply. The change in CNS iron status produces RLS symptoms largely through its effects on the dopaminergic system. Ferritin level was found to correlate with the RLS severity [172]. However, the association of iron metabolism and RLS on a population level has not been clearly established. For example, while in a study of 946 blood donors from Sweden, RLS affected 14.7% of males and 24.7% of females [176], a more recent study on 2,005 blood donors from UK, after controlling for age and sex, found no evidence to suggest that a greater number or frequency of blood donations increased the risk of RLS [177].

Comorbidities

Among health variables, musculoskeletal disease, mental disorders, heart disease and hypertension (treated or not) appear associated with RLS [168]. Presence of OSA and BMI were found to be strong predictors of RLS [168]. Prevalence in end-stage renal disease was reported to vary from 6% to 83% [178]. While data is limited in regard to PD, in a study of 303 patients with Parkinson's disease (PD), 21% fulfilled criteria for RLS and in 2/3 of these patients, RLS began before PD [179]. Peripheral neuropathies such as cryoglobulinemia, Charcot-Marie-Tooth polyneuropathy type 2, diabetic, and amyloid neuropathy tend to frequently develop RLS as an early manifestation [178].

Other Risk Factors

Prevalence of RLS was reported to be higher in widowed, unemployed, retired and homemaker individuals [168].

RESEARCH OUTLOOK

What do we know:

RLS is one of the few disorders that at current time must be assessed through specific questions. The International Restless Legs Syndrome Study Group agreed on four "minimal diagnostic criteria" in 1995, thus paving the way for the development of a standardized questionnaire that can be implemented in epidemiologic studies.

What we don't know:

It remains unclear how to practically conduct surveys using these criteria, *i.e.* how to exactly phrase questions that address the minimal criteria.

Periodic Leg Movements of Sleep and Periodic Leg Movements Disorder (PLMD)

Periodic leg movements of sleep (PLMS) are characterized by periodic episodes of repetitive limb movements caused by contractions of the muscles during sleep, usually in non-REM stages N1 or N2. PLMD is a disorder given when no other cause can be identified for insomnia or hypersomnia. If the affected individual does not have any other related sleep symptom, such as nocturnal awakenings or a bed partner who notices the unusual leg movements, the abnormal movements will remain un-noticed. Consequently, prevalence is likely to be underestimated. In 18,980 subjects (51% women, ages ranged from 15 to 100 years) leg movements occurred at least two or three nights per month in 5.9% of the sample, 5.5% reported having it at least one night per week and 7.8% said it occurred at least two nights or more each week [168]. 3.9% of the sample satisfied minimal criteria for a PLMD according to ICSD classification.

In a community-based sample of 592 participants evaluated with polysomnography, the prevalence of periodic limb movements during sleep (PLMSI > 15) was 7.6% [180]. Subjects with a PLMSI > 15 were approximately 4 times as likely to have reported either "restless or crawling feelings in their legs at night" and almost 4 times as likely to have "repeated leg jerks or twitches during sleep" as those subjects with a PLMSI ≤ 15. In an actigraphic study of 100 community based subjects, the PLMSI (mean of two nights) ranged from 0 to 60.3 and 37% of the sample had a PLMI > 5 [181]. Ten percent of the population had a PLMI ≥ 25.

Risk factors

RLS

Studies have reported a high prevalence of PLMS in RLS patients, reaching 80-100% of subjects [182]. In the above noted actigraphic study of 100 subjects, 67% of those who reported some degree of RLS had a PLMI ≥ 5 [181]. In the above sample of 18,980 subjects, 18.5% of RLS subjects also had PLMD, representing 1.0% of the sample [168]. In RLS patients, the PLM index decreases along NREM sleep stages.

Gender

Studies have reported mixed results, some finding a higher prevalence in women[168] while others reporting higher PLMI's in men (52% vs. 22.0% having a PLMI ≥ 5) [181].

Race

In the above noted community-based sample of 592 participants evaluated with polysomnography, African Americans had a lower prevalence of PLMSI >15 than Caucasians (4.3% vs. 9.3%) [180].

Age

Studies reported an increasing number of subjects with a PLMSI of five events or more per hour with older age. Up to one third of the elderly individuals has a PLMS index >5 events per hour. PLMS index appears to reach a plateau at 15–25 years of age and remains somewhat stable up to 65 years; after this age, it shows a clear increase [183].

Iron Metabolism

In a study of 27 patients with RLS assessed with polysomnography, patients with lower ferritin level (< 50 ng/mL) showed significantly more PLMS with arousal than did those with higher ferritin [172].

Comorbidities

In 79 adult stable outpatients with CHF assessed with overnight polysomnography, 19% had PLMSI >5[184]. In 169 narcolepsy patients compared with controls, more narcoleptics than controls had a PLMSI greater than 5 per hour of sleep (67% versus 37%) and an index greater than 10 (53% versus 21%) [185]. PLMS indices were higher both in NREM and REM sleep in narcoleptic patients. A significant increase of PLMSI was also found with aging in both narcoleptic patients and controls.

Substance Use

Individuals drinking at least three cups of coffee per day appear to be more likely to have PLMD as reported by one study [168], while other studies did not show a relationship between the amount of caffeine consumed and the number of periodic leg movements measured by PSG or Actigraphy [180].

Socio-Economical Factors

Separated or divorced subjects and shift or night workers were reported to have a higher prevalence of PLMD than other individuals [168].

RESEARCH OUTLOOK

What do we know:

The prevalence of periodic leg movements is likely underestimated due to difficulties in recognizing these movements by the affected individual. Periodic leg movements often occur in the context of restless legs syndrome and share many common risk factors.

What we don't know:

The clinical significance of periodic leg movements and association with daytime symptoms are still evolving areas.

EPIDEMIOLOGY OF CIRCADIAN SLEEP DISORDERS

Advanced and Delayed Sleep Phase Syndromes

The most frequent chronotype (14.6% of the population) sleeps on average between 9 min past midnight and 8:18 am [186]. Approximately 35% of the population goes to sleep earlier and 50% later. While only 1% sleep at or before 10:00 pm, 8% fall asleep around 3:00 am or later [186].

Ethnicity, gender, and socio-economic factors were not found to be determinants of morningness/eveningness preference [187]. Work schedules was found to be a predictor of chronotype, with night workers more likely to be evening type [187].

Circadian rhythm sleep disorders require a mismatch between the endogenous circadian sleep tendency and exogenous environmental requirements for sleep timing. In a population 40-64 years old, advance-related complaints (trouble staying awake until bedtime and troubled by waking up early in the morning) were found in 7.4% [188]. Less prevalent were delay-related complaints reported together in 3.1% (trouble falling asleep and trouble waking up in the morning).

Risk Factors:

Age and Gender

Older people show a phase advance of circadian rhythms compared with younger people. In a sample of healthy older adults compared with younger controls, the acrophase of melatonin excretion was advanced by 37 minutes compared with that of young adults, cortisol excretion acrophase was 90-minutes advance and sleep offset was 99-minute advanced [189]. At the other end of the spectrum are teenagers: they tend to have a delay in sleep/wake behavior [190]. The phase of circadian rhythm appears to be moving forward from the young to the older groups [191].

In a sample of almost 9,000 subjects from 10 to 87 yrs of age, sleep-time preference started to shift toward eveningness from the age of 13 yrs [192]. Females reached their peak in eveningness earlier (about 17 yrs of age) than males (about 21 yrs of age). Thereafter, the ideal sleep-time preference advanced in men and women with increasing age, with the gender difference disappearing around the age of 50, which coincides with the average age at menopause [186].

Genetics

Reports of familial aggregation of circadian sleep disorders include a large family with advanced sleep phase syndrome (ASPS) in which an affected member is present in every generation, suggesting that the ASPS phenotype segregates as a single gene with an autosomal dominant mode of inheritance [193].

RESEARCH OUTLOOK

What do we know:

The chronotype (preference to sleep) is dependent on genetic and environmental factors, but also on age. The phase of circadian rhythm appears to be moving forward from the young to the older individual.

What we don't know:

More data is necessary to understand the complex genetic factors contributing to the chronotype and well as the role of sleep deprivation and the environment in shaping a certain chronotype.

Shift Work Syndrome (SWS)

Because 6% of all workers are night or rotating workers, it is estimated that approximately 1% of the working population would meet the criteria for SWS [194].

In 2,570 individuals aged 18 –65 years from a community-based sample including 360 people working rotating shifts, 174 people working nights, 32% of night workers and 26% of rotating workers met the criteria for SWS [194]. When compared with day workers, the differential prevalence of insomnia or excessive sleepiness in the night- and rotating-worker sample was 14% and 8%. The differential corresponding prevalence" of SWS was therefore 10.0% [194].

In another sample of 103 shift workers (2 weeks on 7 nights/7days, 12-h shifts, 4 weeks off), working at an oil rig in the North Sea prevalence for SWS of 23% [195]. In addition, during the 4-week non-work period, individuals with SWS reported significantly poorer sleep quality, as measured by the PQSI, and more subjective health complaints than individuals not having SWSD. In a sample of 775 nursing home caregivers from Japan rotating in a two-shift system, prevalence of difficulty initiating sleep was 38%, insomnia symptoms 43%, and poor quality of sleep 25% [196].

RESEARCH OUTLOOK

What do we know:

Morningness/eveningness preference appears independent of ethnicity, gender, and socio-economic situation, indicating that it is a stable characteristic that may be better explained by endogenous factors.

Reduced or disturbed sleep is a common negative consequence of any occupation that involves shift work due to the disruption of the circadian rhythms

Diagnoses are made in clinical practice taking into account not only sleep timing and complaints, but also individual habits and social life-style. Even if an individual has an unusual sleep schedule, if his activity cycle fits his desires, he may not feel inconvenienced.

What we don't know:

Very little is known about the variability of clock genes in the general population.

We need more longitudinal studies looking at the causal relationship between working under a shift system and greater sleep problems.

REFERENCES

[1]   Young T, Palta M, Dempsey J, Skatrud J, Weber S, Badr S. The occurrence of sleep-disordered breathing among middle-aged adults. N Engl J Med 1993; 328(17): 1230-5.

[2]   Ogden CL, Carroll MD, Curtin LR, McDowell MA, Tabak CJ, Flegal KM. Prevalence of overweight and obesity in the United States, 1999-2004. JAMA 2006; 295(13): 1549-55.

[3]   Bixler EO, Vgontzas AN, Lin HM, *et al.* Prevalence of sleep-disordered breathing in women: effects of gender. Am J Respir Crit Care Med 2001; 163(3 Pt 1): 608-13.

[4]   Bixler EO, Vgontzas AN, Ten Have T, Tyson K, Kales A. Effects of age on sleep apnea in men: I. Prevalence and severity. Am J Respir Crit Care Med 1998; 157(1): 144-8.

[5]   Redline S, Schluchter MD, Larkin EK, Tishler PV. Predictors of longitudinal change in sleep-disordered breathing in a nonclinic population. Sleep 2003; 26(6): 703-9.

[6]   Greenburg DL, Lettieri CJ, Eliasson AH. Effects of surgical weight loss on measures of obstructive sleep apnea: a meta-analysis. Am J Med 2009; 122(6): 535-42.

[7]   Punjabi NM. The epidemiology of adult obstructive sleep apnea. Proc Am Thorac Soc 2008; 5(2): 136-43.

[8]   O'Connor C, Thornley KS, Hanly PJ. Gender differences in the polysomnographic features of obstructive sleep apnea. Am J Respir Crit Care Med 2000; 161(5): 1465-72.

[9]   Netzer NC, Eliasson AH, Strohl KP. Women with sleep apnea have lower levels of sex hormones. Sleep Breath 2003; 7(1): 25-9.

[10]   Ancoli-Israel S, Kripke DF, Klauber MR, Mason WJ, Fell R, Kaplan O. Sleep-disordered breathing in community-dwelling elderly. Sleep 1991; 14(6): 486-95.

[11]   Durán C. Prevalence of obstructive sleep apnea-hypopnea and related clinical features in the elderly: a population-based study in the general population aged 71-100. World Conference 2001 Sleep Odyssey October 21-26, 2001; Montevideo, Uruguay.

[12]   Redline S, Tishler PV, Tosteson TD, *et al.* The familial aggregation of obstructive sleep apnea. Am J Respir Crit Care Med 1995; 151(3 Pt 1): 682-7.

[13]   Carmelli D, Colrain IM, Swan GE, Bliwise DL. Genetic and environmental influences in sleep-disordered breathing in older male twins Sleep 2004; 27(5): 917-22.

[14]   Palmer LJ, Buxbaum SG, Larkin E, *et al.* A whole-genome scan for obstructive sleep apnea and obesity. Am J Hum Genet 2003; 72(2): 340-50.

[15] Palmer LJ, Buxbaum SG, Larkin EK, *et al.* Whole genome scan for obstructive sleep apnea and obesity in African-American families. Am J Respir Crit Care Med 2004; 169(12): 1314-21.

[16] Schwab RJ, Pasirstein M, Kaplan L, *et al.* Family aggregation of upper airway soft tissue structures in normal subjects and patients with sleep apnea. Am J Respir Crit Care Med 2006; 173(4): 453-63.

[17] Cistulli PA. Craniofacial abnormalities in obstructive sleep apnoea: implications for treatment. Respirology 1996; 1(3): 167-74.

[18] Lee RW, Chan AS, Grunstein RR, Cistulli PA. Craniofacial phenotyping in obstructive sleep apnea--a novel quantitative photographic approach. Sleep 2009; 32(1): 37-45.

[19] Miles PG, Vig PS, Weyant RJ, Forrest TD, Rockette HE, Jr. Craniofacial structure and obstructive sleep apnea syndrome--a qualitative analysis and meta-analysis of the literature. Am J Orthod Dentofacial Orthop 1996; 109(2): 163-72.

[20] Wetter DW, Young TB, Bidwell TR, Badr MS, Palta M. Smoking as a risk factor for sleep-disordered breathing. Arch Intern Med 1994; 154(19): 2219-24.

[21] Shaw JE, Punjabi NM, Wilding JP, Alberti KG, Zimmet PZ. Sleep-disordered breathing and type 2 diabetes: a report from the International Diabetes Federation Taskforce on Epidemiology and Prevention. Diabetes Res Clin Pract 2008; 81(1): 2-12.

[22] Elmasry A, Lindberg E, Berne C, *et al.* Sleep-disordered breathing and glucose metabolism in hypertensive men: a population-based study. J Intern Med 2001; 249(2): 153-61.

[23] Meslier N, Gagnadoux F, Giraud P, *et al.* Impaired glucose-insulin metabolism in males with obstructive sleep apnoea syndrome. Eur Respir J 2003; 22(1): 156-60.

[24] Aronsohn RS, Whitmore H, Van Cauter E, Tasali E. Impact of untreated obstructive sleep apnea on glucose control in type 2 diabetes. Am J Respir Crit Care Med 2010; 181(5): 507-13.

[25] West SD, Nicoll DJ, Stradling JR. Prevalence of obstructive sleep apnoea in men with type 2 diabetes. Thorax 2006; 61(11): 945-50.

[26] Botros N, Concato J, Mohsenin V, Selim B, Doctor K, Yaggi HK. Obstructive sleep apnea as a risk factor for type 2 diabetes. Am J Med 2009; 122(12): 1122-7.

[27] Fletcher EC, DeBehnke RD, Lovoi MS, Gorin AB. Undiagnosed sleep apnea in patients with essential hypertension. Ann Intern Med 1985; 103(2): 190-5.

[28] Kales A, Bixler EO, Cadieux RJ, *et al.* Sleep apnoea in a hypertensive population. Lancet. 1984 Nov 3; 2(8410): 1005-8.

[29] Logan AG, Perlikowski SM, Mente A, *et al.* High prevalence of unrecognized sleep apnoea in drug-resistant hypertension. J Hypertens 2001; 19(12): 2271-7.

[30] Mooe T, Rabben T, Wiklund U, Franklin KA, Eriksson P. Sleep-disordered breathing in men with coronary artery disease. Chest 1996; 109(3): 659-63.

[31] Peker Y, Kraiczi H, Hedner J, Loth S, Johansson A, Bende M. An independent association between obstructive sleep apnoea and coronary artery disease. Eur Respir J 1999; 14(1): 179-84.

[32] Garrigue S, Pepin JL, Defaye P, *et al.* High prevalence of sleep apnea syndrome in patients with long-term pacing: the European Multicenter Polysomnographic Study. Circulation 2007; 115(13): 1703-9.

[33] Gami AS, Pressman G, Caples SM, *et al.* Association of atrial fibrillation and obstructive sleep apnea. Circulation 2004; 110(4): 364-7.

[34] MacDonald M, Fang J, Pittman SD, White DP, Malhotra A. The current prevalence of sleep disordered breathing in congestive heart failure patients treated with beta-blockers. J Clin Sleep Med 2008; 4(1): 38-42.

[35] Oldenburg O, Lamp B, Faber L, Teschler H, Horstkotte D, Topfer V. Sleep-disordered breathing in patients with symptomatic heart failure: a contemporary study of prevalence in and characteristics of 700 patients. Eur J Heart Fail 2007; 9(3): 251-7.

[36] Yumino D, Wang H, Floras JS, *et al.* Prevalence and physiological predictors of sleep apnea in patients with heart failure and systolic dysfunction. J Card Fail 2009; 15(4): 279-85.

[37] Chan J, Sanderson J, Chan W, *et al.* Prevalence of sleep-disordered breathing in diastolic heart failure. Chest 1997; 111(6): 1488-93.

[38] Sin DD, Fitzgerald F, Parker JD, Newton G, Floras JS, Bradley TD. Risk factors for central and obstructive sleep apnea in 450 men and women with congestive heart failure. Am J Respir Crit Care Med 1999; 160(4): 1101-6.

[39] Bassetti C, Aldrich MS. Sleep apnea in acute cerebrovascular diseases: final report on 128 patients. Sleep 1999; 22(2): 217-23.

[40] Bassetti C, Aldrich MS, Quint D. Sleep-disordered breathing in patients with acute supra- and infratentorial strokes. A prospective study of 39 patients. Stroke 1997; 28(9): 1765-72.

[41] McArdle N, Riha RL, Vennelle M, *et al.* Sleep-disordered breathing as a risk factor for cerebrovascular disease: a case-control study in patients with transient ischemic attacks. Stroke 2003; 34(12): 2916-21.

[42] Janson C, De Backer W, Gislason T, *et al.* Increased prevalence of sleep disturbances and daytime sleepiness in subjects with bronchial asthma: a population study of young adults in three European countries. Eur Respir J 1996; 9(10): 2132-8.

[43] Knuiman M, James A, Divitini M, Bartholomew H. Longitudinal study of risk factors for habitual snoring in a general adult population: the Busselton Health Study. Chest 2006; 130(6): 1779-83.

[44] Teodorescu M, Consens FB, Bria WF, *et al.* Correlates of daytime sleepiness in patients with asthma. Sleep Med 2006; 7(8): 607-13.

[45] Douglass AB, Bornstein R, Nino-Murcia G, *et al.* The Sleep Disorders Questionnaire. I: Creation and multivariate structure of SDQ. Sleep 1994; 17(2): 160-7.

[46] Yigla M, Tov N, Solomonov A, Rubin AH, Harlev D. Difficult-to-control asthma and obstructive sleep apnea. J Asthma 2003; 40(8): 865-71.

[47] Julien JY, Martin JG, Ernst P, *et al.* Prevalence of obstructive sleep apnea-hypopnea in severe versus moderate asthma. J Allergy Clin Immunol 2009; 124(2): 371-6.

[48] Karachaliou F, Kostikas K, Pastaka C, Bagiatis V, Gourgoulianis KI. Prevalence of sleep-related symptoms in a primary care population - their relation to asthma and COPD. Prim Care Respir J 2007; 16(4): 222-8.

[49] McNicholas WT. COPD and Obstructive Sleep apnea: Overlaps in Pathophysiology, Systemic Inflammation and Cardiovascular Disease. Am J Respir Crit Care Med 2009; 180: 692-700.

[50] Weitzenblum E, Chaouat A, Kessler R, Canuet M. Overlap syndrome: obstructive sleep apnea in patients with chronic obstructive pulmonary disease. Proc Am Thorac Soc 2008; 5(2): 237-41.

[51] Rasche K, Orth M, Kutscha A, Duchna HW. [Pulmonary diseases and heart function]. Internist (Berl). 2007; 48(3): 276-82.

[52] Panossian LA, Avidan AY. Review of sleep disorders. Med Clin North Am 2009; 93(2): 407-25, ix.

[53] Schafer T, Schlafke ME, Westhoff M, *et al.* [Central sleep apnea]. Pneumologie 2009; 63(3): 144-58; quiz 59-62.

[54] Lanfranchi PA, Somers VK, Braghiroli A, Corra U, Eleuteri E, Giannuzzi P. Central sleep apnea in left ventricular dysfunction: prevalence and implications for arrhythmic risk. Circulation 2003; 107(5): 727-32.

[55] Lofaso F, Verschueren P, Rande JL, Harf A, Goldenberg F. Prevalence of sleep-disordered breathing in patients on a heart transplant waiting list. Chest 1994; 106(6): 1689-94.

[56] Javaheri S. Sleep disorders in systolic heart failure: a prospective study of 100 male patients. The final report. Int J Cardiol. 2006; 106(1): 21-8.

[57] Paulino A, Damy T, Margarit L, *et al.* Prevalence of sleep-disordered breathing in a 316-patient French cohort of stable congestive heart failure. Arch Cardiovasc Dis. 2009; 102(3): 169-75.

[58] Carmona-Bernal C, Quintana-Gallego E, Villa-Gil M, Sanchez-Armengol A, Martinez-Martinez A, Capote F. Brain natriuretic peptide in patients with congestive heart failure and central sleep apnea. Chest 2005; 127(5): 1667-73.

[59] Ferrier K, Campbell A, Yee B, *et al.* Sleep-disordered breathing occurs frequently in stable outpatients with congestive heart failure. Chest 2005; 128(4): 2116-22.

[60] BaHammam A, Al-Mobeireek A, Al-Nozha M, Al-Tahan A, Binsaeed A. Behaviour and time-course of sleep disordered breathing in patients with acute coronary syndromes. Int J Clin Pract 2005; 59(8): 874-80.

[61] Brack T, Thuer I, Clarenbach CF, *et al.* Daytime Cheyne-Stokes respiration in ambulatory patients with severe congestive heart failure is associated with increased mortality. Chest 2007; 132(5): 1463-71.

[62] Hermann DM, Siccoli M, Kirov P, Gugger M, Bassetti CL. Central periodic breathing during sleep in acute ischemic stroke. Stroke 2007; 38(3): 1082-4.

[63] Mogri M, Desai H, Webster L, Grant BJ, Mador MJ. Hypoxemia in patients on chronic opiate therapy with and without sleep apnea. Sleep Breath 2009; 13(1): 49-57.

[64] Walker JM, Farney RJ, Rhondeau SM, *et al.* Chronic opioid use is a risk factor for the development of central sleep apnea and ataxic breathing. J Clin Sleep Med 2007; 3(5): 455-61.

[65] Tada T, Kusano KF, Ogawa A, *et al.* The predictors of central and obstructive sleep apnoea in haemodialysis patients. Nephrol Dial Transplant 2007; 22(4): 1190-7.

[66] Dauvilliers Y, Stal V, Abril B, *et al.* Chiari malformation and sleep related breathing disorders. J Neurol Neurosurg Psychiatry 2007; 78(12): 1344-8.

[67] Webster JB, Bell KR, Hussey JD, Natale TK, Lakshminarayan S. Sleep apnea in adults with traumatic brain injury: a preliminary investigation. Arch Phys Med Rehabil 2001; 82(3): 316-21.

[68] Naraine VS, Bradley TD, Singer LG. Prevalence of sleep disordered breathing in lung transplant recipients. J Clin Sleep Med 2009; 5(5): 441-7.

[69] Yaegashi H, Fujimoto K, Abe H, Orii K, Eda S, Kubo K. Characteristics of Japanese patients with complex sleep apnea syndrome: a retrospective comparison with obstructive sleep apnea syndrome. Intern Med 2009; 48(6): 427-32.

[70] Javaheri S, Smith J, Chung E. The prevalence and natural history of complex sleep apnea. J Clin Sleep Med 2009; 5(3): 205-11.

[71] Mokhlesi B, Kryger MH, Grunstein RR. Assessment and management of patients with obesity hypoventilation syndrome. Proc Am Thorac Soc 2008; 5(2): 218-25.

[72] Resta O, Foschino Barbaro MP, Carpagnano GE, *et al.* Diurnal PaCO2 tension in obese women: relationship with sleep disordered breathing. Int J Obes Relat Metab Disord 2003; 27(12): 1453-8.

[73] Laaban JP, Chailleux E. Daytime hypercapnia in adult patients with obstructive sleep apnea syndrome in France, before initiating nocturnal nasal continuous positive airway pressure therapy. Chest 2005; 127(3): 710-5.

[74] Verin E, Tardif C, Pasquis P. Prevalence of daytime hypercapnia or hypoxia in patients with OSAS and normal lung function. Respir Med 2001; 95(8): 693-6.

[75] Sahebjami H, Gartside PS. Pulmonary function in obese subjects with a normal FEV1/FVC ratio. Chest 1996; 110(6): 1425-9.

[76] Yuan X, Hawver LR, Ojo P, *et al.* Bariatric surgery in Medicare patients: greater risks but substantial benefits. Surg Obes Relat Dis 2009; 5: 299-304.

[77] Catheline JM, Bihan H, Le Quang T, *et al.* Preoperative cardiac and pulmonary assessment in bariatric surgery. Obes Surg 2008; 18(3): 271-7.

[78] Nowbar S, Burkart KM, Gonzales R, *et al.* Obesity-associated hypoventilation in hospitalized patients: prevalence, effects, and outcome. Am J Med 2004; 116(1): 1-7.

[79] Ohayon MM. Epidemiology of insomnia: what we know and what we still need to learn. Sleep Med Rev 2002; 6(2): 97-111.

[80] Klink M, Quan SF. Prevalence of reported sleep disturbances in a general adult population and their relationship to obstructive airways diseases. Chest 1987; 91(4): 540-6.

[81] Hale L, Do DP, Basurto-Davila R, *et al.* Does mental health history explain gender disparities in insomnia symptoms among young adults? Sleep Med 2009; 10(10): 1118-23.

[82] Li RH, Wing YK, Ho SC, Fong SY. Gender differences in insomnia--a study in the Hong Kong Chinese population. J Psychosom Res 2002; 53(1): 601-9.

[83] Owens JF, Matthews KA. Sleep disturbance in healthy middle-aged women. Maturitas 1998; 30(1): 41-50.

[84] Ohayon MM, Caulet M, Guilleminault C. How a general population perceives its sleep and how this relates to the complaint of insomnia. Sleep 1997; 20(9): 715-23.

[85] Ohayon MM, Caulet M, Priest RG, Guilleminault C. DSM-IV and ICSD-90 insomnia symptoms and sleep dissatisfaction. Br J Psychiatry 1997; 171: 382-8.

[86] Bixler EO, Kales A, Soldatos CR, Kales JD, Healey S. Prevalence of sleep disorders in the Los Angeles metropolitan area. Am J Psychiatry 1979; 136(10): 1257-62.

[87] Medicine AAoS. International classification of sleep disorders, 2nd edition.: Diagnostic and coding manual. Westchester, Illinois; 2005.

[88] Katz DA, McHorney CA. The relationship between insomnia and health-related quality of life in patients with chronic illness. J Fam Pract 2002; 51(3): 229-35.

[89] Thase ME. Antidepressant treatment of the depressed patient with insomnia. J Clin Psychiatry 1999; 60 Suppl 17: 28-31; discussion 46-8.

[90] Hamilton M. Frequency of symptoms in melancholia (depressive illness). Br J Psychiatry 1989; 154: 201-6.

[91] Reynolds CF, 3rd, Hoch CC, Buysse DJ, *et al.* Sleep in late-life recurrent depression. Changes during early continuation therapy with nortriptyline. Neuropsychopharmacology 1991; 5(2): 85-96.

[92] Lepine JP, Gastpar M, Mendlewicz J, Tylee A. Depression in the community: the first pan-European study DEPRES (Depression Research in European Society). Int Clin Psychopharmacol 1997; 12(1): 19-29.

[93] Livingston G, Blizard B, Mann A. Does sleep disturbance predict depression in elderly people? A study in inner London. Br J Gen Pract 1993; 43(376): 445-8.

[94] Roberts RE, Shema SJ, Kaplan GA, Strawbridge WJ. Sleep complaints and depression in an aging cohort: A prospective perspective. Am J Psychiatry 2000; 157(1): 81-8.

[95] Jackson A, Cavanagh J, Scott J. A systematic review of manic and depressive prodromes. J Affect Disord 2003; 74(3): 209-17.

[96] Kowalski SD, Bondmass MD. Physiological and psychological symptoms of grief in widows. Res Nurs Health 2008; 31(1): 23-30.

[97]   Prigerson HG, Frank E, Kasl SV, *et al.* Complicated grief and bereavement-related depression as distinct disorders: preliminary empirical validation in elderly bereaved spouses. Am J Psychiatry 1995; 152(1): 22-30.

[98]   Monk TH, Begley AE, Billy BD, *et al.* Sleep and circadian rhythms in spousally bereaved seniors. Chronobiol Int 2008; 25(1): 83-98.

[99]   Monti JM, Monti D. Sleep disturbance in generalized anxiety disorder and its treatment. Sleep Med Rev. 2000; 4(3): 263-76.

[100]   Uhde T. Anxiety Disorders. In: Kryger M, Roth T, Dement W, editors. Principles and Practice of Sleep Medicine 3rd ed. Philadelphia: WB Saunders; 2000. p. 1123-39.

[101]   Benca RM, Obermeyer WH, Thisted RA, Gillin JC. Sleep and psychiatric disorders. A meta-analysis. Arch Gen Psychiatry 1992; 49(8): 651-68; discussion 69-70.

[102]   Fuller KH, Waters WF, Binks PG, Anderson T. Generalized anxiety and sleep architecture: a polysomnographic investigation Sleep 1997; 20(5): 370-6.

[103]   Singareddy R, Uhde TW. Nocturnal sleep panic and depression: Relationship to subjective sleep in panic disorder. J Affect Disord 2008 Jun 14.

[104]   Stein MB, Enns MW, Kryger MH. Sleep in nondepressed patients with panic disorder: II. Polysomnographic assessment of sleep architecture and sleep continuity. J Affect Disord 1993; 28(1): 1-6.

[105]   Shapiro CM, Sloan EP. Nocturnal panic--an underrecognized entity. J Psychosom Res 1998; 44(1): 21-3.

[106]   Hauri PJ, Friedman M, Ravaris CL. Sleep in patients with spontaneous panic attacks. Sleep 1989; 12(4): 323-37.

[107]   Mellman TA, Uhde TW. Sleep panic attacks: new clinical findings and theoretical implications. Am J Psychiatry 1989; 146(9): 1204-7.

[108]   Koren D, Arnon I, Lavie P, Klein E. Sleep complaints as early predictors of posttraumatic stress disorder: a 1-year prospective study of injured survivors of motor vehicle accidents. Am J Psychiatry 2002; 159(5): 855-7.

[109]   Mellman TA. Sleep and anxiety disorders. Psychiatr Clin North Am. 2006 Dec; 29(4): 1047-58; abstract x.

[110]   Foley D, Ancoli-Israel S, Britz P, Walsh J. Sleep disturbances and chronic disease in older adults: results of the 2003 National Sleep Foundation Sleep in America Survey. J Psychosom Res 2004; 56(5): 497-502.

[111]   Latham J, Davis BD. The socioeconomic impact of chronic pain. Disabil Rehabil 1994; 16(1): 39-44.

[112]   Rosenberg-Adamsen S, Skarbye M, Wildschiodtz G, Kehlet H, Rosenberg J. Sleep after laparoscopic cholecystectomy. Br J Anaesth 1996; 77(5): 572-5.

[113]   Ellis J HS, Cropley M. Sleep hygiene compensatory sleep practices: an examination of behaviors affecting sleep in older adults. Psychology, Health, & Medicine 2002; 7(2): 157-62.

[114]   Leigh TJ, Hindmarch I, Bird HA, Wright V. Comparison of sleep in osteoarthritic patients and age and sex matched healthy controls. Ann Rheum Dis 1988; 47(1): 40-2.

[115]   Wilcox S, Brenes GA, Levine D, Sevick MA, Shumaker SA, Craven T. Factors related to sleep disturbance in older adults experiencing knee pain or knee pain with radiographic evidence of knee osteoarthritis. J Am Geriatr Soc 2000; 48(10): 1241-51.

[116]   Ancoli-Israel S. The impact and prevalence of chronic insomnia and other sleep disturbances associated with chronic illness. Am J Manag Care 2006; 12(8 Suppl): S221-9.

[117]   Farup C, Kleinman L, Sloan S, *et al.* The impact of nocturnal symptoms associated with gastroesophageal reflux disease on health-related quality of life. Arch Intern Med 2001; 161(1): 45-52.

[118]   Mody R, Bolge SC, Kannan H, Fass R. Effects of gastroesophageal reflux disease on sleep and outcomes. Clin Gastroenterol Hepatol 2009; 7(9): 953-9.

[119]   Prejbisz A, Kabat M, Januszewicz A, *et al.* Characterization of insomnia in patients with essential hypertension. Blood Press 2006; 15(4): 213-9.

[120]   Edell-Gustafsson U, Svanborg E, Swahn E. A gender perspective on sleeplessness behavior, effects of sleep loss, and coping resources in patients with stable coronary artery disease. Heart Lung 2006; 35(2): 75-89.

[121]   Peters RW, Zoble RG, Brooks MM. Onset of acute myocardial infarction during sleep. Clin Cardiol 2002; 25(5): 237-41.

[122]   Brostrom A, Stromberg A, Dahlstrom U, Fridlund B. Sleep difficulties, daytime sleepiness, and health-related quality of life in patients with chronic heart failure. J Cardiovasc Nurs 2004; 19(4): 234-42.

[123]   Principe-Rodriguez K, Strohl KP, Hadziefendic S, Pina IL. Sleep symptoms and clinical markers of illness in patients with heart failure. Sleep Breath 2005; 9(3): 127-33.

[124]   Fleetham J, West P, Mezon B, Conway W, Roth T, Kryger M. Sleep, arousals, and oxygen desaturation in chronic obstructive pulmonary disease. The effect of oxygen therapy. Am Rev Respir Dis 1982; 126(3): 429-33.

[125]   Turner-Warwick M. Epidemiology of nocturnal asthma. Am J Med 1988; 85(1B): 6-8.

[126]   Dethlefsen U, Repgas R. Ein neues Therapieprinzip bei Nachtlichen Asthma. Klin Med 1985; 80: 44-7.

[127] Janson C, Gislason T, Boman G, Hetta J, Roos BE. Sleep disturbances in patients with asthma. Respir Med 1990; 84(1): 37-42.

[128] van Keimpema AR, Ariaansz M, Nauta JJ, Postmus PE. Subjective sleep quality and mental fitness in asthmatic patients. J Asthma 1995; 32(1): 69-74.

[129] Mastronarde JG, Wise RA, Shade DM, Olopade CO, Scharf SM. Sleep quality in asthma: results of a large prospective clinical trial. J Asthma 2008; 45(3): 183-9.

[130] Braido F, Baiardini I, Ghiglione V, *et al.* Sleep disturbances and asthma control: a real life study. Asian Pac J Allergy Immunol 2009; 27(1): 27-33.

[131] Fitzpatrick MF, Engleman H, Whyte KF, Deary IJ, Shapiro CM, Douglas NJ. Morbidity in nocturnal asthma: sleep quality and daytime cognitive performance. Thorax 1991; 46(8): 569-73.

[132] Purdie DW, Empson JA, Crichton C, Macdonald L. Hormone replacement therapy, sleep quality and psychological wellbeing. Br J Obstet Gynaecol 1995; 102(9): 735-9.

[133] Bliwise DL, Foley DJ, Vitiello MV, Ansari FP, Ancoli-Israel S, Walsh JK. Nocturia and disturbed sleep in the elderly. Sleep Med 2009; 10(5): 540-8.

[134] Bing MH, Moller LA, Jennum P, Mortensen S, Lose G. Nocturia and associated morbidity in a Danish population of men and women aged 60-80 years. BJU Int 2008 Jun 17.

[135] Asplund R, Aberg H. Diurnal variation in the levels of antidiuretic hormone in the elderly. J Intern Med 1991; 229(2): 131-4.

[136] Williams SW, Tell GS, Zheng B, Shumaker S, Rocco MV, Sevick MA. Correlates of sleep behavior among hemodialysis patients. The kidney outcomes prediction and evaluation (KOPE) study. Am J Nephrol. 2002; 22(1): 18-28.

[137] Parker KP. Sleep disturbances in dialysis patients. Sleep Med Rev 2003; 7(2): 131-43.

[138] Iliescu EA, Coo H, McMurray MH, *et al.* Quality of sleep and health-related quality of life in haemodialysis patients. Nephrol Dial Transplant 2003; 18(1): 126-32.

[139] Benz RL, Pressman MR, Hovick ET, Peterson DD. A preliminary study of the effects of correction of anemia with recombinant human erythropoietin therapy on sleep, sleep disorders, and daytime sleepiness in hemodialysis patients (The SLEEPO study). Am J Kidney Dis 1999; 34(6): 1089-95.

[140] Savard J, Morin CM. Insomnia in the context of cancer: a review of a neglected problem. J Clin Oncol 2001; 19(3): 895-908.

[141] Davidson JR, Waisberg JL, Brundage MD, MacLean AW. Nonpharmacologic group treatment of insomnia: a preliminary study with cancer survivors. Psychooncology 2001; 10(5): 389-97.

[142] Davidson JR, MacLean AW, Brundage MD, Schulze K. Sleep disturbance in cancer patients. Soc Sci Med 2002; 54(9): 1309-21.

[143] Kozachik SL, Bandeen-Roche K. Predictors of patterns of pain, fatigue, and insomnia during the first year after a cancer diagnosis in the elderly. Cancer Nurs 2008; 31(5): 334-44.

[144] Thorpy MJ. Sleep disorders in Parkinson's disease. Clin Cornerstone 2004; 6 Suppl 1A: S7-15.

[145] Bliwise DL. Sleep disorders in Alzheimer's disease and other dementias. Clin Cornerstone 2004; 6 Suppl 1A: S16-28.

[146] Longstreth WT, Jr., Ton TG, Koepsell T, Gersuk VH, Hendrickson A, Velde S. Prevalence of narcolepsy in King County, Washington, USA. Sleep Med 2009; 10(4): 422-6.

[147] Hublin C, Kaprio J, Partinen M, *et al.* The prevalence of narcolepsy: an epidemiological study of the Finnish Twin Cohort. Ann Neurol 1994; 35(6): 709-16.

[148] Ohayon MM, Priest RG, Zulley J, Smirne S, Paiva T. Prevalence of narcolepsy symptomatology and diagnosis in the European general population. Neurology 2002; 58(12): 1826-33.

[149] Chen L, Fong SY, Lam CW, *et al.* The familial risk and HLA susceptibility among narcolepsy patients in Hong Kong Chinese. Sleep 2007; 30(7): 851-8.

[150] Nishino S, Ripley B, Overeem S, Lammers GJ, Mignot E. Hypocretin (orexin) deficiency in human narcolepsy. Lancet 2000; 355(9197): 39-40.

[151] Nishino S, Ripley B, Overeem S, *et al.* Low cerebrospinal fluid hypocretin (Orexin) and altered energy homeostasis in human narcolepsy. Ann Neurol 2001; 50(3): 381-8.

[152] Kanbayashi T, Inoue Y, Chiba S, *et al.* CSF hypocretin-1 (orexin-A) concentrations in narcolepsy with and without cataplexy and idiopathic hypersomnia. J Sleep Res 2002; 11(1): 91-3.

[153] Mignot E, Lammers GJ, Ripley B, *et al.* The role of cerebrospinal fluid hypocretin measurement in the diagnosis of narcolepsy and other hypersomnias. Arch Neurol 2002; 59(10): 1553-62.

[154] Longstreth WT, Jr., Koepsell TD, Ton TG, Hendrickson AF, van Belle G. The epidemiology of narcolepsy. Sleep 2007; 30(1): 13-26.

[155]   Kok SW, Overeem S, Visscher TL, *et al.* Hypocretin deficiency in narcoleptic humans is associated with abdominal obesity. Obes Res 2003; 11(9): 1147-54.

[156]   Koepsell TD, Longstreth WT, Ton TG. Medical exposures in youth and the frequency of narcolepsy with cataplexy: a population-based case-control study in genetically predisposed people. J Sleep Res 2010; 19: 80-6.

[157]   Smith AJ, Jackson MW, Neufing P, McEvoy RD, Gordon TP. A functional autoantibody in narcolepsy. Lancet 2004; 364(9451): 2122-4.

[158]   Vernet C, Arnulf I. Idiopathic hypersomnia with and without long sleep time: a controlled series of 75 patients. Sleep 2009; 32(6): 753-9.

[159]   Heier MS, Evsiukova T, Vilming S, Gjerstad MD, Schrader H, Gautvik K. CSF hypocretin-1 levels and clinical profiles in narcolepsy and idiopathic CNS hypersomnia in Norway. Sleep 2007; 30(8): 969-73.

[160]   Ohayon MM, Priest RG, Zulley J, Smirne S. The place of confusional arousals in sleep and mental disorders: findings in a general population sample of 13,057 subjects. J Nerv Ment Dis 2000; 188(6): 340-8.

[161]   Ohayon MM, Caulet M, Priest RG. Violent behavior during sleep. J Clin Psychiatry 1997; 58(8): 369-76; quiz 77.

[162]   Gjerstad MD, Boeve B, Wentzel-Larsen T, Aarsland D, Larsen JP. Occurrence and clinical correlates of REM sleep behaviour disorder in patients with Parkinson's disease over time. J Neurol Neurosurg Psychiatry 2008; 79(4): 387-91.

[163]   Arnulf I, Nielsen J, Lohmann E, *et al.* Rapid eye movement sleep disturbances in Huntington disease. Arch Neurol 2008; 65(4): 482-8.

[164]   Teman PT, Tippmann-Peikert M, Silber MH, Slocumb NL, Auger RR. Idiopathic rapid-eye-movement sleep disorder: associations with antidepressants, psychiatric diagnoses, and other factors, in relation to age of onset. Sleep Med 2009; 10(1): 60-5.

[165]   Bonakis A, Howard RS, Ebrahim IO, Merritt S, Williams A. REM sleep behaviour disorder (RBD) and its associations in young patients. Sleep Med 2009; 10(6): 641-5.

[166]   Berger K, Kurth T. RLS epidemiology--frequencies, risk factors and methods in population studies. Mov Disord 2007; 22 Suppl 18: S420-3.

[167]   Allen RP, Walters AS, Montplaisir J, *et al.* Restless legs syndrome prevalence and impact: REST general population study. Arch Intern Med 2005; 165(11): 1286-92.

[168]   Ohayon MM, Roth T. Prevalence of restless legs syndrome and periodic limb movement disorder in the general population. J Psychosom Res 2002; 53(1): 547-54.

[169]   Hening W, Walters AS, Allen RP, Montplaisir J, Myers A, Ferini-Strambi L. Impact, diagnosis and treatment of restless legs syndrome (RLS) in a primary care population: the REST (RLS epidemiology, symptoms, and treatment) primary care study. Sleep Med 2004; 5(3): 237-46.

[170]   Allen RP, La Buda MC, Becker P, Earley CJ. Family history study of the restless legs syndrome. Sleep Med 2002; 3 Suppl: S3-7.

[171]   Kim KW, Yoon IY, Chung S, *et al.* Prevalence, comorbidities and risk factors of restless legs syndrome in the Korean elderly population - results from the Korean Longitudinal Study on Health and Aging. J Sleep Res 2010; 19: 87-92.

[172]   Sun ER, Chen CA, Ho G, Earley CJ, Allen RP. Iron and the restless legs syndrome. Sleep 1998; 21(4): 371-7.

[173]   Sikandar R, Khealani BA, Wasay M. Predictors of restless legs syndrome in pregnancy: a hospital based cross sectional survey from Pakistan. Sleep Med 2009; 10(6): 676-8.

[174]   Suzuki K, Ohida T, Sone T, *et al.* The prevalence of restless legs syndrome among pregnant women in Japan and the relationship between restless legs syndrome and sleep problems. Sleep 2003; 26(6): 673-7.

[175]   Allen RP, Earley CJ. The role of iron in restless legs syndrome. Mov Disord. 2007; 22 Suppl 18: S440-8.

[176]   Ulfberg J, Nystrom B. Restless legs syndrome in blood donors. Sleep Med 2004; 5(2): 115-8.

[177]   Burchell BJ, Allen RP, Miller JK, Hening WA, Earley CJ. RLS and blood donation. Sleep Med 2009; 10(8): 844-9.

[178]   Garcia-Borreguero D, Egatz R, Winkelmann J, Berger K. Epidemiology of restless legs syndrome: the current status. Sleep Med Rev 2006; 10(3): 153-67.

[179]   Ondo WG, Vuong KD, Jankovic J. Exploring the relationship between Parkinson disease and restless legs syndrome. Arch Neurol 2002; 59(3): 421-4.

[180]   Scofield H, Roth T, Drake C. Periodic limb movements during sleep: population prevalence, clinical correlates, and racial differences Sleep. 2008; 31(9): 1221-7.

[181]   Morrish E, King MA, Pilsworth SN, Shneerson JM, Smith IE. Periodic limb movement in a community population detected by a new actigraphy technique. Sleep Med 2002; 3(6): 489-95.

[182]   Wetter TC, Pollmacher T. Restless legs and periodic leg movements in sleep syndromes. J Neurol 1997; 244(4 Suppl 1): S37-45.

[183] Ferri R, Manconi M, Lanuzza B, *et al.* Age-related changes in periodic leg movements during sleep in patients with restless legs syndrome. Sleep Med 2008; 9(7): 790-8.

[184] Skomro R, Silva R, Alves R, Figueiredo A, Lorenzi-Filho G. The prevalence and significance of periodic leg movements during sleep in patients with congestive heart failure. Sleep Breath 2009; 13(1): 43-7.

[185] Dauvilliers Y, Pennestri MH, Petit D, Dang-Vu T, Lavigne G, Montplaisir J. Periodic leg movements during sleep and wakefulness in narcolepsy. J Sleep Res 2007; 16(3): 333-9.

[186] Roenneberg T, Kuehnle T, Juda M, *et al.* Epidemiology of the human circadian clock. Sleep Med Rev 2007; 11(6): 429-38.

[187] Paine SJ, Gander PH, Travier N. The epidemiology of morningness/eveningness: influence of age, gender, ethnicity, and socioeconomic factors in adults (30-49 years). J Biol Rhythms 2006; 21(1): 68-76.

[188] Ando K, Kripke DF, Ancoli-Israel S. Delayed and advanced sleep phase symptoms. Isr J Psychiatry Relat Sci 2002; 39(1): 11-8.

[189] Yoon IY, Kripke DF, Elliott JA, Youngstedt SD, Rex KM, Hauger RL. Age-related changes of circadian rhythms and sleep-wake cycles. J Am Geriatr Soc 2003; 51(8): 1085-91.

[190] Mercer PW, Merritt SL, Cowell JM. Differences in reported sleep need among adolescents. J Adolesc Health 1998; 23(5): 259-63.

[191] Park YM, Matsumoto K, Seo YJ, Shinkoda H, Park KP. Sleep in relation to age, sex, and chronotype in Japanese workers. Percept Mot Skills 1998; 87(1): 199-215.

[192] Tonetti L, Fabbri M, Natale V. Sex difference in sleep-time preference and sleep need: a cross-sectional survey among Italian pre-adolescents, adolescents, and adults. Chronobiol Int 2008; 25(5): 745-59.

[193] Reid KJ, Chang AM, Dubocovich ML, Turek FW, Takahashi JS, Zee PC. Familial advanced sleep phase syndrome. Arch Neurol 2001; 58(7): 1089-94.

[194] Drake CL, Roehrs T, Richardson G, Walsh JK, Roth T. Shift work sleep disorder: prevalence and consequences beyond that of symptomatic day workers. Sleep 2004; 27(8): 1453-62.

[195] Waage S, Moen BE, Pallesen S, *et al.* Shift work disorder among oil rig workers in the North Sea. Sleep 2009; 32(4): 558-65.

[196] Takahashi M, Iwakiri K, Sotoyama M, *et al.* Work schedule differences in sleep problems of nursing home caregivers. Appl Ergon 2008; 39(5): 597-604.

CHAPTER 3

Sleep History and Physical Examination

David A. Schulman*, M.D., M.P.H.

Assistant Professor of Medicine - Emory University, 615 Michael Street, Suite 205, Atlanta, GA 30322, USA

Abstract: Patients afflicted with sleep disorders may have a wide variety of complaints, the majority of which are, generally, nonspecific. It is therefore critically important that providers caring for these patients should be well-versed in the appropriate work-up of snoring, daytime sleepiness, insomnia and nocturnal behaviors. This chapter will briefly review these common complaints and the appropriate evaluation of each.

TOPIC DISCUSSION (CLINICAL OUTLOOK)

While a detailed discussion of the subject of relevant history-taking and physical examination for specific disorders will be found in each chapter within this textbook, it is worthwhile to briefly discuss the evaluation of common sleep-related complaints.

SLEEP HISTORY

In all cases, the initial evaluation of a patient with sleep complaints should begin with the patient's primary reason for presentation; in many cases, the patient's problem is long-standing, in which case it is equally important to determine why the patient has chosen this time to be evaluated. Additional information can often be obtained from family members and bed partners, therefore strong consideration should be given to inviting such individuals to the initial interview, as such a perspective can often shed light on aspects of the patient's disease of which they personally may be unaware. Snoring, apneas, periodic leg movements, bruxism and many nocturnal behaviors are often unrecognized by affected patients until brought to their attention by others, who are often the impetus for having the evaluation completed. Quantification of the frequency, severity and changes in these behaviors over time can also provide useful insight into the patient's condition. Additionally, family may offer a more objective assessment of sleepiness and neurocognitive function, as many patients become habituated to their impairment.

Further information regarding the chief complaint should be sought, including its duration and severity. In most cases, patients describe their symptoms as indolent and progressive, though certain patterns of onset can suggest specific pathologies. Sudden onset of sleeplessness should trigger a search for a stressor that could have precipitated adjustment insomnia. Abrupt onset of excessive daytime somnolence should prompt questions regarding the implementation of medications that could be associated with such symptoms. Other disorders, such as Kleine-Levin syndrome or menstrual-related hypersomnia, are associated with intermittent symptoms. Seasonal variation in symptomatology could suggest nocturnal sleep disruption attributable to asthma or allergies.

The patient should be asked about prior interventions they may have attempted to address the problem, as well as their perceived benefits. Many patients will use over-the-counter aids to treat symptoms of insomnia, or may increase their intake of caffeine to address symptoms of daytime fatigue. Others may have received prescription medications from other care providers for these problems. Patients are also turning to the internet for medical advice in increasing numbers; some may` have already tried easily implemented therapies prior to their visit, such as sleep hygiene for insomnia or melatonin for circadian rhythm problems. We will briefly review below the general framework for the evaluation of the most common sleep complaints.

CHIEF COMPLAINT

Snoring

Patients who snore often present with complaints from others, whose sleep is disturbed by the patients' loud snoring. The most critical aspect of the evaluation of snoring is to distinguish simple snoring from obstructive sleep apnea. One

*Address correspondence to David A. Schulman: Assistant Professor of Medicine - Emory University, 615 Michael Street, Suite 205, Atlanta, GA 30322, USA; E-mail: daschul@emory.edu

Octavian C. Ioachimescu (Ed)

semi-quantitative assessment of snoring that may be useful and may be considered in clinical practice is a grading of snoring intensity (Likert scale 1-5, absent/soft/mild/moderate/severe, softer than/louder than talking/can be heard from outside the room, etc). Specific inquiry with regard to associated symptoms such as witnessed apneas, excessive daytime somnolence, gasping or choking during sleep, frequent nocturnal urination and morning headaches can help in the decision-making process. Other findings in the history that may suggest a need to evaluate for sleep apnea include difficult-to-control hypertension, memory changes, irritability, depression and reduced libido.

Excessive Daytime Sleepiness

Assessment of a patient whose primary complaint is sleepiness should begin by confirming that the patient is indeed sleepy and not just fatigued (lacking physical energy without a proclivity to fall asleep). The use of validated questionnaires, including the Epworth Sleepiness Scale [1], the Pittsburgh Sleep Quality Index [2] and the Stanford Sleepiness Scale (available online at http://www.stanford.edu/~dement/sss.html), can assist in making this distinction. Once confirmed, additional information about the quantity and quality of sleep, as well as the duration and progression of symptomatology can assist the sleep specialist in determining whether formal polysomnography is necessary.

Insomnia

Characterization of the patient with insomnia should include a specific delineation of the onset of symptoms, if possible; this is particularly critical for patients who complain of difficulty with the initiation and maintenance of sleep because a high proportion of cases can be related to a stressful life experience. The comorbid association of mood disorders and insomnia also suggests a utility in screening for underlying depression or anxiety during the interview, if not using a formal validated questionnaire. Additional information regarding the regularity of insomnia, the bedtime routine, the sleep environment and the specific timing of symptoms (at sleep onset versus after sleep onset) can help the care provider determine how best to proceed.

Abnormal Nocturnal Behaviors

Patients reporting abnormal nocturnal behaviors are often personally unaware of the behaviors until they are brought into the open by others in the household. As a result, it is ideal to have affected patients accompanied to their appointments by others, who have witnessed the behaviors. Specific information about the behavior, including the frequency with which it occurs, the time of night at which it occurs, whether its occurrence is related to medication or alcohol use, and whether the behavior itself is stereotypic can occasionally provide a confident diagnosis; alternatively, these features may help to determine whether the patient would benefit from an overnight polysomnogram.

ASSOCIATED SYMPTOMS

Once the chief complaint has been well-characterized, a detailed evaluation of the patient's usual sleep habits should be performed. Information regarding total hours of sleep per day, usual bedtime and rise time, and frequency of nocturnal awakenings should be collected first, as abnormalities in these data are common amongst patients with sleep pathology. A prolonged total sleep time may represent a primary disorder of hypersomnolence when not accompanied by nocturnal awakenings, but is more likely related to an intrinsic abnormality of sleep when frequent nocturnal awakenings are present. Abnormalities in bedtime and rise time may suggest a circadian rhythm disorders or behavioral issues with sleep hygiene. The mechanism of awakening can also be useful, as requiring an external stimulus, such as an alarm clock, to wake each morning may suggest a possible benefit of prolonging the sleep period. If nocturnal awakenings are reported, additional questioning about symptoms at the time of awakening or awareness of external factors that may have contributed to sleep disruption is appropriate. Many of these data can be captured on a sleep log, and it can be quite useful to have such a tool completed for several weeks prior to the initial clinic visit.

The patient's daytime schedule and behaviors should also be delineated; understanding the timing of work and school responsibilities, meals and exercise can often improve the provider's ability to put sleep complaints in the proper context of overall lifestyle. A sleep schedule that varies depending upon the patient's waking responsibilities may suggest a diagnosis of insufficient sleep or shift work syndrome. Meals, caffeine and exercise too close to bedtime may induce insomnia or early nocturnal arousals. Additional focus should be placed upon activities within two hours of bedtime amongst patients with sleep-onset insomnia as stimulating activities and stressful stimuli can lead to prolonged sleep latency.

After detailed information about the patient's sleep and wake schedule has been obtained, it is worthwhile to perform a more complete sleep review of systems. Screening for environmental contributors to sleep discontinuity is also important, as light, noise and disruptive bed partners (pets, children and spouses) can often have significant impact upon sleep quality. Many other symptoms may point the provider in a specific direction. Inquiring specifically about the perception of dream-like scenes in the immediate pre- or post-sleep period, transient paralysis upon awakening and episodes of neuromuscular weakness associated with strong emotions during the day in patients with reported hypersomnolence can suggest a diagnosis of narcolepsy. Symptoms of restless legs syndrome are often under-reported by patients and are worth investigating in patients with reported insomnia. Nocturnal gastro-esophageal reflux, a morning dry mouth and morning headaches may also be seen in patients with sleep-disordered breathing. Frequent nocturnal urination can be seen in prostatism, though this is a non-specific finding that is encountered in other sleep disorders as well.

Review of a patient's other medical problems can shed light upon sleep complaints. Mood disorders and anxiety disorder are frequently associated with insomnia that may improve with therapy of the underlying problem. Respiratory disorders, such as asthma and chronic obstructive pulmonary disease, may be worse at night because of circadian variations in airway caliber as well as the impact of body position upon respiratory function. Congestive heart failure can cause sleep disruption due to the mobilization of dependent fluid that occurs when the patient lies down. Pain is a common cause of sleep disruption, and can be exacerbated by body position. In female patients, determination of menopausal status can shed light upon sleep complaints.

Many medications can induce sleep-related side effects, with insomnia and sleepiness being most common, though restless legs syndrome, parasomnias and sleep-disordered breathing have all been associated with the use of pharmaceuticals. Obtaining a complete list of medications, their duration of use and the timing of their intake may strongly suggest a medication-related sleep disorder. Specific attention should be given to the use of sedative and hypnotic medications, as chronic use of such medications can suggest the diagnosis of hypnotic-dependent sleep-disorder. Over-the-counter medications are also important to review; many commonly-used products, including antihistamines, appetite suppressants and decongestants, may also be associated with sleep complaints.

An appropriate family history should be obtained; genetic contributions have clearly been implicated in the pathophysiology of narcolepsy and restless legs syndrome, while other disorders, such as obstructive sleep apnea, insomnia and parasomnias demonstrating familial patterns suggestive of either an environmental or genetic predisposition. A detailed social history should include frequency (and timing) of tobacco use, ethanol use, and caffeine use, as all of these substances can affect sleep latency and continuity. A history of illicit drug use should also be obtained; a significant history of use can be associated with continued sleep difficulties even after years of abstinence. Job history, including shift work and recent career changes, should be elicited. As previously noted, documentation of any social stressors, including family and spousal relationships and financial issues is important; even if the patient does not believe such issues play a meaningful role in the generation of their sleep complaints.

A complete review of systems should include screening for psychiatric symptoms, including anxiety, a change in appetite and feelings of anhedonia, as underlying psychiatric disturbances can present with a primary sleep-related complaint. Given the association between neurologic disorders and sleep disorders (sleep apnea, parasomnias, restless legs syndrome and periodic limb movements), inquiring about memory changes, tremors, gait difficulty, personality changes and decline in problem solving skills may suggest the need for a more detailed neurologic evaluation. Dyspnea on exertion, palpitations, wheezing, phlegm production, orthopnea and paroxysmal nocturnal dyspnea can indicate an underlying cardiopulmonary disorder causing sleep disruption. The presence of goiter, heat or cold intolerance, changes in body hair and weight changes can suggest an underlying endocrine disorder.

Great care should be taken in assessing the potential short-term risk of a patient's sleep complaint upon their safety and that of others around them. Patients with abnormal sleep behaviors can sometime exhibit violent behavior that can place themselves or others at risk. Patients with abnormal fatigue have an increased risk of motor vehicle accidents due to inattention and an increased risk of falling asleep while driving. Assessing these risks and counseling appropriate patients should occur to avoid potentially dangerous situations. Moving a bed partner to a separate bedroom to avoid harm from a violent parasomniac, moving an affected patient to the ground floor of the home to avoid falling during sleep walking, and advocating for a sleepy patient to avoid driving during the work-up may all be appropriate interventions depending upon the provider's perception of disease impact. Documentation of this counseling in the medical record is advised, given the possibility of legal ramifications if the counseling is ignored by the patient.

PHYSICAL EXAMINATION

Physical examination should begin with collection of vital signs, including height and weight, blood pressure, pulse and pulse oximetry. Morbid obesity can suggest the diagnosis of sleep-disordered breathing; the presence of hypertension may suggest a greater need to treat sleep-disordered breathing if identified, and abnormalities in pulse and blood pressure can also suggest underlying thyroid disease. An abnormally low oxyhemoglobin saturation should indicate the need to screen for cardiac or pulmonary diseases with further questioning or objective testing.

For patients complaining of insomnia, a significant concern should be exclusion of underlying mood disorder. While this is typically accomplished during the history, some patients with depression will demonstrate psychomotor slowing or a flat affect. Other findings on physical examination can suggest hyperthyroidism as a cause of insomnia, including tachycardia, hair loss, hyperreflexia, tremor and exophthalmos. Restless legs syndrome, another common cause of insomnia, can be suggested by physical examination findings of Parkinsonism, including muscle rigidity, resting tremor, a mask-like facies or slowed movements. Pain can be another cause of insomnia; evaluation for arthritis or peripheral neuropathy, both of which can be associated with increasing pain at night, is also important.

Evaluation of the patient complaining of nocturnal behaviors should include a thorough neurologic examination; given the association between REM-sleep behavior disorder (RBD) and neurodegenerative disorders, co-existent parkinsonian features may suggest RBD as a likely diagnosis. A focal motor or sensory defect may indicate the presence of an underlying intracranial lesion that could serve as a nidus for nocturnal seizures. Confusional arousals may sometimes be misinterpreted as parasomnias; it is therefore as important to consider common causes of nocturnal sleep disruption (such as sleep apnea) in patients presenting with abnormal nocturnal behaviors and perform the salient portions of the physical examination, covered in more depth below.

The patient presenting with hypersomnia should be screened for hypothyroidism by looking for bradycardia, hypothermia, dry skin, goiter or myxedema, though sleep apnea is a far more common cause of daytime fatigue. While a patient's body mass index (BMI) was one of the earliest-identified predictors of sleep apnea risk [3], many other physical examination findings can also be of use. Because the upper airway plays a major role in the pathophysiology of obstructive sleep apnea, a number of anatomic abnormalities of the face, neck and airway can suggest this diagnosis. Narrowed upper airway caliber, and specifically enlargement of the lateral peritonsillar tissues, is one of the best predictors of obstructive sleep apnea [4]. Other findings associated with this syndrome include mandibular hypoplasia, an enlarged tongue (with or without tongue ridging), overjet, retrognathia and a low-lying palate. Nasal obstruction, due to boggy mucosa, polyps or septal deviation, can increase the risk of obstructive sleep apnea by increasing the amount of negative pressure needed to inspire against resistance. Neck examination should include notation of thyroid size and a measure of neck circumference (typically at the level of superior border of the cricothyroid cartilage), with a circumference greater than 16 and 17 inches, respectively predicting obstructive sleep apnea in women and men [5].

Several different scales have been developed to quantify airway crowding. The modified Mallampati score [6] is measured with the mouth open and without protrusion of the tongue; based upon the visibility of the base of uvula, the arches in front of and behind the tonsils and the soft palate, the score ranges from 1 (full visibility) to 4 (unable to see any portion of the soft palate or posterior pharynx) (Fig. **1**). Independent of other variables measuring airway anatomy, a score of 4 has been associated with an increased risk of sleep apnea [7]; The Friedman grading system combines Mallampati score, tonsil size and body mass index into an aggregate which yields a very good positive predictive value for moderate-to-severe OSA [8].

Examination of the chest in a patient with excessive daytime somnolence should include inspection for increased antero-posterior diameter and accessory muscle use during respiration, auscultation for expiratory wheezes and percussion for diaphragmatic excursion, as underlying chronic obstructive pulmonary disease is associated with nocturnal hypoventilation and sleep disruption. The rib cage should be examined for signs of kyphoscoliosis or other restrictive abnormality, as restrictive pulmonary diseases can also cause hypoventilation. Long-standing sleep-disordered breathing can lead to *cor pulmonale*; physical findings would include a left parasternal or subxiphoid heave and a prominent fourth heart sound. Tricuspid regurgitation may also be noted, with the classic presentation being a holosystolic murmur heard best at the left middle or lower sternal border when the patient is sitting upright or standing. Abdominal findings consistent with sleep-disordered breathing include manifestations of *cor pulmonale*, including ascites, hepatomegaly and hepato-jugular reflux. Extremities may demonstrate pitting edema in such patients.

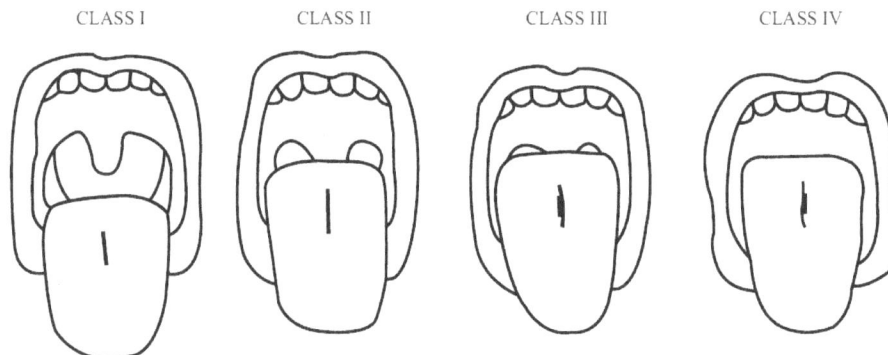

Figure 1: Mallampati's oropharyngeal aperture severity grading. (with permission, courtesy of Jeff Loerch and Dr. Sharon Mace, Cleveland Clinic - Center for Medical Art and Photography).

EPWORTH SLEEPINESS SCALE (ESS)

How likely are you to doze off or fall asleep in the following situations, in contrast to feeling just tired? This refers to your usual way of life in recent times. Even if you have not done some of these activities recently, think about how they would have affected you. Use the following scale to choose the most appropriate number for each situation:

0 = no chance of dozing
1 = slight chance of dozing
2 = moderate chance of dozing
3 = high chance of dozing

Situation	Chance of Dozing or Sleeping
Sitting and reading	_____
Watching TV	_____
Sitting inactive in a public place	_____
Being a passenger in a motor vehicle for an hour or more	_____
Lying down in the afternoon	_____
Sitting and talking to someone	_____
Sitting quietly after lunch (no alcohol)	_____
Stopped for a few minutes in traffic while driving	_____
Total score (add the scores up) (This is your Epworth score)	_____

Score:
0-10 Normal range
10-12 Borderline
12-24 Abnormal

Figure 2: Epworth Sleepiness Scale (ESS) [with permission from American Academy of Sleep Medicine, courtesy of Octavian Ioachimescu, MD, PhD, Atlanta VA Medical Center].

Given the significant data available regarding the role of physical examination in screening for sleep-disordered breathing, a number of different prediction rules have been developed to attempt to distill available data into a composite surrogate [3, 9-11]. For example, Flemons et al. [9] created an adjusted neck circumference calculation, which adjusts neck circumference upwards for reported snoring, witnessed apneas and prevalent hypertension, yielding a value that has a positive predictive value to 81% in the highest risk group. This same group developed the Sleep Apnea Clinical Score (SACS), which combines prevalent hypertension, frequency of snoring, frequency of witnessed apneas and neck measurement into a single metric. This tool, in conjunction with the ESS, demonstrated a 94% positive predictive value for moderate-to-severe OSA. Unfortunately, data demonstrate that such rules have only a reasonable sensitivity and poor specificity for OSA [12]. In addition, they tend to be burdensome to utilize, though they may have some use in identifying certain patients who do not require further evaluation for sleep-disordered breathing (i.e., low likelihood of disease by using a specific instrument with high negative predictive value).

Validated Questionnaires

Many clinical practices find it useful to incorporate standardized questionnaires during the intake of new patients. This may be particularly useful in screening for sleep apnea, since history and physical examination are relatively poor at identifying patients with sleep-disordered breathing. We will briefly summarize a number of such tools and discuss their potential clinical use.

The Stanford Sleepiness Scale (SSS)

Degrees of Sleepiness	Scale Rating
Feeling active, vital, alert or wide awake	1
Functioning at high levels, but not at peak; able to concentrate	2
Awake but relaxed; responsive, but not fully alert	3
Somewhat foggy, let down	4
Foggy, losing interest in remaining awake; slowed down	5
Sleepy, woozy, fighting sleep; prefer to lie down	6
No longer fighting sleep, sleep onset soon; having dream-like thoughts	7
Asleep	x

Figure 3: Stanford Sleepiness Scale (SSS).

The most commonly used questionnaire is the Epworth Sleepiness Scale (ESS), as seen in Fig. **2**, which is intended to measure sleepiness, though there is debate about what constitutes an abnormally high score. In addition, it has a poor sensitivity and specificity for many common sleep disorders, including sleep-disordered breathing, leading some to call for a standard methodology for the clinical use of the ESS [13]. Nevertheless, the tool probably has a role in helping to distinguish the patient who is frankly sleepy from the one who is physically exhausted but has no tendency to fall asleep (and might therefore not require further sleep work-up). Unlike the ESS, which assesses a patient's sleepiness over the last thirty days, the Stanford Sleepiness Scale (Fig. **3**) measures subjective alertness at a given point in time. If administered serially, it can provide information about waxing and waning sleepiness over time, but its most common clinical use is during multiple sleep latency testing (MSLT) and maintenance of wakefulness testing (MWT), both of which attempt to objectively assess sleepiness. Notably, neither questionnaire reliably correlates with these objective metrics of sleep tendency [14, 15]. Other tools, including the Pittsburgh Sleep Quality Index (PSQI) [2], have been designed to assess sleep, but have been used predominantly in the realm of clinical research.

Several questionnaires have been specifically developed to screen for sleep-disordered breathing. The Berlin Questionnaire (BQ), as shown in Fig. **4**, is a ten-item survey which has been well-validated in the primary-care setting. A similar tool, the STOP questionnaire, has been validated in pre-operative surgical patients. However, neither of these tools has been shown to be as reliable as a global, thorough history and a good targeted physical examination, with recent demonstration of positive predictive values of less than 35% and sensitivities of less than 70% for questionnaires such as the ones mentioned above [16].

Berlin Questionnaire

1. Complete the following:

Name_____

Last 4 digits of your SSN _____

Age _____   Gender (M/F) _____

Height _____(ft-in)   Weight _____(lbs)

Category 1

2. Do you snore?

> yes

no
don't know

If you snore:

3. Your snoring is?

> very loud; can be heard in adjacent rooms
> louder than talking

as loud as talking
slightly louder than breathing

4. How often do you snore?

> nearly every day
> 3-4 times a week

1-2 times a week
1-2 times a month
never or nearly never

5. Has your snoring ever bothered other people?

> yes

no

6. Has anyone noticed that you quit breathing during sleep?

> nearly every day
> 3-4 times a week

1-2 times a week
1-2 times a month
never or nearly never

Category 2

7. How often do you feel tired or fatigued after your sleep?

> nearly every day
> 3-4 times a week

1-2 times a week
1-2 times a month
never or nearly never

8. During your wake time, do you feel tired, fatigued or not up to par?

> nearly every day
> 3-4 times a week

1-2 times a week
1-2 times a month
never or nearly never

9. Have you ever nodded off or fallen asleep while driving a vehicle?

> yes

no

If yes, how often does it occur?

> nearly every day
> 3-4 times a week

1-2 times a week
1-2 times a month
never or nearly never

Category 3

10. Do you have high blood pressure?

> yes

no
don't know

BMI = _____ (see the other side)

Scoring Questions: Any answer within a dashed box outline is a positive response.

Scoring categories:

Category 1 is positive if two or more positive responses to questions 2-6
Category 2 is positive if two or more positive responses to questions 7-9
Category 3 is positive if one positive response and/or BMI higher than 30
Final result: 2 or more categories positive: high likelihood of sleep disordered breathing

Figure 4: Berlin Questionnaire (BQ) [with permission from American College of Physicians, courtesy of Octavian Ioachimescu, MD, PhD, Atlanta VA Medical Center].

Patients Already on Therapy for OSA

For patients already on therapy for sleep apnea, some additional points on history, and physical examination should be noted. Regardless of whether the patient is on continuous positive airway pressure (CPAP) or oral appliance therapy (OAT), the frequency of use and the number of hours per night that the device is in place should be determined. For those who report infrequent use, specific questioning regarding the reason for intolerance should follow; patients on CPAP may report discomfort with the facial appliance, a sense of suffocation or noise, whereas patients on OAT may endorse gagging or discomfort at the temporomandibular joint (TMJ).

Physical examination of patients on OAT should include inspecting the preauricular area for redness or swelling. Directly palpation over the joint should follow and should be performed while the patient is opening and closing his mouth in an effort to elicit tenderness. For CPAP patients, inspection of the face for signs of contact dermatitis from their facial appliance or evidence of early skin breakdown related to mask pressure is indicated. Inspection of the conjunctiva is similarly important, as one of the most dangerous repercussions of CPAP mask leak is conjunctivitis, which can become quite severe.

Given the prevalence of sleep-related complaints, affected patients will be commonly seen in medical practice. Because the variety of potential diagnoses that need to be entertained is broad, the clinician needs to be skilled in the performance of a thorough history and physical examination, allowing a narrowing of the list of considerations before proceeding with more involved and expensive diagnostic tests.

RESEARCH OUTLOOK

What do we know:

- Involving the bed partner in the initial evaluation of a patient for sleep pathology can improve the provider's ability to narrow the differential diagnosis and order appropriate diagnostic tests

- Physical findings such as: micronathia, retrognathia, severe dental malocclusions, large neck circumference and body mass index are strong predictors of sleep disordered breathing, especially obstructive sleep apnea, while historical or physical examination findings of congestive heart failure may suggest a higher propensity for central sleep apnea

- Insomnia tends to occur frequently in conjunction with depression, while treatment modalities employed to treat insomnia need to "tackle" both conditions

- The majority of historical risk factors for different sleep conditions are already known, hence a good sleep history and physical examination need to actively look for these predisposing conditions. For example, restless legs syndrome is frequently associated with iron deficiency anemia, hypothyroidism, pregnancy, renal failure, vitamn B12 and folate deficiency, neuropathies, *etc.*

What we don't know:

- In addition to the established, traditional morbid risk factors for various sleep conditions, we currently still don't know which phenotypic characteristics herald morbid consequences; for example why only certain individuals with sleep apnea suffer from the cardiovascular consequences of this condition, why only some of them have daytime symptoms, *etc.*

- What other findings on history and physical examination might obviate the need for diagnostic testing for other disorders, such as periodic limb movement disorder or narcolepsy

- It is still unclear at the present time how can we optimally combine physical examination findings with standardized questionnaires to improve our diagnostic abilities, ameliorate the utilization of both in-laboratory and/ or in-home polysomnography for sleep-disordered breathing diagnosis or to generate diagnostic pathways and algorithms based on outcomes and less so on arbitrary or imperfect metrics (*e.g.*, apnea hyponea index).

REFERENCES

[1] Johns MW. A new method for measuring daytime sleepiness: the Epworth sleepiness scale. Sleep 1991; 14(6): 540-5.
[2] Buysse DJ, Reynolds CF, 3rd, Monk TH, Berman SR, Kupfer DJ. The Pittsburgh Sleep Quality Index: a new instrument for psychiatric practice and research. Psychiatry Res 1989; 28(2): 193-213.
[3] Deegan PC, McNicholas WT. Predictive value of clinical features for the obstructive sleep apnoea syndrome. Eur Respir J 1996; 9(1): 117-24.
[4] Schellenberg JB, Maislin G, Schwab RJ. Physical findings and the risk for obstructive sleep apnea. The importance of oropharyngeal structures. Am J Respir Crit Care Med 2000; 162(2 Pt 1):740-8.
[5] Davies RJ, Stradling JR. The relationship between neck circumference, radiographic pharyngeal anatomy, and the obstructive sleep apnoea syndrome. Eur Respir J 1990; 3(5): 509-14.
[6] Mallampati SR, Gatt SP, Gugino LD, Desai SP, Waraksa B, Freiberger D, *et al.* A clinical sign to predict difficult tracheal intubation: a prospective study. Can Anaesth Soc J 1985; 32(4): 429-34.

[7]   Nuckton TJ, Glidden DV, Browner WS, Claman DM. Physical examination: Mallampati score as an independent predictor of obstructive sleep apnea. Sleep 2006; 29(7): 903-8.

[8]   Friedman M, Tanyeri H, La Rosa M, Landsberg R, Vaidyanathan K, Pieri S, *et al.* Clinical predictors of obstructive sleep apnea. Laryngoscope 1999; 109(12): 1901-7.

[9]   Flemons WW, Whitelaw WA, Brant R, Remmers JE. Likelihood ratios for a sleep apnea clinical prediction rule. Am J Respir Crit Care Med 1994; 150(5 Pt 1): 1279-85.

[10] Viner S, Szalai JP, Hoffstein V. Are history and physical examination a good screening test for sleep apnea? Ann Intern Med 1991; 115(5): 356-9.

[11] Crocker BD, Olson LG, Saunders NA, Hensley MJ, McKeon JL, Allen KM, *et al.* Estimation of the probability of disturbed breathing during sleep before a sleep study. Am Rev Respir Dis 1990; 142(1): 14-8.

[12] Ward Flemons W, McNicholas WT. Clinical prediction of the sleep apnea syndrome. Sleep Med Rev 1997; 1(1): 19-32.

[13] Tachibana N, Taniguchi M. Why do we continue to use Epworth sleepiness scale? Sleep Med 2007; 8(5): 541-2.

[14] Chervin RD, Aldrich MS, Pickett R, Guilleminault C. Comparison of the results of the Epworth Sleepiness Scale and the Multiple Sleep Latency Test. J Psychosom Res 1997; 42(2): 145-55.

[15] Danker-Hopfe H, Kraemer S, Dorn H, Schmidt A, Ehlert I, Herrmann WM. Time-of-day variations in different measures of sleepiness (MSLT, pupillography, and SSS) and their interrelations. Psychophysiology 2001; 38(5): 828-35.

[16] Chung F, Yegneswaran B, Liao P, Chung SA, Vairavanathan S, Islam S, *et al.* STOP questionnaire: a tool to screen patients for obstructive sleep apnea. Anesthesiology 2008; 108(5): 812-21.

CHAPTER 4

Sleep Testing and Monitoring

Kumar S. Budur[*], M.D., M.S.

Associate Medical Director: Clinical Science – Neuroscience, Takeda Global Research and Development Inc., 675 North Field Drive, Lake Forest, IL 60045, USA

Abstract: Sleep testing has evolved over the years and today sleep testing is considered among some of the most sophisticated medical testing modalities. Although the most common sleep test used today is diagnostic polysomnogram, which is generally employed to diagnose sleep apnea, sleep testing today is much more than just-a-tool to diagnose sleep disordered breathing. Various sophisticated tests, with highly standardized processes and technologies, in association with precise diagnostic criteria backed by extensive scientific data, are conducted every day in various sleep centers across the country and the world. The fast pace of technological advancements in this field continues to provide new breakthroughs in the acquisition of various sleep-related physiological variables every day.

Although a nocturnal polysomnogram (PSG) is often used synonymously with the term "sleep test", well-staffed and competent sleep centers are capable of performing a wide array of sleep studies, including: diagnostic PSGs (typically to diagnose sleep apnea), titration studies (*e.g.*, to obtain optimal positive airway pressure setting to treat sleep apnea), PSGs with extended EEG montages (*e.g.*, to diagnose co-existent seizures), PSGs with extended limb leads and video monitoring (*e.g.*, to diagnose REM sleep behavior disorder, etc), nocturnal penile tumescence (NPT, to diagnose erectile impotence), actigraphy tests, etc.

TOPIC DISCUSSION (CLINICAL OUTLOOK)

Introduction

Nocturnal polysomnogram (PSG), commonly referred to as "sleep study", has evolved over the years from a primitive technology, as recently as few decades ago, to one of the most sophisticated tests in medical sciences. The collaboration of specialists, sleep academies and various commercial entities has resulted in phenomenal technological advancements, resulting in the development of miniaturized and patient/health care professional-friendly devices. Nowadays, sleep studies do not have to happen necessarily in the sleep laboratories or in the hospitals. The development and acceptance of portable motoring as a valid testing methodology to diagnose sleep apnea is a relatively new phenomenon that is becoming increasingly popular.

The American Academy of Sleep Medicine (AASM) has published in 2007 new guidelines for acquiring, scoring, and interpreting polysomnographic data [1, 2]. These guidelines were based on the scientific evidence and consensus of experts at that time. Apart from providing minimum standard requirements, these guidelines also help in comparing data from one sleep center to another.

Polysomnography

A nocturnal polysomnogram (PSG) is the most commonly performed sleep test. It is generally an all-night test in a sleep laboratory. The sleep or bed rooms are designed in a way that are not just comfortable for the patients (such as light, noise, temperature, etc.), but these rooms are also expected to meet certain specifications set by the AASM. A trained sleep technologist is in attendance in a "control room" throughout the duration of the recording. A typical overnight PSG consists of at least seven channels or more, including the electroencephalogram (EEG), electro-oculogram (EOG), chin and limb electromyogram (EMG), Electrocardiogram (ECG), nasal pressure transducer/thermistor, chest and abdominal respiratory effort detection (usually by using calibrated or uncalibrated respiratory inductance plethysmography [RIP]), pulse oximetry, snore microphone, body position sensor, video, etc. Depending on the nature of the symptoms and suspected diagnoses, additional features are added including extra limb leads to the arms/legs, expanded EEG, etc.

The EEG, EOG and the chin EMG help with differentiating sleep from wakefulness and in delineating various stages of sleep, *i.e.* NREM (N1, N2 and N3) and REM sleep. The combination of airflow sensors (nasal pressure transducer

---

*Address correspondence to Kumar S. Budur: Associate Medical Director: Clinical Science – Neuroscience, Takeda Global Research and Development Inc., 675 North Field Drive, Lake Forest, IL 60045, USA; E-mail: ksbudur@yahoo.com

and thermistor), respiratory effort sensors (RIP) and pulse oximetry help to identify respiratory events associated with sleep-related breathing disorders. The ECG is primarily used to determine the rate/rhythm and to detect any changes in response to respiratory events. The snore microphone detects the frequency and intensity of the snoring. Body position sensor helps to determine the presence or absence of the positional component to sleep apnea. Video monitoring provides useful information on any abnormal movements, etc occurring during sleep.

The PSG is primarily indicated in the diagnosis of sleep-related breathing disorders, unusual behaviors in sleep, excessive daytime sleepiness (sometimes in combination with a daytime test, Multiple Sleep Latency Test [MSLT]), and to assess efficacy of various treatments for different sleep disorders. It is, however, important to note that PSG is not routinely indicated in conditions such as insomnia or restless legs syndrome (RLS).

Positive Airway Pressure (PAP) Titration

After diagnostic PSGs, Positive Airway Pressure (PAP) titration studies are perhaps the most common types of sleep tests performed in the sleep laboratory. PAP titration studies were traditionally performed to determine optimal PAP settings for treating sleep apnea. However, over the past few years, the tendency to "split" a polysomnogram into diagnostic and PAP titration parts in the presence of significant sleep apnea is becoming increasingly common. The Center for Medicare and Medicaid Services (CMS) has provided guidelines on the criteria to perform split-night polysomnograms [3]. These guidelines include adequate sleep time and respiratory events during the diagnostic portion and adequate time (usually 3 hours) available for the titration part of the study. In the absence of the above, the guidelines suggest to continue the study as a diagnostic nocturnal PSG, and then conduct a separate, full-night PAP titration study.

The goal of PAP titration is to determine optimal PAP setting that is necessary to normalize the apnea hypopnea index (AHI), arousal index (ArI), oxygen saturation, respiratory airflow contour and snoring. PAP therapies have evolved over the years and currently a variety of options are available, including Continuous Positive Airway Pressure (CPAP), Bilevel Positive Airway Pressure (Bilevel PAP), and the Auto/Adaptive/Assisted Servo-Ventilation (ASV). The success of a titration study depends on the use of an appropriate mask, tolerance of the patient to PAP, nature/severity of sleep disordered breathing and the diligence of the sleep technologist in adjusting the PAP.

To date, CPAP is the most common type of PAP device used and, in general, it is well tolerated. Nevertheless, sometimes bilevel PAP is used instead, in order to enhance patient's comfort, especially at higher PAP settings, when it may seem hard to exhale against high pressures. Bilevel PAP has the capability to deliver lower pressure at the beginning of exhalation making it easier for patients to exhale. Recently, Auto/Assisted Servo-Ventilation (ASV) started to be used to treat complex sleep apnea. Complex sleep apnea patients are those who have PAP-induced central apneas, or those events observed for the first time during the titration portion of the study, *i.e.*, before abolishing the obstructive respiratory events with PAP.

Multiple Sleep Latency Test (MSLT)

The Multiple Sleep Latency Test (MSLT) is done to measure/quantify a person's ability to doze off to sleep in a standard setting. Usually performed during the day after an overnight PSG, sometimes this test is performed at night if the major wakefulness period for a particular individual happens to be at night. The preceding PSG is to ensure that the subject gets adequate nocturnal sleep and also to rule out any co-existent sleep disorder (e.g. sleep apnea), contributing to daytime sleepiness.

The "hook-up" (montage) for MSLT is much less extensive than for a PSG and consist of only EEG, EOG, chin EMG and ECG channels.

MSLT consists of 5-nap trials that are separated by 2-hour intervals. The first trial starts after 1.5 hours (but within 3 hours) after the morning awakening. The process of conducting each trial is highly standardized [4]. During each nap, the subject is requested to rest in a quiet, dark room and is instructed to try to fall asleep. Twenty minutes are given for the subject to doze off to sleep with each trial. If the subject remains awake during this period, the particular trial is terminated and lights are turned back on. If sleep is recorded within the 20 minute period, the subject is allowed to sleep for 15 minutes to observe emergence of any REM sleep; the trial is terminated after 15 minutes, regardless of the presence or absence of REM sleep. These trials are repeated 5 times with an interval of 2 hours between each trial. During the period in between trials, the subject is expected not to engage in any stimulating activities including smoking, caffeine consumption or exercise.

The sleep latency (duration of time from lights-out to first epoch of sleep) is calculated for each trial and then averaged over 5 trials, which gives the mean sleep latency (MSL). REM sleep within 15 minutes of sleep onset in of the any trials is noted as a sleep-onset REM period (SOREMP). In general, a MSL less than 5 minutes is abnormal, 5 to 10 minutes is considered borderline, and more than 10 minutes is considered normal. Presence of two or more SOREMPs is supportive of the diagnosis of narcolepsy.

Maintenance of Wakefulness Test (MWT)

The maintenance of wakefulness test (MWT) is performed to measure/quantify a person's ability to stay awake in a standardized environment. Unlike MSLT, MWT does not require a preceding PSG. The MWT comprises of four 40-minute trials which are separated by 2-hour intervals. The first trial also starts after 1.5 hours (but within 3 hours) after the final morning awakening. The "hook-up" for MWT is similar to MSLT and only EEG, EOG, chin EMG and ECG channels are used. The process of conducting each trial is standardized and during each trial the subject is requested to try to remain awake while seated in a dimly lit room [4]. The trials are ended if the patient does not fall asleep in 40 minutes, or if unequivocal sleep is recorded.

Similar to MSLT, the sleep latency (duration of time from lights-out to first epoch of sleep) is calculated for each trial and then averaged over 4 trials, which gives the mean sleep latency (MSL). Although the criteria for "abnormal" MWT are less well established, a subject's ability to stay awake is best supported by absence of sleep in all 4 trials.

Portable Monitoring

With the recent advancements in medical technology, smaller and smarter devices are used to gather physiological data and (fortunately) Sleep Medicine has not been avoided by these trends. Over the past two decades, several small devices have been developed, specifically to diagnose sleep apnea, outside of the sleep lab or the hospital setting (most often in the comfortable setting of home).

In 1994, an attempt was made to classify sleep testing into various types and this is still used as a standard even today. Type I is a an attended full PSG, performed in a sleep laboratory; Type II is an unattended full PSG outside the laboratory setting; Type III is an unattended limited-channel test where at least four cardiopulmonary bioparameters are monitored; and Type IV is an unattended testing with only one or two cardiopulmonary bio-parameters monitored (see Table 1).

Table 1: Types of sleep apnea testing devices (based on Ferber *et al.* Portable recording in the assessment of obstructive sleep apnea [7])

	Type I	Type II	Type III	Type IV
Number of parameters monitored	≥ 7	≥ 7	≥ 4	1-2
Leads	EEG, EOG, EMG, ECG, airflow, effort, oximetry	EEG, EOG, EMG, ECG, airflow, effort, oximetry	airflow, effort, oximetry, ECG	Oximetry and one other lead (usually airflow)
Setting of the study	Usually in a sleep center or hospital setting	Outside a sleep center or a hospital setting	Outside a sleep center or a hospital setting	Outside a sleep center or a hospital setting
Attended/ Unattended	Attended	Unattended	Unattended	Unattended

Portable monitoring (PM) or home sleep testing (as is sometimes called) is a used to conduct sleep studies in a setting outside of the sleep centers or hospitals. Typically these are used to diagnose only sleep apnea and not any other sleep disorders [5-7]. However, with additional monitoring, these devices can be used to diagnose other sleep and neurological disorders. Portable monitoring offers a unique opportunity for those patients who do not have easy access to sleep centers and also to some who do not prefer to spend a night in a sleep laboratory, away from home.

Over the years, the technology for portable monitoring has evolved and the reliability and validity of these devices is well established to diagnose patients who are considered to be at a high risk for moderate or severe sleep apnea. However, it is important to know that these devices have some limitations and, while suitable for the majority of the patients with sleep apnea, these are not for everyone. Patients with significant medical or sleep disorders, which can degrade the quality of recording, are not suitable for portable monitoring. Similarly, it is not to be used to diagnose other sleep disorders, such as narcolepsy, periodic limb movement disorders, etc. Despite some limitations, the acceptance of portable monitoring as a valid test to diagnose sleep apnea has increased over the years. With further advancements in technology, this can only get better.

The AASM guidelines provide an evidence-based summary of the utility of portable monitoring, the recommended training for the personnel involved in testing/interpretation of data and the minimum standards for the monitoring devices [8].

The following is a brief summary of the AASM guidelines on portable monitoring:

(i) PM for the diagnosis of OSA should be done only in conjunction with a comprehensive sleep evaluation. In addition, the AASM states that the clinical evaluation should be performed by a board-certified sleep specialist or an individual who fulfills the eligibility criteria for Sleep Medicine certification examination; the interpretation of the PM study, supervision, and quality assurance are the responsibility of the specialist board certified in Sleep Medicine, as is required for sleep center accreditation.

(ii) PM may be used as an alternative to polysomnography (PSG) for the diagnosis of OSA in patients with a high pretest probability of moderate to severe OSA. However, in the absence of valid predictive models that could reasonable identify subjects with "high pretest probability of moderate to severe sleep apnea", the clinicians are guided by the presence of risk factors such as snoring, witnessed apnea, sleepiness, obesity, large neck circumference, history of hypertension, etc. Although each one of these is associated with increased risk for sleep apnea, there is no linear correlation between the cumulative effects of risk factors and the severity of sleep apnea. Since PM devices can generate false-negative tests, in-lab PSG should be performed in cases where PM shows a negative result or it is technically inadequate in patients with a high pretest probability for sleep apnea.

(iii) PM may also be used in the diagnosis of OSA in patients for whom an in-lab PSG is not possible because of the nature/severity of co-morbid conditions, immobility or for safety issues.

(iv) PM may also be indicated to monitor the response to non-CPAP treatments for sleep apnea. These include upper airway surgery, oral appliances and/or weight loss.

Portable monitoring is not indicated in:

(i) Children

(ii) Significant co-morbid medical conditions that may degrade the accuracy of testing such as significant pulmonary problems, cardiac failure, etc (portable monitoring devices are not validated in these conditions)

(iii) To diagnose other sleep disorders such as Periodic limb movement disorders, REM sleep behavior disorders

Scoring Sleep Studies

The American Academy of Sleep Medicine (AASM) scoring guidelines from 2007, clearly establish criteria on staging sleep and scoring various events observed during sleep [1]. These criteria are based on the best evidence available to date. To start with, sleep staging is done to delineate Wake (W) from sleep and sleep is further staged into Rapid Eye Movement (REM), and the three non-rapid eye movement (NREM) stages N1, N2, and N3. Each of these stages is characterized by specific EEG, EOG, and EMG criteria.

Once the PSG data is acquired, the EEG data is analyzed to differentiate wake from sleep and sleep is further classified into various stages. To understand the staging of sleep, a basic knowledge of the characteristics of EEG is essential. By convention, the EEG waves are classified into alpha, beta, theta and delta waves. In addition, special forms of EEG patterns that occur during sleep (sleep spindles, K-complexes) are also defined. The definitions for each of these wave forms are as follows:

Alpha: Frequency of 8-12 Hz

Beta: Frequency of > 12 Hz

Theta: Frequency of 4-8 Hz

Delta: Frequency of < 2 Hz

Sleep spindles: sinusoidal waves with frequency of 12-14 Hz and lasting for 0.5 to 1.5 sec

K-Complex: high-amplitude, biphasic wave of at least 0.5 second duration; generally, itconsists of a sharp initial negative wave followed by a slow positive wave.

Typically, the data acquired is divided into epochs of 30-second duration and each epoch is assigned a stage depending on the presence of certain EEG characteristics for the majority of that epoch (>15 seconds). Wakefulness is characterized by predominantly alpha waves (50% or more in a 30 second epoch). Sleep is divided into non-rapid eye movement (NREM) and rapid eye movement (REM) sleep. NREM sleep is further divided into N1, N2 and N3, again based on the characteristics of the EEG waves.

An epoch of sleep is scored as N1 when alpha activity occupies less than 50% of an epoch. N1 consists of low-voltage, mixed frequency pattern of theta activity. N2 is defined by the presence of either sleep spindles or K complexes. N3 is characterized by slow waves or delta waves that occupy at least 20% of the epoch. Of note, previously N3 was distinguished as two different stages (stage 3 and stage 4) depending on the proportion of the epoch occupied by the slow waves (*i.e.* 20-50% and >50% of the epoch). However, this distinction is no more recognized. REM sleep is characterized by low-voltage, mixed frequency waves (similar to N1) and has EMG tone (typically chin EMG) that is close to zero micro-volts or at minimum for the study. In addition, rapid eye movements are seen in REM sleep. "Phasic" REM sleep is characterized by rapid eye movements, typically at a frequency of 4 to 6 eye movements per epoch, while "phasic" REM is characterized by the absence of such eye movements (see Fig. **1**).

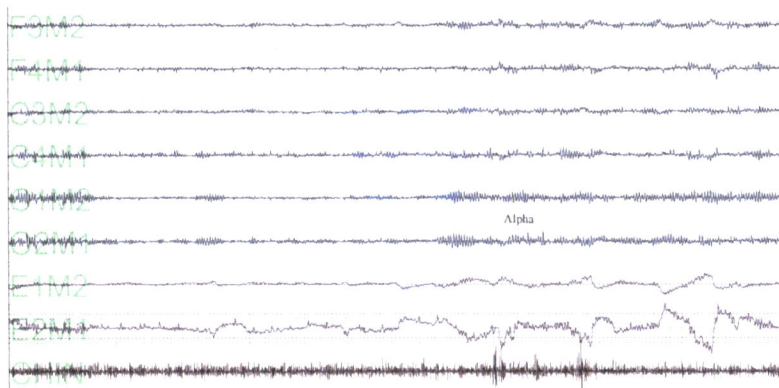

A: Awake (W)

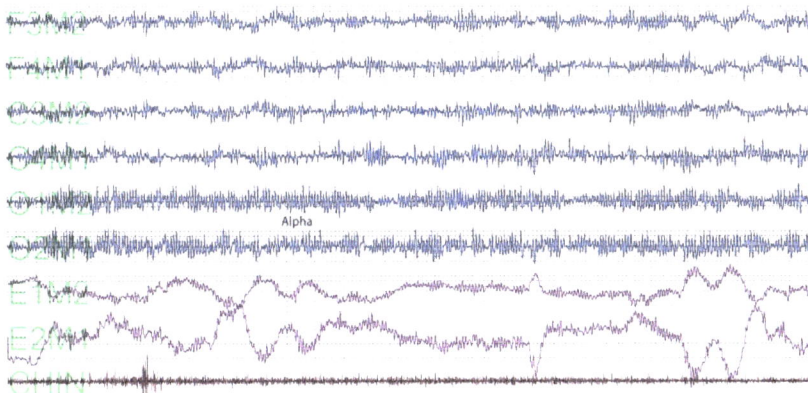

B: Calm Wakefulness (W, eyes closed)

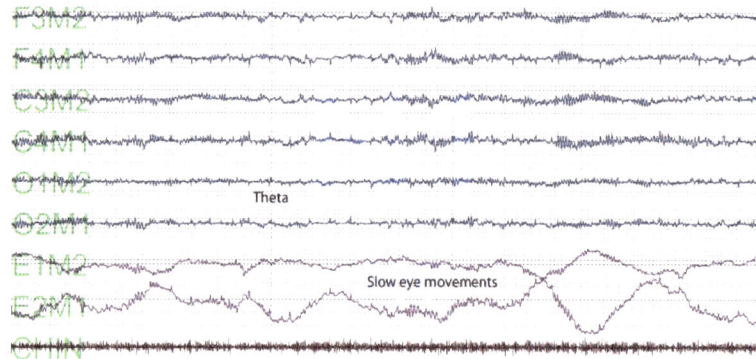

C: Stage 1 (N1, theta waves, alpha reduced, slow eye movements)

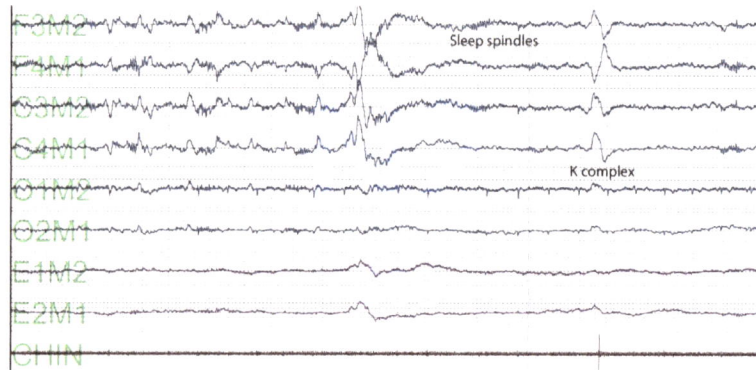

D: Stage 2 (N2, sleep spindles , K complexes)

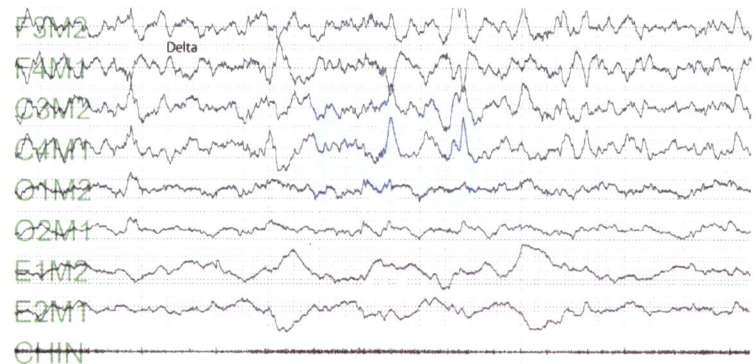

E: Stage 3 (N3, delta waves)

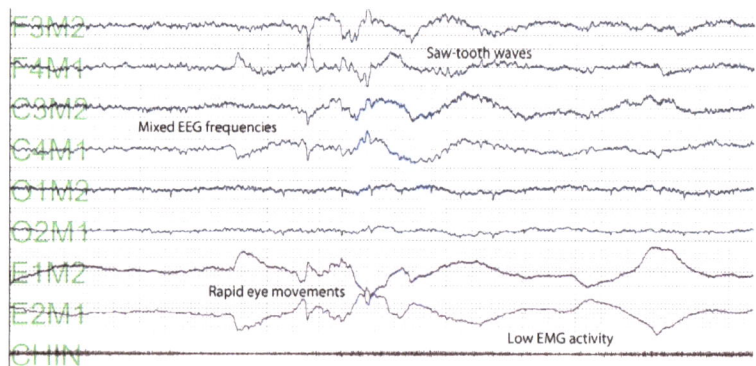

F: Stage REM (R, rapid eye movements, mixed frequencies, saw-tooth waves, low EMG activity)

Figure 1: EEG tracings showing wakefulness and stages of sleep.

Once the sleep staging is accomplished, respiratory events are scored as primarily apneas or hypopneas. An apnea is a 90% or greater reduction of the thermal sensor signal as compared to baseline for 10 seconds or longer. It is classified as obstructive if respiratory effort continues during the cessation of oro-nasal airflow. An apnea is classified as central if there is a cessation of both airflow and respiratory effort. Mixed apneas have both central (initial) and obstructive (later) components. Hypopneas are defined in two different ways: Nasal pressure transducer signal decreases by 30% or more from baseline for at least 10 seconds accompanied by a desaturation that is at least 4% from baseline; or Nasal pressure signal decreases by 50% or more from the baseline for at least 10 seconds and is either associated with either a desaturation of at least 3% or an EEG arousal. The apnea-hypopnea index (AHI) denotes the apneas and hypopneas per hour of the total sleep time recorded (see Fig. **2**).

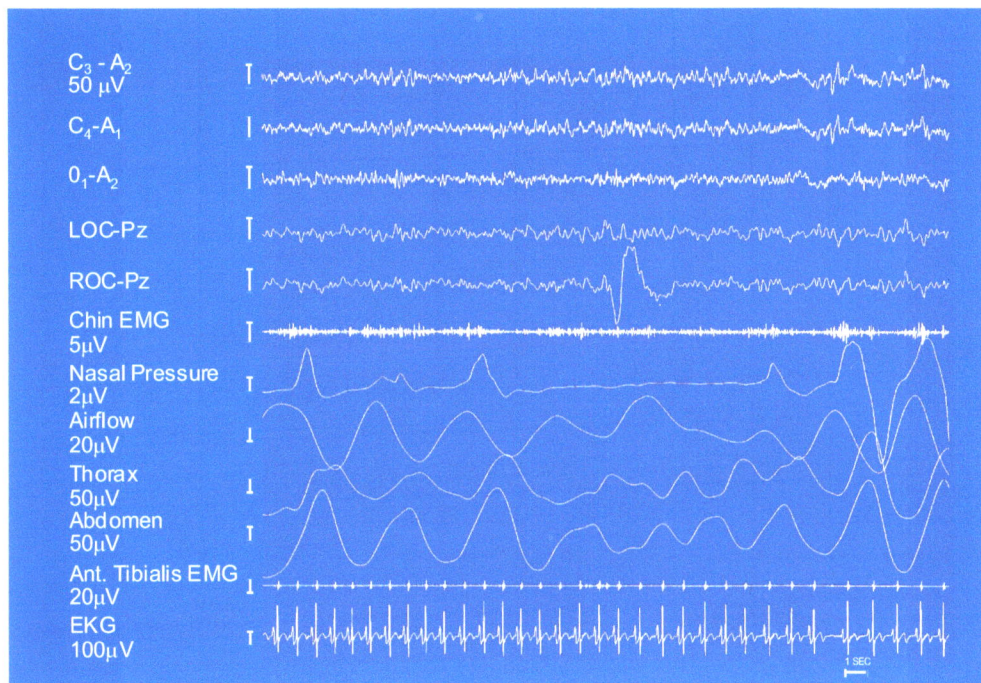

Figure 2: A 30-second epoch showing an obstructive hypopnea *i.e.* reduction in airflow (see nasal pressure and airflow channel) despite effort (see Thorax and Abdomen channels).

An arousal is scored in any stage of sleep when there is an abrupt change in EEG frequencies, including alpha, theta, or frequencies higher than 16 Hz. This definition excludes spindles and requires the frequency shift to persist for at least 3 seconds. For an arousal to be scored during REM sleep, a concomitant increase in chin EMG is also required. To differentiate one arousal from another, a 10 second interval between 2 arousals is required. The arousal index (ArI) denotes the apneas and hypopneas per hour of the total sleep time recorded.

A limb movement is scored when the limb EMG (most commonly, *anterior tibialis*) amplitude increases by 8 microvolts over baseline for at least 0.5 seconds but no longer than 10 seconds. A periodic limb movement (PLM) series is scored if 4 such movements occur in a row, provided each component limb movement occurs within 5 to 90 seconds of its neighbor. The PLM index (PLMI) and the PLM arousal index (PLMArI) denotes the number of PLMs and the number of PLMs associated with arousal per hour of the total sleep time recorded, respectively (see Fig. **3**).

OTHER TESTS

Actigraphy

Actigraph is a small wrist watch-like device that is primarily used to determine the sleep-wake patterns. The actigraph has a motion sensor that monitors rest-activity data. Lack of activity is used as a surrogate for sleep. Over the years, modifications to the actigraph have resulted in monitoring several other parameters such as intensity of exposure to light, data acquisition of up to 15 days and sometimes longer, etc. Actigraphy is most commonly used to study sleep patterns in normal individuals, as well as patients with circadian rhythm disorders. However, the use of actigraphy has expanded recently and it is sometimes used to monitor response to treatments for insomnia, surrogate marker of sleep in Type III portable monitoring devices, etc. Recent studies have shown a good correlation between actigraphy and polysomnography on several sleep parameters such as sleep latency and total sleep time [9].

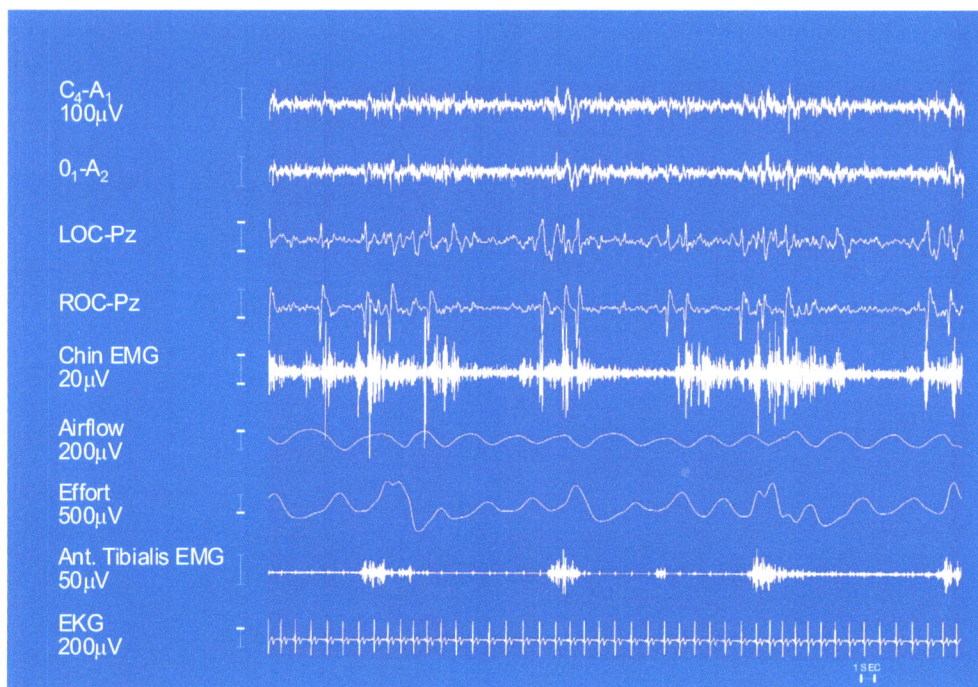

Figure 3: A 60-second epoch with frequent, periodic limb movements (see Anterior Tibialis EMG).

Enhanced/Expanded Polysomnogram

Polysomnogram, as described above, is sometimes modified for the diagnosis of certain sleep disorders such as REM sleep behavior disorder (extra limb leads), and other co-morbid disorders such as seizures (extra EEG electrodes), erectile impotence (Nocturnal Penile Tumescence [NPT] monitors), etc.

RESEARCH OUTLOOK

What do we know:

1. Sleep testing is an advanced medical testing methodology with a very precise measurement of various physiological parameters.

2. Sleep parameter measurement (scoring and interpretation) is standardized and based on strict normative data.

3. Technological advances within the past decade have resulted in devices that are patient-friendly and less intrusive.

What we don't know:

1. Will portable monitoring gain sufficient acceptance within the medical community that uncomplicated sleep apnea is eventually diagnosed and treated in primary care setting rather than wait for long to be assessed and tested at a sleep center?

2. Will auto-titration devices eventually replace manual titration in a sleep lab?

3. Will the technology and algorithms become sophisticated enough to predict appropriate PAP setting based on various demographic, physiological variables with or without the combination with the findings on the diagnostic polysomnograms?

4. Will actigraphy technology be eventually helpful in not just accurately measuring sleep latency and total sleep time but also other parameters such as wake time after sleep onset, etc.

5. Will autonomic testing (such as pupillometry, peripheral arterial tone assessments, etc) be able to quantify/measure day time hypersomnolence, fatigue, etc?

REFERENCES

[1]   Iber C, Ancoli-Israel S, Chesson A, Quan SF, for the American Academy of Sleep Medicine. The AASM manual for the scoring of sleep and associated events: Rules, terminology and technical specifications.1st ed. Westchester, Ill: American Academy of Sleep Medicine; 2007.

[2]   Kushida CA, Littner MR, Morgenthaler T, *et al.* Practice parameters for the indications for polysomnography and related procedures: An update for 2005. Sleep 2005; 28: 499–521.

[3]   Kushida CA, Chediak A, Berry RB, Brown LK, Gozal D, Iber C, Parthasarathy S, Quan SF, Rowley JA. Positive airway pressure titration task force of the American Academy of Sleep Medicine. Clinical guidelines for the manual titration of positive airway pressure in patients with obstructive sleep apnea. J Clin Sleep Med 2008; 4: 157–171.

[4]   Littner MR, Kushida C, Wise M, *et al.* Practice parameters for clinical use of the multiple sleep latency test and the maintenance of wakefulness test. Sleep 2005; 28(1): 113–121.

[5]   Collop N, Anderson WM, Boehlecke B, Claman D, Goldberg R, Gottlieb DJ, Hudgel D, Sateia M, Schwab R. Clinical guidelines for the use of unattended portable monitors in the diagnosis of obstructive sleep apnea in adult patients. J Clin Sleep Med 2007; 3(7): 737–747.

[6]   Ferber R, Millman R, Coppola M, *et al.* ASDA standards of practice: portable recording in the assessment of obstructive sleep apnea. Sleep 1994; 17: 378–392.

[7]   Collop N, Shepard J, Strollo P. Executive summary on the systematic review and practice parameters for portable monitoring in the investigation of suspected sleep apnea in adults. American Thoracic Society Documents. Am J Respir Crit Care Med 2004; 169: 1160–1163.

[8]   Callop NA, Anderson WM, Boehlecke B, *et al.* Clinical guidelines for the use of unattended portable monitors in the diagnosis of obstructive sleep apnea in adult patients. J Clin Sleep Med 2007; 3(7): 737-747.

[9]   Morgenthaler T, Alessi C, Friedman L, Owens J, Kapur V *et al.* Practice parameters for the use of actigraphy in the assessment of sleep and sleep disorders: An update for 2007. Sleep 2007; 30(4): 519–529.

Contemporary Sleep Medicine for Physicians, 2011, 58-70

CHAPTER 5

Snoring and Upper Airway Resistance Syndrome

Kannan Ramar, M.B.B.S., M.D.[1],* and **Eric J. Olson, M.D.[2]**

[1]*Assistant Professor of Medicine, Mayo College of Medicine, Consultant Division of Pulmonary and Critical Care Medicine, Mayo Clinic, Rochester, MN, USA and* [2]*Associate Professor of Medicine, Mayo College of Medicine, Consultant Division of Pulmonary and Critical Care Medicine, Co-Director Center for Sleep Medicine, Mayo Clinic, Rochester, MN, USA*

Abstract: Snoring is a common phenomenon and results from vibration of the soft tissue structures in the upper airway. Snoring may occur alone or as a sign of upper airway resistance syndrome (UARS) or obstructive sleep apnea syndrome (OSA). Snoring carries social consequences and has been linked to increased risk for cardiovascular disease, although this relationship may be confounded by undiagnosed OSA. UARS is characterized by daytime dysfunction and repetitive respiratory effort-related arousals, episodes of increasingly intense breathing efforts that terminate with an arousal from sleep before a hypopnea (episode of partial airflow reduction) or apnea (episode of complete airflow reduction) occur. There is controversy whether UARS is a distinct clinical entity or part of the OSA spectrum. Long-term cardiovascular consequences of UARS are unclear. Risk factors for snoring and UARS are similar and include obesity, nasal congestion, ingestion of pharyngeal relaxing substances before bed such as alcohol, hypnotics, and skeletal muscle relaxants, and abnormalities of the bony and soft tissue structures of the head and neck. Treatment options for snoring and UARS overlap and include risk factor modifications, oral appliances to advance the mandible during sleep, continuous positive airway pressure, and upper airway surgeries.

TOPIC DISCUSSION (CLINICAL OUTLOOK)

Introduction

Snoring is a common occurrence that results from vibration of the upper airway structures during breathing in sleep. Though snoring typically occurs during inhalation, it may also be present exclusively during exhalation, or throughout the respiratory cycle. Snoring may occur during nasal breathing, oral breathing, or oronasal breathing. Nearly everyone has experienced occasional snoring. The estimated prevalence of habitual snoring varies, depending on the method(s) used to capture data. In the Wisconsin Sleep Cohort, a longitudinal study of the epidemiologic aspects of obstructive sleep apnea syndrome (OSA) in middle-age state government employees, 44% of men and 28% of women were habitual snorers [1]. Snoring frequency increases with age, with the prevalence falling after age 75 years [2]. Apart from being disruptive to the bed-partner and socially embarrassing, snoring may indicate the presence of sleep disordered breathing in the form of upper airway resistance syndrome (UARS) or OSA. UARS is generally defined as a condition of daytime dysfunction due to repetitive respiratory effort-related arousals (RERAs) during sleep. RERAs are episodes of increasing respiratory effort in the face of critical upper airway narrowing that do not meet criteria for apneas (episodes of complete airflow reduction) or hypopneas (episodes of partial airflow reduction). These episodes terminate with arousals from sleep, just like many apneas and hypopneas, and similarly result in daytime fatigue and sleepiness. The prevalence of UARS is not known.

Disease History

Snoring has been an ageless occurrence [3]. Until very recently, snoring was generally portrayed as a stereotypic marker of the sleeping state and dismissed as an embarrassing social nuisance without medical significance. However, the recognition of OSA thrust snoring into greater importance. Snoring is a cardinal feature of OSA and thus snoring has drawn greater scrutiny from concerned bed partners and thorough health care providers, and is frequently the trigger for further evaluation of sleep disordered breathing.

The recognition of OSA also ushered in the paradigm that critical upper airway narrowing during sleep leads to recurrent arousals and subsequent daytime sleepiness. Through case series in 1982 [4], 1991 [5] and 1993 [6],

*Address correspondence to Kannan Ramar: Assistant Professor of Medicine, Mayo College of Medicine, Consultant Division of Pulmonary and Critical Care Medicine, Mayo Clinic, Rochester, MN, USA; E-mail: ramar.kannan@mayo.edu

Guilleminault and collaborators at Stanford sought to expand this concept by reporting children and adults with daytime dysfunction in the context of sleep fragmentation from breathing efforts against increased upper airway resistance (*i.e.*, RERAs) without frank apneas or hypopneas, dubbing this condition UARS. Compared to controls, polysomnograms (PSG) with esophageal balloon monitoring of intrathoracic pressure demonstrated increased intrathoracic inspiratory pressure swings during sleep without associated hypoxemia or significant flow amplitude reductions, indicating the need for increased inspiratory effort to overcome heightened upper airway resistive load. The intrathoracic pressure swings returned to baseline with arousal and restoration of upper airway patency. Treatment (tonsillectomy and adenoidectomy in the children; continuous positive airway pressure [CPAP] in adults) decreased the number of arousals and improved daytime alertness, as measured by the multiple sleep latency test (MSLT). A 1993 report detailing 48 patients who had been diagnosed with idiopathic hypersomnia found that 15 of the 48 subjects had PSG findings supportive of UARS, defined as ≥10 arousals per hour immediately following episodes of increased respiratory effort as detected by esophageal pressure monitoring [6]. CPAP decreased the number of arousals and normalized the mean MSLT score after 1 month.

Controversy continues whether UARS is a distinct clinical syndrome or just a variant of OSA because RERAs, apneas, and hypopneas have a shared pathophysiology. A report by the American Academy of Sleep Medicine's (AASM) Task Force on Sleep-Related Breathing Disorders in Adults in 1999 codified the term RERA, but did not name UARS as a distinct sleep disordered breathing syndrome. The Task Force recommended, at least for purposes of standardizing clinical research in adult subjects, that the diagnosis of OSA be based on PSG evidence of ≥ 5 apneas, hypopneas, or RERAs per hour of sleep [7]. Similarly, the International Classification of Sleep Disorders-2nd edition (ICSD-2) recognizes the term RERAs and includes them as discrete PSG events supportive of diagnosis of OSA, but recommends abandoning the term UARS and subsuming it under the heading OSA because of the shared pathophysiology [8]. The latest attempt to standardize the RERA definition came with release of The 2007 AASM manual for PSG scoring [9].

The inclusion of UARS in this chapter is an acknowledgment of the legitimacy of the RERA concept, as well the realization that contemporary clinicians still use the term UARS to describe their fatigued or sleepy patients with respiratory, non-apneic sleep fragmentation on PSG.

Pathophysiology

Snoring and RERAs are consequences of increased airflow resistance in the upper airway during sleep. The upper airway extends from the nares to the larynx and serves several functions, including respiration, phonation and deglutition. The upper airway is highly adapted for vocalization and swallowing in humans by serving not as a simple rigid tube, but as a semi-rigid conduit, but this flexibility leaves the pharynx vulnerable to collapse. With sleep onset, decreased upper airway dilator muscle activity enhances upper airway compliance and, thus, collapsibility and resistance. These developments lead to airflow turbulence and audible soft tissue vibrations in individuals with anatomically and/or functionally susceptible airways. Complex models have been proposed to describe behavior of the upper airway and they predict the pharynx will begin to vibrate during sleep, given certain gas flow, wall compliance and airway dimensions [7]. Integral to the modeling of snoring is the Bernoulli principle which predicts air moving rapidly through the Venturi tube-like upper airway will create a negative pressure at points of critical narrowing, in effect sucking pharyngeal structures inward during inspiration and/or expiration [10]. Whatever site(s) within the upper airway meet the necessary combination of flow, compliance, and dimensions, may generate snoring, including the uvula, soft palate, pharyngeal walls, tongue, and/or epiglottis [11]. Snoring sites vary between persons and may occur at multiple sites within the same individual. Snoring consists of a complex series of sound packets with a fundamental frequency of approximately 600 Hz with the sound spectrum varying depending on the location(s) of snoring generation and nasal versus oral route of breathing [3].

A variety of upper airway imaging techniques have demonstrated that snorers have differences in upper airway configuration compared to non snorers [12], yet the differences are inconsistent, and often based on evaluations of wake/upright rather than sleeping/supine subjects and with incompletely defined control groups. It is also not clear whether these changes are a cause of snoring or a consequence of vibration-induced upper airway mucosal edema and inflammation.

With narrowing of the upper airway and increased upper airway airflow resistance comes a compensatory increase in respiratory effort to maintain ventilation. Gleeson [13] elegantly demonstrated that increasing ventilatory effort to a critical point appears to be a stimulus to arousal from sleep, independent of the source of the heightened drive to breathe. In UARS, an arousal from sleep is triggered once the individual reaches their unique ventilatory effort threshold before the development of apnea or hypopnea, as demonstrated by the progressively negative esophageal pressure deflections immediately preceding arousals. With arousal comes restoration of upper airway patency and reduction in ventilatory effort.

OSA patients have lesions of upper airway motor and sensory pathways, which likely play a role in disease pathogenesis [14, 15]. UARS patients possess normal palatal sensory input using a two-point discrimination test arguing against a similar underlying sensory deficit [16]. Perhaps the absence of an upper airway sensory lesion allows UARS patients a faster response to upper airway narrowing [17], which may provide insight to an additional explanation for the insomnia and fatigue frequently reported by UARS patients.

Upper airway physiologic studies support the concept that snoring, UARS, and OSA are different points along the same spectrum, with the differences in polysomnographic manifestations attributable to gradations in upper airway collapsibility during sleep. The pharyngeal critical airway pressure (Pcrit, or the airway pressure at the flow-limiting site below which this site collapses) has been shown to progressively increase between normal subjects, snorers, and OSA patients, indicating increasingly collapsible airways between the 3 groups [18, 19]. Gold has also shown that the collapsibility of the upper airways of UARS patients is intermediate between that of normal subjects and those with OSA [20].

Risk Factors

Acquired or anatomic factors that increase upper airway collapsibility and/or decrease upper airway caliber will increase risk for snoring (Table **1**). Body weight is a key determinant of upper airway function and configuration with snoring risk varying proportionally with weight gain. Nasal obstruction can increase snoring propensity by leading to greater subatmospheric inspiratory pressures within the upper airway which promote pharyngeal collapse or increasing mouth breathing. Analysis of the Wisconsin Sleep Cohort revealed an odds ratio of 3 for habitual snoring in subjects with chronic nasal obstruction [21]. Adenotonsillar hypertrophy is an important snoring risk factor in children. A variety of commonly ingested substances, including alcohol, opioid analgesics, sedative/hypnotics, and muscle relaxants threaten the stability of the upper airway during sleep by decreasing pharyngeal dilator muscle tone. Smoking, via irritant-induced upper airway inflammation, nightly nicotine withdrawal, or nasal congestion, increases the relative risk for snoring to 2.29 [22]. Snoring becomes louder and more frequent during pregnancy, especially during the third trimester, likely due to a combination of weight gain, upward diaphragm displacement, and increased upper airway edema. A survey of 350 pregnant women and 110 age-matched non pregnant women revealed frequent snoring reported by 14% of the pregnant women versus 4% of controls [23]. Fortunately, pregnant snorers did not report an increased frequency of deliveries with compromised fetal outcomes. Stage N3 sleep is often marked by the loudest and most steady snoring. Because many of the risks for snoring are dynamic, intra- and inter-night snoring variability is common.

Consequences

Snoring is well known for its social consequences, occasionally forcing bed partners to sleep in separate bedrooms. This may solve the marital problems, but provides challenges when traveling or camping. Snoring alone should not be a cause of excessive daytime sleepiness. Excessive daytime sleepiness in a snorer should raise concern for UARS, OSA, or another sleep disorder. The case series of children [4] and adults [6] with UARS demonstrated sleepiness (with MSLT), which improved with treatment, although fatigue may be more prominent in UARS patients than sleepiness.

Evidence continues to mount that OSA is associated with cardiovascular disease [24]. Whether snoring and UARS have similar links to cardiovascular disease is less clear. Lugaresi reported an association between habitual snoring and hypertension occurrence across adult age groups in a general population survey of > 5000 Italians [25]. A survey of 2,001 adult subjects from 4 Canadian family practice units revealed a two-fold increase in hypertension in men and women who snored between the first and 10th decades compared to non-snorers, even when controlling for smoking and obesity [26]. A questionnaire- and record-based study of > 4,000 Finnish men reported relative risks of 2 for ischemic heart disease and stroke amongst habitual and frequent snorers versus non-snorers, and relationship held after adjustment for age, body mass index (BMI), hypertension history, smoking, and alcohol use [27]. Eight-year follow-up of > 71,000 female nurses in the Nurses Health Study demonstrated a relative risk of cardiovascular disease (coronary heart disease and stroke) of 1.20 for occasional snorers and 1.33 for regular snorers after adjustment for smoking, BMI, and other covariates [28]. Similarly, several other epidemiologic surveys have suggested a link between self-reported snoring and stroke [29, 30]. However, a 6-year prospective study of nearly 3,000 middle-aged to elderly Danish men did not show an increased incidence of ischemic heart disease events after multivariant adjustment of potential confounders [31]. While these studies are impressive as far the large number of included subjects is concerned, they are all plagued by dependence on self-reported snoring and lack of PSG data to exclude confounding by occult OSA.

Table 1: Common predisposing and precipitating factors for upper airway obstruction during sleep:

Obesity
Nasal obstruction
Septal deviation
Turbinate enlargement
Chronic rhinitis
Craniofacial structural abnormalities
Micrognathia
Retrognathia
Midface hypoplasia
Craniofacial soft tissue abnormalities
Macroglossia
Adenotonsillar hypertrophy
Low lying soft palate and elongated uvula
Supine sleep posture
Substance ingestion
Alcohol
Sedative/hypnotics
Opioid analgesics
Benzodiazepines
Muscle relaxants
Smoking
Male gender
Pregnancy
Sleep stage
Sleep deprivation
Genetics

There are studies examining cardiovascular sequelae of snoring that include PSG clarification of OSA status, but the data are mixed as well. Bixler and colleagues evaluated with PSG nearly 2,000 subjects randomly culled from a larger community survey examining the epidemiology of OSA; they found snoring without OSA was independently associated with hypertension with an odds ratio of 1.56 (1.09 - 2.20, p=0.01) [32]. On the contrary, Hoffstein *et al* studied 1,415 patients referred to a sleep center with PSG and found no difference in the prevalence of hypertension between heavy snorers and non-snorers [33]. Furthermore, no significant association was found between snoring and hypertension in the large Sleep Heart Health Study cohort [34]. Marin and colleagues examined outcomes in approximately 1,600 men with a baseline PSG over a 10-year follow up period and found that non-apneic snorers did not have an increased incidence of fatal or non fatal cardiovascular events [35].

Heavy snoring may also increase the risk of carotid atherosclerosis, and the increase seems to be independent of other risk factors, including measures of nocturnal hypoxia and AHI. Considering the high prevalence of snoring in the general population, this may have substantial public health implications for the management of carotid atherosclerosis and the prevention of cerebrovascular disease [36].

It is conceivable that, similar to OSA, cyclic changes in intrathoracic pressure and sleep fragmentation during UARS could lead to hypertension. However, such a link remains under-explored. Lofaso examined 105 non-apneic, middle-aged snorers with home PSG and found that the 55 patients with ≥ 10 arousals per hour had a higher prevalence of hypertension compared to the snorers with < 10 arousals per hour, although these patients were not diagnosed with UARS *per se* because esophageal pressure monitoring was not performed [37]. Continuous blood pressure monitoring during sleep in 7 UARS patients demonstrated increases in both diastolic and systolic blood pressures with arousals and within segments of increased respiratory effort [38]. In the same study, 6 UARS patients had daytime hypertension that responded to 1-month of CPAP treatment.

The link between blood pressure and UARS may be modulated by differences in underlying autonomic nervous system activity in UARS versus OSA. The increase in heart rate at the termination of breathing-related arousals appears to be mediated by a drop in parasympathetic tone in UARS versus an increase in sympathetic tone in OSA [39]. Heightened parasympathetic tone has been postulated to be the explanation why approximately 20% of UARS patients conversely have low blood pressure and orthostatic intolerance [40].

OSA patients have shown impaired reaction time on psychomotor vigilance testing [41]. In a recent study by Stoohs and colleagues, 47 UARS patients were found to have worse psychomotor performance on most test metrics compared to age, BMI, and ESS-matched OSA patients [42]. Whether treatment of UARS will lead to improvement in the psychomotor vigilance testing is not known.

Although snoring, UARS, and OSA can be thought of as different aspects of the same spectrum of upper airway narrowing during sleep, it is not clear whether the development of snoring likely or sequentially leads to UARS and OSA. The repetitive vibratory trauma of snoring can lead to upper airway edema and theoretically to contractile dysfunction of the upper airway dilator muscles, loss of sensitivity due to damage to the mechanoreceptors of the upper airway (thereby affecting the negative pressure upper airway reflex), and decreased vascular reactivity in the pharyngeal structures [43-45]. However, a survey of 10-year follow-up of snoring in men indicated 40% of habitual snorers, mostly men older than 50 years, reported resolution rather than worsening of their snoring [46]. A study of essentially untreated UARS patients followed between 43 and 69 months, which included PSG at baseline and at follow-up in 94 patients, demonstrated no longitudinal change in the group mean apnea-hypopnea index (AHI) and respiratory disturbance index (RDI; apneas, hypopneas, and RERAs per hour), but 5 of the patients met criteria for OSA by an increased AHI at follow-up [47].

Assessment

The assessment of the snorer is based on an appropriately focused history and physical examination supplemented by testing in an effort to understand the patient's (and partner's) goals of the evaluation, define the full extent of the sleep disordered breathing, and establish treatment options (see also Chapter 3).

History

As the snorers are usually not aware of their own symptoms or may downplay their snoring, the history is best obtained in the presence of the bed partner or a family member who has observed the patient while sleeping. When obtaining history from the bed partner, the physician should keep in mind the possibilities that the bed partner may be concerned about the impact of the snoring on their own sleep quality, seeking clarification of their partner's OSA status, or that snoring dissatisfaction is a surrogate concern for more profound relationship issues.

The history should not only elucidate the frequency, intensity, position dependency of the snoring, and risk factors for snoring, but also daytime symptoms suggestive of UARS or OSA, and co-morbidities that may increase the OSA risk (ex. hypothyroidism) or be adversely affected, should OSA be present (ex congestive heart failure).

Snoring and daytime sleepiness are classic, but non-specific manifestations of OSA, so clinical impressions based on patient history have limited accuracy for discerning OSA. In the Wisconsin Sleep Cohort, the rates of snoring in men and women were 10 times greater than rates for symptomatic OSA [1]. The positive predictive value and negative predictive value of snoring for OSA in one series were 0.63 and 0.56, respectively [48]. In the Sleep Heart Health Study, snoring of moderate or habitual severity had an odds ratio of only 1.27-2.87 for identifying patients with an AHI≥15 [49]. Eliciting reports of witnessed apneas, gasping or choking episodes, and snort arousals, may increase the diagnostic accuracy. Snoring is not a prerequisite for UARS. In Guilleminault's 1993 [6] series of 15 UARS adult patients that had been previously diagnosed with idiopathic hypersomnia, 2 patients reported no snoring and 3 reported only occasional, light snoring. The history of excessive daytime sleepiness is also a nonspecific marker for OSA because it is commonly due to chronic partial sleep deprivation which is all too prevalent in our society.

Although patients with UARS have symptoms that overlap with OSA, there are some important differences. UARS patients exhibit symptoms of fatigue and tiredness rather than daytime sleepiness, though this distinction may be challenging. UARS is more common in women, compared to the male predominance in OSA. Sleep onset insomnia, headache, irritable bowel syndrome, bruxism, functional somatic syndromes, orthostatic symptoms such as fainting, dizziness, and cold hands/feet are more common among UARS than OSA patients [50, 51]. UARS patients are typically younger, less overweight, and experience less weight gain in the 5 years prior to diagnosis [52].

Physical Examination

The physical examination is generally focused on the conditions that can compromise upper airway patency, yet the discriminating value of physical findings for OSA and UARS is limited. BMI, neck circumference (> 17 inches in men correlates with OSA [53]), and blood pressure should be noted. Nasal inspection, ideally performed with a nasal speculum, focuses on the turbinates, septum, and upper lateral cartilage (the nasal valve area). The presence of a boggy and erythematous inferior nasal turbinate mucosa, deviated nasal septum, and monitoring for collapse of the lateral nasal cartilage by the Cottle test, should be noted. Cottle test is performed by gently applying pressure in a lateral direction using 1-2 fingers over the cheek. If the breathing improves with the Cottle test, it is considered positive and indicates a collapse of the lateral nasal cartilage.

A classification system, such as the Friedman [54] or Mallampati [55], may help standardize the description of the oropharyngeal findings and aid assessment of OSA risk. Every 1-point increase in the Mallampati score increases the odds of OSA by more than 2-fold [56]. The uvula may appear erythematous and edematous from the vibratory trauma of snoring. Other findings to note include tonsillar enlargement (defined as lateral impingement of >50% of the posterior pharyngeal space), reduced posterior oropharyngeal lateral dimensions (defined as encroachment of greater than 25% of the pharyngeal space by peritonsillar tissues excluding the tonsils), micro or retrognathia, maxillary deficiency, inferior displacement of the hyoid bone and high arched palate. Asymmetric tonsillar size may suggest an underlying neoplasm [57]. Macroglossia is usually due to obesity, but may also be a sign of conditions that increase risk for OSA, such as hypothyroidism, acromegaly, and amyloidosis. Laboratory testing for associated conditions such as hypothyroidism should be performed when clinical features are suggestive.

Sleep Laboratory Investigations

Because of the lack of diagnostic accuracy of the history and physical examination for OSA, clinical prediction models that usually include questions about snoring have been created to help hone clinical suspicion for OSA. To date, no clinical model is accepted as optimal to predict severity of OSA [58] and PSG is required to determine if a snorer also has UARS or OSA. Polysomnography is typically a laboratory-based, technologist-conducted, multimodality recording of sleep and breathing. According to standards issued by the AASM in 2007 [9], both oronasal thermal sensor and nasal pressure transducer should be used during PSG to detect apneas and hypopneas, respectively. Recommended sampling rates and filter settings for recording of snoring are provided, but the manual does not specify other aspects of snoring detection, such as preferred sensor location, gradation of snoring intensity, and reporting of snoring. Unattended home PSG with airflow sensors similar to lab-based PSG may also be performed in adult snorers with a high pretest likelihood of moderate to severe OSA without co-morbid cardiopulmonary or sleep disorders [59]. Current evidence does not support the use of overnight oximetry as a singular technique to rule in or out OSA. Overnight oximetry is also insufficient for RERA detection because these events terminate before significant oxyhemoglobin desaturation occurs.

A challenge for UARS has been a lack of standard syndrome definition. While the general concept of symptomatic arousals from increased upper airway resistance without apneas/hypopneas has been consistent, each of the case series by Guilleminault [4, 5, 6] as well as work by others [60, 61] have used different PSG diagnostic criteria. The AASM PSG scoring manual does specify definitions for RERAs in adults and children (Table **2**). While the manual indicates that esophageal pressure monitoring remains the preferred method for assessing respiratory effort, the rules are consistent with the contemporary appreciation of nasal pressure and inductance plethysmography to detect RERAs, and these sensors are easier for patients and polysomnographic technologists to handle. The manual deems the listing of RERAs on the PSG report as "optional". Please also note that ISCD 2nd edition does not parse out UARS, but defines OSA by 15 or more respiratory events (apneas, hypopneas, *or RERAs*) per hour, or 5 or more such events plus symptoms. For clinicians who prefer to continue to use UARS as a diagnosis, a working definition to consider is the combination of ≥ 10 RERAs per hour, AHI < 5, and daytime symptoms.

Table 2: Rules for respiratory effort-related arousals per the American Academy of Sleep Medicine Manual for the Scoring of Sleep and Associated Events, 2007:

Adults:
Score a respiratory effort-related arousal (RERA):
If there is a sequence of breaths lasting at least 10 seconds characterized by increasing respiratory effort or flattening of the nasal pressure waveform leading to an arousal from sleep when the sequence of breaths does not meet criteria for an apnea or hypopnea
With respect to scoring a RERA, use of esophageal pressure is the preferred method of assessing change in respiratory effort, although nasal pressure and inductance plethysmography can be used
Children *(< 18 years, but specialist can choose to use adult criteria in children ≥ 13 years)*:
Score a respiratory effort-related arousal (RERA) event if the conditions in either 1 or 2 are met:
1. When using a nasal pressure sensor all of the following must be met:
a. There is a discernible fall in the amplitude of signal from a nasal pressure sensor, but it is less than 50% in comparison to the baseline level
b. There is flattening of the nasal pressure waveform
c. The event is accompanied by snoring, noisy breathing, elevation in the end-tidal PCO_2, transcutaneous PCO_2 or visual evidence of increased work of breathing
d. The duration of the event is at least 2 breath cycles (or the duration of 2 breaths as determined by baseline breathing pattern)
2. When using an esophageal pressure sensor all of the following must be met:
a. There is a progressive increase in inspiratory effort during the event.
b. The event is accompanied by snoring, noisy breathing, elevation in the end-tidal PCO_2, transcutaneous PCO_2 or visual evidence of increased work of breathing
c. The duration of the event is at least 2 breath cycles (or the duration of 2 breaths as determined by baseline breathing pattern)

Differential Diagnosis

Similar to the statement saying that not all wheezing is asthma, we can safely state that not all sound produced by the sleeping patient is snoring. Stridor is usually a harsh, high-pitched inspiratory sound that occurs due to laryngeal or tracheal obstruction which may indicate neoplasm, relapsing polychondritis, laryngomalacia, vocal cord dysfunction from recurrent laryngeal nerve paralysis or neurologic disease such as Multiple System Atrophy (MSA). Sleep related laryngospasm is characterized by abrupt awakenings from sleep, associated with total or near-total cessation of airflow for a short time (5-45 seconds), followed by choking or stridor for several minutes and may be associated with tachycardia, intense anxiety, sensation of impending death, and/or residual temporary hoarseness [8]. Catathrenia is characterized by recurrent episodes of expiratory groaning or moaning, lasting 2-49 seconds that occurs predominantly during rapid eye movement (REM) sleep [8]. Wheezing is usually an expiratory sound that occurs due to narrow peripheral airways, as in asthma or chronic obstructive pulmonary disease. Sleep talking involves the production of words and speech that may or may not be comprehensible, and is usually reported by the bed partner or observer as the patient is generally unaware [8].

Treatment

When weighing treatment options for snoring and UARS, several issues must be kept in mind. Many studies of snoring treatments rely on subjective reports of treatment response rather than objective measurements, and the 2 outcomes can be quite discrepant. Other methodologic concerns include lack of randomization of subjects and inclusion of OSA patients in some studies. Studies of non-CPAP treatments for UARS are very limited. Third-party payers in the US may not "cover" treatments for isolated snoring or UARS. Currently, the Centers for Medicare and Medicaid Services do not recognize RERAs or UARS in their policies for positive airway pressure coverage. Some snorers may not want treatment for snoring once OSA is ruled out by appropriate tests. Nonetheless, they should be counseled about the potential impact of their snoring on their bed partner's sleep, advised about the risk factors and symptoms/signs of UARS and OSA, and encouraged to seek reevaluation if such features develop. Once treatment is initiated, appropriate follow up visits and tests are needed to assess outcomes.

Lifestyle Modifications

Lifestyle modifications, such as weight loss, smoking cessation, minimizing the use of agents that decrease the airway muscle tone, and avoiding sleeping supine, help decrease upper airway narrowing during sleep. Although the evidence base for these recommendations is limited, they seem to have face validity, are generally inexpensive, and, in the cases of weight loss, smoking cessation and alcohol moderation, are beneficial for overall health as well.

A study of 123 bariatric surgery patients with an average loss of 48% excess body weight, revealed a drop in habitual snoring from 82% of subjects before surgery to 14% at 1 year post-surgery [62] The negative consequences of alcohol on SDB depend on the timing of alcohol intake, amount ingested, and how fast alcohol is metabolized in that particular subject [63]. It is reasonable to advise snorers to eliminate their alcohol consumption at least 2-4 hours before bedtime.

Snoring is generally worse in the supine position and, therefore, sleeping on the side helps to decrease or eliminate snoring [64]. This can be accomplished with special pillows, a position alarm, or a "T-shirt with tennis balls", a tight-fitting night shirt with a pouch on the back panel containing tennis balls. Approximately 50% of OSA patients instructed to avoid supine position sleep will maintain this restriction [65]. Efficacy of position therapy for snorers is not known.

Nasal-Directed Therapy

Nasal obstruction is well known to be associated with sleep disordered breathing [66]. Approximately 50-60% of upper airway resistance is attributable to the nasal valve area (constituted by the nasal septum, anterior part of the inferior nasal turbinate, and caudal lateral nasal cartilage) contributing predominantly to this increased resistance. The resistance from this region can be increased by allergic, chronic non-allergic, and infectious rhinitis, increased collapsibility of the caudal lateral nasal cartilage, and/or presence of deviated nasal septum (either congenital or acquired- *i.e.* trauma). Allergen avoidance and nasal steroids may truncate snoring in the setting of allergic rhinitis. Nasal steroids, oral sympathomimetics, or intranasal ipratropium are options for the snorer with chronic, nonallergic rhinitis. However, the snoring response to intranasal steroids is not a given, as intranasal steroids helped decrease the AHI in a group of OSA patients with rhinitis, but snoring noise was unchanged [67]. Transient (*i.e.* 2-3 days) use of an intranasal topical decongestant may be helpful for snoring associated with the common cold, but longer term use should be avoided because of risk for increased rhinitis (rhinitis medicamentosa). A limitation of intranasal medications is that they have little effect on anatomic abnormalities.

External and internal nasal dilator devices are available to expand the nasal valve area. The Clinical Practice Review Committee of the AASM reviewed the evidence on these products, and concluded that external nasal dilators applied topically to the nose increase the nasal cross sectional area and may be an option in mild, non-apneic snorers, while internal nasal dilators insert into a nostril may decrease snoring intensity but are difficult to use long-term [68]. To date, there are insufficient data for nasal lubricants [68]. Given the benign nature of these interventions, an empirical trial may be worthwhile.

Oral Appliances

Oral appliances (OA) enlarge the upper airway and/or decrease its collapsibility by advancing the mandible and/or the tongue. A systematic review [69] conducted by the Standards of Practice Committee of the AASM in 2006 found that oral appliances decreased the frequency and intensity of snoring in multiple studies, leading the Committee to conclude that oral appliances were "appropriate for use in patients with snoring who do not respond to or are not appropriate candidates for treatment with behavioral measures such as weight loss or sleep-position change" [58]. A case series of 32 patients with UARS based on an AHI<5, an arousal index >10, and Epworth Sleepiness Scale score (ESS)>10, found OA therapy significantly improved the ESS, mean sleep latency, arousal index, sleep efficiency, and minimum oxygen saturation [70].

Side effects of OAs include excessive salivation, xerostomia, teeth and gum discomfort, temporomandibular joint pain, altered sense of morning occlusion, and mild teeth displacement. Although common, these side effects are usually mild. Contraindications to OAs include active dental disease, inadequate number of teeth to anchor the OA, severe TMJ disorder, and minimal mandibular protrusive range. Proper patient selection and assessment, device fabrication and titration, and monitoring for acute and long term side effects must be done in collaboration with a dentist knowledgeable with sleep disordered breathing.

Surgery

Surgical interventions may seem an attractive alternative for snoring or UARS because of the possibility of a 'quick fix' without the need for nightly use of devices such as OA or CPAP, yet the impact of surgery may be limited by the reality of multiple sites of obstruction in the upper airway. Objective outcome data are limited and can differ from subjective reports. Surgeries must be considered on an individual basis, taking into account upper airway anatomy, outcomes of risk factor modification trials, and patient preference.

Nasal Surgery

Nasal surgeries performed for snoring including nasal septoplasty, turbinectomy, nasal polypectomy, and radiofrequency ablation (RFA) of the inferior nasal turbinates Septoplasty has been shown to decrease nasal resistance (albeit not back to normal compared to controls), but not all patients enjoy snoring relief from surgery [36]. The impact of nasal surgery on UARS is under explored.

Palatal Procedures

Uvulopalatopharyngoplasty (UPPP) involves excision of the uvula, a portion of the soft palate, and tonsils (if present). Subjective success may be 80% or greater, but objective and long-term follow-up data are limited. Predicting UPPP outcome is generally difficult. Fiberoptic nasopharyngoscopy is generally performed when a snorer is being considered for UPPP, yet neither this test, nor advanced upper airway imaging studies can fully determine the anatomic snoring generators or reliably predict response to surgery. The major short-term side effect of UPPP is pain, while long-term side effects include velopharyngeal insufficiency, voice change, and globus sensation.

Laser-assisted uvulopalatoplasty (LAUPP) is an office-based, serial procedure that trims the uvula and adjacent soft palate. Subjective snoring improvement rates are similar to UPPP, reported at around 40-90% at varying follow-up lengths. Postprocedure pain and complications are similar to UPPP. An AASM review paper [71] concluded that the "long-term effectiveness of LAUPP on treatment of snoring has not been convincingly established" and that "LAUPP appears comparable to UPPP in relieving snoring".

Radiofrequency ablation, an outpatient procedure involving application of a radiofrequency signal to the soft palate resulting in soft tissue necrosis followed by tissue volume reduction and stiffening has been reported to produce significant subjective improvements in snoring, less painfully than UPPP or LAUPP [72]. Complications include mucosal ulcerations, palatal sloughing, and fistula formation, and snoring can relapse in up to 41% [73].

The pillar procedure is also an outpatient procedure in which three small braided polyester implants are deployed into the soft palate via a specialized hand piece in an effort to stiffen the palate and prevent palatal vibration and collapse. Subjective snoring improvements have been reported [74, 75], but not corroborated by in-home objective monitoring data [74]. In a 1-year follow-up study, the 41% snoring success rate at 90 days dropped to 22% at 1-year [74]. Partial or complete implant extrusion can occur in approximately 10% of implants, causing pain or a foreign-body sensation.

Different types of upper airway surgery have been performed in UARS patients, though none were controlled or provide long-term follow-up. Adenotonsillectomy improved mean sleep latency in 25 pediatric patients with UARS [4]. A variety of upper airway procedures, all including some type of palatal surgery, in 9 UARS patients resulted in a significant reduction in ESS (mean reduction 12 to 3.4) [76]. LAUPP in 11 UARS patients improved daytime sleepiness (for 82% of them), with a reduction in group mean ESS from 13.5 to 8 [77]. Powell and colleagues [78] evaluated soft palate radiofrequency ablation in mild OSA patients, although 14 probably had UARS, and demonstrated improvement in snoring intensity, sleep efficiency and daytime sleepiness.

CONTINUOUS POSITIVE AIRWAY PRESSURE (CPAP)

CPAP serves as a passive pneumatic splint that prevents the upper airway from narrowing during sleep. Though CPAP will eliminate snoring, non-apneic snorers do not find this device practical and third-party payers in the US generally do not cover CPAP for snoring without OSA.

CPAP decreases sleep fragmentation and improves MSLT scores in UARS [5, 6] however compliance with CPAP is a challenge despite apparent clinical benefit. In a study of 98 non apneic snorers as defined by an AHI<15, Krieger [79] found that only 34% initially accepted CPAP and only 60% of these patients remained compliant after 3 years, with an average nightly CPAP use of 5.6 hours. Rauscher [80] reported lower CPAP compliance in their non apneic snorers, defined by an AHI<5 and at least 20 arousals per hour of sleep. Only 19% of patients initially accepted CPAP with an average nightly CPAP use of 2.8 hours after 6 months.

RESEARCH OUTLOOK

Overall, OSA dominates research activity within the spectrum of sleep disordered breathing. With respect to snoring, there was a recent provocative report [81] which challenges the contemporary notion that snoring alone is not associated with increased cardiovascular risk. Heavy snoring, independent of the apnea-hypopnea index and nocturnal hypoxia, was found to significantly increase the risk of carotid atherosclerosis in a PSG-based study of 110 patients with non-hypoxemic, mild OSA [81]. The authors postulated that exposure to chronic snoring vibrations may cause endothelial damage to the nearby carotid vessels, thereby contributing to the pathogenesis of atherosclerosis. An issue with this study is determining the degree of confounding by concurrent OSA that might not be captured by controlling for the AHI and oxygenation parameters.

To date, Guilleminault and collaborators have been responsible for much of the published research on UARS. One uncertainty is the extent of long-term improvements with CPAP therapy for this syndrome. Perhaps further insight will be provided by the Apnea Positive Pressure Long-term Efficacy Study (APPLES) [58], which is a randomized, double-blind, multicenter study of active versus sham CPAP in OSA. The group will include adults with an RDI ≥ 10 by PSG.

What do we know:

1. Snoring is very common in the general population
2. Snoring is a marker of UARS and OSA.
3. Evidence does not conclusively link snorers without OSA to increased risk for adverse cardiovascular outcomes. Therefore, the primary goal of snoring treatment is to reduce noxious noise and social embarrassment or distress.
4. Risk factors for snoring are well established and are listed in Table **1**.
5. Snoring is treatable by lifestyle modifications, oral appliances, or surgical approaches.
6. Due to frequent nocturnal arousals in response to breathing against increased upper airway resistance, UARS patients present with daytime sleepiness and fatigue which improve with treatment.
7. Treatment options for UARS are similar to those for snoring, and also include CPAP.

What we would like to know:

1. The optimal method to measure and quantify snoring.
2. Does treatment of isolated snoring prevent development of UARS or OSA?
3. Cost-effective strategies to separate simple snorers from snorers with OSA.
4. The extent to which the newly reported observation that snoring may lead to carotid atherosclerosis challenge our understanding of the cardiovascular risks of snoring?

5.   Accurate method(s) to predict outcome of different snoring interventions.

6.   The definition of UARS and whether it is a entity distinct from generic OSA

7.   The cardiovascular consequences of untreated UARS.

REFERENCES

[1]   Young T, Palta M, Dempsey J *et al.* The occurrence of sleep-disordered breathing among middle-aged adults. N Engl J Med 1993; 328: 1230-5.

[2]   Enright PL, Newman AB, Wahl PW *et al.* Prevalence and correlates of snoring and observed apneas in 5,201 older adults. Sleep 1996; 19: 531-8.

[3]   Hoffstein V. Snoring. Chest 1996; 109: 201-22.

[4]   Guilleminault C, Winkle R, Korobkin R, Simmons B. Children and nocturnal snoring: evaluation of the effects of sleep related respiratory resistive load and daytime functioning. Eur J Pediatr 1982; 139: 165-71.

[5]   Guilleminault C, Stoohs R, Duncan S. Snoring (I). Daytime sleepiness in regular heavy snorers. Chest 1991; 99: 40-8.

[6]   Guilleminault C, Stoohs R, Clerk A *et al.* A cause of excessive daytime sleepiness. The upper airway resistance syndrome. Chest 1993; 104: 781-7.

[7]   Huang L, Williams JE. Neuromechanical interaction in human snoring and upper airway obstruction. J Appl Physiol 1999; 86: 1759-63.

[8]   American Academy of Sleep Medicine. International Classification of Sleep Disorders: Diagnostic and Coding Manual. Westchester, IL: American Academy of Sleep Medicine; 2005.

[9]   Iber C, Ancoli-Israel S, Chesson A, Quan SF. The AASM Manual for the Scoring of Sleep and Associated Events: Rules, Terminology and technical specifications. Westchester, Illinois: American Academy of Sleep Medicine; 2007.

[10]   Fajdiga I. Snoring imaging: could Bernoulli explain it all? Chest 2005; 128: 896-901.

[11]   Liistro G, Stanescu DC, Veriter C *et al.* Pattern of snoring in obstructive sleep apnea patients and in heavy snorers. Sleep 1991; 14: 517-25.

[12]   Ayappa I, Rapoport DM. The upper airway in sleep: physiology of the pharynx. Sleep Med Rev 2003; 7: 9-33.

[13]   Gleeson K, Zwillich CW, White DP. The influence of increasing ventilatory effort on arousal from sleep. Am Rev Respir Dis 1990; 142: 295-300.

[14]   Edstrom L, Larsson H, Larsson L. Neurogenic effects on the palatopharyngeal muscle in patients with obstructive sleep apnoea: a muscle biopsy study. J Neurol Neurosurg Psychiatry 1992; 55: 916-20.

[15]   Friberg D, Gazelius B, Hokfelt T, Nordlander B. Abnormal afferent nerve endings in the soft palatal mucosa of sleep apnoics and habitual snorers. Regul Pept 1997; 71: 29-36.

[16]   Guilleminault C, Li K, Chen NH, Poyares D. Two-point palatal discrimination in patients with upper airway resistance syndrome, obstructive sleep apnea syndrome, and normal control subjects. Chest 2002; 122: 866-70.

[17]   Guilleminault C, Do Kim Y, Chowdhuri S *et al.* Sleep and daytime sleepiness in upper airway resistance syndrome compared to obstructive sleep apnoea syndrome. Eur Respir J 2001; 17: 838-47.

[18]   Gleadhill IC, Schwartz AR, Schubert N *et al.* Upper airway collapsibility in snorers and in patients with obstructive hypopnea and apnea. Am Rev Respir Dis 1991; 143: 1300-3.

[19]   Schwartz AR, Smith PL, Wise RA *et al.* Induction of upper airway occlusion in sleeping individuals with subatmospheric nasal pressure. J Appl Physiol 1988; 64: 535-42.

[20]   Gold AR, Marcus CL, Dipalo F, Gold MS. Upper airway collapsibility during sleep in upper airway resistance syndrome. Chest 2002; 121: 1531-40.

[21]   Young T, Finn L, Kim H. Nasal obstruction as a risk factor for sleep-disordered breathing. The University of Wisconsin Sleep and Respiratory Research Group. J Allergy Clin Immunol 1997; 99: S757-62.

[22]   Wetter DW, Young TB, Bidwell TR *et al.* Smoking as a risk factor for sleep-disordered breathing. Arch Intern Med 1994; 154: 2219-24.

[23]   Loube DI, Poceta JS, Morales MC *et al.* Self-reported snoring in pregnancy. Association with fetal outcome. Chest 1996; 109: 885-9.

[24]   Lopez-Jimenez F, Sert Kuniyoshi FH, Gami A, Somers VK. Obstructive sleep apnea: implications for cardiac and vascular disease. Chest 2008; 133: 793-804.

[25]   Lugaresi E, Cirignotta F, Coccagna G, Piana C. Some epidemiological data on snoring and cardiocirculatory disturbances. Sleep 1980; 3: 221-4.

[26]   Norton PG, Dunn EV. Snoring as a risk factor for disease: an epidemiological survey. Br Med J (Clin Res Ed) 1985; 291: 630-2.

[27]   Koskenvuo M, Kaprio J, Telakivi T *et al.* Snoring as a risk factor for ischaemic heart disease and stroke in men. Br Med J (Clin Res Ed) 1987; 294: 16-9.

[28]   Hu FB, Willett WC, Manson JE *et al.* Snoring and risk of cardiovascular disease in women. J Am Coll Cardiol 2000; 35: 308-13.

[29]   Neau JP, Meurice JC, Paquereau J *et al.* Habitual snoring as a risk factor for brain infarction. Acta Neurol Scand 1995; 92: 63-8.

[30]   Palomaki H. Snoring and the risk of ischemic brain infarction. Stroke 1991; 22: 1021-5.

[31]   Jennum P, Hein HO, Suadicani P, Gyntelberg F. Risk of ischemic heart disease in self-reported snorers. A prospective study of 2,937 men aged 54 to 74 years: the Copenhagen Male Study. Chest 1995; 108: 138-42.

[32]   Bixler EO, Vgontzas AN, Lin HM *et al.* Association of hypertension and sleep-disordered breathing. Arch Intern Med 2000; 160: 2289-95.

[33]   Hoffstein V. Blood pressure, snoring, obesity, and nocturnal hypoxaemia. Lancet 1994; 344: 643-5.

[34]   Nieto FJ, Young TB, Lind BK *et al.* Association of sleep-disordered breathing, sleep apnea, and hypertension in a large community-based study. Sleep Heart Health Study. JAMA 2000; 283: 1829-36.

[35]   Marin JM, Carrizo SJ, Vicente E, Agusti AG. Long-term cardiovascular outcomes in men with obstructive sleep apnoea-hypopnoea with or without treatment with continuous positive airway pressure: an observational study. Lancet 2005; 365: 1046-53.

[36]   Koutsourelakis I, Georgoulopoulos G, Perraki E *et al.* Randomised trial of nasal surgery for fixed nasal obstruction in obstructive sleep apnoea. Eur Respir J 2008; 31: 110-7.

[37]   Lofaso F, Coste A, Gilain L *et al.* Sleep fragmentation as a risk factor for hypertension in middle-aged nonapneic snorers. Chest 1996; 109: 896-900.

[38]   Guilleminault C, Stoohs R, Shiomi T *et al.* Upper airway resistance syndrome, nocturnal blood pressure monitoring, and borderline hypertension. Chest 1996; 109: 901-8.

[39]   Guilleminault C, Poyares D, Rosa A, Huang YS. Heart rate variability, sympathetic and vagal balance and EEG arousals in upper airway resistance and mild obstructive sleep apnea syndromes. Sleep Med 2005; 6: 451-7.

[40]   Guilleminault C, Faul JL, Stoohs R. Sleep-disordered breathing and hypotension. Am J Respir Crit Care Med 2001; 164: 1242-7.

[41]   Sforza E, Haba-Rubio J, De Bilbao F *et al.* Performance vigilance task and sleepiness in patients with sleep-disordered breathing. Eur Respir J 2004; 24: 279-85.

[42]   Stoohs RA, Philip P, Andries D *et al.* Reaction time performance in upper airway resistance syndrome versus obstructive sleep apnea syndrome. Sleep Med 2009; 10: 1000-4.

[43]   Boyd JH, Petrof BJ, Hamid Q *et al.* Upper airway muscle inflammation and denervation changes in obstructive sleep apnea. Am J Respir Crit Care Med 2004; 170: 541-6.

[44]   Friberg D, Ansved T, Borg K *et al.* Histological indications of a progressive snorers disease in an upper airway muscle. Am J Respir Crit Care Med 1998; 157: 586-93.

[45]   Friberg D, Gazelius B, Lindblad LE, Nordlander B. Habitual snorers and sleep apnoics have abnormal vascular reactions of the soft palatal mucosa on afferent nerve stimulation. Laryngoscope 1998; 108: 431-6.

[46]   Lindberg E, Taube A, Janson C *et al.* A 10-year follow-up of snoring in men. Chest 1998; 114: 1048-55.

[47]   Guilleminault C, Kirisoglu C, Poyares D *et al.* Upper airway resistance syndrome: a long-term outcome study. J Psychiatr Res 2006; 40: 273-9.

[48]   Deegan PC, McNicholas WT. Predictive value of clinical features for the obstructive sleep apnoea syndrome. Eur Respir J 1996; 9: 117-24.

[49]   Young T, Shahar E, Nieto FJ *et al.* Predictors of sleep-disordered breathing in community-dwelling adults: the Sleep Heart Health Study. Arch Intern Med 2002; 162: 893-900.

[50]   Bao G, Guilleminault C. Upper airway resistance syndrome--one decade later. Curr Opin Pulm Med 2004; 10: 461-7.

[51]   Gold AR, Dipalo F, Gold MS, O'Hearn D. The symptoms and signs of upper airway resistance syndrome: a link to the functional somatic syndromes. Chest 2003; 123: 87-95.

[52]   Stoohs RA, Knaack L, Blum HC *et al.* Differences in clinical features of upper airway resistance syndrome, primary snoring, and obstructive sleep apnea/hypopnea syndrome. Sleep Med 2008; 9: 121-8.

[53]   Schellenberg JB, Maislin G, Schwab RJ. Physical findings and the risk for obstructive sleep apnea. The importance of oropharyngeal structures. Am J Respir Crit Care Med 2000; 162: 740-8.

[54]   Friedman M, Ibrahim H, Bass L. Clinical staging for sleep-disordered breathing. Otolaryngol Head Neck Surg 2002; 127: 13-21.

[55]   Mallampati SR. Clinical sign to predict difficult tracheal intubation (hypothesis). Can Anaesth Soc J 1983; 30: 316-7.

[56]   Nuckton TJ, Glidden DV, Browner WS, Claman DM. Physical examination: Mallampati score as an independent predictor of obstructive sleep apnea. Sleep 2006; 29: 903-8.

[57]   Ramar K. Asymmetric tonsillar enlargement and obstructive sleep apnea. Sleep Med 2008; 9: 209-10.

[58]   Kushida CA, Morgenthaler TI, Littner MR *et al.* Practice parameters for the treatment of snoring and Obstructive Sleep Apnea with oral appliances: an update for 2005. Sleep 2006; 29: 240-3.

[59]   Collop NA, Anderson WM, Boehlecke B *et al.* Clinical guidelines for the use of unattended portable monitors in the diagnosis of obstructive sleep apnea in adult patients. Portable Monitoring Task Force of the American Academy of Sleep Medicine. J Clin Sleep Med 2007; 3: 737-47.

[60]   Lofaso F, Goldenberg F, d'Ortho MP *et al.* Arterial blood pressure response to transient arousals from NREM sleep in nonapneic snorers with sleep fragmentation. Chest 1998; 113: 985-91.

[61]   Rees K, Kingshott RN, Wraith PK, Douglas NJ. Frequency and significance of increased upper airway resistance during sleep. Am J Respir Crit Care Med 2000; 162: 1210-4.

[62]   Dixon JB, Schachter LM, O'Brien PE. Sleep disturbance and obesity: changes following surgically induced weight loss. Arch Intern Med 2001; 161: 102-6.

[63]   Issa FG, Sullivan CE. Alcohol, snoring and sleep apnea. J Neurol Neurosurg Psychiatry 1982; 45: 353-9.

[64]   Nakano H, Ikeda T, Hayashi M *et al.* Effects of body position on snoring in apneic and nonapneic snorers. Sleep 2003; 26: 169-72.

[65]   Cartwright R, Ristanovic R, Diaz F *et al.* A comparative study of treatments for positional sleep apnea. Sleep 1991; 14: 546-52.

[66]   Kohler M, Bloch KE, Stradling JR. The role of the nose in the pathogenesis of obstructive sleep apnoea and snoring. Eur Respir J 2007; 30: 1208-15.

[67]   Kiely JL, Nolan P, McNicholas WT. Intranasal corticosteroid therapy for obstructive sleep apnoea in patients with co-existing rhinitis. Thorax 2004; 59: 50-5.

[68]   Meoli AL, Rosen CL, Kristo D *et al.* Nonprescription treatments of snoring or obstructive sleep apnea: an evaluation of products with limited scientific evidence. Sleep 2003; 26: 619-24.

[69]   Ferguson KA, Cartwright R, Rogers R, Schmidt-Nowara W. Oral appliances for snoring and obstructive sleep apnea: a review. Sleep 2006; 29: 244-62.

[70]   Yoshida K. Oral device therapy for the upper airway resistance syndrome patient. J Prosthet Dent 2002; 87: 427-30.

[71]   Littner M, Kushida CA, Hartse K *et al.* Practice parameters for the use of laser-assisted uvulopalatoplasty: an update for 2000. Sleep 2001; 24: 603-19.

[72]   Stuck BA, Maurer JT, Hein G *et al.* Radiofrequency surgery of the soft palate in the treatment of snoring: a review of the literature. Sleep 2004; 27: 551-5.

[73]   Ayappa I, Norman RG, Krieger AC *et al.* Non-Invasive detection of respiratory effort-related arousals (REras) by a nasal cannula/pressure transducer system. Sleep 2000; 23: 763-71.

[74]   Maurer JT, Hein G, Verse T *et al.* Long-term results of palatal implants for primary snoring. Otolaryngol Head Neck Surg 2005; 133: 573-8.

[75]   Romanow JH, Catalano PJ. Initial U.S. pilot study: palatal implants for the treatment of snoring. Otolaryngol Head Neck Surg 2006; 134: 551-7.

[76]   Newman JP, Clerk AA, Moore M *et al.* Recognition and surgical management of the upper airway resistance syndrome. Laryngoscope 1996; 106: 1089-93.

[77]   Utley DS, Shin EJ, Clerk AA, Terris DJ. A cost-effective and rational surgical approach to patients with snoring, upper airway resistance syndrome, or obstructive sleep apnea syndrome. Laryngoscope 1997; 107: 726-34.

[78]   Powell NB, Riley RW, Troell RJ *et al.* Radiofrequency volumetric tissue reduction of the palate in subjects with sleep-disordered breathing. Chest 1998; 113: 1163-74.

[79]   Krieger J, Kurtz D, Petiau C *et al.* Long-term compliance with CPAP therapy in obstructive sleep apnea patients and in snorers. Sleep 1996; 19: S136-43.

[80]   Rauscher H, Formanek D, Zwick H. Nasal continuous positive airway pressure for nonapneic snoring? Chest 1995; 107: 58-61.

[81]   Lee SA, Amis TC, Byth K *et al.* Heavy snoring as a cause of carotid artery atherosclerosis. Sleep 2008; 31: 1207-13.

CHAPTER 6

Obstructive Sleep Apnea

Arman Qamar, M.D.[1,*], Kavitha S. Kotha, M.D.[2] and Octavian C. Ioachimescu, M.D., Ph.D.[3]

[1]*University of Delhi, Delhi, India;* [2]*Senior Fellow, Division of Pulmonary, Allergy, Critical Care and Sleep Medicine, Department of Medicine, Emory University School of Medicine, USA and* [3]*Assistant Professor of Medicine, Division of Pulmonary, Allergy, Critical Care and Sleep Medicine, Department of Medicine, Emory University School of Medicine, USA*

Abstract: Obstructive sleep apnea (OSA) is a condition characterized by repeated episodes of apnea and hypopnea (partial apnea) during sleep. Characteristic symptoms include loud snoring, witnessed apneas, gasping and choking sensations at night, nocturnal awakenings resulting in poor sleep quality, fragmented sleep and excessive daytime sleepiness. Polysomnography is the "gold standard" test for the diagnosis of OSA. The number of apneas and hypopneas per hour of sleep (apnea-hypopnea index, AHI) is the metric most commonly used to determine the severity of OSA. AHI between 5 and 14 represents mild OSA, between 15 and 29 moderate OSA and 30 or higher is severe OSA. Continuous Positive Airway Pressure (CPAP) is the preferred option for the treatment of moderate to severe OSA and optional for mild OSA.

TOPIC DISCUSSION (CLINICAL OUTLOOK)

Introduction

This chapter will review the most salient features of obstructive sleep apnea of the adult; for pediatric aspects of this disease, see Chapter 20, Pediatric Sleep Issues.

Obstructive sleep apnea (OSA) is a condition characterized by repeated episodes of complete or partial cessation of airflow due to upper airway obstruction during sleep [1], *i.e.*, apnea and hypopnea, respectively. OSA associated with excessive daytime sleepiness (EDS) is called obstructive sleep apnea hypopnea *syndrome* (OSAHS) or obstructive sleep apnea *syndrome* (OSAS).

Over the years, the American Academy of Sleep Medicine (AASM) has published multiple sets of Practice Parameters, which list the evidence-based recommendations for different aspects, tests and methodologies used in the diagnosis and management of sleep conditions. Given that these Parameters do not always provide comprehensive reviews of these different topics, in 2007, the Board of Directors of AASM created an Adult Obstructive Sleep Apnea Task Force, charged to review available evidence and to assembly a set of clinical guidelines for evaluation, management and follow-up of these patients. As such, the Clinical Guidelines for the Evaluation, Management and Long-Term Care of Obstructive Sleep Apnea in Adults was published in 2009 [2] in order to better assist primary care physicians, sleep specialists, dentists and surgeons who take care of OSA patients. The levels of recommendation were listed as *Standard*, *Guideline* or *Option*; whenever available, we will list the strength of recommendations for each component of diagnosis and therapy, in the light of this 2009 document.

Review of the literature shows that OSA was recognized as early as 1850s by English physicians. Londonese physician WH Broadbent is credited with the first publication describing obstructive apneas (in fact both obstructive and central apneas) [3-5]. Apneas were very eloquently described in the following fashion:

> *"When a person, especially advanced in years, is lying on his back in heavy sleep and snoring loudly, it very commonly happens that every now and then the inspiration fails to overcome the resistance in the pharynx of which stertor or snoring is the audible sign, and there will be perfect silence through two, three, or four respiratory periods, in which there are ineffectual chest movements; finally, air enters with a loud snort, after which there are several compensatory deep inspirations before the breathing settles down to its usual rhythm" [4].*

[*]**Address correspondence to Arman Qamar:** University of Delhi, Delhi, India; E-mail: armanqamar@gmail.com

Descriptions of periodic breathing (Hunter-Cheyne Stokes respiration) existed even before that [4,6,7]. However, awareness of this condition outside of Sleep Medicine was slow to develop and has evolved in association with the rapid growth of our knowledge about sleep itself.

Epidemiology *(see also Chapter 2, Epidemiology of Sleep Disorders):*

Understanding disease prevalence, that is, the proportion of a population with the condition, is critical to anticipating health care needs and allocating appropriate resources. In addition, comparison of prevalence by demographic factors may yield etiological clues and identify subgroups at particularly high risk for targeted case finding (the essence of screening).

Population-based studies show that up to 5% of adults in western countries are likely to have undiagnosed OSA syndrome [8,9]. However, this does not take into account the large proportion of adults with OSA who do not report sleepiness. This is an area of controversy and the public health significance remains to be determined; however, many studies have shown adverse health outcomes to be associated with OSA, regardless of the presence of sleepiness. Nevertheless, some studies may have underestimated the true prevalence of the disease (*e.g.*, Stradling's study using pulse oximetry and more than 5 desaturations per hour, of more than 4% [10]), while at the other end of the spectrum others may have overestimated it (*e.g.*, including breathholds during wakefulness and/or central apneas during sleep [11]). While the prevalence estimates from different studies done in different countries range between 3-28% for mild OSA and 1-14% for moderate severity, the prevalence estimates with similar design and methodology (Wisconsin, Pennsylvania, Spain, etc) show that roughly 1 of every 5 adults has at least mild OSA and 1 of every 15 has at least moderate OSA [8,9,12-19]. Sleep apnea occurs throughout the human lifespan, from neonatal period until latest decades of life. In adults, there is good evidence that sleep disordered breathing increases in prevalence with age and that it does not correlate well with the presence of daytime [13,14,16,20,21].

While there is good prevalence data from western countries, little is known about incidence, *i.e.*, the occurrence of new cases over a given time interval. A few population studies have looked at OSA progression and focused on changes in apnea hypopnea index (AHI) over time rather than on incidence. Follow up data from Wisconsin Sleep Cohort study showed a significant increase in OSA severity (AHI almost doubled) over an eight-year time interval. Progression was significantly greater in obese, habitual snorers compared to their counterparts. The four-year preliminary data from the same study showed that a 10% increase in weight was associated with 32% increase in AHI and 6-fold risk of developing moderate to severe OSA. Ten percent decrease in weight was associated with a 26% decrease in AHI [9,12]. Cleveland Family Study also showed similar trends [9,22]. However, both studies do not provide insight into disease progression beyond age 65. For this age category, long-term follow-up (18 years) of sleep disordered breathing in older adults showed little change in AHI with aging [9,22].

OSA is even more common in several patient populations, such as those of individuals with known history of hypertension, congestive heart failure, coronary artery disease, stroke, *etc.* As such, about a third of all hypertensive patients seem to have OSA. In a case-control study published in 1998 [23], 38% of the 34 untreated and 38% of the 34 treated people with hypertension had OSA (AHI ≥ 5), versus 4% of the 25 normotensive controls; this relationship stood as significant even after adjusting for age, gender and BMI. In a Canadian study on 41 late-middle-aged patients with drug-resistant hypertension, the prevalence of OSA seemed to be even greater, at 80%; OSA was more prevalent in men than in women (96 versus 65%, p = 0.014) [24].

Additional data suggest that OSA may contribute to the development of hypertension independent of obesity, diabetes, metabolic syndrome or other comobidities. In an analysis of the Wisconsin Sleep Cohort study [25], even mild OSA was associated with a 42% (95% CI: 13%, 78%) increased risk of developing hypertension over a 4-year period. The odds ratio for moderate to severe disease versus those without OSA was 2.9 (95% CI: 1.5, 5.6).

Patients with coronary artery disease (CAD) also seem to have disproportionately high prevalence of OSA. As such, in 1996, Andreas *et al* [26] found OSA (defined as AHI ≥ 10) in 25 of 50 patients with CAD diagnosed by coronary angiography (50% prevalence). Furthermore, among the 6,424 participants in the Sleep Heart Health Study [27], mild to moderate SDB was highly prevalent in the sample (median AHI: 4.4; 25%-75% interquartile range: 1.3-11). A total of 1,023 participants (16%) reported at least one manifestation of cardiovascular disease (myocardial infarction, angina, coronary revascularization, heart failure, or stroke). The multivariate-adjusted relative odds of prevalent cardiovascular disease for the second, third, and fourth quartiles of the AHI (versus the first) were 0.98 (95%CI: 0.7, 1.2; NS), 1.28 (95%CI: 1.01, 1.6), and 1.42 (95%CI: 1.1, 1.7), respectively. SDB was associated more strongly with self-reported heart failure and stroke than with self-reported CAD. The relative odds of heart failure, stroke, and CAD (upper versus lower AHI quartile) were 2.38 (95%CI: 1.2, 4.6), 1.58 (95%CI: 1.02, 2.4), and 1.2 (95%CI: 0.99, 1.6; NS), respectively.

Risk Factors

Despite the fact that OSA has been recognized as a distinct medical condition for many years and data have accumulated with respect to its morbid implications, even today, 70-80% of those affected with OSA remain undiagnosed [28,29]. This is probably due to a lack of awareness in both patients and health care professionals. Some of the important risk factors are discussed below.

Age *(see also Chapter 15, Sleep and Aging)*:

Epidemiological studies have demonstrated an increased number of respiratory events during sleep in elderly subjects, regardless of the methodology, population sample, country of origin and diagnostic criteria used. Remarkably, in individuals over the age 65 years, and asking about 5 frequent sleep complaints (trouble falling asleep, waking up, awaking too early, needing to nap and not feeling rested), the National Institute on Aging's multicentric study entitled "Established Populations for Epidemiologic Studies of the Elderly" (EPESE) showed that more than 50% of these individuals has at least one chronic sleep complaint [30]. Furthermore, the prevalence of SDB ranges from 30-40% in the age group above 65 years, compared to 2-4% in middle-aged adults. In an earlier study, Sonia Ancoli-Israel and collaborators [31] showed that 70% of men and 56% of women between ages of 65 and 99 years have OSA (when defined as AHI ≥ 10). Using the young individuals (20-44 year-old) as controls, the Pennsylvania study investigators found that, for subjects between 65 and 100 years of age, the OR to have SDB (as defined by AHI ≥ 10) was 6.6 (95% CI: 2.6-16.7) [13,14]. Male to female discrepancy also seems to disappears after menopause [32]. Central sleep apnea (CSA) associated with Cheyne-Stokes respiration (CSR) is also common in the elderly, but is out of the scope of this chapter and is usually a consequence of heart failure, stroke or renal failure (for further details, see Chapter 7, Central Sleep Apnea).

With advancing age, sleep is more fragmented with a greater percentage of total sleep time spent in stages N1 and N2 (stages vulnerable for the development of respiratory instability), characterized by periodic breathing and central apneas. Ventilatory control instability seems also to contribute to the pathogenesis of obstructive respiratory events. There seems to be no specific pathophysiological mechanism responsible for the disorder in older subjects compared with middle aged adults, but rather an augmentation of the role played by the well-established causes of SDB.

Obesity

Obesity, particularly central (abdominal) obesity, is a major risk factor for OSA (see also Chapter 18, Sleep and Metabolic Syndrome). Obesity and overweight are becoming significantly more common in the modern world, particularly in the western society [33,34]. There have been many cross-sectional [35-43] and population-based [8,10,15,44-49] studies that reported a strong relationship between obesity and OSA.

The increased risk may be due to obesity-related changes in the upper airway (*i.e.*, fat and/or muscle mass around the collapsible portion of the upper airway, unbalancing the physical forces that keep it open), reductions in functional residual capacity (FRC) and/or vital capacity (with subsequent loss of the "tracheal tug") [50] or to an imbalance between the mechanical load and ventilator drive, as discussed earlier.

In the Wisconsin Sleep Cohort study, which was a population-based prospective study of 602 middle aged adults, investigators found that increments of one standard deviation magnitude in BMI was associated with a 4-fold increase in OSA prevalence [8].

Since obesity is a very important risk factor for OSA, it is not surprising to see very high prevalence of OSA in preoperative bariatric surgery patients. Indeed, available data have shown prevalence rates in this population between 71% and 77% [51-53].

Gender

Between 3 and 4% of females and 6 to 9% of males have OSA, when defined as an AHI of at least 5 and co-existent EDS or a cardiovascular disorder (*e.g.*, hypertension) [54]. While some of the gender differences may be in fact age-related, there is an independent signal regarding a specific predisposition to SDB for males, at least during the ages of 40 to 55 years, while during adolescence and after the age of 50 (or 55), the gender differences seem to be absent [11,54,55].

Overall and at least during adulthood, men seem to have greater vulnerability than women towards developing OSA. The differences may be related to the upper airway structure, with greater fat deposition in the lateral pharyngeal wall in men compared to women, and greater pharyngeal dilator activity in women compared to men. Clinic-based studies show a men to women prevalence ratio of 5-8:1, while epidemiologic studies report a lower range of 2-3:1. These differences may be due to distinct symptom profiles such as snoring in men and fatigue and lack of energy in women and lower threshold for symptom perception and reporting amongst female bed partners of male patients compared to male partners of female patients. Also, it is possible that health care providers have a lower index of suspicion in women than men for OSA.

Hormonal influences likely have an important role in pathogenesis of OSA, as disease prevalence is higher in postmenopausal compared to premenopausal women, while hormonal therapy has been associated with lower prevalence of OSA in epidemiologic studies. In the Wisconsin Sleep Cohort study, post-menopausal women had three times the odds of having moderate or severe OSA compared with premenopausal women, independent of age, BMI and other potential confounding factors. In a Pennsylvania population cohort, there was a 4-fold greater risk of OSA in postmenopausal women not using hormonal therapy versus premenopausal women. While Sleep Heart Health Study showed an association between hormonal therapy and OSA, other studies have found only a weak association.

Familial Aggregation

Although this association may reflect risk factors related to shared lifestyle, there are several studies suggesting a genetic predisposition to snoring and OSA, with a global relative risk factor between 3 and 5, and higher values if both parents are affected [56-62]. The heritability of the AHI has been found to be 30% to 35% in several studies [60,63,64], suggesting one third of the variance is explained by familial factors; approximately 40% of the AHI variance can be explained by obesity, while the rest of the variance can be attributed to genetic and obesity-independent factors [65]. Among anthropometric factors, craniofacial shape and size of the bones and the soft tissues represent another way by which genes may influence predisposition to OSA [66]. Overall, it seems quite clear nowadays that SDB is not the result of one single genetic mutation and the relatively small contribution of the genetic factors may be an acceptable basis for not screening asymptomatic relatives of patients with OSA.

Nevertheless, genetics may explain some ethnic differences in OSA epidemiology [62]. Overall, African Americans and Asians appear to be at higher risk for OSA at a given BMI. A higher prevalence and greater severity of OSA was found in a non-obese Asian population sample versus Caucasian individuals [32]. As such, cephalometric measurements in Asian and Caucasian patients with OSA showed that Asians had a narrower cranial base angle, an anthropometric dimension which may signal a propensity to develop SDB; of note, the disease severity was similar in both groups, although the BMI was higher in Caucasians (30 versus 26) [67]. A more recent study showed that Asians had higher Mallampati grade, smaller thyro-mental distance, and steeper thyromental plane than Caucasian patients, after controlling for BMI and neck circumference [68]. Similarly, some studies have reported a higher prevalence in African American men younger than 35 versus similar-age Caucasians [32,69].

One of the challenges in identifying a relationship between SDB and genetic predisposition is the time factor (*i.e.*, at what age did the disease start) and this has not always been accounted for in epidemiological studies.

Smoking

In the Wisconsin Sleep Cohort study, compared with never smokers, current smokers had a significantly greater risk of snoring (OR 2.3) and of moderate or severe OSA (OR 4.4). Heavy smokers (≥ 40 cigarettes/day) had the greatest risk of mild SDB (OR 6.7) and of moderate or severe OSA (OR 40.5) [70]. Former smoking was not found to be related to snoring and SDB after adjustment for confounders. Hypothesized mechanisms for the role of smoking in

OSA include airway inflammation, smoking related disease as well as effects of declining blood nicotine levels on sleep stability. Furthermore, smoking adds to the cardiovascular risk posed by SDB, complicating even further the issue of cardiovascular morbidity attributable to OSA [71].

Alcohol

Alcohol has a relaxing action, at least on some of the upper airway dilator muscles, thus increasing upper airway resistance; during sleep, this action can lead to OSA in chronic snorers and even in healthy people [72]. It has been shown that ethanol increases the duration and frequency of obstructive respiratory events in patients with OSA [73,74]. Nevertheless, OSA seems to be as common among past alcoholic subjects as among non-alcoholic individuals [75].

Nasal Congestion

In the Wisconsin Sleep Cohort [76], the odds ratio (OR) for polysomnographically identified OSA with chronic versus no nighttime nasal congestion was 1.8. Similar effect size (2-fold increased risk) has been noted in Busselton Health Study [77]. Furthermore, patients with seasonal or allergic rhinitis have been found to have higher AHIs when symptomatic compared to symptom-free periods of time, supporting a role for nasal congestion in OSA [78].

The effect of nasal congestion is probably related to an increase in upper airway resistance to airflow, more negative upper airway pressure produced by inspiratory efforts against a partially closed nasal airway, nasal valve collapsibility, turbulent airflow, nasal reflexes, and snoring causing damage and edema to the upper airway soft tissues [79,80].

Other Risk Factors

A number of conditions have been identified as additional, albeit less important risk factors for OSA. These include endocrine conditions such as polycystic ovary syndrome (PCOS) [81,82], use of exogenous testosterone [83,84], hypothyroidism [85,86] and acromegaly [86-89] (in the case of the latter two conditions, by increasing the amount and density of the soft tissue in the upper airway and through effects on respiratory centers). In the Spanish Acromegaly Registry, out of 1219 patients, 13% were reported to have OSA [89], although significant diagnostic (or lack of ~) bias may exist in this type of retrospective analysis. No large, prospective randomized, trials have been conducted to evaluate specifically the risks and the natural history of these clinical conditions or scenarios with respect to OSA.

Attributed Morbidity

Overall, it is now well known that OSA poses a number of morbid risks, from increased perioperative morbidity [90,91], to hypertension [25], coronary artery disease [92,93], arrhythmias and sudden cardiac death [94], stroke [95,96], pulmonary hypertension [97], deep vein thrombosis [98], *etc.*

Metabolic syndrome is characterized by obesity, hypertension, insulin resistance, hyperlipidemia and oxidative stress. Overall, metabolic syndrome is recognized as an important contributor to the development of atherosclerosis and cardiovascular disease. In the last decades, there has been a growing body of evidence suggesting that OSA is pathogenically linked to altered glucose metabolism. Some investigators have proposed that recurrent hypoxemia and increased sympathetic activity, which are commonly observed in patients with OSA, lead to impaired glucose homeostasis by enhancing glycogen breakdown and gluconeogenesis [99]. OSA has been associated with the metabolic syndrome in many studies and is thought to contribute to and/or modulate the severity of some of the associated metabolic abnormalities (see also Chapter 18, Sleep and Metabolic Syndrome). Data from the Sleep Heart Health Study [100] indicated that the prevalence of abnormal 2-hour glucose tolerance test increased from 9.3% among patients with an AHI <5 to 15% among those with an AHI >15 (OR-1.44). The results also indicated greater insulin resistance among the latter group.

Marin *et al* [101] found that untreated, severe OSA is a significant risk factor for the development of nonfatal myocardial infarction and stroke (odds ratio, OR of 3.17) compared to healthy participants. The authors of Sleep Heart Health Study [102], which is a large, pooled multi-center study, found that the odds ratio for developing hypertension was 1.37 in patients with severe OSA compared to participants without OSA, even after controlling for confounders such as body mass index (BMI), age, alcohol consumption and smoking status. The Wisconsin Sleep Cohort study [103], after only four years of follow up, also found a dose response relationship between the severity of OSA and the presence of hypertension

(OR 2.03 for an AHI 5-15 and 2.89 for an AHI>15). For more details about these relationships, strengths of association and pathogenic implications, see also Chapter 17, Sleep Apnea and Cardiovascular Disorders.

In other studies, OSA has emerged as an independent risk factor for cerebrovascular disease independent of its association with hypertension, age or other known cardiovascular risk factors [96] (see also Chapter 19, Sleep Apnea and Cerebrovascular Disorders). The mechanisms involved in this relation are most likely related to periodic hypoxia/reoxygenation that characteristically occur in OSA, which lead to oxidative stress, endothelial dysfunction and activation of the inflammatory cascade, all of which favoring the development of atherogenesis.

Numerous other prospective and cross-sectional studies have also linked SDB to depression and diminished quality of life [9,104]. On the other hand, SDB-caused sleepiness leads to significant morbidity and mortality on the roads and in the work place. As such, excessive daytime sleepiness has been shown to be a risk factor for motor vehicle crushes [105,106], occupational accidents [105,107] and for impaired cognitive function [108].

Attributed Mortality

Most of the earlier publications linking sleep disordered breathing (SDB) and an increase in mortality have been studies on clinic patient samples; this fact raises a concern for potential referral bias. However, this concern is at least partially counter-balanced by the evidence from two large population-based studies, one from USA and one from Australia.

The Australian study included residents from a small town of Busselton [77], who underwent investigation with a home sleep apnea monitoring device (MESAM IV). Mortality was determined after a mean follow up of 13.4 years and the data was analyzed for a total of 380 participants. Analysis was done after adjustment for age, gender, body mass index (BMI), mean arterial pressure (MAP), total cholesterol, high density lipoprotein (HDL), diabetes and angina. Patients with history of myocardial infarction and stroke were excluded from the study. The investigators found that mild sleep apnea was not an independent risk factor for higher mortality, but moderate to severe sleep apnea was independently associated with greater risk of all cause mortality (hazard ratio, HR = 6.24) compared to non-OSA participants.

Similarly, in the Wisconsin Sleep Cohort (n=1,522) after 18-year follow-up, Young *et al* [109] found that all-cause mortality, after adjustment for age, gender, BMI and other factors, was significantly increased with sleep disordered breathing (SDB) severity. Hazard ratio was 3.0 for participants with severe SDB compared to no SDB.

These two studies found either no or negligible association between mild sleep apnea and mortality. However, mild OSA may have a greater public health significance than moderate-severe OSA, because it is far more common and to determine with certainty this association (*i.e.*, to overcome the dilution of a possible smaller effect), further investigation, in larger cohorts, may be needed.

Symptoms, Signs and Physical Findings

History

The presence of OSA is often initially suspected on the basis of the daytime experience of the patient and the night time experience of the bed partner. Characteristic symptoms include loud snoring, witnessed apneas, gasping or choking at night, nocturnal awakenings resulting in poor sleep quality and excessive daytime sleepiness. In women, fatigue may be a more common symptom. Moodiness, lack of concentration, problems with memory, morning headaches are other common symptoms [110].

Sleepiness, although difficult to define [111], is a symptom that is frequently encountered in patients with sleep apnea. Perhaps one of the best descriptions of sleepiness is as a propensity or tendency to fall asleep during the daytime or activity time of the rest-activity cycle. A useful classification of sleepiness takes into account the time dimension and differentiates between *occasional* sleepiness versus *persistent*, habitual or chronic sleepiness. Whether sleepiness is *physiological* (due to circadian and/or homeostatic pressure) or *pathological* (an expression of sleep disturbances), it is often more difficult to ascertain. The spectrum of clinical descriptions includes several axes:

- Objective:

  o Behavioral – observed yawning, dozing off, inattention, lack of concentration, *etc.*

  o Functional – by assessing activity levels (using accelerometers or actigraphs), performance tests (driving simulators, psychomotor vigilance tests), polygraphic (polysomnography; oligosomnography or limited-channel sleep testing, portable testing; maintenance of wakefulness test, MWT; multiple sleep latency test, MSLT; pupillometry; cerebral evoked potentials, etc)

- Subjective: sleepiness self-assessed on different scales (*e.g.*, at a particular point in time as Stanford Sleepiness Scale, SSS; or pooled over an interval of time, such as Epworth Sleepiness Scale, ESS). Epworth sleepiness scale (ESS) is a validated tool for quantifying excessive daytime sleepiness, which is mainly a subjective measure [112]. A recent analysis of the performance of various parameters in diagnosing SDB [113] has shown that ESS has, unfortunately, an unacceptably high false negative rate (0.71), which may limit its value in screening for sleep apnea (at least in isolation).

Snoring, while associated with a higher prevalence of OSA, has a positive and negative predictive value of only 63% and 56%, respectively.

Witnessed apneas, similarly to hypersomnia, has positive and negative predictive values in the range of 40-60%.

Furthermore, Berlin Questionnaire [114], which is a widely used, integrated questionnaire devised to asses for presence of sleep apnea, has false negative rates up to 38.2% [113], which makes it also an imperfect tool for screening. Nevertheless, in an in-depth analysis of the diagnostic odds ratios (ORs) derived from different studies, Berlin Questionnaire seems to have the highest ORs, while ESS seems to have the lowest, at least in perioperative assessment for SDB.

Nocturia and enuresis generally suggest benign prostatic hypertrophy (BPH) in men and overactive bladder or urinary incontinence in women, but are also common symptoms in elderly individuals with OSA, and generally are reversible (at least partially) with effective treatment.

Dementia and SDB can coexist; cognitive impairment caused by sleep fragmentation and intermittent hypoxia can be misinterpreted as early sign of dementia in elderly subjects. Nocturia, sleepiness and inattention can all increase the risk of accidental falls, particularly in this patient population.

Physical Examination

The most typical patients with OSA are obese males between 40 and 60 years of age [8], although this disorder is common at other ages and in both genders. Most patients are obese (BMI $\geq$ 30 kg/m^2), but not all; obesity is also one of the factors that, upon multiple component analysis, became an important part of the Berlin Questionnaire [114]. Not uncommonly, the OSA patients may have a relatively normal physical examination, except obesity or overweight status, presence of hypertension and the oropharyngeal examination. They typically have a "crowded" oropharyngeal airway [2]. The odds ratio of having OSA increases by 2.5 for every one unit increase in the Mallampati score [115]. Narrow oropharyngeal aperture may be the consequence of retrognathia or micrognathia, macroglossia, enlarged, edematous uvula and soft palate, posterior pharyngeal mucosal edema and "cobblestoned" appearance, adeno-tonsillar lymphoid tissue hypertrophy (especially in children), "kissing" tonsils, high arched palate *etc.* A neck circumference of more than 17 inches in men (43 cm) and 15 inches in women (38 cm) has been associated with an increased risk of OSA [2,116,117]. Some patients may have pulmonary arterial hypertension, but only if OSA co-exists with a condition which leads to daytime hypoxia, such as: hypoventilation (obesity hypoventilation syndrome), parenchymal lung disorders or a cardiovascular condition leading to pulmonary edema.

Diagnosis

The use of home-based nocturnal oximetry alone as a screening tool for OSA has a sensitivity of only about 31% and can lead to significant underestimation of OSA prevalence [10] and/or severity [118]. Derived from pulse oximetry data, the number of oxygen desaturations per hour (oxygen desaturation index, ODI) can be used as a surrogate metric of SDB severity stratification.

Clinical impression or symptom-based diagnosis alone lacks the necessary diagnostic accuracy for the disorder, therefore objective testing by polysomnography is still required in most cases. For more details about different sleep testing technologies and methodologies, see Chapter 4, Sleep Testing and Monitoring.

Polysomnography (PSG)

Polysomnography (PSG) is the gold standard test for the diagnosis of OSA [119]. It is also called type I polysomnographic testing when it is performed in the laboratory, with sleep technologist in attendance throughout the duration of the study. The signals collected during this test are classified into three groups: those related to recognizing sleep (electroencephalogram or EEG, electrooculogram or EOG, submental and extremity electromyogram or EMG), those related to cardiac monitoring (ECG) and those related to respiration (airflow, thoracoabdominal effort, oximetry, capnography, and/or intercostal muscle EMG). Airflow can be monitored either by an oronasal thermistor, nasal pressure transducer system, or inferred from respiratory inductive plethysmography (RIP). For a graphic depiction of the main respiratory events according to AAM definitions, see Fig. **1**.

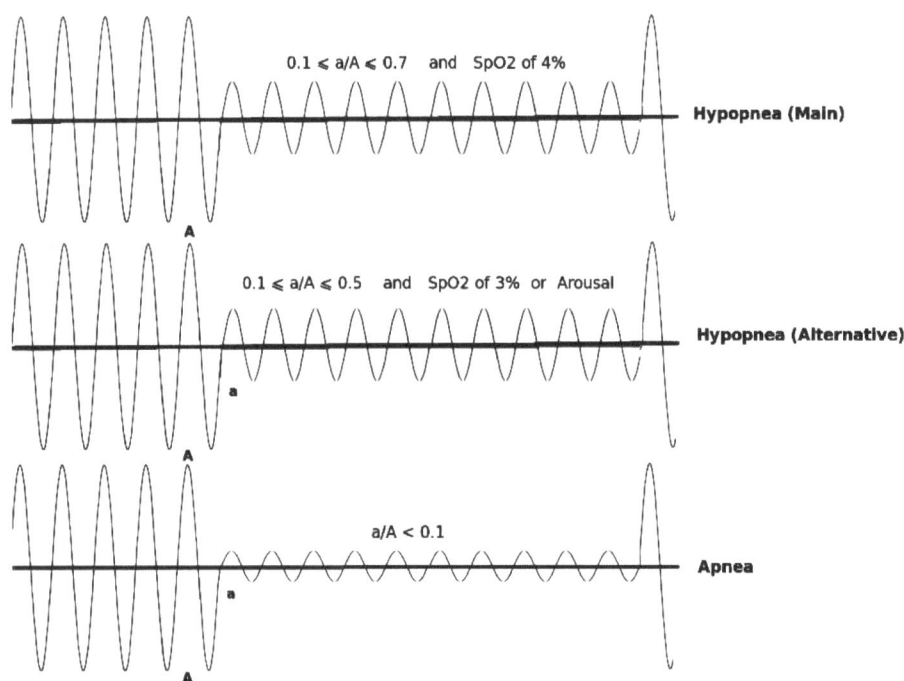

Figure 1: Graphic depiction of the respiratory events (apnea and hyponea), per American Academy of Sleep Medicine (AASM) definitions [120].

By convention, an apnea is characterized by cessation of airflow, *i.e.*, residual flow of less than 10% from baseline flow, for at least 10 seconds in duration (and for at least 90% of the event's duration) [120].

There are currently two definitions for hypopnea [120]:

- The *CMS* definition or the *recommended* AASM definition for hypopnea is as follows: a respiratory event of at least 10 seconds in duration, with reduction in flow for at least 90% of the event's duration, leading to residual flow between 10% and **70%** from baseline flow amplitude either on the thoraco-abdominal effort channels or on the flow channels (preferably, nasal pressure transducer) *and* with an oxygen desaturation of **4%** or more from pre-event baseline.

- The *alternative* definition is a respiratory event of at least 10 seconds in duration, with reduction in flow for at least 90% of the event's duration, leading to residual flow between 10% and **50%** from baseline flow amplitude either on the thoraco-abdominal effort channels or flow channels (preferably, nasal pressure transducer) *and* with an oxygen desaturation of **3%** or more from pre-event baseline *or* post-event **arousal**.

A respiratory effort related arousal (RERA) is defined as a sequence of breaths lasting at least 10 seconds, characterized by increasing respiratory effort or flattening of the nasal pressure waveform leading to an arousal from sleep, as shown by progressively more negative esophageal pressure preceding the arousal and subsequent resumption of normal pressures [120]. RERAs are primarily used to identify patients who may have upper airway resistance syndrome (UARS).

Apneas and hypopneas are considered obstructive if there is evidence of respiratory effort, central if there is no effort and mixed if a respiratory event has both obstructive and central features (the first being the central component).

The number of apneas and hypopneas per hour of sleep (apnea-hypopnea index, AHI, events per hour) is the most commonly used index for severity stratification of OSA. AHI of 5-14/hour indicates mild OSA, 15-29/hour moderate OSA and ≥ 30 severe OSA. Current Medicare criteria require an AHI ≥ 15/hour or an AHI ≥ 5 *with* documented symptoms of excessive daytime sleepiness (EDS), impaired cognition, mood disorders, insomnia, or documented hypertension, ischemic heart disease, or stroke to qualify for treatment with continuous positive airway pressure (CPAP). If RERAs are added to the total number of apneas and hypopneas and divided by total sleep time, the metric resulting from this calculation is called respiratory distress index (RDI). RDI can be used for severity gradation of OSA similarly to the AHI (with the same thresholds). The implications of using RDI versus AHI are relatively straight forward, *i.e.*, AHI may underestimate the OSA severity, or RDI may lead to an overestimation of OSA severity, especially in the absence of esophageal pressure monitoring. Until further data emerge, the current AASM recommendations pertaining to which metric to choose between the above severity indices are to adhere to the recommended definitions and criteria and to maintain consistency throughout scoring and interpretation by reporting the severity linked to the same metric at all times.

Other Sleep Testing Procedures

Oligosomnography (OSG)

Since polysomnography is laborious, time consuming (including time constraints, potential backlogs, etc) and costly, sleep medicine providers started to explore cheaper, easier and less complex diagnostic modalities in the field of sleep testing. A myriad of devices appeared on the market and a significant body of literature reporting about their use in different clinical scenarios. In the face of this mounting literature, the AASM started to monitor on a regular basis the quality of these data and explore the impact and potential changes to the diagnostic decisions that can be made based on the available evidence.

In December 2007, an AASM Task Force published specific guidelines on the use of portable monitoring (PM) for the diagnosis of OSA in adults. These guidelines recommended that PMs can be used in the context of a comprehensive sleep evaluation when supervised by a sleep specialist in an accredited sleep center, utilizing appropriate equipment, technologies and quality control programs [121]. In March 2008, the Center for Medicare and Medicaid Services (CMS) issued its national coverage determination (NCD) policy on CPAP therapy. According to the general statements related to NCD, CMS decided that reimbursement for CPAP will be made if the diagnosis of OSA is made using comprehensive in-laboratory, attended polysomnography (type I testing devices), unattended comprehensive polysomnography (type II testing devices), limited channel PMs (type III devices) or monitors using at least 3 channels (type IV devices). In order to continue eligibility for CPAP therapy, improvement is to be demonstrated within 12 weeks from therapy initiation, or CPAP is no longer "covered".

We prefer to call the portable monitoring (PM types III and IV), home sleep testing (HST) or ambulatory sleep monitoring (ASM), as oligosomnography (OSG), pointing out to the main difference from the traditional polysomnographic recordings: the number of channels and signals is limited by the technical specifications and the technology used by the specific device. As such, the sleep testing can be attended (type I testing device) or unattended PSG (type II testing device, rarely used) or OSG, which are limited-channel, unattended, in-home sleep testing devices, *i.e.*, portable monitors (PM) types III or IV.

OSG is generally recommended to be used in an unattended setting as an alternative to PSG for the diagnosis of OSA in patients with a high pretest probability of moderate to severe OSA (high clinical suspicion) and no co-morbid sleep disorders or other major medical co-morbidities (*e.g.*, COPD, CHF, respiratory failure, etc) [121].

MSLT and MWT

A Multiple Sleep Latency Test (MSLT) may be used if excessive sleepiness persists despite optimal treatment of sleep apnea in order to determine objectively how severe it is and to establish a baseline before further therapy is instituted; alternatively, maintenance of wakefulness test (MWT) can be used to ascertain the capacity to stay awake during the day in patients on optimal therapy [119,122]. Unfortunately, neither of these two tests provides data that correlates very well with subjective, self-rated daytime sleepiness, or with the driving and workplace performance.

These are the main recommendations according to the 2005 AASM Guidelines [123] and Practice Parameters [122] for MSLT and MWT and the strength of evidence at the time of drafting these documents:

1. The Multiple Sleep Latency Test (MSLT) is a validated, objective measure of the ability or tendency to fall asleep. (*Standard*)

2. The Maintenance of Wakefulness Test (MWT) is a validated, objective measure of the ability to stay awake for a defined time. (*Standard*)

3. The MWT is used in association with the clinical history to assess the ability to maintain wakefulness. (*Standard*)

4. The MWT 40-minute protocol is recommended when the sleep clinician requires objective data to assess an individual's ability to remain awake. (*Option*)

5. To provide a valid assessment of sleepiness or wakefulness, the MSLT and MWT must be performed under appropriate conditions, using proper recording techniques and accepted protocols, with interpretation by a qualified and experienced clinician. (*Standard*)

Specific indications for use of the MSLT:

1. The MSLT is indicated as part of the evaluation of patients with suspected narcolepsy to confirm the diagnosis. (*Standard*)

2. The MSLT may be indicated as part of the evaluation of patients with suspected idiopathic hypersomnia to help differentiate idiopathic hypersomnia from narcolepsy. (*Option*)

3. The MSLT is not routinely indicated in the initial evaluation and diagnosis of obstructive sleep apnea syndrome or in assessment of change following treatment with nasal continuous positive airway pressure (CPAP).

4. The MSLT is not routinely indicated for evaluation of sleepiness in medical and neurological disorders (other than narcolepsy), insomnia, or circadian rhythm disorders (*Option*)

5. Repeat MSLT testing may be indicated in the following situations:

    a. When the initial test is affected by extraneous circumstances or when appropriate study conditions were not present during initial testing

    b. When ambiguous or un-interpretable findings are present

    c. When the patient is suspected to have narcolepsy but earlier MSLT evaluation(s) did not provide polysomnographic confirmation (*Standard*)

Specific Indications for Use of the MWT:

1. The MWT 40-minute protocol may be used to assess an individual's ability to remain awake when his or her inability to remain awake constitutes a public or personal safety issue. (*Option*)

2. The MWT may be indicated in patients with excessive sleepiness to assess response to treatment. (*Guideline*)

In general, MSLT and MWT results do not correlate very well, as they seem to measure different dimensions of sleepiness [124]. As such, it seems that MSLT measures underlying arousal as well as propensity to sleep, while MWT assesses the capacity to resist sleep, which may be more relevant clinically when assessing safety, performance and daytime functioning.

Actigraphy

Actigraphy is another useful tool in the diagnostic and monitoring armamentarium of a sleep specialist; it works by determining the activity patterns during the active time as well during sleeping period based on the principle of accelerometry [2,119].

In the AASM Practice Parameters for the use of actigraphy, its use in the diagnosis of OSA is delineated by the following two specific recommendations [125]:

1. Actigraphy is a valid way to assist in determining sleep patterns in normal, healthy adult populations (*Standard*), and in patients suspected of certain sleep disorders. (*Option-Guideline-Standard*; depending on each specific disease)

2. When PSG is not available, actigraphy is indicated as a method to estimate total sleep time in patients with OSA syndrome. Combined with a validated way of monitoring respiratory events, use of actigraphy may improve accuracy in assessing the severity of OSA compared with using time in bed. (*Standard*)

Further details about specific testing protocols, the use of the above diagnostic tests and technologies can be found in Chapter 4, Sleep Testing and Monitoring.

Treatment

OSA is a chronic disease for which there are medical, behavioral and surgical therapeutic options. Although measures that physically increase the size of the upper airway, such as continuous positive airway pressure (CPAP), oral appliances and surgery are the main primary therapeutic modalities in patients with OSA, other medical interventions may play significant roles in management. Among these is weight loss (either through behavioral modifications and/or surgery). When successful, weight loss can ameliorate or completely reverse OSA in obese patients. Because alcohol, hypnotic sedatives and opiates may worsen apnea, such drugs should be avoided as much as possible. Drugs which stimulate breathing, such as progesterone, derivatives or methylxanthines and acetazolamide, do not seem to work in prevention or treatment of SDB. The same holds true for several medications used in an attempt to increase upper airway patency (*e.g.*, antidepressants), but the quest for more selective, more efficacious medications, with effect on different respiratory neurons and/or muscles is underway. Estrogen-progesterone combinations may be effective in selected menopausal patients with sleep apnea, but not as sole treatment, while significant safety concerns remain. The role of such therapy in postmenopausal women has not been studied in large clinical trials yet, and it is not known whether the potential benefits in this group of patients outweigh the risks. Modafinil, a wake-promoting medication, may play a role in treating residual sleepiness in patients compliant with CPAP therapy. Oxygen has been shown to be efficacious as a primary treatment of OSA, and it may have a role in patients with sleep apnea who do not tolerate any other therapy. Oxygen should be used cautiously in this setting because it may prolong the apneic episodes.

A. Behavioral Interventions

Good medical care implies a thorough assessment of the patient's lifestyle and how it may complicate the underlying medical condition. This is particularly true for the patient with OSA. In general, there are a number of lifestyle attributes that place the patient at increased risk. Modification of these behaviors can have a favorable impact on subsequent risks. For purpose of clarity, these behavioral risks are described in separate sub-sections. Nevertheless, it should be kept in mind that multiple interventions, as part of a comprehensive, multidisciplinary approach may be appropriate in a given patient.

Patient Education

Patient education plays an important role in the management of OSA [2]. From the beginning, the patient needs to be actively involved in the planning and implementation of the therapeutic strategies. Treatment options should be discussed in the context of disease severity, as well as co-existent morbid conditions. It should be also emphasized that, as part of the general scaffold for therapy, patient education is of a paramount importance. The successful patient education programs include discussions about the following components:

1. Main findings of the sleep studies; severity of disease

2. Pathophysiology of sleep apnea

3. Explanation of natural course of disease and associated disorders

4. Risk factor identification, explanation of exacerbating factors, and risk factor modification

5. Genetic counseling, when indicated

6. Main treatment modalities and available options

7. What to expect from treatment (set the expectations)

8. Outline the patients' role in treatment, address their concerns, and set goals

9. Consequences of untreated disease

10. Counseling regarding drowsy driving and sleepiness in the workplace

11. Patient overall quality of life assessment and other feedback

Sleep Hygiene and Sleep Deprivation

The statement that we live in a chronically sleep-deprived society became already a truism [126]. In addition to the intuitively obvious adverse impact of sleep deprivation on performance, several lines of evidence suggest that short sleep duration, as well as repetitive sleep disruption, may also predispose to or worsen existing OSA. It is known that sleep deprivation is associated with blunted hypoxic and hypercapnic ventilatory chemoresponsiveness during wakefulness [127,128], and that it may prolong apneas and hypopneas during sleep by depressing the arousal response, with deeper oxyhemoglobin desaturations [127,129]. In one study, for example, Sériès et al [130] have reported that upper airway collapsibility increased after sleep fragmentation, but not after short-term sleep deprivation.

Patients should be encouraged to maintain good sleep hygiene, although this advice is often unheeded because of social and/or financial pressures. It may be useful to remind them that poor sleep hygiene can have an adverse impact on their SDB and contribute to a vicious cycle in which insufficient or fragmented sleep promotes OSA, which in turn perpetuates poor-quality sleep.

Weight Loss

The adverse effect of obesity on upper airway function is in part mediated through a direct mechanical influence on upper airway geometry. Studies on animals have indicated that upper airway resistance is influenced by mass loading of the anterior neck, which may simulatethe clinical scenario of excessive adipose, tissue deposits in this area [131]. Further support for a significant pathophysiologic role of cervical obesity is provided by the observation that changes in pressure surrounding the neck are transmitted to the airway lumen and that cyclic pressure fluctuations in the pharyngeal fat pad coincide with intrapharyngeal pressure fluctuations [131-133]. These data also support the relevance of the observation that patients with OSA have "thick" necks [37] and that increased neck circumference is a predictive factor for OSA [37,39,134]. Furthermore, velophyaryngeal collapsiblility increases with increasing neck circumference, at least in awake patients with OSA [135].

The presence of intrapharyngeal fat deposition may also be of pathophysiologic significance. Several groups of investigators have observed increased intrapharyngeal adipose tissue or increased lateral fat pad size on magnetic resonance imaging of patients with OSA [136,137]. The significance of a space-occupying intrapharyngeal mass on pharyngeal function has been demonstrated in an animal model with increased upper airway resistance that is related to the magnitude of inflation of a balloon catheter in the region of the upper airway lateral fat pad [133,138].

It has been well documented that either medical or surgical weight reduction can have a substantial ameliorative impact on this disorder [139-143]. In a prospective cohort study examining the association between weight change and the severity of sleep-disordered breathing, Young *et al.* demonstrated that a 10% weight loss predicted a 26% reduction in the AHI. Smith and colleagues [142] reported that a relatively modest weight loss may provide a significant benefit for some individuals. Interestingly, besides this subgroup of patients, there is a sub-population of non-obese OSA patients and one of obese OSA patients who do not seem to benefit from weight reduction [142,143]. Nevertheless, obese patients should always be encouraged to lose weight.

A multidisciplinary team approach to weight reduction, encompassing lifestyle and dietary modification, as well as pharmacologic and surgical options, may optimize clinical results [140]. Not only this will have a beneficial impact on overall health, but it also has a high likelihood of reducing the severity of upper airway dysfunction during sleep. Conceivably, the "nonresponders" may be represented by those who have not lost sufficient weight, or have coexistent craniofacial abnormalities. Because of the poor long-term success rate with weight loss in this group, bariatric surgery is being done more frequently in the treatment of these patients, sometimes with excellent results [144]. In fact, most patients referred for bariatric surgery, regardless of whether apnea is suspected, are found to have sleep apnea [53], and it has been suggested that all patients referred for bariatric surgery should have preoperative polysomnography [145,146]. Patients with sleep apnea may have a higher complication rate with such surgery [147,148].

Smith et al [142] found that dietary instructions targeting weight loss resulted in a 47% decrease in the frequency of apneas for a mean weight loss of 9% over a period of few months. Similarly, Schwartz and coworkers [141] compared the effect of weight loss in a small group of 13 obese patients with 13 age and weight matched controls who did not undergo any dietary restriction, with no weight loss over a period of 1.5 years. The found a 60% reduction in the apnea-hypopnea index (AHI) in the intervention group. Additionally, there are several other surgical weight loss studies which showed greater and consistent decreases in weight and associated reductions in AHI [80]. Both non surgical and surgical weight loss studies included small number of patients, while long-term results of weight loss are generally poor, with the only notable exception of the bariatric surgery.

Smoking Cessation

Tobacco use is known to have a detrimental effect on sleep. Cigarette users have more difficulty initiating and maintaining sleep and experience increased daytime sleepiness as well [149]. Although there are a variety of possible explanations for this, including the impact of nicotine withdrawal, it is conceivable that one mechanism is an association between smoking and sleep-disordered breathing. Smokers have an odds ratio that is fourfold to fivefold greater than that of never-smokers for having at least moderate sleep-disordered breathing [70]. Heavy smokers are at greatest risk. Cigarette smoking may contribute to upper airway dysfunction during sleep by eliciting mucosal edema and increased upper airway resistance. It is obvious that tobacco use should be discouraged on the basis of its adverse multisystem effects.

The observation that nicotine administered as gum reduces apnea frequency over the first several hours of sleep [150] is of conceptual if not practical interest. The short duration of action of this mode of delivery precludes effective therapeutic application of nicotine gum for OSAHS. Additional studies have subsequently demonstrated that there was no clinically significant reduction in disordered breathing even frequency after application of transdermal nicotine patches, which have an extended duration of delivery. Apnea duration and snoring intensity were reduced, although the magnitude of the latter was insufficient to be therapeutically useful. Adverse effects were observed in conjunction with the transdermal patch, including reduced total sleep time, sleep efficiency, and rapid gastrointestinal complaints, lightheadedness, and tremor, were also reported.

Alcohol Avoidance

Bed partners and housemates are probably the first to recognize the association between alcohol consumption and upper airway dysfunction during sleep. It is clear that alcohol can elicit obstructive apnea in individuals who otherwise only snore and increase the apnea frequency in patients with preexisting OSA. In addition to increasing the frequency of sleep-disordered breathing events, alcohol consumption increases the duration of these events [151,152].

Alcohol may also have a particularly adverse impact on daytime alertness in patients with OSA. The hypnotic effect of this agent is enhanced in the presence of underlying sleepiness. Alcohol consumption superimposed on sleepiness, as in sleep deprivation, is associated with worse driving simulator test performance compared with sleep deprivation and placebo [153].

To summarize, individuals with OSA, either treated or untreated, would be best served by alcohol abstinence. Although this is a prudent advice, not all patients will follow course. If one is unwilling or unable to discontinue completely the regular alcohol intake, he or she should be advised to limit the alcohol ingestion to small quantities, and not within a few hours from bedtime, allowing thus enough time for the blood alcohol level to fall to near-zero. There is inconsistency in the literature regarding the impact of alcohol on the magnitude of the positive-pressure prescription [151,154]. Patients who are unlikely to alter their habitual alcohol ingestion should have a therapeutic trial under usual lifestyle conditions. Therapy needs to be proven successful despite the presence of exogenous as well as endogenous influences on the pathophysiologic process. This includes not only alcohol consumption, but other factors, such as body position during sleep (some individuals may not be able to sleep in supine position) or unavoidable need for treatment with pharmacologic agents that may adversely affect upper airway stability during sleep (*e.g.*, benzodiazepines).

B. Pharmacological Treatment of OSA

A recent review of the literature pertaining to the use of pharmacologic therapy in OSA has found 33 randomized placebo-controlled trials, investigating the effect of 27 different drugs on either OSA severity or on SDB-associated symptoms [155]. While some of the studies had statistically significant results, they were generally underpowered or ran over short periods of time, with overall small effects on ESS, AHI or ODI (and possibly underestimated the potential long-term benefits).

The main mechanisms by which pharmacological therapy may work in OSA are as follows:

Respiratory Stimulants

Most of the studies that investigated respiratory center stimulants for the treatment of OSA have been essentially negative. Among the drugs studied, methylxanthines (aminophylline [156] and theophylline [157]), carbonic anhydrase inhibitors (acetazolamide [158]) and opioid antagonists (naloxone [159] and naltrexone [160]), all seemed to improve OSA severity to a mild extent (generally, a very small effect), if any. Also, medroxyprogesterone, a synthetic analogue of progesterone, with potential stimulant activity on the respiratory centers, did not change the AHI in 10 male subjects with OSA over one week period trial versus one week of placebo [161].

In the same general category can be included a gas, carbon dioxide (CO_2) that can be used in the therapy of OSA. CO_2 can stimulate ventilation, essentially eliminating hypopneas. It has been used sporadically in OSA [162-164]. Unfortunately, the need for a closed system to administer consistent concentrations, safety aspects and the potential need to monitor both tidal and transcutaneous CO_2 concentrations, make it cumbersome and costly. An alternative to the exogenous administration of CO_2 may be the extension of the circuit (thus adding dead space), which may reset the CO_2 at higher levels.

Muscle Tone Modulators

Based on some physiological data showing that the tone of most of the upper airway muscles is lower in OSA patients during sleep versus non-OSA controls, the more recent pharmacological studies concentrated on the treatment targeting serotoninergic and cholinergic neurons involved in their control, as both neuromediators seem to increase the motor tone of these muscles. Among these, paroxetine [165], mirtazapine [166], physostigmine [167] and donepezil [168,169] seemed to be promising in reducing the OSA severity, but did not really confirm the initial expectations (e.g., mirtazapine [170] and paroxetine [171]) or are still awaiting either confirmatory studies or availability of oral form (e.g., the case of physostigmine) [155]. Donepezil also needs further testing in younger, non-demented patients.

Selective serotonin receptor modulation (*e.g.*, 5-HT3 receptor antagonists [172,173]) has been proposed as a potential future therapeutic target, through action on specific respiratory muscles or on their respiratory center regulatory areas; development of such agents is currently under way.

Given the gender disparities between men and pre-menopausal women in development of SDB, it has been hypothesized that sex hormones may have protective properties on the upper airway. As such, postmenopausal women with reduced genioglossus tone by EMG had a significant improvement after hormone replacement therapy (a combination of estrogen and progesterone) in one study from D.P. White et al [174]. Nevertheless, in a pilot study using estradiol 50 mg patches versus estradiol 50 mg plus progesterone 200 mg capsules versus placebo did not have an impressive effect on AHI in 6 postmenopausal women, except in the arm of estradiol patch [175]. Further results (both short-term and long-term) are awaited for hormone replacement therapy in postmenopausal women, in parallel with long-term potential deleterious effects (malignancy, venous thromboembolic disease, etc).

Antihypertensives

Antihypertensive agents may, at least theoretically, improve OSA by interfering with the baroreceptor chemosensitivity and the respiratory centers' activity. Different classes of antihypertensives have been tried: beta-blockers (BBs), calcium channel blockers (CCBs) and angiotension converting enzyme inhibitors (ACEIs), etc. The available literature reveals very heterogenous results: among BBs, while propranolol can worsen OSA, metoprolol and atenolol may be beneficial [176,177]; among ACEIs, cilazapril and ramipril may also be of use in reducing the AHI of the patients with OSA [176,178]; and among CCBs, isradipine has not been found to be effective in this instance [177]. Although many explanations may exist for these discordant results, the current state of the therapy is that these medications do not have a place in the primary treatment of OSA, but can be used safely in the treatment of co-existent hypertension of these patients.

Topical Therapy

Local application of drugs to the upper airway may be another pathway of pharmacologic delivery; this can work by reducing the local edema, secretions and surface tension or possibly, in the future, by modulating specifically the airway dilator muscle tone. Fluticasone nasal spray [179], xylometazoline [180], topical surfactant [181] and phosphocholinamin [182] have been investigated in various studies and did not pan out so far to be of significant help in reducing the OSA severity.

Oxygen Therapy

In addition to sleep fragmentation, many of the clinically and physiologically evident consequences of OSA are attributable to nocturnal hypoxemia. Prevention of hypoxemia is a worthwhile therapeutic goal in these patients. Several older studies reported that administration of supplemental oxygen to patients with OSA may significantly increase apnea duration with associated hypercapnia and respiratory acidosis [183]. Martin et al [183] observed an initial prolongation of apnea duration in a group of eucapnic patients with OSA, in conjunction with a significant reduction in apnea frequency. There was no change in the mean apnea duration after 30 minutes of oxygen administration compared with a period of room air breathing. This resulted in decreased apnea time and maintenance of satisfactory oxyhemoglobin saturation over the study period. The bradycardia that accompanied apnea was eliminated by supplemental oxygen administration. Gold and coworkers [184] subsequently reported that supplemental oxygen administration was associated with a statistical reduction in apnea frequency, particularly during NREM sleep (although not necessarily a clinical significant reduction), as well as improved oxyhemoglobin saturation. Apnea duration increased slightly by an average of 4 to 7 seconds across the study group. There was no improvement in subjective or objective measures of daytime sleepiness during the period of nocturnal oxygen supplementation.

So far, the evidence suggests that, in itself, supplemental oxygen during sleep is not sufficiently effective in reducing apnea frequency and increasing daytime alertness for most patients. There may be a population of individuals who are symptomatic because of the sleep fragmentation (*i.e.*, hypersomnolent), or have mild OSA, but experience deep oxyhemoglobin desaturations during sleep; in these patients, increasing nocturnal oxyhemoglobin saturation may be a reasonable, if not the only therapeutic goal [185]. Nevertheless, the degree and duration of oxyhemoglobin desaturation that is ultimately harmful remains to be determined [186]. Patients with coronary artery disease or cerebrovascular disease and mild OSA, but with severe oxyhaemoglobin desaturations during the respiratory events might benefit from supplemental oxygen [187,188]. Outcome studies are clearly needed to determine at what hypoxic burden there is cost-benefit advantage for providing oxygen therapy. Consideration should be given to performing initial trials of oxygen therapy during attended monitoring. This may be particularly important in patients with concomitant hypercapnia during wakefulness. Such monitoring is also necessary to determine the flow of supplemental oxygen required for maintenance of acceptable oxyhemoglobin saturation.

In addition to providing sole therapy in selected patients with OSA, oxygen may be a useful adjunct to positive airway pressure (CPAP or bilevel PAP) [189]. Patients with OSA who are sufficiently hypoxemic or borderline hypoxemic during wakefulness to warrant supplemental oxygen therapy usually meet the criteria for this therapy during sleep, even if positive airway pressure treatment maintains upper airway patency [190]. It should be determined if persistent desaturation on CPAP is related to hypoventilation resulting from the high mechanical impedance to expiration or increased dead space-tidal volume ratio that may be associated with this reduction of expiratory pressure to avoid significant hypoventilation and desaturation and obviate the need for supplemental oxygen.

Several studies have described the impact of transtracheal oxygen (TTO) administration to patients with OSA [191,192]. The available data on the clinical utility of this mode of oxygen delivery are limited. If the transtracheal route of oxygen delivery is effective and superior to nasal cannula administration in reducing OSA, it could be the result of stimulation of flow- or temperature-sensitive receptors in the upper airway. Large, well-designed studies are necessary to evaluate the role of this intervention. The frequency and severity of complications resulting from TTO therapy in a predominantly obese patient population have not been well characterized. Availability of this information is essential before this therapeutic modality could be accepted. At present, TTO should be considered investigational in the treatment of patients with OSA.

Central Nervous System (CNS) Stimulants

Some patients with SDB continue to experience EDS despite optimal therapy, *i.e.*, even after normalization of the AHI, hemoglobin saturation, flow contour, and/or arousal index [193]. For this category of patients, after ensuring optimal treatment, good compliance with the primary therapy and after addressing potential co-morbid sleep conditions, adjunctive (secondary) stimulant therapy may be considered for 'residual' EDS [2,194,195]. As the name implies, this therapy is to be added to the primary therapeutic modality and not to replace it, since it targets a symptom (EDS), not the underlying disorder and, potentially, the side effects of this therapy can outweigh the risks of not treating OSA. Prior to initiating secondary therapy with stimulants, repeat PSG (with CPAP, dental appliance or the specific medication used initially as primary therapy) is generally advisable in order to verify the appropriateness of OSA therapy and to rule out other sleep co-morbidities. Since this therapy is tailored to the patient's symptoms, which are poorly correlated to the disease severity, there is no clear-cut threshold for when to treat or when is not necessary to implement it.

Several central nervous system (CNS) stimulants are currently available. While modafinil and R-modafinil are the only agents that have been studied in OSA patients who have residual EDS after optimal primary therapy, alternatives to this are methylphenidate and various amphetamines, which are generally used in the treatment of narcolepsy and idiopathic hypersomnia.

Modafinil acts on the CNS, although the exact mechanism of its effect is still unknown. It is currently considered first-line adjunctive therapy for the treatment of 'residual' EDS after adequate treatment of OSA [2,194]. Its effectiveness has been shown in several randomized trials [196-199], although most of them have been sponsored by the drug's manufacturer. R-modafinil (or Armodafinil) is the R-enantiomer of racemic modafinil, with an apparent longer half-life. It appears to be similarly effective, according to randomized trials [200,201]. Modafinil is generally started at a dose of 100-200 mg orally in the morning and then titrated as needed, up to 400 mg. Patients with persistent afternoon sleepiness may benefit from twice daily administration, *i.e.*, 200 mg in the morning and 200 mg at noon to early afternoon. Although reportedly safer than the other CNS stimulants, modafinil should be used with caution in people with a history of arrhythmias or heart disease [202,203]. Side effects are relatively infrequent, and include headaches, nausea and/or vomiting, diarrhea, anorexia and xerostomia. Addiction related to modafinil has not been unequivocally ruled out, since some emerging data hint that there may be some low-level dependency induced by this medication. Life-threatening side effects are represented by Stevens-Johnson syndrome (SJS) or toxic epidermal necrolysis (TEN), and, consequently, any rash arising while on this therapy should be a strong reason for seeking medical attention right away and for discontinuation of Modafinil or Armodafinil.

Methylphenidate is another CNS stimulant with an unknown mechanism of action. Two actions have been proposed: a sympathomimetic effect (catecholamine re-uptake inhibition?) and stimulation of the brainstem reticular activating system and the cortex. Methylphenidate is commonly used to treat attention deficit hyperactivity disorder (ADHD), narcolepsy, or traumatic brain injury. Although no clinical trials have been performed in patients with OSA, methylphenidate is used sometimes off-label as adjunctive therapy to treat residual EDS despite optimal therapy, especially when a stronger stimulative action is desired. Side effects are about the same, and even more common than those attributed to Modafinil, while the potential o induce addiction is clearly higher. Due to its sympathomimetic effect, it should be used with more caution in patients with heart disease or cardiac dysrrhythmias, if ever.

Amphetamines are also potent CNS stimulants, with strong sympathomimetic action. Similarly, the side effects, addictive potential and unproven clinical efficacy in this clinical setting are similar to the one of methylphenidate.

Amphetamines and their derivatives can lead to irritability, anxiety, tremor, hypertension and cardiac dysrhythmias. There is a strong risk of addiction and illicit use for amphetamine, dextroamphetamine and methamphetamine, hence the controlled substance status and special precautions while monitoring this therapy.

C. Mechanical Therapy

Elevated nasal resistance may promote or aggravate upper airway closure during sleep [204,205]. Although the therapeutic benefit remains somewhat controversial, approximately 10% of patients with snoring and apnea have been reported to improve after administration of mucosal vasoconstrictors. A variety of devices have recently become available that mechanically dilate the anterior nasal valve in order to reduce the nasal airway resistance and putatively decrease the propensity toward OSA.

In one of the few studies to assess objectively the impact of nasal dilation on sleep, breathing, and oxygenation, Hoijer *et al* [206] assessed the impact of an external nasal dilator in 10 snorers, 7 of whom had an apnea index of 5 or higher. Although the average apnea index fell from 18 to 6 and the nadir oxyhemoglobin saturation also improved while asleep with the nasal dilator, the saturation remained severely reduced in those individuals with more severe disease (those with higher baseline hypoxic burden). Snoring intensity was reduced, although there was no subjective effect of the nasal dilator on arousal frequency or on EDS after 10 nights of use. Neither the hypopnea index nor objectively measured arousal frequency were reported in this study, and it is possible that neither the AHI, nor arousal index was favorably affected by this therapy. It is also noteworthy that only four patients expressed a desire to continue to use the nasal dilator. In contrast, Hoffstein *et al* [207] concluded that dilation of the anterior nasal valve using an external dilator has no impact on SDB, nadir desaturation or mean oxyhemoglobin saturation, although a reduction in snoring intensity was noted. As the authors pointed out, it is possible that their results may have been biased by the lack of randomization.

Using an intranasally applied dilator, Scharf et al [208] reported that a significant proportion of their 20 participants had improved Stanford Sleepiness Scale (SSS) scores, morning concentration, and subjective quality of sleep, as well as reduced sleepiness on awakening and number of awakenings. Using a numeric scale, there were no differences in subjective sleep depth, overall sleep quality, refreshing quality of sleep, morning sleepiness, number of awakenings or in subjective parameters. Bed partners reported decreased snoring loudness, but no change in snoring regularity. Unfortunately, in this trial there was no objective assessment of sleep and breathing, either at study onset or during the treatment with a nasal dilator. In another study [209], cyclic alternating pattern (CAP) sequences in non-apneic snorers were diminished during the use of an intranasally applied dilator, suggesting improved sleep continuity.

Nasopharyngeal Airway

Although the concept of nasopharyngeal intubation to maintain upper airway patency during sleep was originally reported in the literature in the 1970s [210], since then, there have been relatively few reports describing its use [211,212].

Overall, nasopharyngeal intubation has limited therapeutic utility. A substantial proportion of patients do not tolerate this intervention; of those who do seem to tolerate it, only about two thirds may have a clinically significant improvement in SDB, as defined by a reduction in respiratory event frequency of 65%, or an apnea index (AI) less than 5 and an AHI less than 10 [212]. Some of these patients continue to have significant hypoxemic burdens when monitored by pulse oximetry, and there seems to be no major improvement in sleep quality and/or architecture. Thus, the limited available data pertaining to this form of therapy suggest that patient tolerance may be suboptimal and many of the apparent responders still have a noteworthy degree of residual SDB, as well as persistently abnormal sleep quality and architecture. In selected patients for whom other therapies have failed, a trial of nasopharyngeal airway may be considered. Alternating nostrils in which the nasoparyngeal airway is placed in conjunction with adequate lubrication (NB: avoiding substances that may cause lipoid pneumonia!), may improve adherence to this therapeutic modality.

Positive Airway Pressure

Positive Airway Pressure (PAP) may be delivered in a continuous (CPAP), bilevel (Bilevel PAP), autotitrating (AutoPAP), 'flexible' CPAP, adaptive servo-ventilation (ASV) modes, *etc.* The positive pressure is applied either through nasal, oral or oro-nasal interface (mask).

First described by Sullivan in 1981 [213], CPAP provides the means of pneumatic splinting or stenting of the upper airway during sleep by providing intraluminal pressure that is positive versus the atmospheric pressure and kept constant throughout the respiratory cycle. Although CPAP therapy for sleep apnea was first described in 1981 [213], it was not until about 1985 that it began to be recognized as a realistic form of long-term therapy in other centers. Despite the fact that initially patients had to use an adhesive to attach the mask, the prompt relief of sleepiness led to an increasing number of users. By 1985, over 100 patients were using this therapy on a regular basis [214,215]. Subsequently, tremendous technical improvements were made in the design of the masks and pressure delivery systems. Over the past 3 decades, the evidence supporting the use of CPAP has accumulated exponentially, attesting the improvement in quality of life and outcomes. This trend was driven, at least in part, by the demands from governmental and private funding agencies, health maintenance organizations and by the availability of industry sponsorship, in parallel with the increasing commercial success of the CPAP equipment and technology [214].

Nasal continuous positive airway pressure (CPAP) is the treatment of choice for moderate to severe OSA syndrome. At an appropriately set pressure, CPAP is very effective for this syndrome, by ameliorating the daytime sleepiness and fatigue. As such, McDaid *et al* [216] scanned the available literature in a recently published systematic review on the effects of CPAP in OSA syndrome and found a pooled effect on Epworth Sleepiness Scale (ESS) of about 2.7 points reduction (95%CI -3.4, -1.9).

Generally, CPAP is very effective is reducing the frequency of respiratory events (*i.e.*, apneas, hypopneas and RERAs), thus normalizing or ameliorating significantly the AHI [217,218]. As a consequence of this therapeutic modality, upper airway muscle tone decreases with the application of the positive pressure (or remains the same). Higher levels of PAP may be required in supine position, in REM sleep, after ingestion of significant amounts of alcohol or after taking different sedative medications. Weight gain may also require an increase in a formerly adequate treatment PAP.

Studies designed to assess and validate a mechanical device such as CPAP have to conform to less stringent requirements and regulatory constraints versus, for example, studies required for registration and market approval of pharmaceutical drugs. Performing true double-blind, randomized, controlled trials of CPAP therapy may also be more problematic. "Sham" CPAP, by its nature, is less efficacious on unavoidably observable variables such as snoring and apnea, with consequent frustration regarding blinding the study participants. It is also quite difficult to effectively blind a CPAP therapist or physician involved in such studies compared with pharmaceutical trials involving placebo medications. The most recent phase in CPAP development has been the advent of automatically titrating CPAP devices (autoPAP or APAP), which have major implications for the delivery of health care to patients with OSA, and for the traditional laboratory titrations. It is important, however, to ensure that use of all new devices for routine CPAP treatment is driven by evidence, not by marketing.   The main limitations to CPAP usage are lack of patient acceptance and lack of tolerance to treatment. Newer modalities of CPAP, such as autotitrating CPAP (APAP), have been advocated to avoid complex and potentially multiple sleep laboratory titrations and to maximize CPAP usage. More research is required before this viewpoint can be fully supported in clinical practice, at least in patients with significant medical or sleep co-morbidities.

CPAP is the preferred option for the treatment of moderate to severe OSA and optional for mild OSA [2]. Bilevel PAP or AutoCPAP (auto-adjusting, APAP) can be considered in patients intolerant of CPAP. Bilevel PAP is also an option when high pressures are required and the patient experiences difficulty in exhaling against a fixed pressure, although there is no proven advantage in using it against CPAP [219]. It is also helpful when there is an element of central hypoventilation, by providing a level of pressure support.

AutoCPAP or APAP devices were developed with two potential uses: (1) to select an effective pressure without the need of an attended PAP titration, and (2) to deliver the lowest effective pressure under any circumstance (body position, sleep stage, weight changes, etc). AutoCPAP algorithms vary among different devices, but in general, pressure changes in response to flow (variations is airflow amplitude, airflow limitation and snoring) or in airway impedance (changes in signal determined by forced oscillation technique). AutoCPAP up-titration may be erroneous in the face of high airflow leaks (mask or mouth leaks), which can simulate respiratory events, and due to the device's inability to differentiate between OSA and CSA (at least by flow-sensing devices). Recently, autoBilevel PAP has been introduced; the settings to be adjusted are: maximum inspiratory PAP (IPAP), minimum expiratory PAP (EPAP), and the maximal level of pressure support (or IPAP-

EPAP difference; in general ≥ 3 cm H20 and ≤ 8 cm H2O, the latter to avoid respiratory center instability). The outcomes related to CPAP versus APAP use are very similar [220,221].

Expiratory pressure modulation ('flexible' CPAP, including C- flex and Expiratory Pressure Relief, EPR) is a recent variant of PAP that was developed to improve patient comfort by allowing the airway pressure to fall below the prescribed PAP in early expiration with return to the prescribed level at end-exhalation. No data exist whether these technological "gadgets" translate into better outcomes.

Adaptive servoventilation (ASV) is another recent variant of PAP which was developed to treat Cheyne Stokes respiration (CSR) in patients with congestive heart failure (CHF). OSA and central breathing disorders such as hypoventilation, CSR and CSA can frequently co-exist. By definition, CSR is represented by a waxing and waning pattern of breathing with a crescendo-decrescendo pattern of respiratory flow amplitude changes (periodic breathing), mainly due to an instability of the respiratory control system. Sleep-related breathing disorders in patients with CHF are associated with impaired clinical outcomes and shorter survival. Therefore, optimal treatment of CSR is critical. While CPAP reduces CSR by roughly 50%, ASV normalizes CSR in most patients. ASV devices apply different levels of pressure support by increasing the levels of inspiratory pressure during periods of hypoventilation and reducing it during periods of hyperventilation. The devices deliver an expiratory pressure to overcome the upper airways obstruction. Pressure support is basically defined as the difference between expiratory and inspiratory pressures. Thus, while the level of pressure support is fixed in bilevel PAP, it varies in ASV (with a "back-up minute ventilation" parameter).

Patients meeting the AASM criteria for the diagnosis of OSA should be treated. The published criteria of the Center for Medicare and Medicaid Services (CMS) are similar to those of the AASM (see Table **1**). The CMS reimburses for CPAP treatment for patients with an AHI of 15 or greater, and AHI greater of 5 or greater *and* concurrent sleepiness or history of hypertension, stroke, ischemic heart disease, *cor pulmonale* or mood disorders.

Table 1: Center for Medicare and Medicaid Services (CMS) criteria for Continuous Positive Airway Pressure (CPAP) reimbursement in patients with Obstructive Sleep Apnea (OSA) [AHI: Apnea Hypopnea Index]

	AHI $\geq$ 15	
CPAP therapy is covered for adults who have sleep-disordered breathing (SDB) and the following findings:	AHI $\geq$ 5 and < 15 *and* any of the following:	Daytime sleepiness
		Hypertension
		Ischemic heart disease
		Stroke
		Insomnia
		Mood disorders

Currently, most patients commence CPAP under supervision, usually in a specialized sleep laboratory. The purposes of the supervision are as follows: to ensure that the patient is appropriately educated about the therapy, to determine the adequacy of CPAP throughout the night, and to evaluate immediate acceptance or problems with the therapy. Nevertheless, economic pressures within the health care systems are challenging this approach and moving in the direction of less intensive staffing, auto-adjustable CPAP, self-titration or even home commencement of CPAP.

Regardless of the location or method of CPAP initiation, there is a need for proper patient assessment (*e.g.*, to determine whether the patient has awake respiratory failure or marked hypoxemia in sleep), and this requires specific physician training and experience. There is no evidence for appropriate safety and efficacy of CPAP titration outside of a medically supervised process [222]. Current evidence supports the use of trained technologists (so-called CPAP coordinators) to provide patient education, technical aspects of titration, and follow-up. However, recent data from small patient groups has challenged the notion of close medical supervision, and this should become a major research focus [223]. The dominant determinants of CPAP usage are patient understanding of the therapy, its impact on symptoms, and close professional support, regardless or mask type, CPAP manufacturer, and delivery.

Additional PAP Features

Several technological improvements to PAP delivery have been developed and implemented over time by device manufacturers, but without very strong data to support their use; nevertheless, some of them became standard, even in the absence of data. We will be listing here the main additional features that are available for PAP delivery:

- Heated humidification. It has been shown that heated humidification can decrease the nasal airway resistance by approximately 50%, whereas cold humidification has little impact [224]. While reduced nasal airway resistance should translate into improved effectiveness, comfort and tolerance for CPA, no clinical studies to date have proven these effects [225,226]. For purpose of tolerance, comfort and patient adherence to CPAP therapy, AASM recommends heated humidification for all patients who receive CPAP [2].

- Pressure ramp. For purpose of better comfort and tolerance, PAP can be initialized at sleep onset at a lower level (usually 4 - 5 cmH2O) and then increased stepwise to the desired level over a period of time specified by the prescriber (*e.g.*, 30-minute ramp). This feature is available with CPAP, AutoPAP, and Bilevel PAP devices and can be used repeatedly with all awakenings from sleep. Similarly to the other additional features, there is no evidence to support this concept at the present time and should be used only when the patient complains specifically about the uncomfortable sensation of a PAP device blowing too high a pressure at sleep onset.

- Expiratory pressure relief (EPR). ERP is based on a brief decrease of the pressure delivered during early exhalatory phase with CPAP and end-inspiratory plus early expiration during bilevel PAP administration [2]. The purpose of EPR was to improve PAP tolerance and adherence by reducing the sensation of breathing against high pressure, although no proven benefit has been shown so far in randomized controlled studies. In one randomized cross-over trial on 104 patients with OSA treated with conventional CPAP versus CPAP-EPR, no differences were noted with regards to follow-up AHI, patient compliance and total sleep time after 7 weeks of therapy [227]. Notwithstanding the lack of evidence for EPR to improve patient compliance, AASM recommends a trial of pressure relief if the patient does not tolerate traditional CPAP [2].

- Altitude compensation. Studies performed using decompression chambers showed that the optimal level of PAP is altitude-dependent, hence may be important for patients who travel at various altitudes [228,229]. The more recent PAP devices include an altitude compensation feature.

- Another interesting way of delivering airway pressure was achieved by a group of investigators by air insufflation through a high-flow nasal cannula, of warm and humidified air, at a constant rate of 20 liters per minute (equivalent of less than 2 cm H_2O); overall, this is a less intrusive, less invasive method of treating OSA [230,231]. This therapeutic modality was found to reduce the frequency of respiratory events both in adults and children [230,231], in all three categories of disease severity.

The Case of the First Night Effect

Sleeping with a nasal mask and air blowing sensation induced by CPAP, although not necessarily uncomfortable, are novel experiences for most patients. Provider explanation and re-assurance, video programs, leaflets and brochures and mask acclimation sessions prior to beginning CPAP all reduce patient anxiety and seem to improve overall acceptance. Current evidence provides support for intensive patient education in CPAP usage [222].

During the first night of treatment, it is important to ensure that the pressure level deemed as optimal is sufficient to prevent not only apneas and oxyhemoglobin desaturations, but also respiratory-related arousals (RERAs) in all stages and in all postures of sleep. It must be ensured that airflow pressure tracings are normalized, with "rounded" flow contour, not "chopped off" (indicative of flow limitation) in order to avoid residual partial airway obstruction and subsequent arousals [214,232]. Many studies have emphasized the importance of proper airflow measurement in CPAP titration using pressure transducers rather than thermistors or other indirect airflow measures. Proper airflow measurement can help determine the optimal pressure level by providing insights regarding the etiology of arousals - for example, whether they are related to respiratory events (respiratory event - related arousals) or whether increasing pressure has a beneficial effect on sleep continuity. Although polysomnographic studies suggest that flow limitation correction may be the optimal target of CPAP titrations, long-term data are still lacking [233].

When the correct pressure level is reached and the airway is fully patent, sleep should no longer be fragmented by repetitive arousals. In this instance, there is often "rebound" slow wave sleep (SWS) and/or rapid eye movement

(REM or R) sleep [234]. This rebound phase of sleep recovery from severe fragmentation seem to last for about a week; during this time and after the initial night of treatment, the duration and intensity of the rebound SWS and/or R sleep follow a fast decrement [234]. However, the improvement in sleep architecture is usually immediate and can be used as a sign of an effective pressure level. Continued frequent arousals may indicate that a critical level of upper airway resistance persists, especially if associated with airflow limitation. Continued snoring is another sign of inadequate PAP pressure.

Other data demonstrate that hysteresis exists in the relationship between CPAP and upper airway resistance. In other words, to eliminate inspiratory flow limitation, higher pressures are required during upward titration of CPAP than with downward titration from higher pressures [235]. This means that patients with OSA may actually normalize their breathing during sleep at a lower pressure level if manual or automatic titration involves both upward titration until airflow is sinusoidal in shape and downward titration until obstructed events re-occur. This may be an important concept in patients with complications of CPAP caused by higher pressure levels, such, as mask or mouth leak, or when an autotitrating CPAP (autoCPAP) does not allow for this up-and-down titration approach.

It appears that a pressure level accurately set on one night of CPAP titration is generally effective on subsequent nights [236]. Early work and clinical experience suggested that this was the case, but the use of autoCPAP technology in the home has provided the research to support this view. For patients who respond immediately to CPAP but then report continued daytime sleepiness on home treatment, one option would be to empirically increase CPAP pressure, assuming that the laboratory study underestimated the pressure requirement. Other factors may have an impact on the therapeutic efficacy of a given CPAP pressure in the home. For example, in time, weight gain may lead to a need for a higher CPAP setting [237]. Heavy (but not moderate) alcohol consumptions may affect CPAP pressure, presumably because alcohol depresses upper airway neuromuscular tone [151,237]. Nasal congestion or a different posture in the home may also lead to different pressure requirements, but this hot been well researched.

Unfortunately, so far, no randomized trial has found that CPAP therapy leads to an improved general and/or cardiovascular mortality, although feasibility of such trials nowadays is seriously questionable.

The Case of the Patient with Respiratory Failure

Patients with heart failure, carbon dioxide (CO_2) retention, and/or extreme nocturnal hypoxemia (*e.g.*, $S_pO_2 \leq 50\%$) require close supervision when initiating CPAP. Such patients may have nigh-time confusion, delirium triggered or worsened by hypoxemia, respiratory acidosis, different environment and/or mask-induced anxiety; additionally, older subjects may experience the so-called "sun-downing", which is also a type of delirium thought to be triggered by some of these factors. The sleep technician must be aware that the patient may try to pull the mask off repeatedly throughout the night. After the first few nights, these patients typically settle down and sleep with the CPAP unit without the need for intensive monitoring.

Previously, the therapy choice for these patients was institution of mechanical ventilation or urgent tracheostomy. While tracheal intubation and ventilation may still be the appropriate option, in trained hands, nasally applied CPAP or noninvasive ventilation (NIV) may be able to control the breathing disturbance during sleep and avoid invasive ventilator assistance. Many of these patients have both upper airway obstruction and hypoventilation, and nasal CPAP may not be adequate to normalize gas exchange. Increasingly, the clinical approach in these patients is to employ bilevel PAP therapy. In general, AutoCPAP approaches are to be avoided in such patients. When possible, hospitalization would be the most reasonable approach in management of patients with severe CO_2 retention due to hypoventilation syndrome, chronic lung disease or CHF until studies showing the safety of ambulatory approaches are available.

The Case of the Split-Night Polysomnogram

It has been suggested that CPAP treatment can be initiated on the same night the diagnosis is established through the so-called "split-night" polysomnograms (with the first part of the night used for diagnosis and the second part for treatment) [238,239]. However, at least in the initial studies, patient selection was not always by randomization, as they tended to be performed in patients with more severe disease and to shorten the time for CPAP therapy initiation. Other studies [134] have identified a subset of patients for whom a split-night study provided insufficient time for CPAP titration to achieve a satisfactory prescription. Patients with milder degrees of SDB (*e.g.*, with an

AHI ≤ 20) in whom the titration was initiated later in the night (because prolonged monitoring was required to establish a diagnosis) were more likely to have unsuccessful split-night titrations.

CPAP titration can potentially be accomplished during the day. In this study, both daytime and nocturnal CPAP titration studies yielded sufficient amounts of REM and non-REM sleep to help determine CPAP settings. The diurnal and nocturnal CPAP titrations resulted in comparable therapeutic pressures, resolution of sleep disordered breathing, and 1-week compliance. Split-night or day studies may appear attractive from a short-term, economic point of view in the United States, but data in larger numbers of unselected patients in different health system are required before this approach is routinely accepted. It is possible that a combination of split-night titration and subsequent home autotitration may be an adequate strategy, but as yet this is speculative.

The Case of CPAP Therapy Initiation at Home

Theoretically, it may be economically advantageous to start CPAP at home and avoid a formal polysomnographic CPAP titration, but outcome studies showing cost utility are not available. Current reviews and guidelines do not advocate home commencement of CPAP, particularly using autotitrating devices [2,240,241]. This is a controversial area, as it implies as major change in practice in sleep centers. One study observed poorer CPAP compliance in patients assessed only with respiratory monitoring [242] but this is not a universal finding [243].Other workers have found reasonable utility with unattended in-hospital CPAP titration in patients with mild to moderate disease but with severe OSA [244]. Other studies have suggested that equations can be determined that would allow an empirical pressure level to be set, potentially preventing the need for any investigation of CPAP efficacy. Recent data in a small group of patients support this empirical method of home CPAP titration instead of laboratory initiation [223]. Again, long-term outcome data are lacking. The ongoing studies in several countries should provide clearer evidence-based guide lines for initiating CPAP. Different predictive models have been developed for optimal CPAP therapy, using either logistic [245] or linear regression models [117,246-262], as well as optical neural networks [263,264]; some of the strongest predictors of the optimal CPAP level seem to be: BMI, neck circumference, baseline AHI; other parameters can add value to these models, although their contribution to the predicted CPAP variance is relatively small.

Problems, Side Effects and Adherence Issues

Many people have problems with their CPAP device, especially at first. It's important to not give up. Often, the problems go away when you get used to wearing the device. It may also be helpful for you to find a support group in your area so that you can talk with other people who have sleep apnea.

The following are some common problems you may have with your CPAP device, and some possible solutions:

- The mask feels uncomfortable. Because everyone's face has a different shape, you may need to try different masks to find one that fits you well.

- Your nose feels dry and stuffy. You can try using a humidifier to moisten the air from the CPAP device.

- Your nose feels blocked up. Some people who have sleep apnea also have nose problems. Ask your doctor if you have a nose problem that can be treated with a nasal spray. Surgery is sometimes also an option. People who breathe through their mouths don't do as well with CPAP nose masks. In this case, a full-face mask that covers both the nose and the mouth may help (see the picture below).

- The mask bothers your skin and nose. Because the mask must fit firmly over your nose and cheeks, it may irritate your skin. A different size or kind of mask may help. There are also special skin moisturizers made for CPAP device users. Some petroleum-based products can damage the mask, so ask your doctor for more information. Some people also benefit from using nasal pillows that fit into the nostrils and relieve pressure on the bridge of the nose (see the picture below). Using a regular CPAP mask one night and nasal pillows the next night may help you feel more comfortable.

- The mask leaks air. Some people can't keep their jaw closed while wearing the mask. A chin strap can help hold up your jaw to keep the air in (see the picture below).

- You don't like the pressure. You may find that breathing out against the air pressure keeps you from sleeping deeply. Your doctor may ask you to use a bi-level machine that lowers the air pressure when you breathe out. The same mask may be used with CPAP and bi-level machines.

- You take the mask off during your sleep or don't wear it every night. Most people can't wear the mask all night long, every night, right from the start. Keep trying, even if you can only use the mask for an hour a night at first. Once you solve your comfort problems, you should be able to increase the time you wear the mask.

- You just can't get used to the mask. Some people find that wearing a dental device that pushes their tongue forward helps. You may want to talk with your doctor about whether throat or jaw surgery could help.

The Case of the Post-CPAP 'Residual' Sleepiness

Sleepiness after initiation of CPAP treatment is common and takes two forms: (1) the case of the patient who had an excellent initial response to therapy and subsequently became sleepy again; and (2) the patient who never had an improvement in sleepiness despite CPAP use, adjustments, interface changes, *etc.* The prevalence of this problem is unknown, but several studies have documented that the mean level of sleepiness does not return to normal in individuals treated with CPAP [198,265]. The first step in evaluating such patients should probably be to obtain some objective measure of compliance, typically accomplished by a meter or a "smart card" on the CPAP machine. Evaluation of the patients for another sleep disorder, particularly shift work sleep disorder, may clarify the issue. Medications and their effects on nocturnal sleep and daytime alertness should be investigated.

Two groups [198,265] have investigated the use in of modafinil in carefully selected, CPAP-compliant patients who were still objective and subjectively sleepy. Each study found improvement in some measure of sleepiness with 400 mg of modafinil a day. Whether and when to use this approach for patients with SDB who are still sleepy is likely to remains controversial. Objective measurements of CPAP compliance and of sleepiness would seem to be minimal prerequisites to such treatment.

Potential causes of 'residual' excessive daytime sleepiness (EDS) despite CPAP therapy:

- Non-compliance or non-adherence

- Inadequate total sleep time (*e.g.* self-imposed sleep restriction)

- Medication effects (especially in an era of polypharmacy)

- Co-existing sleep disorders

- Depression

- Permanent brain damage from untreated SDB (an irreversible effect of hypoxia?)

D. Surgical Management of Sleep Disordered Breathing

Surgical treatment appears to be most effective and logical modality for patients with mild OSA due to surgically correctable obstructing lesions, *e.g.*, adeno-tonsillar lymphoid tissue hypertrophy that is obstructing the pharyngeal airway [2]. In the absence of an identified anatomic obstruction, there is no consensus regarding any potential role of surgery [266]. Uvulopalatopharyngoplasty (UPPP) is one of the most common surgical procedures that is performed in this context and entails resection of the uvula, any redundant retroglossal soft tissue, and palatine tonsillar lymphoid tissue. Laser-assisted ablation (LAA) and radiofrequency ablation (RFA) are less invasive variants of the traditional UPPP. Other common surgical procedures for OSA include septoplasty, rhinoplasty, nasal turbinate reduction, nasal polypectomy, tonsillectomy, adenoidectomy, palatal implants (the so-called "pillar procedure"), tongue reduction (partial glossectomy, lingual tonsillectomy), genioglossal advancement/shortening, and maxillomandibular advancement.

The rationale for surgical therapy in OSA is to eliminate the airway obstruction and diminish the resistance to air flow without impairing the upper airway functions. The main mechanisms by which the surgical procedures work are: (1) by-pass the upper airway, which presents the dynamic collapse during sleep (*e.g.*, tracheostomy); (2) soft tissue removal or 'trimming' [*e.g.*, polypectomy, turbinoplasty, adenotonsillectomy, uvulopalatopharyngoplasty, midline glossectomy, basal tongue reduction); and (3) bony and/or soft tissue modifications (*e.g.*, septoplasty, (mandibulo)maxillary expansion, mandibular advancement, geniglossal advancement or shortening, hyoid myotomy suspension, etc]. The main indications of surgery for SDB are listed in Table **2**.

Table 2: Main indications for surgical therapy in sleep disordered breathing (SDB) patients:

Surgical Indications for SDB	Anatomic abnormalities of the upper airway
	Failure of other therapies
	Excessive daytime sleepiness (EDS)
	Respiratory disturbance index (RDI) ≥ 20
	An RDI <20 *and* severe EDS
	Significant hypoxic burden (sleep time with $S_pO2 < 90\%$)
	Arrhythmia or hypertension
	Esophageal pressure $\leq - 10$ cm H_2O

Relative contraindications to upper airway surgery for SDB are: morbid obesity (except bariatric surgery and tracheostomy), decompensated cardiac or respiratory conditions, alcohol or drug abuse, psychosis and other unstable mental disorders [267].

Only a few trials have compared surgery to either conservative management or a nonsurgical therapy [268]. Overall, there is no consistent benefit proven by the available trials in favor of surgical therapy. While this could be a true effect, it may also be due to small sample sizes, heterogeneous patient populations, or short-term follow-ups. As such, one study investigated 32 patients with OSA and more than 50% obstruction at the palatal level; they were randomized to receive either conservative management or UPPP, with or without mandibular osteotomy [269]. At one year, there was improvement of subjective daytime sleepiness with UPPP compared to conservative treatment, according to a non-validated sleepiness scale. More patients in the UPPP group had a normal ODI, but the surgical complication rate was 22%. In another trial, 90 patients with OSA (mean AHI 20) were randomly assigned to receive CPAP, RFA, or sham RFA [270]. RFA improved EDS and quality of life compared to sham RFA, while the AHI was unchanged. In contrast, RFA had no effect on EDS or quality of life compared to CPAP, and AHI was better in the CPAP group. There was no increase in complications in the RFA group in this trial. Usual complications of RFA include: palatal mucosal breakdown, pain (transient neuralgias), tongue base abscesses, airway compromise due to edema [271-274].

The most commonly used technique is the uvulo-palato-pharyngoplasty (UPPP, U3P). In general, this procedure is effective in about half of the patients. Interestingly, it improves the symptoms of OSA but minimal improvement in the apnea pattern. UPPP appears to achieve a surgical cure (*i.e.*, a postoperative AHI of less than 5) in only a minority of patients [275], and may compromise subsequent CPAP therapy by promoting mouth leaking and reducing the maximal level of pressure tolerated by many patients treated subsequently with CPAP [276].

Hyoid suspension, genioglossus advancement are some of the other surgical procedures. Riley *et al.* have taken a progressive approach to the surgical treatment of OSA. A UPPP was performed for retropalatal obstruction alone, genioglossus advancement and hyoid suspension without UPPP for patients with hypopharyngeal obstruction and for obstruction at both sites, all three procedures are done.

If these surgical procedures fail, then a maxillary or mandibular advancement could be considered. Tracheostomy is probably the most definitive surgical procedure for OSA but it carries its own risks and, understandably, is less preferred by the patients.

E. Dental Appliances in the Treatment of OSA

The 50-60% compliance rate with CPAP therapy inexorably led to development of other therapeutic modalities, such as dental or oral appliances, designed to maintain the airway patency during sleep. They fall into two general categories: (1) mandibular advancement devices (MAD), which work by protruding the mandible forward, hence increasing the luminal area of the airway during sleep, and (2) tongue retaining devices (TRD), which seem to work by holding the tongue in place and preventing it to fall backwards, into the upper airway.

Oral appliances are to be prescribed and followed by specialized providers (dentists, orthodontists), experienced in slowly adjusting forward the device (over weeks and months) and in ensuring best outcomes and tolerance to therapy. The specific algorithms of adjustment take into account the maximal protrusion (maximal mandibular advancement, MAA) and then step-wise advancements of the lower jaw as fractions of the MAA, so that the protrusive titration would not compromise patient's comfort and tolerance for the device.

So far, oral appliances have been shown to decrease the frequency of respiratory events, arousals, and episodes of oxyhemoglobin desaturation, compared to no treatment or a sham intervention. They may also improve daytime sleepiness, quality of life, and neurocognitive function. Their impact on mortality is currently unknown. Most of the trials conducted so far have evaluated the effects of MADs, and less so the effects and tolerability of TRDs.

From available evidence, MADs seem to reduce the frequency of respiratory events and arousals during sleep, improve oxygenation and diminish significantly snoring [277-279]. Several studies have suggested that complete resolution of OSA can be obtained, especially in patients with mild or moderate OSA (AHI < 30), and less so in severe OSA (AHI ≥30) [2,279], while others have not confirmed the same findings [277,278]. Until further large-scale studies are conducted, the gold standard for primary therapy for OSA patients remains CPAP therapy [2].

MADs have also been shown to be effective in short-term symptomatic improvement, by decreasing the level of EDS [279,280], although it is hard to discern how much this is a placebo-effect or an ascertainment bias. One randomized cross-over trial on 68 patients with OSA (RDI ≥10 *and* at least two symptoms or signs of OSA) investigated the efficacy of a MAD versus a control device and showed after 4 weeks of therapy a statistically significant improvement in mean sleep latency (10 versus 9 minutes) and ESS (7 versus 9) [278]. When an oral appliance was compared to CPAP therapy, a French group found that both therapies reduced daytime sleepiness versus baseline (assessed by ESS and OSLER test) [281]. Both treatments significantly improved subjective and objective sleepiness, cognitive tests and health-related quality of life. The reported compliance was higher for MAD, with more than 70% of patients preferring this treatment. Although overall less effective than CPAP, successfully titrated MAD was very effective at reducing the AHI and was associated with a higher reported compliance. Furthermore, one-night MAD titration had a low negative predictive value for treatment success [281]. Oral appliances have also been reported to improve driving simulator performance, with a magnitude of effect similar to that seen after successful CPAP therapy [282].

Several studies have reported hemodynamic (reductions of blood pressure), neurocognitive, and quality of life improvements [278,280,283,284]. In one Australian study [278], the effect of a MAD was a reduction in the awake mean systolic and diastolic blood pressures, with the peak effect (approximately 3 mmHg) noted during the late sleeping period and early morning. In a more recent study by Andren *et al* [284], at 3 years of therapy with a dental appliance, systolic and diastolic blood pressure improved by 25 and 10 mm Hg, respectively, a magnitude of effect which is very high and may input other contributors over time.

The subjective and objective favorable effects of MAD seem to be persistent in the long run for many patients, although it is currently unclear which exact category of patients benefits the most [279,285-287]. In one observational study on 619 patients [287], treatment was successful (defined as an AHI < 10) at one year in 54% of patients and 24% discontinued the treatment with a MAD. Female gender predicted treatment success, defined as an AHI of less than 10 in both supine and lateral positions, with an OR of 2.4 (p = 0.01). In women, the ORs for treatment success were 12 for mild sleep apnea (p = 0.04), and 0.1 for complaints of nasal obstruction (p = 0.03). In men, the OR for treatment success were 6.0 for supine-dependent sleep apneas (p<0.001), 2.5 for mild sleep apnea (p = 0.04), 1.3 for each millimeter of mandibular advancement (p = 0.03), and 0.8 for each kilogram of weight increase (p = 0.001). In an earlier observational study from the same group, on 33 consecutive patients with OSA (mean AHI 22) treated with MAD [286]. Among the 19 patients who returned for follow-up at 5 years from inception, treatment was successful (defined as an AHI <10) in 84% of them.

Not surprisingly, most clinical trials which compared MADs to CPAP found that PAP is superior in normalizing AHI and sleep oxygenation, but not necessarily in improving symptoms (*e.g.*, EDS), arousal index, or overall sleep architecture [218,280-282,288]. For reasons probably related to ease of use and comfort, patients generally comply better with the dental appliance therapy.

Recently, in an interesting cross-over polysomnographic study from Japan [289], in which both oral appliances and CPAP therapy were used for therapy, the median baseline AHI was reduced with the oral appliances from 36 to 12 in thirty-five patients. In this study, OSA patients with an optimal CPAP of 10.5 cm H_2O or higher were unlikely to respond to oral appliance therapy. This type of predictive model may become in the future clinically useful for identifying the optimal categories of patients who could benefit from oral appliances for the therapy of OSA.

On the other hand, clinical studies comparing oral appliances with surgical interventions are very scarce. In one study done in Sweden, patients with OSA (AHI 5-25) were randomly assigned to receive UPPP or a MAD that protruded the mandible to 50% of the maximum [290]. At 1 year, the success rate (% of patients with at least 50% reduction in AI) in the MAD group was 81%, versus 53% in the UPPP group (p < 0.05). After 4 years of therapy, normalization (AI < 5 or AHI < 10) was observed in 63% of the MAD group and 33% in the UPPP group, while the compliance rate for MAD was only 62%. Pronounced complaints of nasopharyngeal regurgitation of fluid and difficulty with swallowing after UPPP were reported by 8% and 10%, respectively. Overall, the dental appliances had few adverse effects on the stomatognathic system and required only moderate adjustments.

The side effects of dental appliances are generally encountered early during therapy and are represented by dental discomfort (in upper or lower incisors), temporomandibular joint pain, either xerostomia or hypersalivation, gingival irritation, and, occasionally, bruxism [279]. These side effects are generally mild and self-limited to several weeks or less and do not seem to be frequent reasons for therapy discontinuation. In the medium-long term (> 2 years of therapy), occlusal changes can occur due to dental appliance therapy, *e.g.*, retroposition of the upper incisors and forward movement of the lower teeth and jaw, ranging from 0.4 to 3 mm [291,292]. In one observational study on 70 patients, with an average follow-up of 7 years, occlusal changes were diagnosed in 86% of patients treated with dental appliances [293]. Nevertheless, further research is needed to define the factors that can predict long-term outcomes and complications.

In summary, dental appliances can be used in mild and moderate OSA, if the patient's opts for this therapeutic modality, or if the patient cannot tolerate CPAP therapy. In severe OSA oral appliances should not be used as first line therapy, unless major contraindications or intolerance to CPAP is encountered.

RESEARCH OUTLOOK

What do we know:

Pathophysiology of OSA

OSA is a common disorder, characterized by repetitive narrowing or collapse of the pharyngeal airway during sleep. During sleep, important physiologic changes occur pertaining to breathing, neurologic control of ventilation, cardiovascular and autonomic tone, hormonal milieu, *etc.* These changes, corroborated with different anatomic factors and environmental contributions, pave the way to the development of sleep disordered breathing (SDB). This encompasses a spectrum of conditions which are listed here in crescendo order of severity (and without implying a continuum of progression) as follows: primary snoring and upper airway resistance syndrome (PS and UARS, see Chapter 5), obstructive sleep apnea (OSA), central sleep apnea (CSA, see Chapter 7) and obesity hypoventilation syndrome (OHS, see Chapter 8).

Understanding the normal sleep-wake cycle is important in the elucidation of the OSA pathogenesis. The sleep-wake cycle is thought to be regulated through interactions between multiple sets of neurons and various neuromodulators [80]. Recent evidence suggests that during wakefulness, adenosine accumulates extracellularly (especially in the basal forebrain), and this probably constitutes the main homeostatic drive to sleep (or the biomarker of sleep debt) [294]. Increasing levels of extracellular adenosine is thought to inhibit specific wake-active neurons (noradrenergic, serotonergic and histaminergic neurons), resulting in activation of ventrolateral preoptic neurons (VLPO), which may be the "master switch" that turns on the sleep process [295]. VLPO neurons are silent during wakefulness and start firing at sleep onset and allow NREM sleep to set in. As firing of the monoaminergic neurons decreases during NREM sleep, cholinergic neurons start firing and REM sleep sets in. This cycle of NREM and REM sleep repeats generally every 90-120 min. The sleep stages have different effects on respiratory physiology, hence they have different propensity to generate SDB.

Research indicates that both anatomic and neuromuscular factors are important in predisposing the pharynx to collapse. As such, several major theories have been proposed to explain the pathogenesis of OSA:

The Anatomical Theory

It is possible that most patients with OSA have an anatomically small pharyngeal airway. This concept is supported by studies done by Haponik and colleagues [296], who reported a reduced cross sectional airway size in the nasopharynx, oropharynx and hypopharynx of patients with OSA. They compared 10 normal subjects with 20 apneic patients during wakefulness and measured airway luminal size using CT imaging. Similar studies, done by Schwab *et al* [136,137,297], reported that large tongue and lateral pharyngeal wall size independently increased the risk for sleep apnea. The difference between these two groups was that while Haponik *et al* measured the airway luminal size, Schwab measured the actual size of the pharyngeal structures, rather than the endoluminal opening. This concept was yet again supported by the work done by Isono and Remmers [298,299], who studied patients under general anesthesia and complete muscle paralysis. They showed that patients with apnea have higher collapsing pressures and a smaller airway size than normal control subjects. This shows that true anatomical differences are present and that the results of the study are not confounded by the contribution from dilator muscle activity.

Women tend to have a smaller pharynx and oropharyngeal junctions compared to men, but overall tend to have a lower prevalence of OSA, suggesting that anatomical factors may not be sufficient to produce pharyngeal collapse during sleep. Thus, neuromuscular factors must play a role in protecting the patency of the airway.

In the Starling resistor model [300-302], the pharynx is considered a collapsible segment, which is bound by an upstream (Pus) and downstream (Pds) pressure and resistance. Pus is technically the atmospheric barometric pressure and Pds as the tracheal pressure. According to this model, Pcrit is the pressure surrounding the collapsible segment of the pharynx [302] (see Fig. 2). Occlusion in the collapsible segment of the upper airway occurs when the surrounding pressure (Pcrit) becomes greater than the intraluminal pressure. Flow normally occurs when Pus>Pds>Pcrit. Complete occlusion of the upper airway occurs when Pcrit>Pus>Pds. Flow limitation occurs when Pus>Pcrit>Pds. Flow limitation is seen in cases of snoring, hypopneas or upper airway resistance syndrome (UARS). Measurements of Pcrit have shown to range from < -10cm H2O in normal breathing, -10 to -5 cm of H2O in primary snoring, -5 to 0 cm H2O in obstructive hypopneas, and, finally, > 0 cm H2O in apneas during sleep [301]. Pcrit depends on the relative contributions of the anatomically imposed mechanical loads and the dynamic neuromuscular responses.

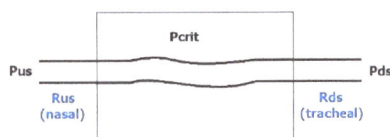

Figure 2: Starling resistor model of the upper airway, where the pharynx is considered a collapsible segment, with an upstream (P_{us}) and downstream (P_{ds}) pressure and R_{us} and R_{ds} resistances. P_{us} is technically the atmospheric barometric pressure and P_{ds} as the tracheal pressure. According to this model, P_{crit} is the pressure surrounding the collapsible segment of the pharynx.

The Neurological Control Theory

There are more than 20 muscles in the human pharynx. To better study the effects of sleep-wake cycle on these muscles, these are further grouped as phasic (*e.g.*, genioglossus) and tonic or postural muscles (*e.g.*, *tensor palatini*). Among oropharyngeal muscles, genioglossus muscle has been studied more extensively, mainly due to its airway dilator activity.

The activity of the pharyngeal dilator muscles is controlled by many factors [80,303,304]:

1) Input from respiratory neurons in medulla, which leads to inspiratory phasic activation of the genioglossus, preparing the upper airway for negative inspiratory pressure even before the inspiratory

flow begins; this suggests coordination at the level of central nervous system between upper airway and diaphragm;

2)   Rising PaCO2 and falling PaO2, as potent stimuli for the central drive to the upper airway and decreasing pharyngeal collapsibility;

3)   Negative intrapharyngeal pressure - the most important local stimulus for the activation of the pharyngeal muscles during wakefulness, which is supported by the evidence that topical anesthesia substantially reduces this reflex and positive pressure (CPAP) reduces the genioglossus EMG tonus to nearly normal levels in patients with OSA, but has little effect in controls (suggesting that increased upper airway dilator muscle activity even during wake state compensates for a more anatomically narrow upper airway in the OSA patient);

4)   State-sensitive activity of the muscles - transition from wake to sleep is associated with initial fall but with subsequent recovery of genioglossus activity and continued fall in the activity of *tensor palatini* muscle activity during sleep (20-30% of wake activity during stage N3 of sleep). During sleep, the negative pressure reflex is also substantially diminished or lost completely, more so in patients with apnea. This decrease in muscle activity in patients who have anatomically small and collapsible airway leads to pharyngeal collapse resulting in apnea.

Other Factors Involved in Pathogenesis (Other Theories)

It has also been hypothesized that repetitive opening and closing of the upper airway and vibratory trauma lead to muscle and neuronal fiber injury with subsequent functional sensorimotor dysfunction of these muscles. This could attenuate the response of the muscles to the markedly negative airway pressures generated during periods of airway obstruction.

Respiratory instability may also play a role in the pathogenesis of OSA and "loop gain" (a concept from engineering) is the current best model explaining it. Respiratory instability is likely to be more important in patients with only a mild pharyngeal anatomical deficiency. Loop gain is basically a measurement of the tendency of the ventilator control system to amplify respiration in response to a stimulus or perturbation. Techniques have been developed to measure loop gain of the respiratory system, such as proportional assist ventilation technique (PAV) [303,304]. Patients with high loop gain (>1) have a more unstable respiratory control system, as seen in patients with OSA compared with people with loop gain of <1 who can stabilize the airway in response to the same perturbation.

Reduction in lung volume during sleep due to decreased functional residual capacity (FRC) may also lead to loss of "tracheal tug" on the upper airway, resulting in decreased airway size and increased airway resistance. This potentially increases the risk of airway collapse during sleep.

What we don't know:

*   Currently, nasal CPAP is the gold standard of treatment of moderate to severe OSA [2]. However, many patients do not use it at all, or they use it infrequently. Comparative, intention-to-treat trials involving all degrees of OSA severity are still needed to delineate specific treatment pathways and necessary interventions. The studies, which will focus on comparative treatments and how to obtain better acceptance of and compliance with CPAP, will form the next phase in the developing of this treatment. A viable pharmacologic therapy for sleep apnea [214] does not appear to be in the near-future, although the strides made by pharmaceutical industry in this field may make it closer than we previously thought.

*   Although acceptable CPAP compliance is often defined as use of at least 4 hours per night, optimal CPAP use for individual patients is not known. More refined risk stratification may be needed and risk reduction may be a function of more specific prescription and/or use.

*   What is the role and efficacy of alternative therapies – such as mandibular advancing devices and surgical procedures in moderate and severe OSA?

*   To what extent hypoxia versus re-oxygenation are deleterious and to try to find markers of susceptibility to hypoxia (endocrine, cardiovascular, neurologic, etc)?

- Air insufflation by nasal cannula has been shown to be useful in reducing the SDB severity [230,231]; we still need to clarify if this can be useful in our therapeutic armamentarium and to what degree the achieved reduction in the AHI translates into better long-term outcomes.

- So far, the role of oxygen in the SDB therapy has not been clearly elucidated (neither alone nor in combination with PAP); future research needs to clarify what is the "dangerous level" of hypoxic burden and to better characterize surrogate markers of succeptibility to hypoxia and consequently to poor outcomes in SDB

- It is still unclear if transtracheal route of oxygen delivery is effective and superior to nasal cannula administration in reducing OSA severity

- It is currently still unclear what is the optimal algorithm for SDB therapy (targeting the best outcomes) that would incorporate the available modalities (CPAP, dental appliances and surgery)

REFERENCES

[1]   Guilleminault C, Tilkian A, Dement WC. The sleep apnea syndromes. Annu Rev Med 1976; 27: 465-84.

[2]   Epstein LJ, Kristo D, Strollo PJ, Jr., Friedman N, Malhotra A, Patil SP *et al.* Clinical guideline for the evaluation, management and long-term care of obstructive sleep apnea in adults. J Clin Sleep Med 2009; 5(3): 263-76.

[3]   Broadbent WH. Cheyne Stokes respiration in cerebral hemorrhage. Lancet 1877; 3: 307-9.

[4]   Lavie P. Restless Nights: Understanding Snoring and Sleep Apnea. New Haven, CT: Yale University Press. 2003.

[5]   Lavie P. Nothing new under the moon. Historical accounts of sleep apnea syndrome. Arch Intern Med 1984; 144(10): 2025-8.

[6]   Cheyne J. A case of apoplexy in which the fleshy part of the heart was connected to fat. Dublin Hospital Report 1818; 2: 216-23.

[7]   Stokes W. The Diseases of the Heart and Aorta. Dublin: 1854.

[8]   Young T, Palta M, Dempsey J, Skatrud J, Weber S, Badr S. The occurrence of sleep-disordered breathing among middle-aged adults. N Engl J Med 1993; 328(17): 1230-5.

[9]   Young T, Peppard PE, Gottlieb DJ. Epidemiology of obstructive sleep apnea: a population health perspective. Am J Respir Crit Care Med 2002; 165(9): 1217-39.

[10]   Stradling JR, Crosby JH. Predictors and prevalence of obstructive sleep apnoea and snoring in 1001 middle aged men. Thorax 1991; 46(2): 85-90.

[11]   Jennum P, Sjol A. Epidemiology of snoring and obstructive sleep apnoea in a Danish population, age 30-60. J Sleep Res 1992; 1(4): 240-4.

[12]   Punjabi NM. The epidemiology of adult obstructive sleep apnea. Proc Am Thorac Soc 2008; 5(2): 136-43.

[13]   Bixler EO, Vgontzas AN, Ten HT, Tyson K, Kales A. Effects of age on sleep apnea in men: I. Prevalence and severity. Am J Respir Crit Care Med 1998; 157(1): 144-8.

[14]   Bixler EO, Vgontzas AN, Lin HM, Ten HT, Rein J, Vela-Bueno A, Kales A. Prevalence of sleep-disordered breathing in women: effects of gender. Am J Respir Crit Care Med 2001; 163(3 Pt 1): 608-13.

[15]   Bearpark H, Elliott L, Grunstein R, Cullen S, Schneider H, Althaus W, Sullivan C. Snoring and sleep apnea. A population study in Australian men. Am J Respir Crit Care Med 1995; 151(5): 1459-65.

[16]   Duran J, Esnaola S, Rubio R, Iztueta A. Obstructive sleep apnea-hypopnea and related clinical features in a population-based sample of subjects aged 30 to 70 yr. Am J Respir Crit Care Med 2001; 163(3 Pt 1): 685-9.

[17]   Ip MS, Lam B, Lauder IJ, Tsang KW, Chung KF, Mok YW, Lam WK. A community study of sleep-disordered breathing in middle-aged Chinese men in Hong Kong. Chest 2001; 119(1): 62-9.

[18]   Ip MS, Lam B, Tang LC, Lauder IJ, Ip TY, Lam WK. A community study of sleep-disordered breathing in middle-aged Chinese women in Hong Kong: prevalence and gender differences. Chest 2004; 125(1): 127-34.

[19]   Udwadia ZF, Doshi AV, Lonkar SG, Singh CI. Prevalence of sleep-disordered breathing and sleep apnea in middle-aged urban Indian men. Am J Respir Crit Care Med 2004; 169(2): 168-73.

[20]   Puvanendran K, Goh KL. From snoring to sleep apnea in a Singapore population. Sleep Res Online 1999; 2(1): 11-4.

[21]   Gislason T, Almqvist M, Eriksson G, Taube A, Boman G. Prevalence of sleep apnea syndrome among Swedish men--an epidemiological study. J Clin Epidemiol 1988; 41(6): 571-6.

[22]   Tishler PV, Larkin EK, Schluchter MD, Redline S. Incidence of sleep-disordered breathing in an urban adult population: the relative importance of risk factors in the development of sleep-disordered breathing. JAMA 2003; 289(17): 2230-7.

[23]   Worsnop CJ, Naughton MT, Barter CE, Morgan TO, Anderson AI, Pierce RJ. The prevalence of obstructive sleep apnea in hypertensives. Am J Respir Crit Care Med 1998; 157(1): 111-5.

[24] Logan AG, Perlikowski SM, Mente A, Tisler A, Tkacova R, Niroumand M *et al.* High prevalence of unrecognized sleep apnoea in drug-resistant hypertension. J Hypertens 2001; 19(12): 2271-7.

[25] Peppard PE, Young T, Palta M, Skatrud J. Prospective study of the association between sleep-disordered breathing and hypertension. N Engl J Med 2000; 342(19): 1378-84.

[26] Andreas S, Schulz R, Werner GS, Kreuzer H. Prevalence of obstructive sleep apnoea in patients with coronary artery disease. Coron Artery Dis 1996; 7(7): 541-5.

[27] Shahar E, Whitney CW, Redline S, Lee ET, Newman AB, Javier NF *et al.* Sleep-disordered breathing and cardiovascular disease: cross-sectional results of the Sleep Heart Health Study. Am J Respir Crit Care Med 2001; 163(1): 19-25.

[28] Young T, Evans L, Finn L, Palta M. Estimation of the clinically diagnosed proportion of sleep apnea syndrome in middle-aged men and women. Sleep 1997; 20(9): 705-6.

[29] Kapur V, Strohl KP, Redline S, Iber C, O'Connor G, Nieto J. Underdiagnosis of sleep apnea syndrome in U.S. communities. Sleep Breath 2002; 6(2): 49-54.

[30] Foley DJ, Monjan AA, Brown SL, Simonsick EM, Wallace RB, Blazer DG. Sleep complaints among elderly persons: an epidemiologic study of three communities. Sleep 1995; 18(6): 425-32.

[31] Ancoli-Israel S, Kripke DF, Klauber MR, Mason WJ, Fell R, Kaplan O. Sleep-disordered breathing in community-dwelling elderly. Sleep 1991; 14(6): 486-95.

[32] Young T, Skatrud J, Peppard PE. Risk factors for obstructive sleep apnea in adults. JAMA 2004; 291(16): 2013-6.

[33] Obesity and overweight, 2006. World Health Organization. Available online at: www.who.int/mediacentre/factsheets/fs311/en/index.html.

[34] Obesity in US Adults: 2007. American Obesity Association. 2007. Available online at: http://www.obesity.org/statistics/.

[35] Katz I, Stradling J, Slutsky AS, Zamel N, Hoffstein V. Do patients with obstructive sleep apnea have thick necks? Am Rev Respir Dis 1990; 141(5 Pt 1): 1228-31.

[36] Grunstein R, Wilcox I, Yang TS, Gould Y, Hedner J. Snoring and sleep apnoea in men: association with central obesity and hypertension. Int J Obes Relat Metab Disord 1993; 17(9): 533-40.

[37] Davies RJ, Stradling JR. The relationship between neck circumference, radiographic pharyngeal anatomy, and the obstructive sleep apnoea syndrome. Eur Respir J 1990; 3(5): 509-14.

[38] Davies RJ, Ali NJ, Stradling JR. Neck circumference and other clinical features in the diagnosis of the obstructive sleep apnoea syndrome. Thorax 1992; 47(2): 101-5.

[39] Hoffstein V, Mateika S. Differences in abdominal and neck circumferences in patients with and without obstructive sleep apnoea. Eur Respir J 1992; 5(4): 377-81.

[40] Levinson PD, McGarvey ST, Carlisle CC, Eveloff SE, Herbert PN, Millman RP. Adiposity and cardiovascular risk factors in men with obstructive sleep apnea. Chest 1993; 103(5): 1336-42.

[41] Millman RP, Carlisle CC, McGarvey ST, Eveloff SE, Levinson PD. Body fat distribution and sleep apnea severity in women. Chest 1995; 107(2): 362-6.

[42] Shelton KE, Woodson H, Gay S, Suratt PM. Pharyngeal fat in obstructive sleep apnea. Am Rev Respir Dis 1993; 148(2): 462-6.

[43] Shinohara E, Kihara S, Yamashita S, Yamane M, Nishida M, Arai T *et al.* Visceral fat accumulation as an important risk factor for obstructive sleep apnoea syndrome in obese subjects. J Intern Med 1997; 241(1): 11-8.

[44] Ferini-Strambi L, Zucconi M, Palazzi S, Castronovo V, Oldani A, Della MG, Smirne S. Snoring and nocturnal oxygen desaturations in an Italian middle-aged male population. Epidemiologic study with an ambulatory device. Chest 1994; 105(6): 1759-64.

[45] Newman AB, Nieto FJ, Guidry U, Lind BK, Redline S, Pickering TG, Quan SF. Relation of sleep-disordered breathing to cardiovascular disease risk factors: the Sleep Heart Health Study. Am J Epidemiol 2001; 154(1): 50-9.

[46] Olson LG, King MT, Hensley MJ, Saunders NA. A community study of snoring and sleep-disordered breathing. Prevalence. Am J Respir Crit Care Med 1995; 152(2): 711-6.

[47] Jennum P, Hein HO, Suadicani P, Gyntelberg F. Cardiovascular risk factors in snorers. A cross-sectional study of 3,323 men aged 54 to 74 years: the Copenhagen Male Study. Chest 1992; 102(5): 1371-6.

[48] Jennum P, Sjol A. Snoring, sleep apnoea and cardiovascular risk factors: the MONICA II Study. Int J Epidemiol 1993; 22(3): 439-44.

[49] Schmidt-Nowara WW, Coultas DB, Wiggins C, Skipper BE, Samet JM. Snoring in a Hispanic-American population. Risk factors and association with hypertension and other morbidity. Arch Intern Med 1990; 150(3): 597-601.

[50] Bliwise DL. Epidemiology of age-dependence in sleep disordered breathing (SDB) in old age: The Bay Area Sleep Cohort (BASC). Sleep Med Clin 2009; 4(1): 57-64.

[51] Frey WC, Pilcher J. Obstructive sleep-related breathing disorders in patients evaluated for bariatric surgery. Obes Surg 2003; 13(5): 676-83.

[52]   O'Keeffe T, Patterson EJ. Evidence supporting routine polysomnography before bariatric surgery. Obes Surg 2004; 14(1): 23-6.

[53]   Bae C, Schauer P, Chand B, Ioachimescu OC, Foldvary-Schaefer N. Clinical and polysomnographic features of bariatric surgery candidates with suspected sleep apnea. Sleep 29[Abstract Supplement], A215. 2006.

[54]   Jennum P, Riha RL. Epidemiology of sleep apnoea/hypopnoea syndrome and sleep-disordered breathing. Eur Respir J 2009; 33(4): 907-14.

[55]   Flemons WW. Clinical practice. Obstructive sleep apnea. N Engl J Med 2002; 347(7): 498-504.

[56]   Pillar G, Lavie P. Assessment of the role of inheritance in sleep apnea syndrome. Am J Respir Crit Care Med 1995; 151(3 Pt 1): 688-91.

[57]   Mathur R, Douglas NJ. Family studies in patients with the sleep apnea-hypopnea syndrome. Ann Intern Med 1995; 122(3): 174-8.

[58]   Redline S, Tishler PV, Tosteson TD, Williamson J, Kump K, Browner I *et al.* The familial aggregation of obstructive sleep apnea. Am J Respir Crit Care Med 1995; 151(3 Pt 1): 682-7.

[59]   Ovchinsky A, Rao M, Lotwin I, Goldstein NA. The familial aggregation of pediatric obstructive sleep apnea syndrome. Arch Otolaryngol Head Neck Surg 2002; 128(7): 815-8.

[60]   Carmelli D, Bliwise DL, Swan GE, Reed T. Genetic factors in self-reported snoring and excessive daytime sleepiness: a twin study. Am J Respir Crit Care Med 2001; 164(6): 949-52.

[61]   Jennum P, Hein HO, Suadicani P, Sorensen H, Gyntelberg F. Snoring, family history, and genetic markers in men. The Copenhagen Male Study. Chest 1995; 107(5): 1289-93.

[62]   Riha RL, Gislasson T, Diefenbach K. The phenotype and genotype of adult obstructive sleep apnoea/hypopnoea syndrome. Eur Respir J 2009; 33(3): 646-55.

[63]   Palmer LJ, Buxbaum SG, Larkin E, Patel SR, Elston RC, Tishler PV, Redline S. A whole-genome scan for obstructive sleep apnea and obesity. Am J Hum Genet 2003; 72(2): 340-50.

[64]   Palmer LJ, Buxbaum SG, Larkin EK, Patel SR, Elston RC, Tishler PV, Redline S. Whole genome scan for obstructive sleep apnea and obesity in African-American families. Am J Respir Crit Care Med 2004; 169(12): 1314-21.

[65]   Patel SR, Larkin EK, Redline S. Shared genetic basis for obstructive sleep apnea and adiposity measures. Int J Obes (Lond) 2008; 32(5): 795-800.

[66]   Schwab RJ, Pasirstein M, Kaplan L, Pierson R, Mackley A, Hachadoorian R *et al.* Family aggregation of upper airway soft tissue structures in normal subjects and patients with sleep apnea. Am J Respir Crit Care Med 2006; 173(4): 453-63.

[67]   Li KK, Powell NB, Kushida C, Riley RW, Adornato B, Guilleminault C. A comparison of Asian and white patients with obstructive sleep apnea syndrome. Laryngoscope 1999; 109(12): 1937-40.

[68]   Lam B, Ip MS, Tench E, Ryan CF. Craniofacial profile in Asian and white subjects with obstructive sleep apnoea. Thorax 2005; 60(6): 504-10.

[69]   Wellman A, Jordan AS, Malhotra A, Fogel RB, Katz ES, Schory K *et al.* Ventilatory control and airway anatomy in obstructive sleep apnea. Am J Respir Crit Care Med 2004; 170(11): 1225-32.

[70]   Wetter DW, Young TB, Bidwell TR, Badr MS, Palta M. Smoking as a risk factor for sleep-disordered breathing. Arch Intern Med 1994; 154(19): 2219-24.

[71]   Lavie L, Lavie P. Smoking interacts with sleep apnea to increase cardiovascular risk. Sleep Med 2008; 9(3): 247-53.

[72]   Mitler MM, Dawson A, Henriksen SJ, Sobers M, Bloom FE. Bedtime ethanol increases resistance of upper airways and produces sleep apneas in asymptomatic snorers. Alcohol Clin Exp Res 1988; 12(6): 801-5.

[73]   Berry RB, Bonnet MH, Light RW. Effect of ethanol on the arousal response to airway occlusion during sleep in normal subjects. Am Rev Respir Dis 1992; 145(2 Pt 1): 445-52.

[74]   Scanlan MF, Roebuck T, Little PJ, Redman JR, Naughton MT. Effect of moderate alcohol upon obstructive sleep apnoea. Eur Respir J 2000; 16(5): 909-13.

[75]   Al Lawati NM, Patel SR, Ayas NT. Epidemiology, risk factors, and consequences of obstructive sleep apnea and short sleep duration. Prog Cardiovasc Dis 2009; 51(4): 285-93.

[76]   Young T, Finn L, Kim H. Nasal obstruction as a risk factor for sleep-disordered breathing. The University of Wisconsin Sleep and Respiratory Research Group. J Allergy Clin Immunol 1997; 99(2): S757-S762.

[77]   Marshall NS, Wong KK, Liu PY, Cullen SR, Knuiman MW, Grunstein RR. Sleep apnea as an independent risk factor for all-cause mortality: the Busselton Health Study. Sleep 2008; 31(8): 1079-85.

[78]   McNicholas WT, Tarlo S, Cole P, Zamel N, Rutherford R, Griffin D, Phillipson EA. Obstructive apneas during sleep in patients with seasonal allergic rhinitis. Am Rev Respir Dis 1982; 126(4): 625-8.

[79]   Mirza N, Lanza DC. The nasal airway and obstructed breathing during sleep. Otolaryngol Clin North Am 1999; 32(2): 243-62.

[80]   White DP. The pathogenesis of obstructive sleep apnea: advances in the past 100 years. Am J Respir Cell Mol Biol 2006; 34(1): 1-6.

[81]   Fogel RB, Malhotra A, Pillar G, Pittman SD, Dunaif A, White DP. Increased prevalence of obstructive sleep apnea syndrome in obese women with polycystic ovary syndrome. J Clin Endocrinol Metab 2001; 86(3): 1175-80.

[82]   Vgontzas AN, Legro RS, Bixler EO, Grayev A, Kales A, Chrousos GP. Polycystic ovary syndrome is associated with obstructive sleep apnea and daytime sleepiness: role of insulin resistance. J Clin Endocrinol Metab 2001; 86(2): 517-20.

[83]   Schneider BK, Pickett CK, Zwillich CW, Weil JV, McDermott MT, Santen RJ *et al.* Influence of testosterone on breathing during sleep. J Appl Physiol 1986; 61(2): 618-23.

[84]   Liu PY, Yee B, Wishart SM, Jimenez M, Jung DG, Grunstein RR, Handelsman DJ. The short-term effects of high-dose testosterone on sleep, breathing, and function in older men. J Clin Endocrinol Metab 2003; 88(8): 3605-13.

[85]   Winkelman JW, Goldman H, Piscatelli N, Lukas SE, Dorsey CM, Cunningham S. Are thyroid function tests necessary in patients with suspected sleep apnea? Sleep 1996; 19(10): 790-3.

[86]   Lanfranco F, Motta G, Minetto MA, Baldi M, Balbo M, Ghigo E *et al.* Neuroendocrine alterations in obese patients with sleep apnea syndrome. Int J Endocrinol 2010; 2010: 474518.

[87]   Grunstein RR, Ho KY, Sullivan CE. Sleep apnea in acromegaly. Ann Intern Med 1991; 115(7): 527-32.

[88]   Fatti LM, Scacchi M, Pincelli AI, Lavezzi E, Cavagnini F. Prevalence and pathogenesis of sleep apnea and lung disease in acromegaly. Pituitary 2001; 4(4): 259-62.

[89]   Mestron A, Webb SM, Astorga R, Benito P, Catala M, Gaztambide S *et al.* Epidemiology, clinical characteristics, outcome, morbidity and mortality in acromegaly based on the Spanish Acromegaly Registry (Registro Espanol de Acromegalia, REA). Eur J Endocrinol 2004; 151(4): 439-46.

[90]   Gupta RM, Parvizi J, Hanssen AD, Gay PC. Postoperative complications in patients with obstructive sleep apnea syndrome undergoing hip or knee replacement: a case-control study. Mayo Clin Proc 2001; 76(9): 897-905.

[91]   Kaw R, Golish J, Ghamande S, Burgess R, Foldvary N, Walker E. Incremental risk of obstructive sleep apnea on cardiac surgical outcomes. J Cardiovasc Surg (Torino) 2006; 47(6): 683-9.

[92]   Schafer H, Koehler U, Ewig S, Hasper E, Tasci S, Luderitz B. Obstructive sleep apnea as a risk marker in coronary artery disease. Cardiology 1999; 92(2): 79-84.

[93]   Peker Y, Kraiczi H, Hedner J, Loth S, Johansson A, Bende M. An independent association between obstructive sleep apnoea and coronary artery disease. Eur Respir J 1999; 14(1): 179-84.

[94]   Gami AS, Howard DE, Olson EJ, Somers VK. Day-night pattern of sudden death in obstructive sleep apnea. N Engl J Med 2005; 352(12): 1206-14.

[95]   Arzt M, Young T, Finn L, Skatrud JB, Bradley TD. Association of sleep-disordered breathing and the occurrence of stroke. Am J Respir Crit Care Med 2005; 172(11): 1447-51.

[96]   Yaggi HK, Concato J, Kernan WN, Lichtman JH, Brass LM, Mohsenin V. Obstructive sleep apnea as a risk factor for stroke and death. N Engl J Med 2005; 353(19): 2034-41.

[97]   Krieger J, Sforza E, Apprill M, Lampert E, Weitzenblum E, Ratomaharo J. Pulmonary hypertension, hypoxemia, and hypercapnia in obstructive sleep apnea patients. Chest 1989; 96(4): 729-37.

[98]   Ambrosetti M, Lucioni A, Ageno W, Conti S, Neri M. Is venous thromboembolism more frequent in patients with obstructive sleep apnea syndrome? J Thromb Haemost 2004; 2(10): 1858-60.

[99]   Jean-Louis G, Zizi F, Clark LT, Brown CD, McFarlane SI. Obstructive sleep apnea and cardiovascular disease: role of the metabolic syndrome and its components. J Clin Sleep Med 2008; 4(3): 261-72.

[100] Punjabi NM, Shahar E, Redline S, Gottlieb DJ, Givelber R, Resnick HE. Sleep-disordered breathing, glucose intolerance, and insulin resistance: the Sleep Heart Health Study. Am J Epidemiol 2004; 160(6): 521-30.

[101] Marin JM, Carrizo SJ, Vicente E, Agusti AG. Long-term cardiovascular outcomes in men with obstructive sleep apnoea-hypopnoea with or without treatment with continuous positive airway pressure: an observational study. Lancet 2005; 365(9464): 1046-53.

[102] Nieto FJ, Young TB, Lind BK, Shahar E, Samet JM, Redline S *et al.* Association of sleep-disordered breathing, sleep apnea, and hypertension in a large community-based study. Sleep Heart Health Study. JAMA 2000; 283(14): 1829-36.

[103] Peppard PE, Young T, Palta M, Dempsey J, Skatrud J. Longitudinal study of moderate weight change and sleep-disordered breathing. JAMA 2000; 284(23): 3015-21.

[104] Moyer CA, Sonnad SS, Garetz SL, Helman JI, Chervin RD. Quality of life in obstructive sleep apnea: a systematic review of the literature. Sleep Med 2001; 2(6): 477-91.

[105] Engleman HM, Douglas NJ. Sleep, driving and the workplace. Clin Med 2005; 5(2): 113-7.

[106] Sassani A, Findley LJ, Kryger M, Goldlust E, George C, Davidson TM. Reducing motor-vehicle collisions, costs, and fatalities by treating obstructive sleep apnea syndrome. Sleep 2004; 27(3): 453-8.

[107] Lindberg E, Carter N, Gislason T, Janson C. Role of snoring and daytime sleepiness in occupational accidents. Am J Respir Crit Care Med 2001; 164(11): 2031-5.

[108] Saunamaki T, Jehkonen M. A review of executive functions in obstructive sleep apnea syndrome. Acta Neurol Scand 2007; 115(1): 1-11.

[109] Young T, Finn L, Peppard PE, Szklo-Coxe M, Austin D, Nieto FJ *et al.* Sleep disordered breathing and mortality: eighteen-year follow-up of the Wisconsin sleep cohort. Sleep 2008; 31(8): 1071-8.

[110] Wenner JB, Cheema R, Ayas NT. Clinical manifestations and consequences of obstructive sleep apnea. J Cardiopulm Rehabil Prev 2009; 29(2): 76-83.

[111] Cluydts R, De VE, Verstraeten E, Theys P. Daytime sleepiness and its evaluation. Sleep Med Rev 2002; 6(2): 83-96.

[112] Johns MW. A new method for measuring daytime sleepiness: the Epworth sleepiness scale. Sleep 1991; 14(6): 540-5.

[113] Ramachandran SK, Josephs LA. A meta-analysis of clinical screening tests for obstructive sleep apnea. Anesthesiology 2009; 110(4): 928-39.

[114] Netzer NC, Stoohs RA, Netzer CM, Clark K, Strohl KP. Using the Berlin Questionnaire to identify patients at risk for the sleep apnea syndrome. Ann Intern Med 1999; 131(7): 485-91.

[115] Nuckton TJ, Glidden DV, Browner WS, Claman DM. Physical examination: Mallampati score as an independent predictor of obstructive sleep apnea. Sleep 2006; 29(7): 903-8.

[116] Waite PD. Obstructive sleep apnea: a review of the pathophysiology and surgical management. Oral Surg Oral Med Oral Pathol Oral Radiol Endod 1998; 85(4): 352-61.

[117] Ioachimescu OC. The diagnosis and severity of obstructive sleep apnea (OSA): a comprehensive analysis of different predictive models. Sleep (APSS), Minneapolis, June 2007 (Personal Communication).

[118] Netzer N, Eliasson AH, Netzer C, Kristo DA. Overnight pulse oximetry for sleep-disordered breathing in adults: a review. Chest 2001; 120(2): 625-33.

[119] ICSD-2 - The International Classification of Sleep Disorders - Diagnostic and Coding Manual. Second Edition ed. Westchester,IL: American Academy of Sleep Medicine. 2005.

[120] Iber C, Ancoli-Israel S, Chesson A, Quan SF. The AASM Manual for the Scoring of Sleep and Associated Events - Rules, Terminology and Technical Specifications. 1 ed. Westchester, IL: American Academy of Sleep Medicine. 2007.

[121] Collop NA, Anderson WM, Boehlecke B, Claman D, Goldberg R, Gottlieb DJ *et al.* Clinical guidelines for the use of unattended portable monitors in the diagnosis of obstructive sleep apnea in adult patients. Portable Monitoring Task Force of the American Academy of Sleep Medicine. J Clin Sleep Med 2007; 3(7): 737-47.

[122] Littner MR, Kushida C, Wise M, Davila DG, Morgenthaler T, Lee-Chiong T *et al.* Practice parameters for clinical use of the multiple sleep latency test and the maintenance of wakefulness test. Sleep 2005; 28(1): 113-21.

[123] Arand D, Bonnet M, Hurwitz T, Mitler M, Rosa R, Sangal RB. The clinical use of the MSLT and MWT. Sleep 2005; 28(1): 123-44.

[124] Bonnet MH. ACNS clinical controversy: MSLT and MWT have limited clinical utility. J Clin Neurophysiol 2006; 23(1): 50-8.

[125] Morgenthaler T, Alessi C, Friedman L, Owens J, Kapur V, Boehlecke B *et al.* Practice parameters for the use of actigraphy in the assessment of sleep and sleep disorders: an update for 2007. Sleep 2007; 30(4): 519-29.

[126] Bonnet MH, Arand DL. We are chronically sleep deprived. Sleep 1995; 18(10): 908-11.

[127] Guilleminault C, Rosekind M. The arousal threshold: sleep deprivation, sleep fragmentation, and obstructive sleep apnea syndrome. Bull Eur Physiopathol Respir 1981; 17(3): 341-9.

[128] White DP, Douglas NJ, Pickett CK, Zwillich CW, Weil JV. Sleep deprivation and the control of ventilation. Am Rev Respir Dis 1983; 128(6): 984-6.

[129] Bowes G, Woolf GM, Sullivan CE, Phillipson EA. Effect of sleep fragmentation on ventilatory and arousal responses of sleeping dogs to respiratory stimuli. Am Rev Respir Dis 1980; 122(6): 899-908.

[130] Series F, Cormier Y, La FJ, Desmeules M. Mechanisms of the effectiveness of continuous positive airway pressure in obstructive sleep apnea. Sleep 1992; 15(6 Suppl): S47-S49.

[131] Koenig JS, Thach BT. Effects of mass loading on the upper airway. J Appl Physiol 1988; 64(6): 2294-9.

[132] Wolin AD, Strohl KP, Acree BN, Fouke JM. Responses to negative pressure surrounding the neck in anesthetized animals. J Appl Physiol 1990; 68(1): 154-60.

[133] Winter WC, Gampper T, Gay SB, Suratt PM. Lateral pharyngeal fat pad pressure during breathing. Sleep 1996; 19(10 Suppl): S178-S179.

[134] Hoffstein V, Mateika S. Predicting nasal continuous positive airway pressure. Am J Respir Crit Care Med 1994; 150(2): 486-8.

[135] Ryan CF, Love LL. Mechanical properties of the velopharynx in obese patients with obstructive sleep apnea. Am J Respir Crit Care Med 1996; 154(3 Pt 1): 806-12.

[136] Schwab RJ, Gefter WB, Pack AI, Hoffman EA. Dynamic imaging of the upper airway during respiration in normal subjects. J Appl Physiol 1993; 74(4): 1504-14.

[137] Schwab RJ, Gefter WB, Hoffman EA, Gupta KB, Pack AI. Dynamic upper airway imaging during awake respiration in normal subjects and patients with sleep disordered breathing. Am Rev Respir Dis 1993; 148(5): 1385-400.

[138] Winter WC, Gampper T, Gay SB, Suratt PM. Enlargement of the lateral pharyngeal fat pad space in pigs increases upper airway resistance. J Appl Physiol 1995; 79(3): 726-31.

[139] Harman EM, Wynne JW, Block AJ. The effect of weight loss on sleep-disordered breathing and oxygen desaturation in morbidly obese men. Chest 1982; 82(3): 291-4.

[140] Kajaste S, Brander PE, Telakivi T, Partinen M, Mustajoki P. A cognitive-behavioral weight reduction program in the treatment of obstructive sleep apnea syndrome with or without initial nasal CPAP: a randomized study. Sleep Med 2004; 5(2): 125-31.

[141] Schwartz AR, Gold AR, Schubert N, Stryzak A, Wise RA, Permutt S, Smith PL. Effect of weight loss on upper airway collapsibility in obstructive sleep apnea. Am Rev Respir Dis 1991; 144(3 Pt 1): 494-8.

[142] Smith PL, Gold AR, Meyers DA, Haponik EF, Bleecker ER. Weight loss in mildly to moderately obese patients with obstructive sleep apnea. Ann Intern Med 1985; 103(6 (Pt 1)): 850-5.

[143] Suratt PM, McTier RF, Findley LJ, Pohl SL, Wilhoit SC. Changes in breathing and the pharynx after weight loss in obstructive sleep apnea. Chest 1987; 92(4): 631-7.

[144] Buchwald H, Avidor Y, Braunwald E, Jensen MD, Pories W, Fahrbach K, Schoelles K. Bariatric surgery: a systematic review and meta-analysis. JAMA 2004; 292(14): 1724-37.

[145] Frey WC, Pilcher J. Obstructive sleep-related breathing disorders in patients evaluated for bariatric surgery. Obes Surg 2003; 13(5): 676-83.

[146] O'Keeffe T, Patterson EJ. Evidence supporting routine polysomnography before bariatric surgery. Obes Surg 2004; 14(1): 23-6.

[147] Fernandez AZ, Jr., DeMaria EJ, Tichansky DS, Kellum JM, Wolfe LG, Meador J, Sugerman HJ. Experience with over 3,000 open and laparoscopic bariatric procedures: multivariate analysis of factors related to leak and resultant mortality. Surg Endosc 2004; 18(2): 193-7.

[148] Perugini RA, Mason R, Czerniach DR, Novitsky YW, Baker S, Litwin DE, Kelly JJ. Predictors of complication and suboptimal weight loss after laparoscopic Roux-en-Y gastric bypass: a series of 188 patients. Arch Surg 2003; 138(5): 541-5.

[149] Phillips BA, Danner FJ. Cigarette smoking and sleep disturbance. Arch Intern Med 1995; 155(7): 734-7.

[150] Gothe B, Strohl KP, Levin S, Cherniack NS. Nicotine: a different approach to treatment of obstructive sleep apnea. Chest 1985; 87(1): 11-7.

[151] Berry RB, Desa MM, Light RW. Effect of ethanol on the efficacy of nasal continuous positive airway pressure as a treatment for obstructive sleep apnea. Chest 1991; 99(2): 339-43.

[152] Gleeson K, Zwillich CW, White DP. The influence of increasing ventilatory effort on arousal from sleep. Am Rev Respir Dis 1990; 142(2): 295-300.

[153] Roehrs T, Beare D, Zorick F, Roth T. Sleepiness and ethanol effects on simulated driving. Alcohol Clin Exp Res 1994; 18(1): 154-8.

[154] Teschler H, Berthon-Jones M, Wessendorf T, Meyer HJ, Konietzko N. Influence of moderate alcohol consumption on obstructive sleep apnoea with and without AutoSet nasal CPAP therapy. Eur Respir J 1996; 9(11): 2371-7.

[155] Kohler M, Bloch KE, Stradling JR. Pharmacological approaches to the treatment of obstructive sleep apnoea. Expert Opin Investig Drugs 2009; 18(5): 647-56.

[156] Espinoza H, Antic R, Thornton AT, McEvoy RD. The effects of aminophylline on sleep and sleep-disordered breathing in patients with obstructive sleep apnea syndrome. Am Rev Respir Dis 1987; 136(1): 80-4.

[157] Mulloy E, McNicholas WT. Theophylline in obstructive sleep apnea. A double-blind evaluation. Chest 1992; 101(3): 753-7.

[158] Whyte KF, Gould GA, Airlie MA, Shapiro CM, Douglas NJ. Role of protriptyline and acetazolamide in the sleep apnea/hypopnea syndrome. Sleep 1988; 11(5): 463-72.

[159] Atkinson RL, Suratt PM, Wilhoit SC, Recant L. Naloxone improves sleep apnea in obese humans. Int J Obes 1985; 9(4): 233-9.

[160] Ferber C, Duclaux R, Mouret J. Naltrexone improves blood gas patterns in obstructive sleep apnoea syndrome through its influence on sleep. J Sleep Res 1993; 2(3): 149-55.

[161] Cook WR, Benich JJ, Wooten SA. Indices of severity of obstructive sleep apnea syndrome do not change during medroxyprogesterone acetate therapy. Chest 1989; 96(2): 262-6.

[162] Hudgel DW, Hendricks C, Dadley A. Alteration in obstructive apnea pattern induced by changes in oxygen- and carbon-dioxide-inspired concentrations. Am Rev Respir Dis 1988; 138(1): 16-9.

[163] Villiger PM, Hess CW, Reinhart WH. Beneficial effect of inhaled CO2 in a patient with non-obstructive sleep apnoea. J Neurol 1993; 241(1): 45-8.

[164] Badr MS, Grossman JE, Weber SA. Treatment of refractory sleep apnea with supplemental carbon dioxide. Am J Respir Crit Care Med 1994; 150(2): 561-4.

[165] Sunderram J, Parisi RA, Strobel RJ. Serotonergic stimulation of the genioglossus and the response to nasal continuous positive airway pressure. Am J Respir Crit Care Med 2000; 162(3 Pt 1): 925-9.

[166] Carley DW, Olopade C, Ruigt GS, Radulovacki M. Efficacy of mirtazapine in obstructive sleep apnea syndrome. Sleep 2007; 30(1): 35-41.

[167] Hedner J, Kraiczi H, Peker Y, Murphy P. Reduction of sleep-disordered breathing after physostigmine. Am J Respir Crit Care Med 2003; 168(10): 1246-51.

[168] Moraes W, Poyares D, Sukys-Claudino L, Guilleminault C, Tufik S. Donepezil improves obstructive sleep apnea in Alzheimer disease: a double-blind, placebo-controlled study. Chest 2008; 133(3): 677-83.

[169] Hedner J, Kraiczi H, Peker Y. Reducation of sleep apnea after orally available cholinesterase inhibitor donepezil. Sleep Med 6, S54-S55. 2005.

[170] Marshall NS, Yee BJ, Desai AV, Buchanan PR, Wong KK, Crompton R *et al.* Two randomized placebo-controlled trials to evaluate the efficacy and tolerability of mirtazapine for the treatment of obstructive sleep apnea. Sleep 2008; 31(6): 824-31.

[171] Kraiczi H, Hedner J, Dahlof P, Ejnell H, Carlson J. Effect of serotonin uptake inhibition on breathing during sleep and daytime symptoms in obstructive sleep apnea. Sleep 1999; 22(1): 61-7.

[172] Stradling J, Smith D, Radulovacki M, Carley D. Effect of ondansetron on moderate obstructive sleep apnoea, a single night, placebo-controlled trial. J Sleep Res 2003; 12(2): 169-70.

[173] Veasey SC, Chachkes J, Fenik P, Hendricks JC. The effects of ondansetron on sleep-disordered breathing in the English bulldog. Sleep 2001; 24(2): 155-60.

[174] Popovic RM, White DP. Upper airway muscle activity in normal women: influence of hormonal status. J Appl Physiol 1998; 84(3): 1055-62.

[175] Manber R, Kuo TF, Cataldo N, Colrain IM. The effects of hormone replacement therapy on sleep-disordered breathing in postmenopausal women: a pilot study. Sleep 2003; 26(2): 163-8.

[176] Weichler U, Herres-Mayer B, Mayer J, Weber K, Hoffmann R, Peter JH. Influence of antihypertensive drug therapy on sleep pattern and sleep apnea activity. Cardiology 1991; 78(2): 124-30.

[177] Salo TM, Kantola I, Voipio-Pulkki LM, Pelttari L, Viikari JS. The effect of four different antihypertensive medications on cardiovascular regulation in hypertensive sleep apneic patients--assessment by spectral analysis of heart rate and blood pressure variability. Eur J Clin Pharmacol 1999; 55(3): 191-8.

[178] Salo TM, Metsala TH, Kantola IM, Jalonen JO, Voipio-Pulkki LM, Valimaki IA, Viikari JS. Ramipril Enhances Autonomic Control in Essential Hypertension: A Study Employing Spectral Analysis of Heart Rate Variation. Am J Ther 1994; 1(3): 191-7.

[179] Kiely JL, Nolan P, McNicholas WT. Intranasal corticosteroid therapy for obstructive sleep apnoea in patients with co-existing rhinitis. Thorax 2004; 59(1): 50-5.

[180] Clarenbach CF, Kohler M, Senn O, Thurnheer R, Bloch KE. Does nasal decongestion improve obstructive sleep apnea? J Sleep Res 2008; 17(4): 444-9.

[181] Morrell MJ, Arabi Y, Zahn BR, Meyer KC, Skatrud JB, Badr MS. Effect of surfactant on pharyngeal mechanics in sleeping humans: implications for sleep apnoea. Eur Respir J 2002; 20(2): 451-7.

[182] Jokic R, Klimaszewski A, Mink J, Fitzpatrick MF. Surface tension forces in sleep apnea: the role of a soft tissue lubricant: a randomized double-blind, placebo-controlled trial. Am J Respir Crit Care Med 1998; 157(5 Pt 1): 1522-5.

[183] Martin RJ, Sanders MH, Gray BA, Pennock BE. Acute and long-term ventilatory effects of hyperoxia in the adult sleep apnea syndrome. Am Rev Respir Dis 1982; 125(2): 175-80.

[184] Gold AR, Schwartz AR, Bleecker ER, Smith PL. The effect of chronic nocturnal oxygen administration upon sleep apnea. Am Rev Respir Dis 1986; 134(5): 925-9.

[185] Strollo PJ, Jr. Indications for treatment of obstructive sleep apnea in adults. Clin Chest Med 2003; 24(2): 307-13, vii.

[186] Sanders MH, Rogers RM. Sleep apnea: when does better become benefit? Chest 1985; 88(3): 320-1.

[187] Hanly P, Sasson Z, Zuberi N, Lunn K. ST-segment depression during sleep in obstructive sleep apnea. Am J Cardiol 1993; 71(15): 1341-5.

[188] Franklin KA, Nilsson JB, Sahlin C, Naslund U. Sleep apnoea and nocturnal angina. Lancet 1995; 345(8957): 1085-7.

[189] Sanders MH, Kern N. Obstructive sleep apnea treated by independently adjusted inspiratory and expiratory positive airway pressures via nasal mask. Physiologic and clinical implications. Chest 1990; 98(2): 317-24.

[190] Piper AJ, Sullivan CE. Effects of short-term NIPPV in the treatment of patients with severe obstructive sleep apnea and hypercapnia. Chest 1994; 105(2): 434-40.

[191] Chauncey JB, Aldrich MS. Preliminary findings in the treatment of obstructive sleep apnea with transtracheal oxygen. Sleep 1990; 13(2): 167-74.

[192] Farney RJ, Walker JM, Elmer JC, Viscomi VA, Ord RJ. Transtracheal oxygen, nasal CPAP and nasal oxygen in five patients with obstructive sleep apnea. Chest 1992; 101(5): 1228-35.

[193] Pepin JL, Viot-Blanc V, Escourrou P, Racineux JL, Sapene M, Levy P *et al.* Prevalence of residual excessive sleepiness in CPAP-treated sleep apnoea patients: the French multicentre study. Eur Respir J 2009; 33(5): 1062-7.

[194] Morgenthaler TI, Kapen S, Lee-Chiong T, Alessi C, Boehlecke B, Brown T *et al.* Practice parameters for the medical therapy of obstructive sleep apnea. Sleep 2006; 29(8): 1031-5.

[195] Veasey SC, Guilleminault C, Strohl KP, Sanders MH, Ballard RD, Magalang UJ. Medical therapy for obstructive sleep apnea: a review by the Medical Therapy for Obstructive Sleep Apnea Task Force of the Standards of Practice Committee of the American Academy of Sleep Medicine. Sleep 2006; 29(8): 1036-44.

[196] Black JE, Hirshkowitz M. Modafinil for treatment of residual excessive sleepiness in nasal continuous positive airway pressure-treated obstructive sleep apnea/hypopnea syndrome. Sleep 2005; 28(4): 464-71.

[197] Kingshott RN, Vennelle M, Coleman EL, Engleman HM, Mackay TW, Douglas NJ. Randomized, double-blind, placebo-controlled crossover trial of modafinil in the treatment of residual excessive daytime sleepiness in the sleep apnea/hypopnea syndrome. Am J Respir Crit Care Med 2001; 163(4): 918-23.

[198] Pack AI, Black JE, Schwartz JR, Matheson JK. Modafinil as adjunct therapy for daytime sleepiness in obstructive sleep apnea. Am J Respir Crit Care Med 2001; 164(9): 1675-81.

[199] Schwartz JR, Hirshkowitz M, Erman MK, Schmidt-Nowara W. Modafinil as adjunct therapy for daytime sleepiness in obstructive sleep apnea: a 12-week, open-label study. Chest 2003; 124(6): 2192-9.

[200] Roth T, White D, Schmidt-Nowara W, Wesnes KA, Niebler G, Arora S, Black J. Effects of armodafinil in the treatment of residual excessive sleepiness associated with obstructive sleep apnea/hypopnea syndrome: a 12-week, multicenter, double-blind, randomized, placebo-controlled study in nCPAP-adherent adults. Clin Ther 2006; 28(5): 689-706.

[201] Hirshkowitz M, Black JE, Wesnes K, Niebler G, Arora S, Roth T. Adjunct armodafinil improves wakefulness and memory in obstructive sleep apnea/hypopnea syndrome. Respir Med 2007; 101(3): 616-27.

[202] Hou RH, Langley RW, Szabadi E, Bradshaw CM. Comparison of diphenhydramine and modafinil on arousal and autonomic functions in healthy volunteers. J Psychopharmacol 2007; 21(6): 567-78.

[203] Wong YN, Simcoe D, Hartman LN, Laughton WB, King SP, McCormick GC, Grebow PE. A double-blind, placebo-controlled, ascending-dose evaluation of the pharmacokinetics and tolerability of modafinil tablets in healthy male volunteers. J Clin Pharmacol 1999; 39(1): 30-40.

[204] Lavie P, Fischel N, Zomer J, Eliaschar I. The effects of partial and complete mechanical occlusion of the nasal passages on sleep structure and breathing in sleep. Acta Otolaryngol 1983; 95(1-2): 161-6.

[205] Suratt PM, Turner BL, Wilhoit SC. Effect of intranasal obstruction on breathing during sleep. Chest 1986; 90(3): 324-9.

[206] Hoijer U, Ejnell H, Hedner J, Petruson B, Eng LB. The effects of nasal dilation on snoring and obstructive sleep apnea. Arch Otolaryngol Head Neck Surg 1992; 118(3): 281-4.

[207] Hoffstein V, Mateika S, Metes A. Effect of nasal dilation on snoring and apneas during different stages of sleep. Sleep 1993; 16(4): 360-5.

[208] Scharf MB, Brannen DE, McDannold M. A subjective evaluation of a nasal dilator on sleep & snoring. Ear Nose Throat J 1994; 73(6): 395-401.

[209] Scharf MB, McDannold MD, Zaretsky NT, Hux GT, Brannen DE, Berkowitz DV. Cyclic alternating pattern sequences in non-apneic snorers with and without nasal dilation. Ear Nose Throat J 1996; 75(9): 617-9.

[210] Cornblatt B, Obuchowski M, Roberts S, Pollack S, Erlenmeyer-Kimling L. Cognitive and behavioral precursors of schizophrenia. Dev Psychopathol 1999; 11(3): 487-508.

[211] Afzelius LE, Elmqvist D, Hougaard K, Laurin S, Nilsson B, Risberg AM. Sleep apnea syndrome--an alternative treatment to tracheostomy. Laryngoscope 1981; 91(2): 285-91.

[212] Nahmias JS, Karetzky MS. Treatment of the obstructive sleep apnea syndrome using a nasopharyngeal tube. Chest 1988; 94(6): 1142-7.

[213] Sullivan CE, Issa FG, Berthon-Jones M, Eves L. Reversal of obstructive sleep apnoea by continuous positive airway pressure applied through the nares. Lancet 1981; 1(8225): 862-5.

[214] Grunstein RR. Sleep-related breathing disorders. 5. Nasal continuous positive airway pressure treatment for obstructive sleep apnoea. Thorax 1995; 50(10): 1106-13.

[215] Grunstein RR, Hedner J, Grote L. Treatment options for sleep apnoea. Drugs 2001; 61(2): 237-51.

[216] McDaid C, Duree KH, Griffin SC, Weatherly HL, Stradling JR, Davies RJ *et al.* A systematic review of continuous positive airway pressure for obstructive sleep apnoea-hypopnoea syndrome. Sleep Med Rev 2009; 13(6): 427-36.

[217] Patel SR, White DP, Malhotra A, Stanchina ML, Ayas NT. Continuous positive airway pressure therapy for treating sleepiness in a diverse population with obstructive sleep apnea: results of a meta-analysis. Arch Intern Med 2003; 163(5): 565-71.

[218] Giles TL, Lasserson TJ, Smith BH, White J, Wright J, Cates CJ. Continuous positive airways pressure for obstructive sleep apnoea in adults. Cochrane Database Syst Rev 2006; 3: CD001106.

[219] Reeves-Hoche MK, Hudgel DW, Meck R, Witteman R, Ross A, Zwillich CW. Continuous versus bilevel positive airway pressure for obstructive sleep apnea. Am J Respir Crit Care Med 1995; 151(2 Pt 1): 443-9.

[220] Fietze I, Glos M, Moebus I, Witt C, Penzel T, Baumann G. Automatic pressure titration with APAP is as effective as manual titration with CPAP in patients with obstructive sleep apnea. Respiration 2007; 74(3): 279-86.

[221] Nussbaumer Y, Bloch KE, Genser T, Thurnheer R. Equivalence of autoadjusted and constant continuous positive airway pressure in home treatment of sleep apnea. Chest 2006; 129(3): 638-43.

[222] Zozula R, Rosen R. Compliance with continuous positive airway pressure therapy: assessing and improving treatment outcomes. Curr Opin Pulm Med 2001; 7(6): 391-8.

[223] Fitzpatrick MF, Alloway CE, Wakeford TM, MacLean AW, Munt PW, Day AG. Can patients with obstructive sleep apnea titrate their own continuous positive airway pressure? Am J Respir Crit Care Med 2003; 167(5): 716-22.

[224] Richards GN, Cistulli PA, Ungar RG, Berthon-Jones M, Sullivan CE. Mouth leak with nasal continuous positive airway pressure increases nasal airway resistance. Am J Respir Crit Care Med 1996; 154(1): 182-6.

[225] Wiest GH, Harsch IA, Fuchs FS, Kitzbichler S, Bogner K, Brueckl WM *et al.* Initiation of CPAP therapy for OSA: does prophylactic humidification during CPAP pressure titration improve initial patient acceptance and comfort? Respiration 2002; 69(5): 406-12.

[226] Mador MJ, Krauza M, Pervez A, Pierce D, Braun M. Effect of heated humidification on compliance and quality of life in patients with sleep apnea using nasal continuous positive airway pressure. Chest 2005; 128(4): 2151-8.

[227] Nilius G, Happel A, Domanski U, Ruhle KH. Pressure-relief continuous positive airway pressure vs constant continuous positive airway pressure: a comparison of efficacy and compliance. Chest 2006; 130(4): 1018-24.

[228] Fromm RE, Jr., Varon J, Lechin AE, Hirshkowitz M. CPAP machine performance and altitude. Chest 1995; 108(6): 1577-80.

[229] Indications and standards for use of nasal continuous positive airway pressure (CPAP) in sleep apnea syndromes. American Thoracic Society. Official statement adopted March 1944. Am J Respir Crit Care Med 1994; 150(6 Pt 1): 1738-45.

[230] McGinley BM, Patil SP, Kirkness JP, Smith PL, Schwartz AR, Schneider H. A nasal cannula can be used to treat obstructive sleep apnea. Am J Respir Crit Care Med 2007; 176(2): 194-200.

[231] McGinley B, Halbower A, Schwartz AR, Smith PL, Patil SP, Schneider H. Effect of a high-flow open nasal cannula system on obstructive sleep apnea in children. Pediatrics 2009; 124(1): 179-88.

[232] Montserrat JM, Ballester E, Olivi H, Reolid A, Lloberes P, Morello A, Rodriguez-Roisin R. Time-course of stepwise CPAP titration. Behavior of respiratory and neurological variables. Am J Respir Crit Care Med 1995; 152(6 Pt 1): 1854-9.

[233] Meurice JC, Paquereau J, Denjean A, Patte F, Series F. Influence of correction of flow limitation on continuous positive airway pressure efficiency in sleep apnoea/hypopnoea syndrome. Eur Respir J 1998; 11(5): 1121-7.

[234] Issa FG, Sullivan CE. The immediate effects of nasal continuous positive airway pressure treatment on sleep pattern in patients with obstructive sleep apnea syndrome. Electroencephalogr Clin Neurophysiol 1986; 63(1): 10-7.

[235] Condos R, Norman RG, Krishnasamy I, Peduzzi N, Goldring RM, Rapoport DM. Flow limitation as a noninvasive assessment of residual upper-airway resistance during continuous positive airway pressure therapy of obstructive sleep apnea. Am J Respir Crit Care Med 1994; 150(2): 475-80.

[236] Jokic R, Klimaszewski A, Sridhar G, Fitzpatrick MF. Continuous positive airway pressure requirement during the first month of treatment in patients with severe obstructive sleep apnea. Chest 1998; 114(4): 1061-9.

[237] Miljeteig H, Hoffstein V. Determinants of continuous positive airway pressure level for treatment of obstructive sleep apnea. Am Rev Respir Dis 1993; 147(6 Pt 1): 1526-30.

[238] Sanders MH, Kern NB, Costantino JP, Stiller RA, Studnicki K, Coates J *et al.* Adequacy of prescribing positive airway pressure therapy by mask for sleep apnea on the basis of a partial-night trial. Am Rev Respir Dis 1993; 147(5): 1169-74.

[239] McArdle N, Grove A, Devereux G, Mackay-Brown L, Mackay T, Douglas NJ. Split-night versus full-night studies for sleep apnoea/hypopnoea syndrome. Eur Respir J 2000; 15(4): 670-5.

[240] Littner M, Hirshkowitz M, Davila D, Anderson WM, Kushida CA, Woodson BT *et al.* Practice parameters for the use of auto-titrating continuous positive airway pressure devices for titrating pressures and treating adult patients with obstructive sleep apnea syndrome. An American Academy of Sleep Medicine report. Sleep 2002; 25(2): 143-7.

[241] Morgenthaler TI, Aurora RN, Brown T, Zak R, Alessi C, Boehlecke B *et al.* Practice parameters for the use of autotitrating continuous positive airway pressure devices for titrating pressures and treating adult patients with obstructive sleep apnea syndrome: an update for 2007. An American Academy of Sleep Medicine report. Sleep 2008; 31(1): 141-7.

[242] Krieger J, Sforza E, Petiau C, Weiss T. Simplified diagnostic procedure for obstructive sleep apnoea syndrome: lower subsequent compliance with CPAP. Eur Respir J 1998; 12(4): 776-9.

[243] White DP, Gibb TJ. Evaluation of the Healthdyne NightWatch system to titrate CPAP in the home. Sleep 1998; 21(2): 198-204.

[244] Juhasz J, Schillen J, Urbigkeit A, Ploch T, Penzel T, Peter JH. Unattended continuous positive airway pressure titration. Clinical relevance and cardiorespiratory hazards of the method. Am J Respir Crit Care Med 1996; 154(2 Pt 1): 359-65.

[245] Flemons WW, Whitelaw WA, Brant R, Remmers JE. Likelihood ratios for a sleep apnea clinical prediction rule. Am J Respir Crit Care Med 1994; 150(5 Pt 1): 1279-85.

[246] Ioachimescu O, Bedford T, Stephenson L., Foldvary-Schaefer N., Golish J. A Large Cohort Validation of CPAP Setting Predictions Based on Demographic, Anthropometric and Polysomnographic Data. Am J Respir Crit Care Med 2007; 175: A708.

[247] Ioachimescu O, Bedford T, Bae C, Foldvary-Schaefer N, AL, Golish J. Continuous positive airway pressure (CPAP) level in obstructive sleep apnea (OSA): the aftermath of various mathematical models. Sleep 2006; 28: 456.

[248] Ioachimescu OC, Bedford T, Stephenson L., Foldvary-Schaefer N, Golish J. A Large Cohort Validation of CPAP Setting Predictions Based on Demographic, Anthropometric and Polysomnographic Data. Am J.Respir.Crit Care Med 2007; 175[Suppl]: A708.

[249] Ioachimescu OC, Bedford T, Bae C, Foldvary-Schaefer N, Aboussouan L, Golish J. Continuous positive airway pressure (CPAP) level in obstructive sleep apnea (OSA): the aftermath of various mathematical models. Sleep 2006; 29[Suppl]: A203.

[250] Hoffstein V, Szalai JP. Predictive value of clinical features in diagnosing obstructive sleep apnea. Sleep 1993; 16(2): 118-22.

[251] Hoffstein V, Mateika S. Predicting nasal continuous positive airway pressure. Am J Respir Crit Care Med 1994; 150(2): 486-8.

[252] Hoffstein V. Accuracy of CPAP predicted from anthropometric and polysomnographic indices. Sleep 1997; 20(3): 237-8.

[253] Lin IF, Chuang ML, Liao YF, Chen NH, Li HY. Predicting effective continuous positive airway pressure in Taiwanese patients with obstructive sleep apnea syndrome. J Formos Med Assoc 2003; 102(4): 215-21.

[254] Masa JF, Jimenez A, Duran J, Capote F, Monasterio C, Mayos M *et al.* Alternative methods of titrating continuous positive airway pressure: a large multicenter study. Am J Respir Crit Care Med 2004; 170(11): 1218-24.

[255] Fitzpatrick MF, Alloway CE, Wakeford TM, MacLean AW, Munt PW, Day AG. Can patients with obstructive sleep apnea titrate their own continuous positive airway pressure? Am J Respir Crit Care Med 2003; 167(5): 716-22.

[256] Stradling JR, Hardinge M, Paxton J, Smith DM. Relative accuracy of algorithm-based prescription of nasal CPAP in OSA. Respir Med 2004; 98(2): 152-4.

[257] Stradling JR, Hardinge M, Smith DM. A novel, simplified approach to starting nasal CPAP therapy in OSA. Respir Med 2004; 98(2): 155-8.

[258] Rowley JA, Tarbichi AG, Badr MS. The use of a predicted CPAP equation improves CPAP titration success. Sleep Breath 2005; 9(1): 26-32.

[259] Zeng Y, Zhong N. [Prediction of the level of continuous positive airway pressure in the management of obstructive sleep apnea syndrome via nasal mask]. Zhonghua Jie He He Hu Xi Za Zhi 1996; 19(5): 269-72.

[260] Viner S, Szalai JP, Hoffstein V. Are history and physical examination a good screening test for sleep apnea? Ann Intern Med 1991; 115(5): 356-9.

[261] Maislin G, Pack AI, Kribbs NB, Smith PL, Schwartz AR, Kline LR *et al.* A survey screen for prediction of apnea. Sleep 1995; 18(3): 158-66.

[262] Roche N, Herer B, Roig C, Huchon G. Prospective testing of two models based on clinical and oximetric variables for prediction of obstructive sleep apnea Chest 2002; 121(3): 747-52.

[263] Ioachimescu OC, Bedford T. Aftermath of optimal CPAP prediction models using various linear, logistic regression and artificial neural networks (ANN) in OSA. Eur.Respir J. 2010; 36(Suppl 54):P975.

[264] El Solh A, Akinnusi M, Patel A, Bhat A, TenBrock R. Predicting optimal CPAP by neural network reduces titration failure: a randomized study. Sleep Breath 2009; 13(4): 325-30.

[265] Lamphere J, Roehrs T, Wittig R, Zorick F, Conway WA, Roth T. Recovery of alertness after CPAP in apnea. Chest 1989; 96(6): 1364-7.

[266] Loube DI, Gay PC, Strohl KP, Pack AI, White DP, Collop NA. Indications for positive airway pressure treatment of adult obstructive sleep apnea patients: a consensus statement. Chest 1999; 115(3): 863-6.

[267] Holty JE, Guilleminault C. Surgical options for the treatment of obstructive sleep apnea. Med Clin North Am 2010; 94(3): 479-515.

[268] Sundaram S, Bridgman SA, Lim J, Lasserson TJ. Surgery for obstructive sleep apnoea. Cochrane Database Syst Rev 2005;(4): CD001004.

[269] Lojander J, Maasilta P, Partinen M, Brander PE, Salmi T, Lehtonen H. Nasal-CPAP, surgery, and conservative management for treatment of obstructive sleep apnea syndrome. A randomized study. Chest 1996; 110(1): 114-9.

[270] Woodson BT, Steward DL, Weaver EM, Javaheri S. A randomized trial of temperature-controlled radiofrequency, continuous positive airway pressure, and placebo for obstructive sleep apnea syndrome. Otolaryngol Head Neck Surg 2003; 128(6): 848-61.

[271] Brown DJ, Kerr P, Kryger M. Radiofrequency tissue reduction of the palate in patients with moderate sleep-disordered breathing. J Otolaryngol 2001; 30(4): 193-8.

[272] Woodson BT, Nelson L, Mickelson S, Huntley T, Sher A. A multi-institutional study of radiofrequency volumetric tissue reduction for OSAS. Otolaryngol Head Neck Surg 2001; 125(4): 303-11.

[273] Pazos G, Mair EA. Complications of radiofrequency ablation in the treatment of sleep-disordered breathing. Otolaryngol Head Neck Surg 2001; 125(5): 462-6.

[274] Terris DJ, Chen V. Occult mucosal injuries with radiofrequency ablation of the palate. Otolaryngol Head Neck Surg 2001; 125(5): 468-72.

[275] Khan A, Ramar K, Maddirala S, Friedman O, Pallanch JF, Olson EJ. Uvulopalatopharyngoplasty in the management of obstructive sleep apnea: the mayo clinic experience. Mayo Clin Proc 2009; 84(9): 795-800.

[276] Mortimore IL, Bradley PA, Murray JA, Douglas NJ. Uvulopalatopharyngoplasty may compromise nasal CPAP therapy in sleep apnea syndrome. Am J Respir Crit Care Med 1996; 154(6 Pt 1): 1759-62.

[277] Mehta A, Qian J, Petocz P, Darendeliler MA, Cistulli PA. A randomized, controlled study of a mandibular advancement splint for obstructive sleep apnea. Am J Respir Crit Care Med 2001; 163(6): 1457-61.

[278] Gotsopoulos H, Chen C, Qian J, Cistulli PA. Oral appliance therapy improves symptoms in obstructive sleep apnea: a randomized, controlled trial. Am J Respir Crit Care Med 2002; 166(5): 743-8.

[279] Cistulli PA, Gotsopoulos H, Marklund M, Lowe AA. Treatment of snoring and obstructive sleep apnea with mandibular repositioning appliances. Sleep Med Rev 2004; 8(6): 443-57.

[280] Ferguson KA, Cartwright R, Rogers R, Schmidt-Nowara W. Oral appliances for snoring and obstructive sleep apnea: a review. Sleep 2006; 29(2): 244-62.

[281] Gagnadoux F, Fleury B, Vielle B, Petelle B, Meslier N, N'Guyen XL *et al.* Titrated mandibular advancement versus positive airway pressure for sleep apnoea. Eur Respir J 2009; 34(4): 914-20.

[282] Hoekema A, Stegenga B, Bakker M, Brouwer WH, de Bont LG, Wijkstra PJ, van der Hoeven JH. Simulated driving in obstructive sleep apnoea-hypopnoea; effects of oral appliances and continuous positive airway pressure. Sleep Breath 2007; 11(3): 129-38.

[283] Barnes M, McEvoy RD, Banks S, Tarquinio N, Murray CG, Vowles N, Pierce RJ. Efficacy of positive airway pressure and oral appliance in mild to moderate obstructive sleep apnea. Am J Respir Crit Care Med 2004; 170(6): 656-64.

[284] Andren A, Sjoquist M, Tegelberg A. Effects on blood pressure after treatment of obstructive sleep apnoea with a mandibular advancement appliance - a three-year follow-up. J Oral Rehabil 2009; 36(10): 719-25.

[285] Schmidt-Nowara W, Lowe A, Wiegand L, Cartwright R, Perez-Guerra F, Menn S. Oral appliances for the treatment of snoring and obstructive sleep apnea: a review. Sleep 1995; 18(6): 501-10.

[286] Marklund M, Sahlin C, Stenlund H, Persson M, Franklin KA. Mandibular advancement device in patients with obstructive sleep apnea : long-term effects on apnea and sleep. Chest 2001; 120(1): 162-9.

[287] Marklund M, Stenlund H, Franklin KA. Mandibular advancement devices in 630 men and women with obstructive sleep apnea and snoring: tolerability and predictors of treatment success. Chest 2004; 125(4): 1270-8.

[288] Lim J, Lasserson TJ, Fleetham J, Wright J. Oral appliances for obstructive sleep apnoea. Cochrane Database Syst Rev 2006;(1): CD004435.

[289] Tsuiki S, Kobayashi M, Namba K, Oka Y, Komada Y, Kagimura T, Inoue Y. Optimal positive airway pressure predicts oral appliance response to sleep apnoea. Eur Respir J 2010; 35(5): 1098-105.

[290] Walker-Engstrom ML, Tegelberg A, Wilhelmsson B, Ringqvist I. 4-year follow-up of treatment with dental appliance or uvulopalatopharyngoplasty in patients with obstructive sleep apnea: a randomized study. Chest 2002; 121(3): 739-46.

[291] Pantin CC, Hillman DR, Tennant M. Dental side effects of an oral device to treat snoring and obstructive sleep apnea. Sleep 1999; 22(2): 237-40.

[292] Rose EC, Staats R, Virchow C, Jr., Jonas IE. Occlusal and skeletal effects of an oral appliance in the treatment of obstructive sleep apnea. Chest 2002; 122(3): 871-7.

[293] Almeida FR, Lowe AA, Otsuka R, Fastlicht S, Farbood M, Tsuiki S. Long-term sequellae of oral appliance therapy in obstructive sleep apnea patients: Part 2. Study-model analysis. Am J Orthod Dentofacial Orthop 2006; 129(2): 205-13.

[294] Porkka-Heiskanen T, Strecker RE, Thakkar M, Bjorkum AA, Greene RW, McCarley RW. Adenosine: a mediator of the sleep-inducing effects of prolonged wakefulness. Science 1997; 276(5316): 1265-8.

[295] Sherin JE, Shiromani PJ, McCarley RW, Saper CB. Activation of ventrolateral preoptic neurons during sleep. Science 1996; 271(5246): 216-9.

[296] Haponik EF, Smith PL, Bohlman ME, Allen RP, Goldman SM, Bleecker ER. Computerized tomography in obstructive sleep apnea. Correlation of airway size with physiology during sleep and wakefulness. Am Rev Respir Dis 1983; 127(2): 221-6.

[297] Schwab RJ, Gupta KB, Gefter WB, Metzger LJ, Hoffman EA, Pack AI. Upper airway and soft tissue anatomy in normal subjects and patients with sleep-disordered breathing. Significance of the lateral pharyngeal walls. Am J Respir Crit Care Med 1995; 152(5 Pt 1): 1673-89.

[298] Remmers JE, Anch AM, deGroot WJ, Baker JP, Jr., Sauerland EK. Oropharyngeal muscle tone in obstructive sleep apnea before and after strychnine. Sleep 1980; 3(3-4): 447-53.

[299] Isono S, Feroah TR, Hajduk EA, Brant R, Whitelaw WA, Remmers JE. Interaction of cross-sectional area, driving pressure, and airflow of passive velopharynx. J Appl Physiol 1997; 83(3): 851-9.

[300] Smith PL, Wise RA, Gold AR, Schwartz AR, Permutt S. Upper airway pressure-flow relationships in obstructive sleep apnea. J Appl Physiol 1988; 64(2): 789-95.

[301] Patil SP, Schneider H, Schwartz AR, Smith PL. Adult obstructive sleep apnea: pathophysiology and diagnosis. Chest 2007; 132(1): 325-37.

[302] Gold AR, Schwartz AR. The pharyngeal critical pressure. The whys and hows of using nasal continuous positive airway pressure diagnostically. Chest 1996; 110(4): 1077-88.

[303] Fogel RB, Malhotra A, White DP. Sleep. 2: pathophysiology of obstructive sleep apnoea/hypopnoea syndrome. Thorax 2004; 59(2): 159-63.

[304] Dempsey JA, Veasey SC, Morgan BJ, O'Donnell CP. Pathophysiology of sleep apnea. Physiol Rev 2010; 90(1): 47-112.

CHAPTER 7

Central Sleep Apnea

Naveen Kanathur, M.D.[*], John Harrington, M.D., Vipin Malik, M.D. and Teofilo Lee-Chiong, M.D.

National Jewish Health, 1400 Jackson Street, Denver, CO 80213, USA

Abstract: Central sleep apnea (CSA) is a sleep-related breathing disorder that is characterized by repetitive cessation of airflow due to diminished or absent ventilatory effort. There are several types of CSA, and these can be classified into two general types, namely hypercapnic (central alveolar hypoventilation, secondary to neuromuscular disorders or chronic use of long-acting opioids) or non-hypercapnic forms (idiopathic CSA, CSA due to heart failure, sleep-onset periodic breathing, high-altitude central apneas, and continuous positive airway pressure-emergent CSA). Whatever its cause(s), CSA can give rise to sleep disturbance, repetitive awakenings, insomnia or excessive sleepiness. Definitive diagnosis of CSA requires polysomnography. Therapy should be individualized depending on the nature and severity of central apnea; this may include use of oxygen supplementation, drug therapy or positive airway pressure.

TOPIC DISCUSSION (CLINICAL OUTLOOK)

Introduction

Central sleep apnea (CSA) is a sleep-related breathing disorder that is characterized by repetitive cessation of airflow due to diminished or absent ventilatory effort. There are several types of CSA, and these can be classified into two general types, namely hypercapnic or non-hypercapnic forms. Hypercapnic CSA, including those due to central alveolar hypoventilation, or secondary to neuromuscular disorders or chronic use of long-acting opioids, is characterized by relative hypoventilation during sleep and higher levels of partial pressure of arterial carbon dioxide (P_aCO_2) during sleep compared to waking. In many instances, hypercapnic CSA is accompanied by high waking P_aCO_2 levels.

Non-hypercapnic CSA, on the other hand, is associated with increased ventilatory responsiveness to hypercapnia and presents with normal or low waking P_aCO_2 levels. Central apneas during sleep are produced when rising P_aCO_2 levels associated with sleep trigger a hyperventilatory overshoot during brief arousals that, in turn, causes P_aCO_2 to fall below its apneic threshold. Apnea threshold is defined as the arterial PCO_2 below which breathing ceases or becomes dysrhythmic, and is generally 2-6 mmHg below eupneic sleeping P_aCO_2 levels. Causes of non-hypercapnic CSA include idiopathic CSA, CSA due to heart failure, sleep-onset periodic breathing, high-altitude central apneas, and continuous positive airway pressure-emergent CSA (complex sleep apnea; CompSA). Transient episodes of central apneas may develop at the onset of sleep when levels of P_aCO_2, which are typically higher during sleep and lower during wakefulness, fluctuate above or below the apnea threshold; these tend to resolve as sleep progresses and respiration stabilizes. High-altitude periodic breathing is also more prominent at sleep onset and non-rapid eye movement (NREM) sleep compared to rapid eye movement (REM) sleep; it is characterized by cycles of central apneas and hyperpneas developing following ascent to high altitude, generally at elevations greater than 4,000-7,600 meters. Risk factors for high-altitude central apneas include male gender, greater intrinsic hypoxic ventilatory drive, higher elevation reached, and rapidity of ascent. It is believed that high-altitude central apneas arise as a result of hypoxia-induced hyperventilation that, in turn, leads to hypocapnic alkalosis and central apneas.

Whatever its cause(s), CSA can give rise to sleep disturbance, repetitive awakenings, insomnia or excessive sleepiness. Many patients with CSA remain asymptomatic.

Definitive diagnosis of CSA requires polysomnography (PSG), which demonstrates recurrent periods of cessation of respiration and ventilatory effort lasting at least 10 seconds. Snoring may be present, but is generally less prominent than in obstructive sleep apnea (OSA). Measures of airflow, including thermal sensors and pressure transducers, demonstrate no fluctuations. This is accompanied by the absence of chest and abdominal movement in the respiratory inductance plethysmography or strain gauge channels, no respiratory muscle activity in the diaphragmatic electromyogram (EMG), or no change in the esophageal pressure monitor (if used).

*Address correspondence to Naveen Kanathur: National Jewish Health, 1400 Jackson Street, Denver, CO 80213, USA; E-mail: kanathurnaveen@hotmail.com

Idiopathic Central Sleep Apnea

Idiopathic CSA is an uncommon condition that is distinct from other forms of central apneas. It is present in less than 5% of patients undergoing PSG. It affects predominantly males, as well as middle-aged and older adults. The pathophysiology of idiopathic CSA is not completely understood. Arterial partial pressure of CO_2 (P_aCO_2) is a major pathophysiologic variable in this disorder. Other factors that are important in the genesis and persistence of CSA include apnea threshold, loop gain, circulation time and hypercapnic sensitivity [1, 2]. Low hypercapnic sensitivity or ventilatory response is associated with dampening of the loop gain. High hypercapnic sensitivity is associated with amplified loop gain that causes oscillation around the apneic threshold and perpetuates the cyclical breathing pattern.

Ventilation has both metabolic and behavioral control processes. Metabolic control involves carotid chemoreceptors that are sensitive to hypoxia and hypercapnia, as well as medullary chemoreceptors that respond to hypercapnia. In addition, vagally-mediated intrapulmonary and other brainstem mechanisms process peripheral stimuli and have important roles in controlling respiratory patterns. These pathways are active during waking and sleep, although there is greater dampening of physiologic ventilatory responses to hypercapnia during sleep compared to responsiveness to hypoxia. Behavioral control is active only during waking, when it likely involves input from the descending reticular activating system. The sleep-state transition is prone to ventilatory destabilization; at the onset of NREM stages N1 or N2 sleep, apneas may develop when P_aCO_2 falls below the apneic threshold due to sleep onset dysrhythmic breathing. Eventually, P_aCO_2 rises above the apneic threshold and respiration resumes. This cycle of hyperventilation and apneas may recur until "deeper" stages of NREM sleep (generally N2) are reached. Reduction in upper airway dilator muscle tone at sleep onset may also contribute to higher P_aCO_2 levels due to the heightened work of breathing required to compensate for greater airflow resistance.

Clinical manifestations primarily include insomnia, frequent nighttime awakenings, hypersomnolence and mild intermittent snoring. Males appear to be affected more frequently than females, and unlike OSA, patients generally have a normal body habitus. Hemodynamic consequences include elevation in pulmonary and systemic blood pressures due to hypoxia.

Polysomnography demonstrates more than five central apneas per hour of recorded sleep time. If both central and obstructive events are present, CSA is suggested if central apneas constitute more than 80% of respiratory events. Idiopathic CSA is mostly observed during NREM stages N1 and N2 sleep.

There are several important polysomnographic differences between idiopathic CSA and Cheyne-Stokes respiration (CSR). Compared to the latter, cycle duration is typically shorter (20-40 seconds vs. 60-90 seconds), oxygen desaturation is less severe, arousals occur earlier (at the termination of apnea vs. at mid-cycle during the peak of ventilatory effort), and resumption of breathing is more abrupt with a large breath (vs. gradual increment in respiration with CSR).

Therapy of idiopathic CSA should be tailored based on likely causes contributing to apneas. Idiopathic CSA resolves spontaneously in about 20% of patients; watchful waiting, therefore, may be considered if the patient does not have any clinically significant symptoms. Treating upper airway obstruction, such as nasal congestion, might benefit some patients, but its efficacy should be confirmed with repeat sleep studies.

Supplemental oxygen has also been used in treatment of idiopathic CSA [3]. The presence of hypoxia seen in some patients with this disorder can induce hyperventilation and, as a consequence, hypocapnia and cyclic ventilation. Supplemental oxygen is believed to attenuate this response and, thus, can regularize the breathing pattern. Administration of small amounts of supplemental carbon dioxide or introduction of dead space has also been shown in some studies to reduce central events [4]. The efficacy of nasal CPAP and bi-level positive airway pressure (BPAP) to treat idiopathic CSA has been reported and is attributed to positive airway pressure-induced increase in arterial P_aCO_2 above apnea threshold as well as to an increase in oxygen stores [5, 6]. Finally, the use of both zolpidem, a benzodiazepine receptor agonist, and acetazolamide, a carbonic anhydrase inhibitor that induces metabolic acidosis by increasing loss of urinary bicarbonate, and which can be used to lower the apnea threshold, have been described [7, 8].

Central Sleep Apnea in Heart Failure

Both CSA and CSR can develop in persons with heart failure (HF). An early study evaluating the prevalence of sleep disordered breathing in patients with HF was reported by Javaheri et al in 1998 [9]. Eighty-one male patients prospectively enrolled from the cardiology and primary care clinics underwent overnight PSG and 51% of them were noted to have sleep disordered breathing with an apnea-hypopnea index (AHI) of at least 15 per hour, with 40% of subjects having CSA and 11% with OSA. Patients with sleep disordered breathing had a high prevalence of atrial fibrillation and ventricular arrhythmias compared to controls [9].

A later, large retrospective study that involved 450 patients with HF who were referred to a sleep laboratory for evaluation of sleep disordered breathing demonstrated the presence of CSA in 33% and OSA in 38% of patients (AHI >10) [10]. Risk factors for CSA were male gender [odds ratio (OR) 3.5], presence of atrial fibrillation (OR 4.1), age greater than 60 years (OR 2.4) and hypocapnia with P_aCO_2 38 mmHg (OR 4.3). Significant advances in treatment of HF were made in the several years following these initial studies specifically with the widespread use of beta-blockers and aldosterone antagonists. It was anticipated that these treatment changes would result in decrease in prevalence of CSA in this patient population. However, recent studies from France, Germany and the United States (as listed in Table **1**), continue to show high prevalence rates of CSA, in the range of 30-40%. The reason(s) for this is (are) still unclear.

Table 1: Central Sleep Apnea in Heart Failure patients in different published studies [ACEIs/ARBs – (patients taking) angiotensin converting enzyme inhibitors or angiotensin receptor blockers, Asympt – asymptomatic, BBs – (patients taking) beta-blockers, CSA – central sleep apnea, LVEF – left ventricular ejection fraction, n – number of individuals studied, NA- not available, NYHA – New York Heart Association (heart failure class), OSA – obstructive sleep apnea, Prev – prevalence, PSG – polysomnography, SDB AHI – sleep disordered breathing (overall) apnea hypopnea index]

Reference	n	Age	NYHA	Mean LVEF	BBs	ACEIs /ARBs	Aldosteron antagonists	PSG	SDB AHI	OSA prev	CSA prev
Javaheri *et al* 1998 [9]	81	64	I-III	25	NA	NA	NA	attended	≥ 15	11%	40%
Sin *et al* 1999 [10]	450	60	II-IV	27	NA	NA	NA	attended	>10	38%	33%
Lanfranchi *et al* 2003 [11]	47	59	Asympt	27	36%	83%	NA	unattended	≥ 15	11%	55%
Ferrier *et al* 2005 [12]	53	60	I-II	23	31%	97%	30%	attended	>10	53%	15%
Wang *et al* 2007 [13]	218	55	II-III	25	81%	93%	NA	attended	≥ 15	26%	21%
Schulz *et al* 2007 [14]	203	65	II-III	28	90%	91%	46%	unattended	>10	43%	28%
Oldenburg *et al* 2007 [15]	700	64.5	II-III	28	62%	95%	64%	unattended	≥ 15	19%	32%
Vazir *et al* 2007 [16]	55	61	II	31	78%	98%	49%	attended	>15	15%	38%
Hagenah *et al* 2009 [17]	50	63	II,III	26	100%	100%	36%	attended	≥ 15	20%	44%
Paulino *et al* 2009 [18]	316	59	II-III	30	82%	98%	58%	unattended	≥ 10	56%	25%
Macdonald *et al* 2008 [19]	108	57	II-IV	20	82%	83%	36%	unattended	≥ 15	30%	31%

Cheyne - Stokes Respiration

Cheyne-Stokes respiration is defined as periodic breathing with recurring episodes of waxing and waning ventilation separated by central apneas or hypopneas. Cheyne-Stokes respiration is generally observed during NREM (N) sleep, and improves or resolves during REM (R) sleep.

A large randomized controlled trial evaluating the effectiveness of continuous positive airway pressure (CPAP) in patients who have CSA and systolic HF failed to show any benefit in improving the survival rate (Canadian Positive Airway Pressure, CANPAP trial) [20]. In this multicentric trial, 258 patients who were on optimal medical treatment for HF were randomly assigned to receive either CPAP (128 patients) or no CPAP (130 patients), and were followed for a mean of 2 years. Continuous positive airway pressure was started at an initial setting of 5 cmH20 and increased by 2-3 cm H20 over one or two nights to a maximum pressure of 10 cm H20 or to the highest pressure tolerated. Polysomnography was performed at baseline and repeated at 3 and 24 months. Left ventricular ejection fraction (LVEF), 6-min walk distance, quality of life, and levels of plasma epinephrine and atrial natriuretic peptide were evaluated at baseline, and at 3, 6 and 24 months. The primary outcome was the combined rate of death from all causes and rate of heart transplantation. The mean AHI at baseline was 40 per hour. The average daily use of CPAP was 4.3 hours during the first three months and decreased to 3.6 hours subsequently. There were 28 deaths and four patients who required heart transplantation in the control group versus 27 deaths and five heart transplantations in the CPAP group. There was a divergence of event rates in the first 18 months favoring the control group, but reversed at 18 months in favor of the CPAP group. Overall, death, transplant free survival and hospitalization rates did not differ significantly between the two groups. Continuous positive airway pressure reduced AHI by about 50%, improved mean oxygen saturation and LVEF, and reduced levels of plasma norepinephrine.

Due to improvements in medical therapy during this trial period (December 1998- May 2004), with greater widespread use of beta-blockers and spironolactone, the trial was felt to be underpowered to determine CPAP benefit in this patient population. The other criticism of this trial was that CPAP did not effectively treat CSA, as it reduced the mean apnea-hypopnea index to only 19 events per hour, which was higher than the inclusion threshold of 15 events per hour. In a post-hoc analysis of this trial, patients who had their CSA suppressed effectively by CPAP at 3 months (AHI <15) had better transplant-free survival than the control group [21].

Newer forms of positive airway pressure devices which may also be effective in suppressing CSA in patients with HF are being studied [22]. In a group of 15 patients with Cheyne-Stokes respiration (CSR) and HF, treatment with adaptive servo ventilation (ASV) reduced sleepiness and improved plasma brain natriuretic peptide and urinary metanephrine excretion [23]. Compared to CPAP, in 25 patients with CSR and HF, ASV was more effective in decreasing AHI and in correcting the latter to below 10 events per hour. At six months, compliance, LVEF improvement and quality of life were better with ASV [24]. Randomized trials involving larger number of patients and with long-term follow up are required to demonstrate the utility of ASV treatment in controlling CSR and, possibly, improving survival in patients with HF.

Acromegaly and Central Sleep Apnea

Acromegaly is caused by overproduction and secretion of growth hormone, often due to benign pituitary adenomas. Sleep-related breathing disorders, including OSA and CSA, are commonly reported in these patients. These respiratory complications may be important because of the associated cardiovascular abnormalities in acromegalic patients [25]. The prevalence of OSA is more common in acromegaly than is CSA [26, 27]. The pathogenesis of CSA in patients with acromegaly is poorly defined, but may be related to upper airway narrowing and reflex inhibition of the respiratory center, as well as increased ventilatory responsiveness to hypercapnia associated with hypersecretion of growth hormone [25, 26, 28].

Somatostatin analogs therapy in acromegaly can induce tumor shrinkage and reduce symptoms in patients not considered surgical candidates. Due to the persistence of skeletal abnormalities in these patients, sleep-disordered breathing may persist [29]. Grunstein *et al* evaluated the effect of treatment with octreotide, a somatostatin analog, on sleep apnea in 19 patients with active acromegaly. After 6 months of therapy, the severity of both OSA and CSA improved, but sleep apnea was not eliminated in most subjects [30]. Surgical therapy of acromegaly can also improve CSA. Trans-sphenoidal adenomectomy improves CSA by decreasing chemosensitivity to hypoxia [28]. Pelttari *et al*, however, noted persistence of periodic breathing in 10 of 11 acromegalic patients who had undergone adenomectomy with or without radiotherapy [31] and others have reported similarly limited improvement after surgery [32].

Chronic Renal Disease and Central Sleep Apnea

Sleep disorders, including obstructive and central sleep apneas, are frequently associated with chronic renal disease (CRD) and end-stage renal disease (ESRD) [33-36]. Pathophysiologic factors thought to contribute to the increased prevalence of sleep disordered breathing in this population include volume overload, uremia, pharyngeal airway narrowing, and altered chemoreflex responsiveness during sleep [36-39]. The prevalence of central and obstructive sleep apnea among patients with ESRD varies among studies but obstructive component appears to be more prevalent in most [36, 39, 40].

The development of hypocapnia and subsequent periodic breathing in patients with CRD may be related to respiratory compensation to chronic metabolic acidosis [41, 42]. Nocturnal hemodialysis (HD) has been shown to improve CSA as well as OSA in patients with CRD, supporting the notion that sleep apnea incidence in this population is related to ventilatory destabilization and upper airway occlusion [43]. In an earlier study by Jean and colleagues, the influence of dialysis buffer (either acetate or bicarbonate) on sleep apnea incidence was assessed via polysomnography. Each group was randomly assigned to use the same buffer solution over a series of HD sessions. The rates of OSA were not different between groups, but those using acetate had significantly more CSA [44].

Tada and colleagues investigated predictors of OSA and CSA among HD patients. Factors associated with CSA included higher prevalence of atrial fibrillation, decreased apnea-hypopnea index on HD nights, and increased cardiothoracic ratio. A possible mechanism for CSA relates to volume overload leading to pulmonary vagal irritation and resultant hyperventilation. Whereas OSA may be related to uremic toxins and metabolic acidosis, contributors to CSA included fluid status, hypoxia, hypocapnia, and atrial fibrillation [36].

The treatment of ESRD and its effect on sleep apnea frequency and severity were evaluated in several studies. In a recent report, Beecroft *et al* evaluated 58 ESRD patients undergoing either HD or peritoneal dialysis (PD), and assessed basal ventilation and ventilatory sensitivity and threshold (modified Read re-breathing technique) before and after overnight polysomnographic recording. Subjects with sleep apnea were noted to have increased ventilatory sensitivity mediated by altered central and peripheral chemoreceptor responsiveness, which may destabilize respiratory control and increase loop gain, and contribute to the pathogenesis of CSA [40, 45]. Tang *et al.* have recently demonstrated that reduced uremic waste elimination may be related to a significantly increased severity of CSA in peritoneal dialysis patients following conversion to continuous peritoneal dialysis (CPD) from nocturnal peritoneal dialysis (NPD) [46]. Finally, cases involving improvements in sleep apnea following renal transplantation have been reported [47, 48].

Opioid-Related Central Sleep Apnea

Opioid use in the management of chronic pain has been on the rise over the last decade or so [49]. Emphasis on aggressive pain management has led to increasing use of sustained-release opioids and long-acting agents, such as methadone, in the treatment of both malignant and non-malignant pain [50]. Sleep disordered breathing in the form of CSA can emerge in patients on long-term opioid therapy [50-55] (see Table **2**). Other irregular respiratory patterns, including Biot's, ataxic and cluster breathing, have also been described in relation to opioid use. Central sleep apnea due to opioid use differs from CSR – it is not crescendo-decrescendo in character and has a shorter cycle time. Blunted central (medullary) and elevated peripheral (carotid) chemoreceptor responses have been described in patients on chronic stable doses of methadone; it is possible that an unstable breathing pattern or periodic respiration may develop when carotid chemoreceptor stimulation becomes the main input for ventilatory drive [56].

Opioids are known to cause changes in sleep architecture. Reduced NREM N3 and REM (R) sleep with increased arousals can develop, but tend to normalize with chronic use. Excessive daytime sleepiness and fatigue are also seen [56]. Prevalence of CSA is high among long-term opioid users and is dose related. The prevalence of CSA was 30% in one large cohort of patients enrolled in a methadone maintenance program [54].

Continuous positive airway pressure therapy is effective in controlling obstructive sleep disordered breathing in patients on long-term opioid therapy, but tends to worsen CSA. Two studies testing the use of ASV for treatment of central sleep apnea associated with opioid therapy have recently been published [57]. In a study by Javaheri *et al* [57] that included 5 patients with a baseline mean AHI of 70 per hour, mean AHI was reduced to 42 per hour on CPAP and to 13 per hour on ASV. The mean central apnea index (CAI) was 26 (baseline), 33 (on CPAP) and 0 per hour (on ASV). Thus, it appears that ASV is effective in controlling sleep disordered breathing in patients on chronic opioid therapy. Contrasting results were noted in another study [58] of 22 patients who had been on opioid therapy for at least 6 months. Baseline mean AHI and CAI were 66.6 and 26.4 per hour, respectively and on ASV were 54.2 and 15.6 per hour. In this study, oxygen saturation did not improve on ASV. The authors concluded that ASV was insufficient therapy, but added that their suboptimal results could have been related to the use of default settings on the ASV in a majority of patients, which potentially may have left untreated residual upper airway obstruction. Both event frequency and desaturation severity improved in patients in whom end-expiratory pressure was titrated. Further studies with ASV are required to determine its effectiveness and studies with long-term follow up are needed to know if treatment of sleep disordered breathing in this patient population would affect outcomes. Finally, acetazolamide has been reported to be effective as an adjunct to CPAP treatment in a patient on opioid therapy [59].

Table 2: Opioid-Related Central Sleep Apnea, CSA (BMI – body mass index, F – females, M – males, N – number of subjects studied)

Reference	Subjects	Medication/s	Central apnea index (CAI)	Comments
Wang *et al*, 2005 [54]	N=50 M:F= 1:1 Age: 35±9 yr BMI: 27	Previous heroin addicts on Methadone maintenance	CAI ≥ 5: 15 (30%)	Methadone blood concentration was the only significant variable associated with CSA. Awake P_aCO_2 was >45 in only 10 patients (20%). Average peak overnight PtcCO2 was 46.6±5 mmHg.
Walker *et al*, 2007 [53]	N=60 M:F= 3:2 Age: 52.7±13yr BMI: 31.8	98% on opioids for non-malignant pain and 2% for malignant pain. Medications: hydrocodone, methadone, oxycodone, fentanyl, morphine and propoxyphene. Mean morphine dose equivalent :144 mg (range : 7.5 to 750 mg)	CAI 12.8 vs. 2.1 in control	Ataxic breathing pattern was seen in 70% of patients. Each 100 mg morphine dose equivalent increased the rate of central apneas by 29%
Webster *et al*, 2008 [55]	N=140 M:F=1:1.5 Age: 51 yr	Opioids for chronic pain. Median morphine dose equivalent : 266 mg	CAI ≥ 5: 33%	Significant relation between CAI and the daily dosage of methadone

Complex Sleep Apnea Syndrome

Upon acute application of CPAP, some patients with OSA develop frequent central apneas or a periodic breathing pattern, a phenomenon referred to as CPAP-emergent central apnea or complex sleep apnea (CompSA). The long-term clinical consequences of this type of sleep disordered breathing are still poorly understood. Several case series have characterized its prevalence, clinical course and associated risk factors [60-65] (Table **3**). The prevalence is estimated at 5-6% based on large retrospective studies [61, 63].

The natural course of CompSA has been detailed in several retrospective studies [60, 62, 63]. In a larger and more recent study, Jahaveri *et al* [62] performed a second full-night attended CPAP titration on patients who had CompSA on their initial study. Eighty four of 1,286 patients had CAI of at least 5 per hour on their initial study and 42 of these 84 patients underwent a second CPAP titration about 5 to 6 weeks after being on CPAP therapy. CompSA resolved in 33 patients, but persisted in 9 patients, in whom the average CAI was 13 per hour. Thus, it appears that CompSA is generally transitory with a prevalence of 1.5% for chronic disease. For symptomatic, persistent CompSA, therapy using ASV could be considered [62]. In a prospective randomized crossover trial comparing noninvasive positive pressure ventilation (NPPV) and ASV on subjects with central, mixed and complex sleep apnea, mean AHI was 49.4 ± 25.4 (diagnostic study), 41.9 ± 28.1 (on CPAP), 6.8 ± 6.8 (on NPPV) and 1.6 ± 3.6 (on ASV). Adaptive servo ventilation was more effective in improving the AHI and decreasing the respiratory effort-related arousals [66].

Table 3: Complex Sleep Apnea (AHI – apnea hypopnea index, OSA – obstructive sleep apnea, CAD – coronary artery disease, CAI – central apnea index, CHF – congestive heart failure, CPAP – continuous positive airway pressure, N – number of individuals)

Reference	N	N with CompSA (Prevalence)	Risk factors
Morgenthaler *et al*, 2006 [65]	233	31 (15%)	-
Dernaika *et al*, 2007 [60]	116	23(19.8%)	-
Lehman *et al*, 2007 [64]	99	13 (13%)	Higher AHI during baseline, history of CHF or CAD
Endo *et al*, 2008 [61]	1232	14 (5%)	Higher AHI during baseline
Javaheri *et al*, 2009 [62]	1,286	84 (6.5%)	Severity of OSA, CAI ≥ 5, use of opioids Prevalence of CPAP persistent CSA was 1.5%

RESEARCH OUTLOOK

Central sleep apnea is not a single entity, but rather several disorders that share clinical features and polysomnographic findings. It is important to characterize each specific condition's risk factors, natural clinical course, response to various treatment modalities, prognosis, and to develop more accurate diagnostic methods that can distinguish one disorder from another.

What We Don't Know:

- What factors increase the risk of developing CSA? Clinical risk factors for central sleep apnea secondary to heart failure and high-altitude periodic breathing have been described. Still uncertain are those that relate to complex sleep apnea and sleep-onset central apneas.

- What is the role of portable sleep monitoring in the evaluation of CSA? What is the role, if any, of automated positive airway pressure devices in the treatment of CSA? Advances in technology have made possible the use of portable, unmonitored devices for the diagnosis and treatment of obstructive sleep apnea. Currently, these devices are not recommended for use among patients with predominantly central apneas. Would new algorithms endorse the use of devices capable to detect central apneas and allow non-laboratory based management of patients with this disorder?

- What is the role, if any, of pharmacologic therapy for the treatment of CSA? There are limited data on the use of medications for treating central apneas. As the neurochemistry responsible for the control of respiration is better understood, are there specific pharmacological targets that can reverse CSA in certain defined patient subgroups?

- What are the long-term beneficial effects associated with positive airway pressure (PAP) therapy for central sleep apnea? Should mild CSA be treated? Should complex sleep apnea (CompSA) be treated? Unless we understand the natural history of these disorders and until we determine the long-term outcomes of therapy, it would remain difficult to provide meaningful recommendations regarding treatment to patients presenting with central sleep apnea.

- What are the indications for bilevel positive airway pressure or adaptive servo-ventilation therapy in patients with central sleep apnea? Are there significant advantages to using newer positive airway pressure modalities in treating CSA? There are few published studies comparing these difference devices in patients with central sleep apnea.

- What factors influence compliance to PAP therapy? The use of heated humidification and systematic education improve PAP compliance in patients with obstructive sleep apnea (OSA), but do these measures provide similar advantages in those with CSA?

- How effective is oxygen or carbon dioxide therapy for CSA? What are their risks and long-term consequences? Acute application of low-flow oxygen or carbon dioxide has been shown to reduce the frequency of central apneas, but the effects on cardiovascular and neurocognitive functions are still unclear.

REFERENCES

[1]   Xie A, Wong B, Phillipson EA, *et al.* Interaction of hyperventilation and arousal in the pathogenesis of idiopathic central sleep apnea. Am J Respir Crit Care Med 1994; 150: 489-95.

[2]   Xie A, Rutherford R, Rankin F, *et al.* Hypocapnia and increased ventilatory responsiveness in patients with idiopathic central sleep apnea. Am J Respir Crit Care Med 1995; 152: 1950-5.

[3]   Franklin KA, Eriksson P, Sahlin C, Lundgren R. Reversal of central sleep apnea with oxygen. Chest 1997; 111: 163-9.

[4]   Szollosi I, Jones M, Morrell MJ, *et al.* Effect of CO2 inhalation on central sleep apnea and arousals from sleep. Respiration 2004; 71: 493-8.

[5]   Hommura F, Nishimura M, Oguri M, *et al.* Continuous versus bilevel positive airway pressure in a patient with idiopathic central sleep apnea. Am J Respir Crit Care Med 1997; 155: 1482-5.

[6]   Issa FG, Sullivan CE. Reversal of central sleep apnea using nasal CPAP. Chest 1986; 90: 165-71.

[7]   DeBacker WA, Verbraecken J, Willemen M, *et al.* Central apnea index decreases after prolonged treatment with acetazolamide. Am J Respir Crit Care Med 1995; 151: 87-91.

[8]   Quadri S, Drake C, Hudgel DW. Improvement of idiopathic central sleep apnea with zolpidem. J Clin Sleep Med 2009; 5: 122-9.

[9]   Javaheri S, Parker TJ, Liming JD, *et al.* Sleep apnea in 81 ambulatory male patients with stable heart failure. Types and their prevalences, consequences, and presentations. Circulation 1998; 97: 2154-9.

[10]   Sin DD, Fitzgerald F, Parker JD, *et al.* Risk factors for central and obstructive sleep apnea in 450 men and women with congestive heart failure. Am J Respir Crit Care Med 1999; 160: 1101-6.

[11]   Lanfranchi PA, Somers VK, Braghiroli A, *et al.* Central sleep apnea in left ventricular dysfunction: prevalence and implications for arrhythmic risk. Circulation 2003; 107: 727-32.

[12]   Ferrier K, Campbell A, Yee B, *et al.* Sleep-disordered breathing occurs frequently in stable outpatients with congestive heart failure. Chest 2005; 128: 2116-22.

[13]   Wang H, Parker JD, Newton GE, *et al.* Influence of obstructive sleep apnea on mortality in patients with heart failure. J Am Coll Cardiol 2007; 49: 1625-31.

[14]   Schulz R, Blau A, Borgel J, *et al.* Sleep apnoea in heart failure. Eur Respir J 2007; 29: 1201-5.

[15]   Oldenburg O, Lamp B, Faber L, *et al.* Sleep-disordered breathing in patients with symptomatic heart failure: a contemporary study of prevalence in and characteristics of 700 patients. Eur J Heart Fail 2007; 9: 251-7.

[16]   Vazir A, Hastings PC, Dayer M, *et al.* A high prevalence of sleep disordered breathing in men with mild symptomatic chronic heart failure due to left ventricular systolic dysfunction. Eur J Heart Fail 2007; 9: 243-50.

[17]   Hagenah G, Beil D. Prevalence of Cheyne-Stokes respiration in modern treated congestive heart failure. Sleep Breath 2009; 13: 181-5.

[18]   Paulino A, Damy T, Margarit L, *et al.* Prevalence of sleep-disordered breathing in a 316-patient French cohort of stable congestive heart failure. Arch Cardiovasc Dis 2009; 102: 169-75.

[19]   MacDonald M, Fang J, Pittman SD, *et al.* The current prevalence of sleep disordered breathing in congestive heart failure patients treated with beta-blockers. J Clin Sleep Med 2008; 4: 38-42.

[20]   Bradley TD, Logan AG, Kimoff RJ, *et al.* Continuous positive airway pressure for central sleep apnea and heart failure. N Engl J Med 2005; 353: 2025-33.

[21]   Arzt M, Floras JS, Logan AG, *et al.* Suppression of central sleep apnea by continuous positive airway pressure and transplant-free survival in heart failure: a post hoc analysis of the Canadian Continuous Positive Airway Pressure for Patients with Central Sleep Apnea and Heart Failure Trial (CANPAP). Circulation 2007; 115: 3173-80.

[22]   Teschler H, Dohring J, Wang YM, Berthon-Jones M. Adaptive pressure support servo-ventilation: a novel treatment for Cheyne-Stokes respiration in heart failure. Am J Respir Crit Care Med 2001; 164: 614-9.

[23]   Pepperell JC, Maskell NA, Jones DR, *et al.* A randomized controlled trial of adaptive ventilation for Cheyne-Stokes breathing in heart failure. Am J Respir Crit Care Med 2003; 168: 1109-14.

[24]   Philippe C, Stoica-Herman M, Drouot X, *et al.* Compliance with and effectiveness of adaptive servoventilation versus continuous positive airway pressure in the treatment of Cheyne-Stokes respiration in heart failure over a six month period. Heart 2006; 92: 337-42.

[25]   Fatti LM, Scacchi M, Pincelli AI, *et al.* Prevalence and pathogenesis of sleep apnea and lung disease in acromegaly. Pituitary 2001; 4: 259-62.

[26]   Grunstein RR, Ho KY, Berthon-Jones M, *et al.* Central sleep apnea is associated with increased ventilatory response to carbon dioxide and hypersecretion of growth hormone in patients with acromegaly. Am J Respir Crit Care Med 1994; 150: 496-502.

[27]   Weiss V, Sonka K, Pretl M, *et al.* Prevalence of the sleep apnea syndrome in acromegaly population. J Endocrinol Invest 2000; 23: 515-9.

[28]   Sze L, Schmid C, Bloch KE, *et al.* Effect of transsphenoidal surgery on sleep apnoea in acromegaly. Eur J Endocrinol 2007; 156: 321-9.

[29]   Tolis G, Angelopoulos NG, Katounda E, *et al.* Medical treatment of acromegaly: comorbidities and their reversibility by somatostatin analogs. Neuroendocrinology 2006; 83: 249-57.

[30]   Grunstein RR, Ho KK, Sullivan CE. Effect of octreotide, a somatostatin analog, on sleep apnea in patients with acromegaly. Ann Intern Med 1994; 121: 478-83.

[31]   Pelttari L, Polo O, Rauhala E, *et al.* Nocturnal breathing abnormalities in acromegaly after adenomectomy. Clin Endocrinol (Oxf) 1995; 43: 175-82.

[32]   Pekkarinen T, Partinen M, Pelkonen R, Iivanainen M. Sleep apnoea and daytime sleepiness in acromegaly: relationship to endocrinological factors. Clin Endocrinol (Oxf) 1987; 27: 649-54.

[33]   Di Iorio B, Bartiromo M, Cesare MC, De Santo RM. Do sleep disorders start in dialysis or in early chronic kidney disease? Nephrol Dial Transplant 2006; 21: 1731; author reply 1732.

[34]   Kimmel PL, Miller G, Mendelson WB. Sleep apnea syndrome in chronic renal disease. Am J Med 1989; 86: 308-14.

[35]   Merlino G, Piani A, Dolso P, *et al.* Sleep disorders in patients with end-stage renal disease undergoing dialysis therapy. Nephrol Dial Transplant 2006; 21: 184-90.

[36]   Tada T, Kusano KF, Ogawa A, *et al.* The predictors of central and obstructive sleep apnoea in haemodialysis patients. Nephrol Dial Transplant 2007; 22: 1190-7.

[37]   Beecroft JM, Duffin J, Pierratos A, *et al.* Decreased chemosensitivity and improvement of sleep apnea by nocturnal hemodialysis. Sleep Med 2009; 10: 47-54.

[38]   Beecroft JM, Hoffstein V, Pierratos A, *et al.* Nocturnal haemodialysis increases pharyngeal size in patients with sleep apnoea and end-stage renal disease. Nephrol Dial Transplant 2008; 23: 673-9.

[39]   de Oliveira Rodrigues CJ, Marson O, Tufic S, *et al.* Relationship among end-stage renal disease, hypertension, and sleep apnea in nondiabetic dialysis patients. Am J Hypertens 2005; 18: 152-7.

[40]   Beecroft J, Duffin J, Pierratos A, *et al.* Enhanced chemo-responsiveness in patients with sleep apnoea and end-stage renal disease. Eur Respir J 2006; 28: 151-8.

[41]   Hamilton RW, Epstein PE, Henderson LW, *et al.* Control of breathing in uremia: ventilatory response to CO2 after hemodialysis. J Appl Physiol 1976; 41: 216-22.

[42]   Wilcox I, McNamara SG, Dodd MJ, Sullivan CE. Ventilatory control in patients with sleep apnoea and left ventricular dysfunction: comparison of obstructive and central sleep apnoea. Eur Respir J 1998; 11:7-13.

[43]   Hanly PJ, Pierratos A. Improvement of sleep apnea in patients with chronic renal failure who undergo nocturnal hemodialysis. N Engl J Med 2001; 344: 102-7.

[44]   Jean G, Piperno D, Francois B, Charra B. Sleep apnea incidence in maintenance hemodialysis patients: influence of dialysate buffer. Nephron 1995; 71: 138-42.

[45]   Khoo MC. Determinants of ventilatory instability and variability. Respir Physiol 2000; 122: 167-82.

[46]   Tang SC, Lam B, Lai AS, *et al.* Improvement in sleep apnea during nocturnal peritoneal dialysis is associated with reduced airway congestion and better uremic clearance. Clin J Am Soc Nephrol 2009; 4: 410-8.

[47]   Beecroft JM, Zaltzman J, Prasad R, *et al.* Impact of kidney transplantation on sleep apnoea in patients with end-stage renal disease. Nephrol Dial Transplant 2007; 22: 3028-33.

[48]   Langevin B, Fouque D, Leger P, Robert D. Sleep apnea syndrome and end-stage renal disease. Cure after renal transplantation. Chest 1993; 103: 1330-5.

[49]   Novak S, Nemeth WC, Lawson KA. Trends in medical use and abuse of sustained-release opioid analgesics: a revisit. Pain Med 2004; 5: 59-65.

[50]   Porucznik C. Increased mortality rate associated with prescribed opioid medications: is there a link with sleep disordered breathing? In: European Respiratory Society. European Respiratory Journal; 2005.

[51]　Teichtahl H, Prodromidis A, Miller B, *et al.* Sleep-disordered breathing in stable methadone programme patients: a pilot study. Addiction 2001; 96: 395-403.

[52]　Teichtahl H, Wang D, Cunnington D, *et al.* Ventilatory responses to hypoxia and hypercapnia in stable methadone maintenance treatment patients. Chest 2005; 128: 1339-47.

[53]　Walker JM, Farney RJ, Rhondeau SM, *et al.* Chronic opioid use is a risk factor for the development of central sleep apnea and ataxic breathing. J Clin Sleep Med 2007; 3: 455-61.

[54]　Wang D, Teichtahl H, Drummer O, *et al.* Central sleep apnea in stable methadone maintenance treatment patients. Chest 2005; 128: 1348-56.

[55]　Webster LR, Choi Y, Desai H, *et al.* Sleep-disordered breathing and chronic opioid therapy. Pain Med 2008; 9: 425-32.

[56]　Wang D, Teichtahl H. Opioids, sleep architecture and sleep-disordered breathing. Sleep Med Rev 2007; 11: 35-46.

[57]　Javaheri S, Malik A, Smith J, Chung E. Adaptive pressure support servoventilation: a novel treatment for sleep apnea associated with use of opioids. J Clin Sleep Med 2008; 4: 305-10.

[58]　Farney RJ, Walker JM, Boyle KM, *et al.* Adaptive servoventilation (ASV) in patients with sleep disordered breathing associated with chronic opioid medications for non-malignant pain. J Clin Sleep Med 2008; 4: 311-9.

[59]　Glidewell RN, Orr WC, Imes N. Acetazolamide as an adjunct to CPAP treatment: a case of complex sleep apnea in a patient on long-acting opioid therapy. J Clin Sleep Med 2009; 5: 63-4.

[60]　Dernaika T, Tawk M, Nazir S, *et al.* The significance and outcome of continuous positive airway pressure-related central sleep apnea during split-night sleep studies. Chest 2007; 132: 81-7.

[61]　Endo Y, Suzuki M, Inoue Y, *et al.* Prevalence of complex sleep apnea among Japanese patients with sleep apnea syndrome. Tohoku J Exp Med 2008; 215: 349-54.

[62]　Javaheri S, Smith J, Chung E. The prevalence and natural history of complex sleep apnea. J Clin Sleep Med 2009; 5: 205-11.

[63]　Kuzniar TJ, Pusalavidyasagar S, Gay PC, Morgenthaler TI. Natural course of complex sleep apnea--a retrospective study. Sleep Breath 2008; 12: 135-9.

[64]　Lehman S, Antic NA, Thompson C, *et al.* Central sleep apnea on commencement of continuous positive airway pressure in patients with a primary diagnosis of obstructive sleep apnea-hypopnea. J Clin Sleep Med 2007; 3: 462-6.

[65]　Morgenthaler TI, Kagramanov V, Hanak V, Decker PA. Complex sleep apnea syndrome: is it a unique clinical syndrome? Sleep 2006; 29: 1203-9.

[66]　Morgenthaler TI, Gay PC, Gordon N, Brown LK. Adaptive servoventilation versus noninvasive positive pressure ventilation for central, mixed, and complex sleep apnea syndromes. Sleep 2007; 30: 468-75.

CHAPTER 8

Obesity Hypoventilation Syndrome

Stephen W. Littleton, M.D.[1,*] and Babak Mokhlesi, M.D., M.Sc.[2]

[1]*Attending Physician, John H. Stroger Jr. Hospital of Cook County, Assistant Professor, Rush University Medical Center, 1900 W. Polk St. Room 1416 Chicago, IL 60612, USA and* [2]*Associate Professor of Medicine, Section of Pulmonary and Critical Care Medicine, Director, Sleep Disorders Center and Sleep Medicine Fellowship Program, University of Chicago Pritzker School of Medicine, 5841 S. Maryland Ave, MC0999, Room L11B, Chicago, IL 60637, USA*

Abstract: Obesity Hypoventilation syndrome (OHS) is defined as the triad of obesity, daytime hypoventilation, and sleep disordered breathing in the absence of an alternative explanation for hypoventilation. Among patients with obstructive sleep apnea (OSA), those who are more obese and have more severe OSA are more likely to have the syndrome. It is unclear why some patients with OSA develop OHS and others do not. It is important to identify the syndrome early, as these patients may have a significantly increased risk of mortality if left untreated. The authors describe current understanding of the pathogenesis of the disorder and optimal treatment modalities.

TOPIC DISCUSSION (CLINICAL OUTLOOK)

Among patients with OSA, those who are severely obese (BMI >40 kg/m^2) or have more severe obstructive sleep apnea (apnea-hypopnea index, or AHI>60) seem to be at a higher risk of having OHS. A useful clinical predictor of OHS may be >45% of total sleep time with an oxygen saturation by pulse oximetry (SpO$_2$) <90%. By definition, sleep disordered breathing must be present, and the syndrome improves or completely resolves with proper treatment. Leptin resistance and a long bicarbonate excretion time-constant may play a role in the pathogenesis of the disorder. In a patient suspected of having OHS, other causes of hypoventilation need to be ruled out. Treatment consists of positive airway pressure (PAP) therapy, either in the form of continuous positive airway pressure (CPAP) or bilevel positive airway pressure (bilevel PAP), with or without supplemental oxygen. Response to therapy should be monitored closely. The need for daytime or nocturnal oxygen supplementation should be re-assessed a few weeks to months after therapy, as it is temporary in a significant proportion of these patients.

Definition

Obesity Hypoventilation syndrome (OHS) is defined as daytime hypercapnia and hypoxemia (P$_a$CO$_2$ > 45 mm Hg and P$_a$O$_2$ < 70 mm Hg) in an obese patient (BMI ≥ 30 kg/m^2) with sleep disordered breathing, in the absence of any other cause of hypoventilation [1]. In 90% of patients with OHS, the sleep-disordered breathing is simply OSA. The remaining 10% have sleep hypoventilation, which is defined as an increase in P$_a$CO$_2$ of >10 mm Hg above that of wakefulness, or significant oxygen desaturations, neither of which are the result of obstructive apneas or hypopneas. There is no accurate way to predict the form of sleep disordered breathing in a particular patient; polysomnography must be performed.

Other conditions that mimic OHS are the overlap syndrome and adult onset of congenital central hypoventilation syndrome. The **overlap syndrome** is the term used to describe patients with chronic obstructive pulmonary disease (COPD) and OSA. It has been reported that 10-15% of patients with OSA have the overlap syndrome [2-4]. Patients with OSA are no more likely to have COPD than the general population [5]. Patients with the overlap syndrome, when compared to patients with simple OSA, are more likely to be hypoxemic, hypercapnic, and have pulmonary hypertension [2, 3, 6]. Patients with the overlap syndrome develop hypercapnia at a lower BMI and AHI than that of patients with OHS without an obstructive defect on spirometry, and at a higher forced expiratory volume in one second (FEV$_1$) than hypercapnic patients with pure COPD. The **congenital central hypoventilation syndrome** is a disorder of ventilatory control that typically presents in newborns and — in 90% of the cases — is caused by a polyalanine repeat expansion mutation in the PHOX2B gene [7]. Symptomatic and asymptomatic children have

*Address correspondence to Stephan W. Littleton:** Attending Physician, John H. Stroger Jr. Hospital of Cook County, Assistant Professor, Rush University Medical Center, 1900 W. Polk St. Room 1416 Chicago, IL 60612, USA; E-mail: slittleton@cchil.org

Octavian C. Ioachimescu (Ed)

survived to adulthood without ventilatory support [8]. These patients are heterozygous for the mildest of the PHOX2B polyalanine expansion mutations [9, 10]. Transmission of late-onset congenital central hypoventilation syndrome in an autosomal dominant fashion has been well described in the recent literature [8].

Epidemiology

Numerous studies have reported a prevalence of OHS between 10-20% in obese patients with OSA. A recent meta-analysis of 4,250 patients with obesity and OSA (who did not have COPD) reported a 19% prevalence of hypercapnia [11]. Although the prevalence of OHS in a community-based cohort is unknown, its prevalence can be estimated amongst the general adult population in the US. If approximately 3% of the general US population has severe obesity (body mass index or BMI $\geq$ 40 kg/m^2) [12] and half of patients with severe obesity have OSA [13], and 10-20% of the severely obese patients with OSA have OHS, then a conservative estimated prevalence of OHS in the general adult population is anywhere between 0.15-0.3% (1.5 to 3 individuals out of 1000 adults) [14].

Many studies have sought risk factors or predictors of hypercapnia (*i.e.* likely OHS) in cohorts of patients with OSA [15-23]. Results have been mixed, but in a recent meta-analysis, Kaw *et al* were able to identify three significant predictors: 1) severity of obesity as measured by the BMI; 2) severity of OSA measured by either AHI or hypoxia during sleep; and 3) degree of restrictive chest physiology. The mean AHI in the hypercapnic group was 63.7 (CI 51.9-75.5) vs. 51.19 in eucapnic group (CI 42.3-60.1, difference between groups p<0.0001). In two studies, the authors found the prevalence of OHS in patients with an AHI > 60 to be 25-30% [14, 23]. Likewise, Kaw found the mean BMI in the hypercapnic group to be 38.94 kg/m^2 (CI 34.2-43.9) vs. 35.81 kg/m^2 in the simple OSA group (CI 31.1-41.2, difference between groups p<0.00001). In patients with OSA who have a BMI of >40 kg/m^2, the prevalence of hypercapnia is between 20-25%. Age and sex were not found to be significant in the meta-analysis. Although increasing BMI and a higher AHI are correlated with hypercapnia, there is significant overlap in the hypercapnic and eucapnic groups, so these parameters cannot be relied upon as predictors in a particular patient. Additionally, patients who were hypercapnic had a more severe restrictive ventilatory pattern on their pulmonary function tests (Table 1).

Table 1: Weighted averages of individual determinants between hypercapnic and eucapnic patients with OSA

Weighted Mean (95% CI)

Variable	Hypercapnic	Eucapnic	MD (95% CI)	P value
BMI	38.9 (34 to 44)	35.8 (31 to 41)	3.1 (1.8 to 4.4)	< 0.00001
AHI	63.7 (52 to 76)	51.2 (42 to 60)	12.5 (6.6 to 18.4)	< 0.0001
FEV$_1$ %	70.8 (63 to 79)	82.1 (75 to 89)	-11.2 (-15.7 to 6.8)	< 0.00001
VC %	84.9 (72 to 98)	93.1 (82 to 104)	-8.1 (11.3 to 4.9)	< 0.00001
FEV$_1$/FVC	78.5 (74 to 83)	80.1 (77 to 84)	-1.7 (-4.6 to 0.8)	< 0.02
TLC %	77.4 (70 to 85)	83.8 (79 to 89)	-6.4 (10.0 to -2.7)	< 0.0006
% TST spo$_2$ < 90%	56.1 (42 to 70)	18.8 (-9.8 to 47)	37.4 (29.7 to 44.9)	< 0.00001

From Kaw R, Hernandez A, Walker E, Aboussouan L, Mokhlesi B. Determinants of Hypercapnia in Obese Patients with Obstructive Sleep Apnea. *Chest* 136 (3); 787-796. MD=mean difference, CI= confidence interval, BMI= body mass index, AHI= apnea-hypopnea index, FEV$_1$%= percent of predicted forced expiratory volume in one second, VC%= percent of predicted vital capacity, TLC%= percent of predicted total lung capacity, %TST SpO$_2$ < 90% = percent of total sleep time with oxygen saturation of less than 90%. Used with permission.

One parameter in Kaw's meta-analysis that seemed to clearly delineate between the two groups was % of total sleep time [TST] during polysomnography with oxygen saturation by pulse oximetry (SpO$_2$) below 90%. The eucapnic group spent 18.8% of TST with an SpO$_2$ < 90% (CI -9.86-47.47), whereas this parameter was an impressive 56.16% in the hypercapnic group (CI 42.47-69.87, difference between groups p<0.00001).

Pathophysiology

A variety of physiologic derangements has been described in patients with obesity and OHS, and has been thought to contribute to or cause the syndrome. These include: increased upper airway resistance [24], ventilation/perfusion mismatching secondary to pulmonary edema [25] or low lung volumes/atelectasis [26], respiratory muscle dysfunction [27], and decreased pulmonary and chest wall compliance [28]. Although these are undoubtedly present, the most convincing evidence for the pathogenesis lies behind the universal presence of sleep-disordered breathing and a blunted central response to hypercapnia and hypoxia.

Sleep Disordered Breathing: Sleep-disordered breathing is considered integral to OHS. When it is treated with either PAP therapy or tracheostomy, daytime hypercapnia either improves substantially or completely resolves in the vast majority of patients without any significant change in the BMI [4, 6, 29-33]. The degree of correction also correlates with the degree of usage of PAP [6, 30]. Since a minority of patients with severe sleep disordered breathing develop OHS, this alone is not sufficient for the development of the syndrome.

Blunted ventilatory response: Patients with OHS are able to voluntarily hyperventilate to eucapnia [34]. This is probably the simplest evidence for a defective central respiratory drive, although there is plenty of additional evidence. Patients with OHS do not hyperventilate to the same degree as morbidly obese patients when rebreathing CO_2 [29, 35, 36]. This deficit corrects in most patients after therapy with PAP [29, 37, 38]. In patients with severe OSA but without hypercapnia, the hypercapnic ventilatory response does not change with PAP therapy [38]. In addition, patients with OHS do not augment their minute ventilation to the same degree as when forced to breathe a hypoxic gas mixture [29, 38, 39]. This blunted hypoxic drive also corrects with PAP therapy [29, 38]. The reversibility of these defects suggest that they are secondary effects of the syndrome (and necessary for its persistence), but not the origin of it. There are a few hypotheses as to the origin of these defects.

Hypoxemia: It has long been recognized that patients with hypoxemia from COPD have a blunted hypoxemic respiratory drive [40]. There is some evidence that the recurrent nocturnal hypoxemia in OHS can blunt respiratory drive as well [26]. There are no controlled studies in humans, as they would likely be unethical. Patients with OHS have much more profound hypoxemia than those with OSA, which supports this hypothesis [11, 26].

Leptin: Leptin's contribution to OHS and central respiratory drive is complex but the evidence is convincing. Obesity leads to an increase in the CO_2 production and load. Leptin is an adipokine, *i.e.*, a cytokine secreted by adipocytes which acts as a satiety hormone on hypothalamic receptors. It also stimulates ventilation [41]. Therefore, with worsening obesity, the excess adipose tissue leads to increasing levels of leptin, which in turn, increase ventilation to compensate for the additional CO_2 load. This could be the reason why the vast majority of humans with significant obesity do not develop hypercapnia. Mice that have mutations in the *ob* gene are deficient in leptin and develop obesity as well as a blunted hypercapnic response, much like patients with OHS. The blunted hypercapnic response occurs before overt weight gain, and leptin therapy corrects these abnormalities. Interestingly, the respiratory drive is corrected before any significant weight loss, suggesting that the central respiratory stimulant effect, not weight loss, leads to the correction of hypercapnia [42].

Leptin physiology in humans is not as simple. There is a direct correlation between serum leptin and body fat, the opposite of what is seen in *ob/ob* mice [43]. Patients with OHS and OSA have significantly higher leptin levels compared to lean or BMI matched subjects without OSA. Moreover, patients with OHS have higher leptin levels than BMI and AHI matched patients with OSA[45, 46]. It remains unclear why the higher leptin levels do not lead to an increase in ventilation, hence the concept of leptin resistance was born. Evidence suggests that some obese patients have lower cerebrospinal fluid levels of leptin than lean patients [44]. Individual differences in leptin CSF penetration may explain why some patients with severe OSA develop OHS and others do not [45]. After treatment with PAP therapy, leptin levels drop [46].

Transition of acute to chronic hypercapnia: Norman and colleagues have proposed an elegant model that explains how OSA can lead to daytime hypercapnia. In most patients with OSA, the hyperventilation after an apnea eliminates all CO_2 accumulated during the apnea [47]. But if the inter-apnea hyperventilation is inadequate or the ventilator response to the accumulated CO_2 is blunted, it could lead to an increase in P_aCO_2 during sleep (Fig. **1**). Even in this acute setting during sleep, the kidneys can retain bicarbonate to buffer the decrease in pH. If the time constant for the excretion of the small amount of accumulated bicarbonate is slow, and the patient falls asleep before this bicarbonate is eliminated, then the patient will have a net gain of bicarbonate, and retain some CO_2 during wakefulness to compensate for this retained bicarbonate [48]. Therefore, the combination of a decreased response to CO_2 and a slow rate of bicarbonate excretion will lead to a blunted respiratory drive during the next sleep cycle.

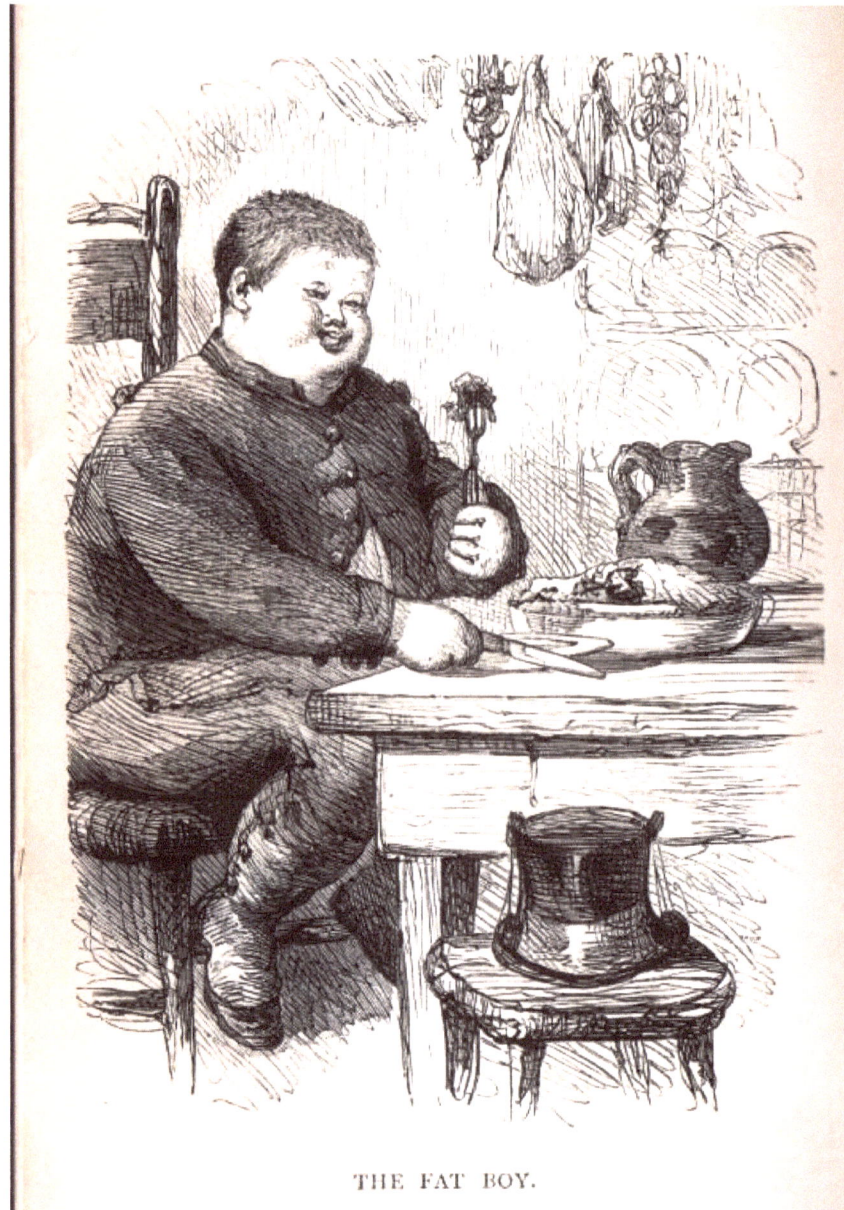

THE FAT BOY.

Figure 1: Joe the "Fat Boy". Illustration by S. Etyinge, Jr. (From: Dickens C. The Posthumous Papers of the Pickwick Club. Boston: Ticknor and Fields, 1867).

Signs and Symptoms

Symptoms of OHS generally overlap the classic symptoms of OSA: daytime hypersomnolence, nocturnal choking episodes, morning headaches, and loud snoring. Signs that can distinguish OHS from simple OSA are low room air pulse oximetry during wakefulness, erythrocytosis, or elevated serum bicarbonate [45]. If any of these signs are present the clinician should obtain an arterial blood gas (ABG) to confirm the presence of hypercapnia and hypoxemia. In severe cases, signs can include cyanosis, pulmonary hypertension, and cor pulmonale. Pretibial edema should raise suspicion for pulmonary hypertension in patients with OSA, especially in the severely obese [49].

Diagnosis

Any patient in whom OHS is suspected should undergo an overnight polysomnogram. A split night study is usually sufficient, as these patients tend to have severe sleep apnea that is readily apparent in the first half of the night. Continuous Positive Airway Pressure (CPAP) titrations in these patients can be difficult, however, and a full night titration may be necessary after the initial study if CPAP fails to correct the sleep disordered breathing and sleep hypoventilation.

In order to confirm OHS in a patient with known OSA, they should have: 1) obesity (BMI > 30 kg/m^2); 2) sleep disordered breathing; 3) P_aCO_2 > 45mmHg and P_aO_2 < 70 mm Hg on arterial blood gas (ABG) obtained on room air during wakefulness and while resting; and 4) other causes of hypoventilation excluded. Additional testing should include chest radiograph to look for interstitial lung diseases and chest wall deformities such as kyphoscoliosis, pulmonary function testing to examine for obstructive lung disease (a mild to moderate restrictive defect would be expected in the more severely obese), and thyroid stimulating hormone serum level to rule out severe hypothyroidism. Other entities that could be considered are neuromuscular weakness and central hypoventilation syndromes (such as Arnold-Chiari type II malformations or late onset central hypoventilation syndrome) [1].

Providers should suspect OHS in obese patients with abnormal room air pulse oximetry during a routine outpatient clinic visit. Elevated serum bicarbonate has also been shown to be a useful screening tool for OHS. Approximately 50% of patients with a serum bicarbonate level of > 27 mEq/L, obesity (BMI ≥ 30 kg/m^2), and OSA have OHS [22]. It is important to note that a low oxygen saturation during wakefulness and/or an elevated serum bicarbonate should lead to a confirmatory test with the measurement of arterial blood gases.

A useful tool for a sleep physician interpreting a polysomnogram of a patient they have not seen in clinic may be the % of total sleep time (TST) with SpO2 spent below 90%. In a recent meta-analysis, the mean difference of %TST with SpO2 spent below 90% was 37.4% (56.2% for hypercapnic patients, 18.8% for eucapnic patients), with very little overlap in the 95% confidence intervals[11]. Table **2** provides a summary of 757 patients with OHS reported in the literature [1].

Table 2: Clinical features of patients with obesity hypoventilation syndrome

Variables	Mean (range)
Age, *year*	52 (42-61)
Men, *%*	60 (49-90)
Body mass index, *kg/m²*	44 (35-56)
Neck circumference, *cm*	46.5 (45-47)
pH	7.38 (7.34-7.40)
PaCO₂, *mm Hg*	53 (47-61)
PaO₂, *mm Hg*	56 (46-74)
Serum bicarbonate, *mEq/L*	32 (31-33)
Hemoglobin, *g/dL*	15
Apnea-Hypopnea Index	66 (20-100)
Oxygen nadir during sleep, *%*	65 (59-76)
Percent time SaO₂ < 90%, *%*	50 (46-56)
FVC, *% of predicted*	68 (57-102)
FEV₁, *% of predicted*	64 (53-92)
FEV₁/FVC	77 (74-88)
Medical Research Council dyspnea class 3 and 4, *%*	69
Epworth Sleepiness Scale	14 (12-16)

Data presented as mean (range) of the 16 studies and includes a total of 757 patients with obesity hypoventilation syndrome [1]. Reprinted from reference 2 with permission of the American Thoracic Society. Copyright © American Thoracic Society.

Morbidity and Mortality

The majority of patients with OHS are severely obese and have severe OSA [1]. Severe obesity [50] and severe OSA (defined as an apnea-hypopnea index of ≥30 events per hour) [51], independent of hypercapnia, are known to negatively affect quality of life, morbidity, and mortality. OHS seems to present an additional burden on these patients above and beyond that of severe obesity and severe OSA.

Quality of Life: The data on the syndrome's effect on quality of life is scarce. Hida *et al* matched patients with OHS to patients with eucapnic OSA by age, BMI and lung function, and assessed quality of life with the short form 36 (SF-36) questionnaire [52]. There was no significant difference between the two groups with the exception of social functioning, those with OHS being worse (p < 0.01). The authors hypothesized this was because the patients with OHS were sleepier (Epworth Sleepiness Scale 14.6 ± 4.9 vs. 12.5 ± 4.6, p < 0.05). Quality of life improved after 6 months of treatment with CPAP in both groups, but the authors did not examine whether the patients with OHS had a significantly greater improvement. In another study, Patients with OHS had a better quality of life than those with other causes of chronic hypercapnic respiratory failure, despite being significantly more obese than the other groups [53].

Morbidity: It is also unclear whether patients with OHS experience higher morbidity than patients who are similarly obese and have OSA, as no studies have been performed to date. Berg et al performed a study where 26 patients with OHS were matched with patients of similar BMI, age, gender, and postal code (to control for socio-economic factors) [30]. The group with OHS was significantly more obese, although both groups were severely obese. The group with OHS was found to be more likely to carry a diagnosis of congestive heart failure (odds ratio [OR] 9, 95% CI 2.3-35) angina pectoris (OR 9; 95% CI 1.4-57.10) or cor pulmonale (OR 9; 95% CI 1.4-57.1). Patients with OHS were more likely to be hospitalized and more likely to be admitted to the intensive care unit. Rates of hospital admission decreased and were equivalent with the control group two years after treatment was instituted. In another prospective study, 47 patients with OHS had higher rates of admission to the intensive care unit (40% vs. 6%) and need for invasive mechanical ventilation (6% vs. 0%) when compared to 103 patients with similar degree of obesity but without hypoventilation [54].

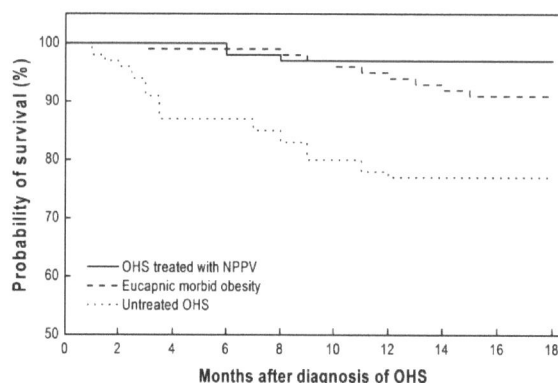

Figure 2: Survival curves for patients with untreated OHS (n=47; mean age 55±14; mean BMI 45±9 kg/m^2; mean P$_a$CO$_2$ 52±7 mm Hg) and eucapnic morbidly obese patients (n=103; mean age 53±13; mean BMI 42±8 kg/m^2) as reported by Nowbar et al [54] compared to patients with OHS treated with NPPV therapy (n=126; mean age 55.6±10.6; mean BMI 44.6±7.8 kg/m^2; mean baseline P$_a$CO$_2$ 55.5±7.7 mm Hg; mean adherence to NPPV of 6.5±2.3 h/day). Data for OHS patients treated with NPPV was provided courtesy of Dr. Stephan Budweiser and colleagues from the University of Regensburg, Germany [55]. Reprinted from reference 2 with permission of the American Thoracic Society. Copyright © American Thoracic Society.

Mortality: The data on mortality is also scarce, but suggests untreated OHS leads to a significantly increased risk of mortality. Budweiser and colleagues conducted a retrospective analysis of 126 patients with OHS and found the 1, 2 and 5 - year survival rates to be 97%, 92%, and 70%, respectively [55]. Patients in this study were adherent to noninvasive positive airway pressure therapy (>6 hours/night). Patients with untreated OHS have a significant risk of death. A prospective study by Nowbar et al followed a group of 47 severely obese patients after hospital discharge [54]. The 18-month mortality rate for patients with untreated OHS was higher than the control cohort of 103 patients with obesity alone (23% vs. 9%), despite the fact that the groups were well-matched for BMI, age, and a number of co-morbid conditions (the exception being that OSA was more prevalent in the OHS group). When adjusted for age, sex, BMI, and renal function, the hazard ratio of death in the OHS group was 4.0 in the 18-month period. Only 13% of the 47 patients were treated for OHS after hospital discharge. A retrospective study of 126 patients with OHS who were highly adherent to noninvasive positive pressure ventilation (NPPV) therapy in the form of bilevel PAP, reported an 18-month mortality of 3% [1, 55]. Together, these two studies suggest that adherence to PAP therapy may lower the short term mortality of patients with OHS (Fig. **2**).

TREATMENT

Positive Airway Pressure (PAP) Therapy

Positive airway pressure (PAP) is the first line therapy for treatment of OHS. Treatment of sleep disordered breathing with PAP therapy leads to a significant improvement or normalization of daytime blood gases in most patients [45]. Improvement in blood gases is directly correlated with duration of usage of the PAP device [6], and can be seen within one month of instituting therapy [6, 29, 56].

PAP therapy can be delivered in the form of CPAP or bilevel PAP therapy. CPAP therapy alone is effective in treating nocturnal hypoxemia and sleep disordered breathing in approximately half of the patients, particularly those who have concomitant OSA [57]. A recent prospective controlled study compared the impact of a full night of CPAP titration— without supplemental oxygen therapy or bilevel PAP — on 23 patients with OHS and 23 patients with eucapnic OSA matched for BMI, AHI, and lung function. Both patient groups were extremely obese, had severe OSA and those with OHS had significant daytime hypercapnia. In more than half of patients with OHS (57%) CPAP significantly improved OSA and nocturnal hypoxemia. The optimal CPAP pressure of 13.9±3.1 cm H_2O was reached within one hour of sleep onset. Ten patients with OHS (43%), however, had refractory hypoxemia during CPAP titration. The fact that more than half of the patients with stable, but extreme cases of OHS (based on BMI, AHI, and the level of daytime hypercapnia) were successfully titrated with CPAP—without requiring bilevel PAP or supplemental oxygen — suggests that the majority of patients with milder forms of OHS can be successfully titrated with CPAP as well [58].

A recent prospective randomized study found that CPAP therapy is no more effective than bilevel PAP in improving daytime blood gases when the initial CPAP titration was successful [59]. Therefore, CPAP is not inferior to bilevel PAP *a priori*. However, bilevel PAP therapy may be necessary to eliminate desaturations and obstructive events in a particular patient. Fig. **3** describes a therapeutic algorithm for PAP titration in patients with OHS.

Average volume-assured pressure support ventilation (AVAPS) is a mode that is a hybrid mode of pressure support and volume controlled ventilation that delivers a more consistent tidal volume with the comfort of pressure support ventilation. AVAPS ensures a preset tidal volume during bilevel-S/T mode and the expiratory tidal volume is estimated based on pneumotachographic inspiratory and expiratory flows. The inspiratory positive airway pressure (IPAP) support is then titrated in steps of 1 cm H_2O/min in order to achieve the preset tidal volume. As a result, the IPAP is variable. The EPAP, on the other hand, is set between 4 and 8 cm H_2O and the respiratory "back-up rate" can be set at 12-18/min, with an I:E ratio of 1:2. The role of a "back-up rate" remains unclear, since patients with OHS are typically tachypneic during sleep with respiratory rates ranging between 15-30 breaths per minute. However, it is conceivable that during titration, central apneas could develop with pressure support ventilation and in those instances a "back-up rate" would be useful. Although significantly more expensive than CPAP or bilevel PAP therapy, it has been shown effective in a randomized controlled study of OHS patients with milder degrees of hypercapnia [60].

The improvement in chronic daytime hypercapnia in patients who adhere to PAP therapy is neither universal nor complete. In two studies [6, 59], the P_aCO_2 did not improve significantly in approximately a quarter of patients that had undergone successful PAP titration in the laboratory and were highly adherent (> 6 hours/night) with either CPAP or bilevel PAP therapy (personal communication by Amanda Piper). This lack of response to PAP therapy combined with reports of persistent hypoventilation after tracheostomy [30] suggests that in a subset of patients with OHS, factors other than sleep disordered breathing are the driving force behind the pathogenesis of hypoventilation. These patients will most likely need more aggressive nocturnal mechanical ventilation with or without respiratory stimulants (see below).

```
┌─────────────────────────────────────────────┐
│      Increase CPAP to eliminate obstructive  │
│      apneas, hypopneas, and flow limitation  │
└─────────────────────────────────────────────┘
                      │
                      ▼
┌─────────────────────────────────────────────┐
│      SpO₂ persistently below 90% in the absence│
│      of obstructive apneas or hypopneas       │
└─────────────────────────────────────────────┘
                      │
                      ▼
┌─────────────────────────────────────────────┐
│      Switch to bi-level PAP and increase IPAP │
│      over the last CPAP pressure that eliminated│
│      obstructive apneas until SpO₂ > 90%      │
└─────────────────────────────────────────────┘
                      │
                      ▼
┌─────────────────────────────────────────────┐
│      Add supplemental oxygen if SpO₂ is       │
│      persistently < 90% despite an IPAP to EPAP│
│      delta of at least 8-10 cm H₂O            │
└─────────────────────────────────────────────┘
                      │
                      ▼
┌─────────────────────────────────────────────┐
│      Weight loss surgery or tracheostomy with or without│
│      mechanical ventilation and/or respiratory stimulants in patients│
│      that fail positive airway pressure therapy│
└─────────────────────────────────────────────┘
```

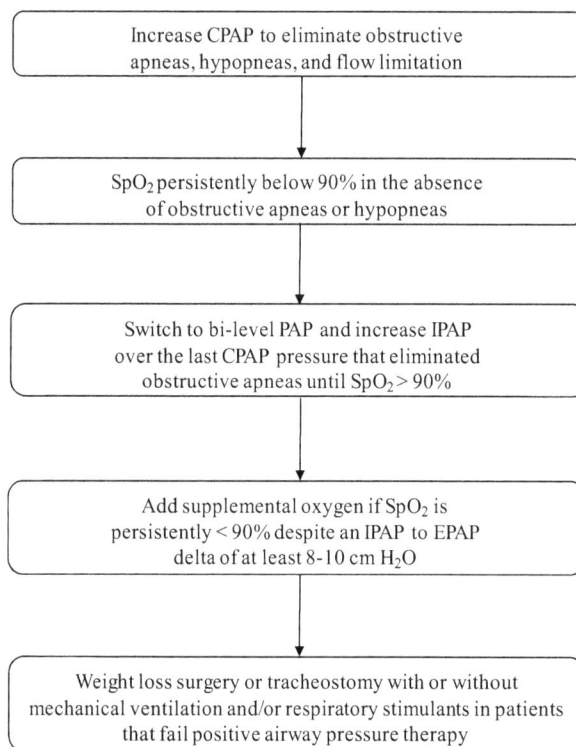

Figure 3: Suggested therapeutic algorithm during PAP titration in patients with OHS. Adapted from Mokhlesi et al [45]. IPAP = inspiratory positive airway pressure; EPAP = expiratory positive airway pressure.

Oxygen Therapy

In up to 50% of patients with OHS, oxygen therapy (in addition to PAP therapy) is necessary to keep $S_pO_2 > 90\%$ in the absence of hypopneas and apneas [57]. The need for nocturnal oxygen may abate with regular PAP usage. One retrospective cohort study found that the need for daytime supplemental oxygen decreased from 30% to 6% in patients who were adherent to PAP therapy [6]. Therefore, patients should be reassessed for both diurnal and nocturnal oxygen requirements a few weeks to months after PAP therapy is instituted since oxygen therapy is costly.

Tracheostomy

Tracheostomy was the first therapy described for the treatment of OHS [61]. In a retrospective study of 13 patients with OHS, tracheostomy was associated with significant improvement in OSA. With the tracheostomy closed the mean non-REM AHI and REM AHI were 64 and 46, respectively and with the tracheostomy open the non-REM AHI and REM AHI decreased to 31 and 39, respectively. In seven patients the AHI remained above 20. These residual respiratory events were associated with persistent respiratory effort, suggesting that sleep disordered breathing was caused by hypoventilation through an open tracheostomy rather than central apneas. However, the overall improvement in the severity of sleep-disordered breathing after tracheostomy led to the resolution of hypercapnia in the majority of the patients [62].

Today tracheostomy is generally reserved for patients who are intolerant of or not adherent with PAP therapy. It is also an option for that minority of patients who do not have a significant improvement in daytime blood gases despite adherence to PAP therapy, especially those patients who have signs or symptoms of cor pulmonale. Patients with tracheostomy may require nocturnal ventilation, as it does not treat any central hypoventilation that may be present [45]. A polysomnogram with the tracheostomy open is necessary to determine whether nocturnal ventilation is required [30].

Weight Reduction Surgery

Bariatric surgery has variable long-term efficacy in treating OSA, and the same is probably true of OHS. One study of patients undergoing Roux-en-Y montage showed that those with severe OSA had a reduction in AHI from 80 to 20 an average of 11 months after surgery [63]. Although this drastic reduction in sleep disordered breathing would likely be enough to normalize daytime blood gases, these patients still have moderate OSA and would benefit from continued PAP therapy. In another study, approximately half of the patients who had mild residual OSA after bariatric surgery developed severe OSA seven years post-operatively, despite no significant change in their weight [64]. A recently published meta-analysis that included 12 studies with 342 patients that underwent PSG before bariatric surgery and after maximum weight loss, reported that there was a 71% reduction in the AHI, with a reduction from a baseline of 55 (95% CI 49-60) to 16 (95% CI 13-19). Only 38% achieved cure, defined as AHI < 5. In contrast, 62% of patients had residual disease with the mean residual AHI of 16 events per hour. Many of these patients had persistent moderate OSA, defined as AHI ≥ 15 events per hour [65]. It is also known that in the 6-8 years after weight reduction surgery, patients tend to gain a mean of 7% of the pre-operative weight back [66]. Therefore, patients with OHS who undergo bariatric surgery should be monitored closely for recurrence of sleep disordered breathing.

Only one study has examined the impact of bariatric surgery in patients with OHS. Initially, blood gases improved: in 31 patients, preoperative P_aO_2 increased from 53 to 73 mm Hg one year after surgery, and P_aCO_2 decreased from 53 to 44 mm Hg. In the 12 patients in whom arterial blood gas measurements were available 5 years after surgery, values had worsened, with the mean P_aO_2 dropping to 68 mm Hg and P_aCO_2 increasing to 47 mm Hg [67]. In these 12 patients, BMI had hardly increased from 1 to 5 years postoperatively (38 to 40 kg/m^2). The worsening in daytime blood gases is likely from the re-development of sleep-disordered breathing.

Bariatric surgery is associated with significant risks. The perioperative mortality is between 0.5% and 1.5%. Patients with OHS may have an even higher operative mortality [67]. The independent risk factors associated with mortality are: intestinal leak, pulmonary embolism, pre-operative weight, and hypertension. Depending on the type of the surgery, intestinal leak occurs in 2-4% of patients and pulmonary embolism occurs in about 1% of patients [68]. Ideally, patients with OHS should be treated with PAP therapy (or tracheostomy in cases of PAP failure) before undergoing surgical intervention, in order to decrease perioperative morbidity and mortality. Moreover, PAP therapy should be initiated immediately after extubation to avoid postoperative respiratory failure [69-71], particularly since PAP therapy initiated postoperatively does not lead to anastomotic disruption or leakage [70, 72].

Pharmacotherapy

Respiratory stimulants can theoretically increase respiratory drive and improve daytime hypercapnia, but the data are very limited.

Medroxyprogesterone acts as a respiratory stimulant at the hypothalamic level [73]. The results of treatment in patients with OHS have been contradictory. In an observational series of 10 men with OHS treated with high doses of oral medroxyprogesterone (60 mg/day) for one month, the P_aCO_2 decreased from 51 mm Hg to 38 mm Hg and the P_aO_2 increased from 49 mm Hg to 62 mm Hg [74]. All these patients were able to normalize their P_aCO_2 with 1-2 minutes of voluntary hyperventilation, suggesting that there was no limitation to ventilation. Of note, polysomnographic data was not available on these 10 men with OHS, so it remains unclear whether they had concomitant OSA as well. In contrast, medroxyprogestrone did not improve P_aCO_2, minute ventilation, and ventilatory response to hypercapnia in three OHS patients that remained hypercapnic after tracheostomy [75]. Administration of a medication that may increase the risk of venous thromboembolism [76, 77] to a population whose mobility is limited may be unwise. In addition, high doses of medroxyprogesterone can lead to breakthrough uterine bleeding in women and to decreased libido and erectile dysfunction in men.

Acetazolamide induces metabolic acidosis through carbonic anhydrase inhibition, which increases minute ventilation in normal subjects. There is only one published case report describing normalization of blood gases after tracheostomy [75], although, interestingly, the agent also reduces the AHI in patients with moderate to severe OSA [78, 79]. Most, but not all patients with OHS can normalize their P_aCO_2 with voluntary hyperventilation [34]. The inability to eliminate CO_2 with voluntary hyperventilation may be due to mechanical impairment. In one study the ability to drop the P_aCO_2 by at least 5 mm Hg with voluntary hyperventilation was the main predictor of a favorable response to medroxyprogesterone [80]. Therefore, a respiratory stimulant in a patient who cannot normalize their P_aCO_2 with voluntary hyperventilation — due to limited ventilation and/or mechanical impairment — can lead to an increase in dyspnea or even worsening of acidosis with acetazolamide.

RESEARCH OUTLOOK

OHS is more prevalent in populations with increasingly severe OSA (AHI>60) and severe obesity (BMI $\geq$ 40 kg/m^2), but there is significant overlap between OHS and OSA populations in these two characteristics. Helpful clinical predictors of OHS in a population of patients with OSA need to be identified. Patients with OHS may be at an increased risk of mortality, but this topic and which co-morbidities are common in OHS need further study. Two theories of the pathogenesis of OHS have been described, leptin resistance and bicarbonate excretion with a long time-constant. Many alterations in respiratory mechanics have been described in OHS, but these do not seem to contribute to its pathogenesis. PAP therapy is the mainstay of treatment, but the best approach for those who do not respond to this modality is unknown and may include a combination of PAP therapy and pharmacotherapy with respiratory stimulants.

What do we know:

- Patients with severe obesity and more severe sleep disordered breathing are more likely to have OHS.

The most recent large study performed by Kawata and colleagues found that of 1,227 patients who presented to a sleep clinic with OSA, 14% were hypercapnic. Patients that were hypercapnic had a significantly higher AHI (39.3 $\pm$ 0.8 vs. 58.8 $\pm$ 2.0, p<0.01) and BMI (28.2 kg/m^2 vs. 31.1 kg/m^2, p< 0.01). Logistic regression analysis showed that a higher AHI was a strong predictor of hypercapnia (p < 0.001) and a higher BMI was a borderline predictor (p = 0.051) [23]. Of the eight other studies reported in the literature, seven have found a significant correlation between BMI and OHS in patients with OSA [15, 17-21, 81, 82]. Only five of these studies found a significant correlation between increasing AHI and hypercapnia in OSA. A recent meta-analysis (using these same studies) found that AHI was significantly associated with hypercapnia [11].

- Patients with untreated OHS may have a significant risk of mortality.

Nowbar and colleagues performed a prospective study and found that patients with obesity-associated hypoventilation had an 18-month post-hospitalization mortality rate of 23% compared with 9% of those with simple obesity. It is notable that polysomnograms were not performed and sleep disordered breathing was confirmed by history only. Only 13% of the hypoventilation patients received PAP therapy after discharge. The groups were well matched for age and several co-morbid conditions, but the hypercapnic group was more obese (BMI of 42 $\pm$ 8 kg/m^2 in the simple obesity group vs. 45 $\pm$ 9 kg/m^2 in the hypercapnic group). Further supporting this idea is a retrospective study performed by Budweiser and associates of 126 patients with a similar BMI, age and P_aCO_2 levels (adjusted for Denver's higher altitude) than the Nowbar study. They found the 18-month mortality rate of those patients highly adherent to PAP therapy to be only 3% [1, 55].

- Patients with OHS have altered respiratory mechanics, but this does not seem to significantly contribute to the derangements in blood gases.

Patients with OHS have significantly worsened chest wall and lung compliance than equally obese patients [28]. They have a decreased FEV_1 and forced vital capacity (FVC) when compared to significantly obese patients, although the ratio of the two remains normal [26]. Obesity increases the oxygen cost of breathing at rest [83]. Obese patients also develop intrinsic positive end-expiratory pressure in the supine position [84]. When the respiratory muscles are unable to compensate for the increased load, hypoventilation occurs. But, to date, there is no evidence that the inability of the respiratory muscles to compensate leads to hypoventilation.

The simplest evidence that respiratory muscles function normally in OHS is that these patients are able to voluntarily hyperventilate to eucapnia [34]. When presented with a hypercapnic ventilatory challenge, patients with OHS do not generate the same level of change in transdiaphragmatic pressure (Pdi), a measure of diaphragmatic work, as equally obese patients. This was because of decreased electrical stimulation of the diaphragm, or respiratory drive (Edi). When the ratio of Edi/Pdi was compared, the two groups were equivalent [35]. If the ratio had increased, this would have suggested respiratory muscle fatigue (*i.e.* decreased output relative to drive). But since the ratio was equal in the two groups, this suggests that the muscles were functioning equally as effectively, and the defect was in an inadequate input, or Edi. Other studies examining respiratory muscle strength in obesity have shown mixed results [26]. In addition, many patients with OHS normalize their blood gases with PAP therapy alone, without losing significant amounts of weight [29, 37, 38].

- Positive airway pressure therapy (with or without supplemental oxygen) is the most effective treatment.

Since it was first described in 1982 [31], PAP has emerged as the leading treatment for OHS. Multiple studies have confirmed its efficacy [6, 57, 82, 85-87], and there is a direct dose-response effect. In a study of 75 outpatients with OHS, P_aCO_2 decreased by 1.8 mm Hg and P_aO_2 increased by 3 mm Hg for each daily hour of PAP usage in the last thirty days before a repeat measurement of arterial blood gases. Those patients who used their devices for more than 4.5 hours daily had a greater improvement in daytime blood gases than those who did not (ΔP_aCO_2 7.7 vs. 2.4 mm Hg [p<0.001], ΔP_aO_2 9.2 vs. 1.8 mm Hg [p < 0.001]). Prior to the initiation of PAP therapy, 30% of the adherent patients needed daytime oxygen therapy, but this decreased to only 6% after PAP therapy [6]. On the initial PAP titration, up to 50% of patients may require nocturnal supplemental oxygen [57].

CPAP was the first described form of PAP therapy, but since there are CPAP treatment failures, there was some question as to whether bilevel PAP therapy was more appropriate for all patients. A recent prospective randomized study by Piper and colleagues examined this question. Out of 45 patients enrolled only 9 were excluded because of a priori failure of CPAP titration due to persistent hypoxemia defined arbitrarily as 10 continuous minutes with SpO_2 below 80% on the best CPAP pressure. Thirty six patients were then randomized to 3 months of either CPAP or bilevel PAP usage. Interestingly, the residual AHI on the long term therapy was 22 in the CPAP group and 13 in the bilevel PAP group. Regardless, there was no significant difference in any of the measured parameters after 3 months, including improvement in daytime awake SpO_2, P_aCO_2, Epworth Sleepiness Scale, measures of quality of life, and adherence to PAP therapy [59].

What we don't know:

- What are useful clinical predictors of OHS?

Patients with higher AHI and BMI are more likely to be hypercapnic, but there is much overlap between the two groups. Two studies showed the prevalence of hypercapnia in those with only moderate OSA (AHI 15-30) to be between 7.5 and 15% [14, 22, 23]. Three studies showed the prevalence of hypercapnia in those with a BMI of 30-34 kg/m^2 to be approximately 7.5% [14, 16, 22]. Clinicians should have a lower index of suspicion for OHS in patients with moderate OSA and (relatively) mild obesity. As patients with untreated OHS have a much higher mortality rate than those who are treated, it is important to identify those with OHS to objectively monitor adherence to PAP therapy and demonstrate improvement or resolution of hypercapnia [6, 45].

A useful tool for a sleep physician interpreting a polysomnogram of a patient they have not seen in clinic may be the % of TST with SpO_2 spent below 90%. The previously mentioned meta-analysis showed that obese OSA patients with hypercapnia spend a mean of 56.2% (95% CI 42.4 to 69.8) of TST with an SpO_2 below 90%, while patients with OSA spend 18.8% (95% CI 9.8 to 47.4) below 90% [11]. This may be a useful way to distinguish these two groups as there is very little overlap in the 95% confidence intervals. It would be interesting to see if this variable is predictive in a prospective fashion, and if so, at what %TST.

- How does OHS affect morbidity and mortality independent of OSA and obesity?

There has not yet been a study of morbidity and mortality that matches a group of OHS patients to a group with a similar degree of both obesity and OSA severity. One retrospective study performed by Berg and colleagues matched patients with OHS with controls with similar degrees of obesity with the goal of determining how health-care utilization differed between the two groups. Because of the extreme obesity seen in the OHS group, the BMI of the two groups differed significantly (47.3 ± 11.0 kg/m^2 in the OHS group, 43.4 ± 5.1 kg/m^2 in the group with obesity). Those with OHS were more likely to carry a diagnosis of congestive heart failure, angina, and cor pulmonale. They were also more likely to be hospitalized prior to diagnosis. After they were diagnosed, health-care utilization decreased [88]. This study supports the intuitive notion that patients with OHS have high levels of cardiovascular morbidity, but a more carefully controlled study would be helpful to distinguish common co-morbidities that clinicians should suspect in patients with OHS.

- Why do some patients with OSA develop OHS and others do not?

Currently, there are two viable hypotheses: leptin resistance and a model that incorporates nighttime hypercapnia and decreased bicarbonate excretion leading to chronic daytime hypercapnia.

Leptin acts as a central respiratory stimulant and increases as adiposity increases [43]. Leptin levels are directly correlated with BMI in patients with OHS as well [89]. Theoretically, obese patients produce more CO_2 than lean individuals, and the increased serum leptin increases ventilation to maintain eucapnia. Serum leptin levels drop in patients with OHS after effective treatment is instituted [46]. A recent study by Makinodan showed that serum leptin levels correlated with hypercapnic ventilatory response in control subjects and in patients with OSA, but not in those with OHS [90]. This suggests that, when leptin fails to stimulate ventilation, OHS could result. The suggested mechanism of leptin resistance is decreased leptin CSF penetration [44]. A study that examined CSF leptin levels in patients with OHS vs. an equally obese control group with equally severe OSA would be very helpful in answering this question. Individual variance in CSF leptin penetration could explain why some patients with severe obesity and severe OSA develop OHS and others do not.

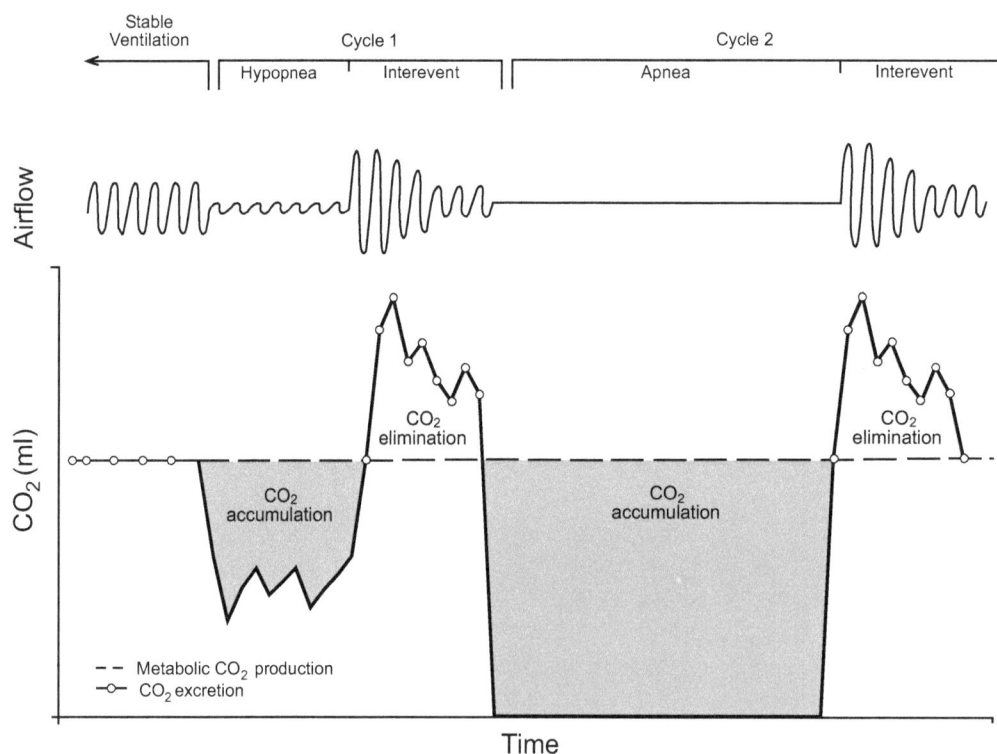

Figure 4: Schematic demonstrating how CO_2 excretion is dependent upon inter-event hyperventilation. In the first cycle, the interevent hyperpnea is sufficient to excrete the CO_2 accumulated during the hypopnea. In the second cycle, much more CO_2 is accumulated during the apnea than is excreted after the event. Reprinted from reference [91] with permission of the American Physiological Society. Copyright © American Physiological Society.

The second hypothesis was proposed by Norman and colleagues. Most patients with OSA are able to hyperventilate between apneas and remain eucapnic. However, if the inter-event hyperpnea is inadequate, a small net increase in P_aCO_2 would develop [91]. The kidneys would then retain a small amount of bicarbonate to compensate, even in an acute setting. When the subject awakens, the hypercapnia would resolve and the kidneys would then excrete the accumulated bicarbonate. But, if the subject falls asleep before the accumulated bicarbonate is excreted, then a small net increase in serum bicarbonate would result. With a mathematical model these investigators ran simulations under several conditions. Only the combination of a decreased hypercapnic ventilatory response and decreased bicarbonate excretion produced a daytime increase of P_aCO_2 like that seen in OHS **(Fig. 4)**.

The two hypotheses are not mutually exclusive. Exactly what leads to the inadequate inter-event hyperventilation in the second model is unclear. Is it leptin resistance? Is the duration of the hyperventilation simply inadequate because the upper airway is so likely to collapse that it does so before hyperventilation is complete? In the second model, individual variance in upper airway collapsibility and/or bicarbonate excretion could explain why some OSA patients develop OHS and others do not.

- Why do some patients fail to respond to PAP therapy, and how are they best managed?

Some possibilities include: inadequate treatment of sleep-disordered breathing (poor adherence or inadequate PAP titration), unrecognized sleep hypoventilation (requiring oxygen therapy or AVAPS therapy), unidentified pulmonary disease such as concomitant COPD, unidentified neuromuscular weakness (leading to sleep hypoventilation), or metabolic alkalosis (secondary to excessive loop diuretic usage or other culprits) [45]. After all of these potential causes have been ruled out, it is unclear how these patients are best managed, as there is little literature on the topic. The improvement in chronic daytime hypercapnia in patients that are adherent to PAP therapy is neither universal nor complete. In two studies [6, 59], the $PaCO_2$ did not improve significantly in approximately a quarter of patients that had undergone successful PAP titration in the laboratory and were highly adherent (> 6 h/night) with either CPAP or bilevel PAP therapy (personal communication by Amanda Piper). This lack of response to PAP therapy combined with reports of persistent hypoventilation after tracheostomy [30] suggests that in a subset of patients with OHS factors other than OSA are the driving force behind the pathogenesis of hypoventilation. In these patients tracheostomy and nocturnal (volume controlled) ventilation with or without respiratory stimulants may be necessary. The few studies examining medroxyprogesterone and acetazolamide included very few patients in an observational fashion and showed variable results [74, 75, 92]. Bariatric surgery would also be beneficial, although cardiopulmonary optimization preoperatively would likely require tracheostomy and nocturnal ventilation which can later be discontinued once significant weight loss occurred.

REFERENCES

[1]   Mokhlesi B, Kryger MH, Grunstein RR. Assessment and management of patients with obesity hypoventilation syndrome. Proc Am Thorac Soc 2008; 5: 218-25.

[2]   Resta O, Foschino Barbaro MP, Brindicci C, *et al.* Hypercapnia in overlap syndrome: possible determinant factors. Sleep Breath 2002; 6: 11-8.

[3]   Chaouat A, Weitzenblum E, Krieger J, *et al.* Association of chronic obstructive pulmonary disease and sleep apnea syndrome. Am J Respir Crit Care Med 1995; 151: 82-6.

[4]   Perez de Llano LA, Golpe R, Ortiz Piquer M, *et al.* Short-term and long-term effects of nasal intermittent positive pressure ventilation in patients with obesity-hypoventilation syndrome. Chest 2005; 128: 587-94.

[5]   Bednarek M, Plywaczewski R, Jonczak L, Zielinski J. There is no relationship between chronic obstructive pulmonary disease and obstructive sleep apnea syndrome: a population study. Respiration 2005; 72: 142-9.

[6]   Mokhlesi B, Tulaimat A, Evans AT, *et al.* Impact of adherence with positive airway pressure therapy on hypercapnia in obstructive sleep apnea. J Clin Sleep Med 2006; 2: 57-62.

[7]   Berry-Kravis EM, Zhou L, Rand CM, Weese-Mayer DE. Congenital central hypoventilation syndrome: PHOX2B mutations and phenotype. Am J Respir Crit Care Med 2006; 174: 1139-44.

[8]   Doherty LS, Kiely JL, Deegan PC, *et al.* Late-onset central hypoventilation syndrome: a family genetic study. Eur Respir J 2007; 29: 312-6.

[9]   Weese-Mayer DE, Berry-Kravis EM, Zhou L. Adult identified with congenital central hypoventilation syndrome--mutation in PHOX2b gene and late-onset CHS. Am J Respir Crit Care Med 2005; 171: 88.

[10]   Antic NA, Malow BA, Lange N, *et al.* PHOX2B mutation-confirmed congenital central hypoventilation syndrome: presentation in adulthood. Am J Respir Crit Care Med 2006; 174: 923-7.

[11]   Kaw R, Hernandez AV, Walker E, *et al.* Determinants of hypercapnia in obese patients with obstructive sleep apnea: a systematic review and metaanalysis of cohort studies. Chest 2009; 136: 787-96.

[12]   Sturm R. Increases in morbid obesity in the USA: 2000-2005. Public Health 2007; 121: 492-6.

[13]   Lee W, Nagubadi S, Kryger MH, Mokhlesi B. Epidemiology of Obstructive Sleep Apnea: a Population-based Perspective. Expert Rev Respir Med 2008; 2: 349-364.

[14]   Littleton SW, Mokhlesi B. The Pickwickian Syndrome-Obesity Hypoventilation Syndrome. Clin Chest Med 2009; 30:467-78, vii-viii.

[15]   Verin E, Tardif C, Pasquis P. Prevalence of daytime hypercapnia or hypoxia in patients with OSAS and normal lung function. Respir Med 2001; 95: 693-6.

[16]   Laaban JP, Chailleux E. Daytime hypercapnia in adult patients with obstructive sleep apnea syndrome in France, before initiating nocturnal nasal continuous positive airway pressure therapy. Chest 2005; 127: 710-5.

[17]   Kessler R, Chaouat A, Schinkewitch P, *et al.* The obesity-hypoventilation syndrome revisited: a prospective study of 34 consecutive cases. Chest 2001; 120: 369-76.

[18]   Resta O, Foschino Barbaro MP, Bonfitto P, *et al.* Hypercapnia in obstructive sleep apnoea syndrome. Neth J Med 2000; 56: 215-22.

[19]   Golpe R, Jimenez A, Carpizo R. Diurnal hypercapnia in patients with obstructive sleep apnea syndrome. Chest 2002; 122: 1100-1.

[20]   Akashiba T, Akahoshi T, Kawahara S, *et al.* Clinical characteristics of obesity-hypoventilation syndrome in Japan: a multi-center study. Intern Med 2006; 45: 1121-5.

[21]   Leech JA, Onal E, Baer P, Lopata M. Determinants of hypercapnia in occlusive sleep apnea syndrome. Chest 1987; 92: 807-13.

[22]   Mokhlesi B, Tulaimat A, Faibussowitsch I , *et al.* Obesity hypoventilation syndrome: prevalence and predictors in patients with obstructive sleep apnea. Sleep Breath 2007; 11: 117-24.

[23]   Kawata N, Tatsumi K, Terada J, *et al.* Daytime hypercapnia in obstructive sleep apnea syndrome. Chest 2007; 132: 1832-8.

[24]   Lin CC, Wu KM, Chou CS, Liaw SF. Oral airway resistance during wakefulness in eucapnic and hypercapnic sleep apnea syndrome. Respir Physiol Neurobiol 2004; 139: 215-24.

[25]   Kaltman AJ, Goldring RM. Role of circulatory congestion in the cardiorespiratory failure of obesity. Am J Med 1976; 60:645-53.

[26]   Piper AJ, Grunstein RR. Big Breathing - the complex interaction of obesity, hypoventilation, weight loss and respiratory function. J Appl Physiol 2009.

[27]   Koenig SM. Pulmonary complications of obesity. Am J Med Sci 2001; 321: 249-79.

[28]   Sharp JT, Henry JP, Sweany SK , *et al.* The Total Work of Breathing in Normal and Obese Men. J Clin Invest 1964; 43: 728-39.

[29]   Han F, Chen E, Wei H , *et al.* Treatment effects on carbon dioxide retention in patients with obstructive sleep apnea-hypopnea syndrome. Chest 2001; 119: 1814-9.

[30]   Berger KI, Ayappa I, Chatr-Amontri B, *et al.* Obesity hypoventilation syndrome as a spectrum of respiratory disturbances during sleep. Chest 2001; 120: 1231-8.

[31]   Rapoport DM, Sorkin B, Garay SM, Goldring RM. Reversal of the "Pickwickian syndrome" by long-term use of nocturnal nasal-airway pressure. N Engl J Med 1982; 307:931-3.

[32]   Masa JF, Celli BR, Riesco JA, *et al.* The obesity hypoventilation syndrome can be treated with noninvasive mechanical ventilation. Chest 2001; 119: 1102-7.

[33]   Leech JA, Onal E, Lopata M. Nasal CPAP continues to improve sleep-disordered breathing and daytime oxygenation over long-term follow-up of occlusive sleep apnea syndrome. Chest 1992; 102: 1651-5.

[34]   Leech J, Onal E, Aronson R, Lopata M. Voluntary hyperventilation in obesity hypoventilation. Chest 1991; 100: 1334-8.

[35]   Sampson MG, Grassino K. Neuromechanical properties in obese patients during carbon dioxide rebreathing. Am J Med 1983; 75: 81-90.

[36]   Lopata M, Freilich RA, Onal E, *et al.* Ventilatory control and the obesity hypoventilation syndrome. Am Rev Respir Dis 1979; 119: 165-8.

[37]   Berthon-Jones M, Sullivan CE. Time course of change in ventilatory response to CO_2 with long-term CPAP therapy for obstructive sleep apnea. Am Rev Respir Dis 1987; 135: 144-7.

[38]   Lin CC. Effect of nasal CPAP on ventilatory drive in normocapnic and hypercapnic patients with obstructive sleep apnoea syndrome. Eur Respir J 1994; 7: 2005-10.

[39]   Zwillich CW, Sutton FD, Pierson DJ, *et al.* Decreased hypoxic ventilatory drive in the obesity-hypoventilation syndrome. Am J Med 1975; 59: 343-8.

[40]   Bradley CA, Fleetham JA, Anthonisen NR. Ventilatory control in patients with hypoxemia due to obstructive lung disease. Am Rev Respir Dis 1979; 120:21-30.

[41]   Kalra SP. Central leptin insufficiency syndrome: an interactive etiology for obesity, metabolic and neural diseases and for designing new therapeutic interventions. Peptides 2008; 29: 127-38.

[42]   Tankersley CG, O'Donnell C, Daood MJ, *et al.* Leptin attenuates respiratory complications associated with the obese phenotype. J Appl Physiol 1998; 85: 2261-9.

[43]   Considine RV, Sinha MK, Heiman ML, *et al.* Serum immunoreactive-leptin concentrations in normal-weight and obese humans. N Engl J Med 1996; 334:292-5.

[44]   Caro JF, Kolaczynski JW, Nyce MR, *et al.* Decreased cerebrospinal-fluid/serum leptin ratio in obesity: a possible mechanism for leptin resistance. Lancet 1996; 348: 159-61.

[45]   Mokhlesi B, Tulaimat A. Recent advances in obesity hypoventilation syndrome. Chest 2007; 132: 1322-36.

[46]   Yee BJ, Cheung J, Phipps P, *et al.* Treatment of obesity hypoventilation syndrome and serum leptin. Respiration 2006; 73: 209-12.

[47]   Ayappa I, Berger KI, Norman RG, *et al.* Hypercapnia and ventilatory periodicity in obstructive sleep apnea syndrome. Am J Respir Crit Care Med 2002; 166: 1112-5.

[48]   Norman RG, Goldring RM, Clain JM, *et al.* Transition from acute to chronic hypercapnia in patients with periodic breathing: predictions from a computer model. J Appl Physiol 2006; 100: 1733-41.

[49]   O'Hearn DJ, Gold AR, Gold MS , *et al.* Lower extremity edema and pulmonary hypertension in morbidly obese patients with obstructive sleep apnea. Sleep Breath 2009; 13: 25-34.

[50]   Flegal KM, Graubard BI, Williamson DF, Gail MH. Excess deaths associated with underweight, overweight, and obesity. JAMA 2005; 293: 1861-7.

[51]   Young T, Finn L, Peppard PE, *et al.* Sleep disordered breathing and mortality: eighteen-year follow-up of the Wisconsin sleep cohort. Sleep 2008; 31: 1071-8.

[52]   Hida W. Quality of life in obesity hypoventilation syndrome. Sleep Breath 2003; 7: 1-2.

[53]   Budweiser S, Hitzl AP, Jorres RA, *et al.* Health-related quality of life and long-term prognosis in chronic hypercapnic respiratory failure: a prospective survival analysis. Respir Res 2007; 8: 92.

[54]   Nowbar S, Burkart KM, Gonzales R, *et al.* Obesity-associated hypoventilation in hospitalized patients: prevalence, effects, and outcome. Am J Med 2004; 116: 1-7.

[55]   Budweiser S, Riedl SG, Jorres RA, *et al.* Mortality and prognostic factors in patients with obesity-hypoventilation syndrome undergoing noninvasive ventilation. J Intern Med 2007; 261: 375-83.

[56]   Piper AJ, Sullivan CE. Effects of short-term NIPPV in the treatment of patients with severe obstructive sleep apnea and hypercapnia. Chest 1994; 105: 434-40.

[57]   Banerjee D, Yee BJ, Piper AJ, *et al.* Obesity hypoventilation syndrome: hypoxemia during continuous positive airway pressure. Chest 2007; 131: 1678-84.

[58]   Mokhlesi B. Positive airway pressure titration in obesity hypoventilation syndrome: continuous positive airway pressure or bilevel positive airway pressure. Chest 2007; 131: 1624-6.

[59]   Piper AJ, Wang D, Yee BJ , *et al.* Randomised trial of CPAP vs bilevel support in the treatment of obesity hypoventilation syndrome without severe nocturnal desaturation. Thorax 2008; 63: 395-401.

[60]   Storre JH, Seuthe B, Fiechter R, *et al.* Average volume-assured pressure support in obesity hypoventilation: A randomized crossover trial. Chest 2006; 130: 815-21.

[61]   Hensley MJ, Read DJ. Intemittent obstruction of the upper airway during sleep causing profound hypoxaemia. A neglected mechanism exacerbating chronic respiratory failure. Aust N Z J Med 1976; 6: 481-6.

[62]   Kim SH, Eisele DW, Smith PL, *et al.* Evaluation of patients with sleep apnea after tracheotomy. Arch Otolaryngol Head Neck Surg 1998; 124: 996-1000.

[63]   Haines KL, Nelson LG, Gonzalez R, *et al.* Objective evidence that bariatric surgery improves obesity-related obstructive sleep apnea. Surgery 2007; 141: 354-8.

[64]   Pillar G, Peled R, Lavie P. Recurrence of sleep apnea without concomitant weight increase 7.5 years after weight reduction surgery. Chest 1994; 106: 1702-4.

[65]   Greenburg DL, Lettieri CJ, Eliasson AH. Effects of surgical weight loss on measures of obstructive sleep apnea: a meta-analysis. Am J Med 2009; 122: 535-42.

[66]   Sjostrom L, Lindroos AK, Peltonen M, *et al.* Lifestyle, diabetes, and cardiovascular risk factors 10 years after bariatric surgery. N Engl J Med 2004; 351: 2683-93.

[67]   Sugerman HJ, Fairman RP, Sood RK, *et al.* Long-term effects of gastric surgery for treating respiratory insufficiency of obesity. Am J Clin Nutr 1992; 55: 597S-601S.

[68]   Fernandez AZ, Jr., Demaria EJ, Tichansky DS, *et al.* Multivariate analysis of risk factors for death following gastric bypass for treatment of morbid obesity. Ann Surg 2004; 239: 698-702; discussion 702-3.

[69]   Squadrone V, Coha M, Cerutti E, *et al.* Continuous positive airway pressure for treatment of postoperative hypoxemia: a randomized controlled trial. JAMA 2005; 293: 589-95.

[70]   Ebeo CT, Benotti PN, Byrd RP, Jr., *et al.* The effect of bi-level positive airway pressure on postoperative pulmonary function following gastric surgery for obesity. Respir Med 2002; 96: 672-6.

[71]   El-Solh AA, Aquilina A, Pineda L, *et al.* Noninvasive ventilation for prevention of post-extubation respiratory failure in obese patients. Eur Respir J 2006; 28: 588-95.

[72]   Huerta S, DeShields S, Shpiner R, *et al.* Safety and efficacy of postoperative continuous positive airway pressure to prevent pulmonary complications after Roux-en-Y gastric bypass. J Gastrointest Surg 2002; 6: 354-8.

[73]   Bayliss DA, Millhorn DE. Central neural mechanisms of progesterone action: application to the respiratory system. J Appl Physiol 1992; 73: 393-404.

[74]   Sutton FD, Jr., Zwillich CW, Creagh CE, *et al.* Progesterone for outpatient treatment of Pickwickian syndrome. Ann Intern Med 1975; 83: 476-9.

[75]   Rapoport DM, Garay SM, Epstein H, Goldring RM. Hypercapnia in the obstructive sleep apnea syndrome. A reevaluation of the "Pickwickian syndrome". Chest 1986; 89: 627-35.

[76]   Poulter NR, Chang CL, Farley TM, Meirik O. Risk of cardiovascular diseases associated with oral progestagen preparations with therapeutic indications. Lancet 1999; 354: 1610.

[77]   Douketis JD, Julian JA, Kearon C, *et al.* Does the type of hormone replacement therapy influence the risk of deep vein thrombosis? A prospective case-control study. J Thromb Haemost 2005; 3: 943-8.

[78]   Tojima H, Kunitomo F, Kimura H, *et al.* Effects of acetazolamide in patients with the sleep apnoea syndrome. Thorax 1988; 43: 113-9.

[79]   Whyte KF, Gould GA, Airlie MA, *et al.* Role of protriptyline and acetazolamide in the sleep apnea/hypopnea syndrome. Sleep 1988; 11: 463-72.

[80]   Skatrud JB, Dempsey JA, Bhansali P, Irvin C. Determinants of chronic carbon dioxide retention and its correction in humans. J Clin Invest 1980; 65: 813-21.

[81]   Akashiba T, Kawahara S, Kosaka N, *et al.* Determinants of chronic hypercapnia in Japanese men with obstructive sleep apnea syndrome. Chest 2002; 121: 415-21.

[82]   Laaban JP, Orvoen-Frija E, Cassuto D, *et al.* Mechanisms of diurnal hypercapnia in sleep apnea syndromes associated with morbid obesity. Presse Med 1996; 25: 12-6.

[83]   Kress JP, Pohlman AS, Alverdy J, Hall JB. The impact of morbid obesity on oxygen cost of breathing (VO2RESP) at rest. Am J Respir Crit Care Med 1999; 160: 883-6.

[84]   Steier J, Jolley CJ, Seymour J, *et al.* Neural respiratory drive in obesity. Thorax 2009; 64: 719-25.

[85]   Sullivan CE, Berthon-Jones M, Issa FG. Remission of severe obesity-hypoventilation syndrome after short-term treatment during sleep with nasal continuous positive airway pressure. Am Rev Respir Dis 1983; 128: 177-81.

[86]   Hida W, Okabe S, Tatsumi K, *et al.* Nasal continuous positive airway pressure improves quality of life in obesity hypoventilation syndrome. Sleep Breath 2003; 7: 3-12.

[87]   Shivaram U, Cash ME, Beal A. Nasal continuous positive airway pressure in decompensated hypercapnic respiratory failure as a complication of sleep apnea. Chest 1993; 104: 770-4.

[88]   Berg G, Delaive K, Manfreda J, *et al.* The use of health-care resources in obesity-hypoventilation syndrome. Chest 2001; 120: 377-83.

[89]   Shimura R, Tatsumi K, Nakamura A, *et al.* Fat accumulation, leptin, and hypercapnia in obstructive sleep apnea-hypopnea syndrome. Chest 2005; 127: 543-9.

[90]   Makinodan K, Yoshikawa M, Fukuoka A, *et al.* Effect of serum leptin levels on hypercapnic ventilatory response in obstructive sleep apnea. Respiration 2008; 75: 257-64.

[91]   Berger KI, Ayappa I, Sorkin IB, *et al.* Postevent ventilation as a function of CO(2) load during respiratory events in obstructive sleep apnea. J Appl Physiol 2002; 93: 917-24.

[92]   Lyons HA, Huang CT. Therapeutic use of progesterone in alveolar hypoventilation associated with obesity. Am J Med 1968; 44: 881-8.

CHAPTER 9

Insomnia

Lina Fine, M.D.[2,*], **Boris Dubrovsky Ph.D.**[3] **and Arthur J. Spielman, Ph.D.**[1,2,3]

[1]Cognitive Neuroscience Doctoral Program, Department of Psychology, The City College of New York, City University of New York, New York, NY, USA; [2]Center for Sleep Medicine, Department of Neurology, New York Presbyterian Hospital, Weill Cornell Medical College, New York, NY, USA and [3]Center for Sleep Disorders Medicine and Research, Department of Pulmonary Medicine, New York Methodist Hospital, Brooklyn, NY, USA

Abstract: Insomnia is a common health complaint that produces a significant impairment in quality of life and involves difficulty in initiating sleep, maintaining sleep, waking too early, non-restorative sleep, and daytime functional deficits. Insomnia is associated with a disturbance in one or more of the three systems that regulate sleep: homeostatic, circadian and arousal. A disturbance may result from genetic/dispositional issues, from acute life events, from habitual behaviors and attitudes, or from any combination of these three types of issues. A number of treatment methods have been developed that use behavior modification and cognitive restructuring to facilitate homeostatic and circadian mechanisms of sleep, and to reduce arousal during bedtime. These methods actively engage the patient to implement life style changes, attitudes and beliefs that promote sleep.

TOPIC DISCUSSION (CLINICAL OUTLOOK)

Insomnia: Definition and Prevalence

Insomnia is one of the most common health complaints, often leading to significant impairment in quality of life. In addition to difficulty initiating sleep, maintaining sleep, waking too early, and/or the experience that sleep in not restorative, sleep complaints must be accompanied by some daytime deficit to qualify for the diagnosis of insomnia. In the context of an adequate opportunity to sleep, the daytime consequences of insomnia include fatigue, malaise, impairment in attention, concentration or memory, mood disturbance or irritability, sleepiness, functional impairment, reduced motivation, headaches and sleep worries [1]. Insomnia is classified as primary - when there is no other diagnosable condition that may be causing sleep disturbance, or secondary, if insomnia is directly precipitated by another condition. Sleep apnea, restless legs syndrome, periodic limb movement disorder, circadian rhythm disorders and a wide array of medical conditions and medications are among other causes of secondary insomnia. Although secondary insomnia is used in current nosology (with the descriptor "due to"), many investigators and clinicians feel more comfortable with the term "insomnia associated with a disorder", without assuming direct causality.

Several diagnostic classification systems are used to categorize symptoms and related functions of insomnia (see Table **1**). These include Diagnostic and Statistical Manual – IV (Fourth Edition - Text Revision, DSM-IV-TR), the International Classification of Sleep Disorders – 2 (Second version, or ICSD-2), International Classification of Diseases – 10th Revision (ICD-10) and the Research Diagnostic Criteria (RDC). DSM-IV-TR and ICSD-2 have proven to have moderate agreement between clinicians using the criteria for insomnia [2-4].

Causes of Insomnia

Neurophysiological model of sleep regulation: Homeostatic process, circadian rhythmicity, and arousal

In considering the etiology of insomnia, two broad approaches have been proposed. Insomnia can be viewed as a manifestation, or a symptom, of a physiological disturbance that creates malfunction in the sleep process. Alternatively, insomnia can be understood as a lifestyle problem whose course of development is closely related to the person's overall functioning. While recognizing that these two approaches overlap as well as complement each other, we will discuss their main tenets separately.

Address correspondence to Lina Fine: Center for Sleep Medicine, Department of Neurology, New York Presbyterian Hospital, Weill Cornell Medical College, New York, NY, USA; E-mail: linefine@yahoo.com

Table 1: Comparison of Insomnia Diagnostic Criteria (Harvey & Spielman) [97]

ICSD-2 Insomnia Categories	DSM-IV-TR Insomnia Categories	ICD-10 Insomnia Categories	RDC Insomnia Categories
I. Insomnias	307.42 Primary Insomnia	F51.0 Nonorganic insomnia G47.0 Disorders of initiating and maintaining sleep [insomnias]	Primary Insomnia
307.41 Adjustment Sleep Disorder			
307.42 Psychophysiologic Insomnia			Psychophysiological Insomnia
307.42 Paradoxical Insomnia			Paradoxical Insomnia
327.02 Insomnia due to a mental disorder	Insomnia related to Another Mental Disorder		Insomnia due to a Mental Disorder
307.42 Idiopathic Insomnia			Idiopathic (Childhood Onset) Insomnia
V69.4 Inadequate Sleep Hygiene			
V69.5 Behavioral Insomnia of Childhood			
292.85 Insomnia due to a drug or substance	291.89/ Substance-Induced Sleep 292.89 Disorder, Insomnia Type		Insomnia due to Drug or Substance
327.01 Insomnia due to a medical condition	Sleep Disorder Due to a General Medical Condition, Insomnia Type		Insomnia due to Medical Condition
780.52 Other insomnia not due to a substance or physiological condition, unspecified			

The view that considers insomnia a result of a physiological disturbance can be termed a neurophysiological model. The model conceptualizes sleep as the result of the interplay of three major systems or processes: homeostatic, circadian, and arousal [5-9]. The homeostatic process, or Process S (or sleep debt, pressure to sleep, etc), is what gradually increases the sleep propensity over time during wakefulness [5]. The process is nearly linear: the longer someone is awake, the greater the sleep propensity or sleep potential. Homeostasis generally produces similar amounts of sleep each night. For example, homeostasis compensates for sleep deprivation or a short night's sleep with a greater sleep drive to generate a longer sleep period, if behaviorally allowed. On the other hand, extending one's sleep on a given night, or taking a nap, leads to a diminished homeostatic propensity for sleep, and shorter or lighter sleep on the following night. The homeostatic process keeps an account of the amount of wakefulness and sleep.

The circadian system, or Process C, produces rhythmic fluctuations in sleep and wakefulness by governing a number of physiological functions intimately tied with sleep, such as the cycles of melatonin secretion and body temperature. The ubiquitous rhythmic pattern is presumed to have developed as a result of the daily environmental changes in light and darkness on the Earth, and follows an approximately 24-hour period [6]. In contrast to the homeostatic process, the circadian process generates the alternating sleep and wakefulness potential regardless of the amount of sleep and wakefulness obtained. The circadian system works in concert (see The opponent process model [7]) with the homeostatic system in order to consolidate sleep at night time and maintain even levels of alertness during the day [8]. In the morning, after a full night's sleep, the homeostatic sleep drive is at its lowest, and the circadian system generates just enough activation to promote adaptive function at the start of the day. During the first part of the day, homeostatic sleep propensity is still low, and the circadian system does not produce much activation. As the day proceeds, the homeostatic sleep potential increases in a nearly linear fashion. Similarly, the circadian system gradually increases its activating output, which results in the maintenance of alertness throughout the day and prevents sleep from occurring too early in the day. In the evening, the circadian activation system starts to wane, no longer countering the heightened homeostatic sleep potential. At bedtime, the readiness for sleep generated by the homeostatic sleep drive begins to be experienced and discharged and sleep onset results.

The arousal system's name aptly reflects the nature of its effect: it produces physiological arousal and increased alertness, which, of course, are incompatible with sleep [9]. This is essentially a stress response or "fight-or-flight" system, and both environmental and internal triggers can set it off. The physiological markers of arousal include such responses as elevated respiratory and heart rates, higher oxygen consumption, muscle tension and body temperature, and increased circulating levels of cortisol and epinephrine [10, 11]. Individuals with insomnia may also demonstrate a greater spectral power of faster "wake" EEG frequencies during sleep [12]. Subjectively, people may report worries, emotional tension and feeling of nervousness or anxiety, as well as racing thoughts, overactive mind or the inability to stop thinking about a problem, especially at bedtime or during a midnight awakening. An articulated cognitive perspective on arousal and insomnia has been advanced by a number of theorists and includes dysfunctions in the individual's attending to sleep, intending to sleep, efforts to sleep, ideas about sleep and general cognitive hyperarousal [13-16]. While increased arousal in response to a significant event is normal, prolonged or chronic hyper-arousal may override homeostatic sleep drive and serve as a major factor in difficulty sleeping.

A balance between homeostatic, circadian and arousal systems is required to maintain good sleep from night to night. A disturbance of one of these systems will upset the balance and lead to insomnia. Such a disturbance may be constitutional in nature, may be due to a medical or psychiatric illness, or may be a result of stress or the individual's behavior. Constitutional problems include weak homeostatic sleep drive, over-reactive arousal mechanisms, and endogenous circadian rhythmicity that is substantially different from the environmental 24-hour cycle or is too rigid to be entrained easily. Some people may be "light sleepers" or "short sleepers" even under the best conditions, simply because their homeostatic need for sleep is low. People whose personality is such that they respond strongly to environmental events have very active minds, or frequently experience somatic tension, may keep their arousal system working overtime, which may prevent them from sleeping well, even when they feel tired and sleepy. And people who are born "night owls" or "morning larks" or have some other rare form of circadian rhythm dysregulation, are at a risk of not being able to sleep during the typical sleep hours, although they may sleep well at non-preferred times.

A medical illness may upset the balance between the three systems and lead to insomnia. Discomfort or pain may undermine the homeostatic discharge of the sleep drive. Elimination of bright light by staying indoors and a variable sleep-wake schedule interferes with circadian regulation. Worry about illness may create stress and elevate arousal levels. Apart from these general features, there are multiple medical conditions, including endocrine and neurological disorders, which may directly affect one's ability to sleep at night or to maintain his/her alertness during the day. These conditions are listed in Table **2**. Psychiatric disorders that involve elevated arousal, such as anxiety disorders and mood disorders, may also have insomnia as an associated feature. These conditions are listed in Table **3**.

Table 2: Common Medical Disorders Comorbid with Insomnia

Category	Examples
Neurological	Stroke, dementia, Parkinson's, seizures, headache, TBI, neuropathy, pain, neuromuscular
Cardiovascular	Angina, CHF, dyspnea, dysrhythmias
Pulmonary	COPD, emphysema, asthma, laryngospasm
Digestive	Reflux, ulcer, colitis, irritable bowel syndrome
Genitourinary	Incontinence, benign prostatic hypertrophy, nocturia, enuresis, interstitial cystitis
Endocrine	Hypothyroidism, hyperthyroidism, diabetes
Musculoskeletal	Arthritis, fibromyalgia, Sjogren's, kyphosis
Reproductive	Pregnancy, menopause, menstrual variations

Table 3: Common Psychiatric Disorders Comorbid with Insomnia

Category	Examples
Mood disorders	Major depressive, bipolar mood, dysthymia
Anxiety disorders	Generalized anxiety, panic, post-traumatic stress, OCD
Psychotic disorders	Schizophrenia, schizoaffective
Amnestic disorders	Alzheimer's, other dementias
Seen in childhood	Attention deficit disorder
Other disorders and symptoms	Adjustment, personality, bereavement, stress

Medications may also be the culprit. Taking activating medications late in the day will create sleep onset difficulty. Medications that negatively impact alertness during the day may produce dozing, which reduces homeostatic sleep drive at night. Table **4** shows medications that may contribute to the etiology of insomnia.

Table 4: Common Medications and Substances Contributing to Insomnia

Category	Examples
Antidepressants	SSRIs (fluoxetine, paroxetine, sertraline, citalopram, escitalopram, fluvoxamine), venlafaxine, duloxetine, MAOIs
Stimulants	Caffeine, methylphenidate, amphetamine derivatives, ephedrine, cocaine
Decongestants	Pseudoephedrine, phenylephrine, phenylpropanolamine
Narcotic analgesics	Oxycodone, codeine, propoxyphene
Cardiovascular	Beta blockers, alpha receptor agonists/antagonists, diuretics, lipid-lowering agents
Pulmonary	Theophylline, albuterol
Alcohol	

Finally, certain behavioral patterns work against the homeostatic or circadian systems, or activate the arousal system at inopportune times. Irregular bedtimes and lack of bright light exposure at the right time will make the circadian system dysregulated, which in turn may lead to poor sleep consolidation at night, or inappropriate daytime sleepiness. Sedentary life style, daytime naps, or "vegging out (dozing)" in front of TV in the evening may reduce homeostatic drive for sleep at night. Engaging in stressful activities, such as working or paying bills close to bedtime or even in bed may create a state of arousal non-conducive to sleep.

The 3P Model of Insomnia

A heuristic model of insomnia, called the 3P model, categorizes contributions to sleep difficulties as Predisposing, Precipitating, and Perpetuating Factors [17, 18]. This overview of causes suggests that insomnia may be associated with a genetically determined issue that changes little throughout one's life, such as being a "night owl." In contrast, a relatively circumscribed issue, such as a medical illness, may trigger an insomnia that can be addressed in a short time. Another cause of insomnia may be a pervasive lifestyle issue, such as trying to cope with multiple responsibilities at the expense of sleep. It is clear in clinical practice that multiple types of issues affecting sleep may be present in one person and interact with one another in numerous ways. To account for the dynamic nature of the contributions to insomnia, the 3P model was developed [17, 18]. The model has been devised to elucidate the course of insomnia and to help guide the clinician's attention to the facets of insomnia that may be more pertinent at different points in time.

Predisposing factors encompass all parts of the personality and the genetic endowment of an individual that, while not necessarily pathological, place the individual at a higher risk for poor sleep. These include being a reactive person who is prone to worrying, a hard-driving person who strives on stress, someone with an elevated metabolic rate or an over-active hypothalamic-pituitary-adrenal axis, or a person prone to somatic tension. Predisposing factors also include weak homeostatic drive, e.g., being a short or light sleeper by constitution, as well as the tendency for the endogenous circadian cycle to be "misaligned" with the exogenous clock, as in "night owls" or "morning larks." A person with one or multiple predisposing characteristics is at a greater risk for difficulty sleeping, but may not develop a full-blown insomnia without a precipitating event.

Precipitating events trigger the insomnia. Any event associated with stress or changes in daily routine, such as marriage, a job promotion, a cold, or a trip, may cause some difficulty sleeping. An event that has a known direct effect on sleep mechanisms, e.g., jet lag or menopause, may also trigger insomnia. A significant life event may also be unexpected and involve extended psychological and physiological ramifications, including a serious illness or death of a loved one. It is expected that a person will not sleep well for some time after such an event. In many instances, normal sleep patterns return as time passes and the event becomes the thing of the past. However, in substantial number of cases insomnia lingers on, now fueled by perpetuating maladaptive practices and beliefs.

Perpetuating behavioral factors enter the clinical picture after the insomnia has begun. To compensate for poor sleep individuals may spend extra time in bed "trying" to sleep, change bedtimes erratically based on how they feel, watch TV or listen to the radio, often performed in bed in the hope that sleep will come "unobserved." These new strategies to help summon sleep may be counterproductive and perpetuate the sleep disturbance. These changes may create a mismatch between the biological propensity for sleep (partially determined by circadian time) and the imposed new sleep schedule. Alternatively, perpetuating practices, such as spending time in bed watching TV or listening to the radio, may weaken the connection between cues (the bed, lying down with eyes closed without focused attention) that elicit or control sleep behavior. It is probably universally understood that taking daytime naps or consuming caffeine to overcome daytime tiredness and sleepiness may interfere with sleep. However, the pressure to perform, function well or just feel good motivates insomnia sufferers to try and cope by way of an extra coffee or brief snooze in the afternoon. Drinking alcohol in the evening to "wind down" works to hasten sleep onset but may produce awakenings during the night which disturb the continuity of sleep.

Numerous perpetuating behaviors often develop together, interact with one another, and involve cognitive and attitudinal factors. For example, a person who is concerned about "abusing" a hypnotic decides to start the night by hoping to fall asleep "naturally", but after not being able to fall asleep takes a sleep aid too late in the night, which makes the person feel groggy the next day and sets the stage for excessive caffeine consumption. The following night the person decides to try to go to bed earlier to "compensate" for the short sleep the night before and hoping that the tiredness will do the trick. However, going to bed too early while still having caffeine in the system may not lead to the relief of sleep but rather to aggravated tossing and turning awake in bed. To continue this saga, the person may start worrying about being unable to sleep without a medication and about poor performance the next day. To pass the time and to distract oneself from worry, she/he starts to watch TV in bed, and begins to doze on and off, while the program is still on. Upon turning off the TV, the person feels even more awake after the incidental dozing has occurred, and, out of frustration, takes the medication again in the middle of the night, and the cycle repeats itself.

The maladaptive nature of perpetuating behaviors is not apparent at first, especially to the insomnia sufferer. On the contrary, the pervasive and problematic nature of the perpetuating factors stems from the fact that at least some of these practices may have provided some relief. A person who has developed difficulty falling asleep, for example, may decide to sleep longer in the morning as a way to "catch up" and feel better during the day. Or the person may try to go to bed earlier, reasoning that if it takes a couple of hours to fall asleep it might help to start "trying" sooner rather than later. Both of these "strategies" may be helpful on occasion, but then over the long run they will make sleep worse by compromising both the circadian and homeostatic sleep systems. The poor sleeper, however, may decide to stick to these practices because they episodically have been helpful. In addition, since the quality of sleep typically fluctuates from night to night, these maladaptive behaviors may happen to have been instituted on night's of better sleep, thus further strengthening the maladaptive belief of their effectiveness in the person's mind.

The hypothetical examples above, whose variants are seen only too often in clinical practice, underscore the intimate connection that develops between the maladaptive behaviors and maladaptive beliefs in patients with insomnia. On the one hand, patients do things they believe are helpful because it gives them the sense of control over their problem. Although maladaptive behaviors hurt their sleep in the long run, they continue to engage in them because they believe these behaviors worked for them in the past or may provide help going forward. On the other hand, due to the persistent nature of sleep difficulty, patients develop beliefs that reflect the lack of control: the fear of bedtime and the expectation of wakefulness at night, the anticipation of daytime performance decrements and deleterious effects on health, the search for "organic" causes of sleeplessness and preoccupation with the amount of sleep obtained. Both cognitive and behavioral factors work together over time to produce a learned activation of the arousal system at night.

From the perspective of the 3P model, the cognitive-behavioral approach to insomnia treatment is essential, and the majority of non-pharmacological treatment modalities discussed in detail below focus on identifying and eliminating the perpetuating practices and beliefs. However, the predisposing and precipitating factors should also be addressed. Predisposing factors are relatively constant throughout the life span and as such present a continuous risk. They should be the target of both the immediate treatment and prospective counseling, such as the reduction of arousal using relaxation techniques, or entraining the endogenous circadian rhythms using light exposure. Precipitating events identified in the course of clinical evaluation are often labeled as the "cause" of insomnia. Although these events are typically too remote to be dealt with directly by the time the patient seeks treatment for the sleep problem, depending on the nature and current saliency of the precipitating event, there may still be a need for specific treatment. For example, if a divorce was the initial trigger for insomnia and it is difficult for the patient to get on with his/her life, psychological counseling may be useful.

Non-Pharmacological Treatment Modalities for Insomnia

Cognitive and behavioral approaches to the treatment of insomnia address putative causes of the sleep disturbance, the three components of the neurophysiological model of sleep regulation as well as the cognitive and behavioral aspects emphasized in the 3P model of insomnia. It should be noted, however, that there is a degree of overlap between different treatment methods, both in terms of specific recommendations and in terms of the mechanisms of therapeutic change. In addition, as all behavioral treatments require that the patient follow detailed instructions, some of which may be initially counter-intuitive, all treatments involve cognitive restructuring aimed to provide evidence to the patient of the usefulness of the recommendations. Therefore, we will discuss the cognitive elements of behavioral techniques in the section on cognitive therapy.

Behavioral Therapy

Stimulus Control Therapy

Stimulus Control Therapy (SCT; formerly called Stimulus Control Instructions) is a technique based on learning principles [19, 20]. The underlying assumption is that a person with chronic insomnia has learned to associate pre-sleep cues such as retiring time, the bedroom environment, and lying in bed with sleeplessness, frustration, and worry. As a result, the pre-sleep cues no longer reliably lead to sleep. In contrast, the person with insomnia has learned a state of heightened physiological and cognitive arousal in anticipation of nighttime aggravations "on cue." The two goals of the SCT are to extinguish the maladaptive association between the bed and arousal and to condition an association between the bed and rapid sleep onset. To achieve these goals, two basic behaviors are prescribed. First, the patient must use the bed and, living space permitting, the bedroom only for sleep and sex; any other activity, such as reading, watching TV, computer work, etc., must be performed out of bed and ideally out of the bedroom. Second, the patient must not spend more than approximately 20 minutes at a stretch in bed without sleep. If sleep does not occur within 20 minutes, the patient must get out of bed and ideally out of the bedroom.

To ensure an adequate sleep onset trial, the patient should be instructed not to go to bed if not feeling sufficiently sleepy; this direction should be followed both in the evening and after getting up in the middle of the night. Setting an alarm clock for the same time every morning is also part of the SCT intervention. Patients should choose an appropriate activity for the time when they are out of bed in the middle of the night. The activity should not be too stimulating, since the specific aim for this time is to wait for sleepiness to build. Reading a boring book is typically the best choice. Relaxation exercises and meditation tapes may also be helpful. Obviously, any activity that may be associated with stress, such as work-related projects or paying bills, should be avoided at this time. The summary of SCT procedures is presented in Table **5**.

Table 5: Stimulus Control Instructions (Bootzin, 1972; Bootzin *et al,* 1991) [19, 20]

1.	Go to sleep only when you feel sleepy.
2.	Do not use your bed or bedroom for anything except sleep (sexual activity is the only exception).
3.	If you have not fallen asleep within approximately 20 minutes, get up and go into another room. Engage in relaxing activities, such as non-work related light reading, and go back to bed when you feel sleepy or ready for sleep.
4.	If you cannot fall back to sleep, repeat step 3.
5.	Set the alarm for the same time each morning.

Sleep Restriction Therapy

Sleep Restriction Therapy (SRT) is a behavioral technique that aims to promote both homeostatic and circadian sleep processes [21, 22]. The main element of SRT is based on the observation that patients with insomnia typically spend substantially more time in bed than they actually sleep. Hoping for some sleep to occur, patients commonly go to bed earlier than usual, lie awake in bed during night awakenings, and stay in bed later than their final awakening. All these behaviors weaken both the homeostatic and circadian regulation of sleep. To create a better match between the amount of time spent in bed and the amount of sleep accrued and to consolidate the patient's sleep at night, SRT prescribes spending the same amount of time in bed as the average amount of sleep per night. Thus, a substantial reduction of time in bed is the basic initial recommendation of SRT. Initially, patients do not sleep as much as usual and are more fatigued. However, this short-term sleep loss is rewarded in the long run by more reliable and quicker sleep onset and more continuous and deeper sleep.

SRT begins with the patient filling out a sleep log for 1-2 weeks to obtain the average amount of sleep per night and the time of the night when sleep is the best. After this information is obtained, the amount of time allowed in bed should closely match the average self-reported amount of sleep per night. However, if the patient reports only a few hours of sleep or no sleep at all, at least 5 hours in bed should be allowed to prevent severe sleep deprivation and help minimize compliance problems. The specific bedtime and the rising time are set through negotiations with the patient, taking into consideration the patient's daytime obligations and the time of night when the log indicates that the patient is most likely to sleep. A person who has substantial difficulty falling asleep, for example, would be instructed to go to bed at a later time, whereas a person who wakes up too early would be scheduled to rise earlier.

After the initial restriction of the time in bed, the patient continues to fill out sleep logs to monitor subjective sleep efficiency (SE), which is defined as the percentage of the total sleep time (TST) relative to the time in bed (TIB; SE% = TST / TIB x 100). The amount of time allowed in bed is adjusted weekly. There are two alternative methods for the adjustment of the TIB. The original method [21] uses a target SE of 90% or greater (85% for elderly individuals). The TIB is adjusted based on the reported SE in relation to the target value: it is increased by 15 minutes if the target SE is reached, kept unchanged if the reported SE is no more than 5% below the target, and reduced by 15 minutes if the reported SE is below the target by more than 5%. According to the more recent method [21], the TIB is increased every week by 15 or 30 minutes, unless the patient reports more than 45 minutes of wakefulness in bed per night. When the TIB reaches 7 hours, further adjustments are based on considerations of the patient's daytime functioning and reported levels of sleepiness and fatigue. The summary of the SRT procedures is presented in Table **6**.

In addition to restricting the amount of time in bed at night, the patient is required to keep to the prescribed bedtimes, which helps regulate the circadian system. It is necessary to eliminate any daytime napping and dozing. Exercise may be used to prevent nodding during the mid-afternoon alertness trough. In the evening, less strenuous physical activity is helpful, such as walking or stretching, or minor household chores. Early evening is a danger zone for inadvertent nodding or "vegging out", which often creates a "second wind" when it is time to go to bed. This pattern is typical in patients for whom a later bedtime is scheduled. These patients should be taught to gauge their sleepiness and stay sufficiently physically and mentally engaged in the early evening to prevent premature discharge of sleepiness through nodding in front of the TV, "resting with eyes closed", or even mindlessly browsing through channels in a state of diminished alertness.

Table 6: Sleep Restriction Therapy (Spielman et al, 1987; Glovinsky and Spielman, 2006) [21, 22]

1.	From information provided on a sleep log completed for at least one week, set the initial time in bed equal to the reported average total sleep time.
Version 1:	
2.	Increase time in bed by 15 to 30 minutes when the average reported sleep efficiency (sleep efficiency = average sleep time/time in bed x 100%) for five days is ≥ 90% (85% in older individuals)
3.	When sleep efficiency from five days documented on a sleep log is < 85% (80% in older individuals) decrease time in bed by 15 minutes.
4.	When sleep efficiency from five days documented on a sleep log is ≥ 85% and <90% (≥80 to <85% in older individuals) keep time in bed the same
Version 2:	
2.	Following the original restriction increase time in bed progressively by 15 or 30 minutes each week until the patient is spending 7 hours in bed. Further changes are made based on daytime functioning, fatigue, and sleepiness

Circadian Entrainment

Light Therapy Bright light is the most powerful zeitgeber (stimulus) that entrains and shifts circadian rhythms [23-25]. Bright light exposure has a direct physiological effect on the "master clock" of the brain, located in the suprachiasmatic nucleus (SCN) of the hypothalamus, SCN regulates sleep-wake, melatonin, body temperature, and other physiological cycles that endogenously recur on a near-24-hour schedule [23-29]. The effect of light on the circadian system depends on the time when the light exposure takes place within the circadian cycle [30, 31]. Light exposure in the morning produces a phase advance of circadian rhythms, that is, a shift of the internal clock to an earlier time. A phase advance will help an individual fall asleep faster and/or earlier in the evening. Morning light induces a phase advance and will also produce an earlier wake-up time in the morning. As the circadian system in humans typically runs on a schedule that is slightly longer than 24 hours, exposure to bright light at the same time every morning helps entrain the endogenous cycle to the real clock time. In contrast, exposure to bright light in the evening produces a phase delay of endogenous rhythms, producing longer sleep latency or a later sleep onset time. In addition, evening light induced phase delay will produce a later wake-up time in the morning.

The sleep disturbance in circadian rhythm disorders, while distinct, shares some features with insomnia. For example, in delayed sleep phase syndrome (DSPS), the patient experiences significant difficulties falling asleep at the desired time in the evening and waking up in the morning. In advanced sleep phase syndrome (ASPS), the opposite pattern is evident: the patient falls asleep readily in the early evening, sometimes too early, and wakes up too early ready to start the day. However, unlike patients with insomnia, patients with circadian sleep disorders typically sleep well, especially if allowed to live on their preferred schedule.

Bright light exposure in the morning is used to produce circadian phase advance in patients with DSPS [32]. The patient is instructed to get up at the same time every day and initiate light exposure soon after rising. The initial scheduled rising time should be close to the patient's self-selected time, even if it means early afternoon. The timing of waking up and light exposure is gradually adjusted to an earlier time, e.g., in the increments of 30-60 minutes every 5-7 days, until the target wake-up time is reached. The following parameters of light exposure are crucial for the success of the treatment: (i) light exposure should occur as soon as possible after rising; (ii) light exposure should occur every day; (iii) light exposure should occur at the same time of day until the shift to an earlier time is scheduled; (iv) light should be bright and (v) exposure should be sufficiently long. Natural sunlight always provides sufficient brightness (well in excess of 10,000 lux even on a cloudy day). Artificial light sources that are specifically designed for this purpose can also be used successfully if the patient is sitting at the correct distance from the light source that the manufacturer recommends (typically about 18 inches) and gazes in the direction of the source to achieve sufficient brightness at the eye level (2,500-10,000 lux). The duration of exposure depends on the brightness of the source; with the natural sunlight 30-60 minutes is typically sufficient, whereas artificial sources may require as little as 15 minutes (with blue light sources) or up to 60-90 minutes.

Essentially the same principles of bright light exposure in the morning can be used to help alleviate difficulty falling asleep in the evening in a patient with insomnia, even if there is no dramatic misalignment between patient's preferred sleep time and the external clock time. As mentioned in the sections on SCT and SRT, insomnia patients tend to spend too much time in bed and stay in bed during late morning hours, which weakens the circadian system regulation of sleep at night. Light exposure in the morning creates a strong circadian sleep propensity in the evening and has an added benefit of increased alertness in the morning.

Bright light exposure in the evening, typically with an artificial light source, has been used for patients with ASPS as well as for patients with insomnia who complain of early morning awakenings [33-35]. The light exposure should stop at least 1 hour prior to the scheduled bedtime to prevent the alerting effect of bright light interfering with sleep onset.

It should be noted that bright light exposure may precipitate manic episodes in bipolar patients [36], and therefore should be used with caution in patients who are at risk. Light in the blue wavelength of the visible spectrum has been recently shown to have the most potent effect on the circadian clock [37]. Several new devices have become commercially available which use less intense blue light over shorter periods of exposure. As exposure to very bright full-spectrum light or narrow spectrum blue light may be hazardous to the eye, it is important to follow manufacturer's instructions carefully, and a consultation with an ophthalmologist may be prudent in some cases prior to using such a device. In a similar fashion, sunglasses that are designed to block the blue portion of the spectrum may be used in the evening during summer months by patients with sleep onset difficulty to help them fall asleep [38], or in the morning by patients with early morning awakenings to avoid phase advance.

Chronotherapy This is a behavioral technique that was specifically developed to treat patients with DSPS [39, 40]. The patient is instructed to stabilize their delayed sleep schedule, and then delay it further in increments of 2-3 hours every day until the desired bedtime is reached. The treatment capitalizes on these patients' natural tendency to delay their circadian rhythms. Preparations need to be made for the few days when the patient is sleeping in the middle of the day and up all night. When the individual's schedule approaches the desired time to fall asleep the last few days should delay bedtime more gradually, by an hour instead of 2-3. After achieving the desired bedtime the individual should strictly adhere to a rigid sleep period for several weeks. During the first couple of months after the treatment, the individual should adhere to the target wake up time even if the bedtime is delayed.

Sleep Hygiene

Sleep hygiene is a method of managing insomnia by encouraging behaviors that may promote sleep and avoidance of practices that make falling and staying asleep a challenge [41]. The recommendations may be auxiliary to other approaches to treatment of insomnia or stand independently as a regimen that aims at promoting sleep. The suggestions to the patient include avoidance of alcohol, caffeine, daytime naps, late hot showers, not looking at the clock during the night, and maintaining consistent sleep and wake times. The patient may be encouraged to keep his or her bedroom cool, dark and quiet as much as possible. Many individuals may state that they find alcohol to be helpful in facilitating sleep onset. However, alcohol leads to fragmentation of sleep during the night, resulting in minimally restorative sleep and early morning awakenings [42]. Caffeine is a stimulant that markedly disrupts sleep and should be avoided entirely or consumed no later than early afternoon (and preferably only in the morning). Napping during the day leads to reduced sleep at night by decreasing the sleep need that accumulates over the course of the day. For many people hot showers or baths are a relaxing evening ritual that may alleviate muscle tension. However, the resulting increase in body temperature if it occurs too close to bedtime may conflict with the natural decrease in temperature that occurs in the late evening before bedtime. Removal of time clocks from the bedroom targets the potential anxiety and obsessive thinking that may accompany one's sleepless hours. Consistent sleep and wake hours are helpful in adhering to a sleep schedule that closely correlates with the biological clock. Limiting time in bed is the mode of treatment that fits under the rubric of sleep restriction – an important modality described in a separate section. It has been shown that sleep hygiene education combined with stimulus control reduced sleep onset latency from 87 to 56 minutes while sleep hygiene education and relaxation showed similar efficacy reducing sleep onset latency from 71 minutes to 51 minutes [43].

Cognitive Therapy

As a person tries to cope with sleeping difficulties, faulty cognitions develop and further perpetuate the insomnia by providing the rationale for maladaptive behaviors and fueling anticipatory arousal and anxiety that interfere with sleep [44-46]. The goal of cognitive therapy for insomnia is to identify and eliminate dysfunctional beliefs about sleep. In addition, cognitive restructuring is directly or indirectly involved in behavioral techniques aimed to improve sleep. In this section, we will first discuss the principles of cognitive therapy proper, and then examine some of the common misconceptions that interfere with the implementation of different behavioral techniques.

Charles Morin [13] identifies five categories of dysfunctional cognitions: misconceptions concerning the causes of insomnia, misattributions or amplifications of its consequences, unrealistic sleep expectations, diminished perceptions of control, and mistaken beliefs about the predictability of sleep. For example, patients may believe that a malfunction in the brain is the cause of their insomnia, or that the difficulty sleeping is caused by stress at work, or by their bedroom environment being too noisy, *etc.* The common theme is that the cause of insomnia is perceived to be entirely outside of the patient's control, or any attempt to control the alleged cause would involve dramatic and essentially impossible measures. Similarly, many patients with insomnia hold unrealistic beliefs that it is imperative to fall asleep quickly at their selected bedtime and sleep continuously for 8 hours every night. The deleterious effects of poor sleep on health, work performance, cognitive capacity, mood, and the general sense of well-being are frequently in the foreground of the patient's thinking, especially at night.

These notions and concerns may be volunteered freely, sometimes in a repetitive fashion, during the initial clinical interview, or may begin to emerge after the clinician begins to suggest some avenues for possible improvement. In the evaluation phase of cognitive therapy, the clinician works with the patient on identifying such dysfunctional cognitions. In addition to an interview, a scale can be administered to obtain the information on the patient's sleep-related beliefs (Dysfunctional Beliefs and Attitudes about Sleep scale, DBAS [45]).

In the treatment phase, maladaptive beliefs are challenged, tested and gradually replaced with more realistic conceptions about normal sleep patterns, causes and consequences of insomnia, and the patient's active role in establishing a healthy sleep routine. Three main approaches are followed. First, the patient is provided with as much knowledge as feasible about normal sleep and circadian rhythm physiology and the interplay between homeostatic, circadian, and arousal forces. Second, the patient is asked to collect prospective evidence *via* sleep logs and daily observations. This information is used in follow up sessions to examine the validity of the patient's dysfunctional cognitions and to suggest more constructive ways of thinking about the problem. And third, the patient is encouraged to develop the sense of control over insomnia, in other words, to re-conceptualize oneself as a good sleeper, or at least a sleeper who "knows how to do it."

For example, a patient who spends 10 hours in bed while only obtaining 5 hours of light, unrefreshing sleep punctuated by long awakenings may be surprised to find out that any "normal" sleeper would start having fragmented sleep when spending substantially more time in bed than required. The opportunity should be seized to discuss how fruitlessly lying in bed for hours both degrades homeostatic and circadian mechanisms that drive healthy sleep and at the same time tremendously increases the arousal due to frustration. The patient may reply that spending all this time in bed "trying" to sleep helps ensure that some sleep, albeit light, does eventually occur. To show how this "solution" may be counter-productive in the long run, the patient should fill out sleep logs daily and examine them with the clinician on a weekly or bi-weekly basis. Over the course of several weeks a pattern often emerges that after a few nights that were shorter, e.g., due to work demands, a better night emerges when the patient falls asleep faster or sleeps more continuously or deeply. On the other hand, "catch-up" nights, e.g., when the patient stays in bed late on weekends, are often followed by especially poor nights. Once the patient understands the dysfunctional cycle, a suggestion can be made for the patient to try to control one's sleep by voluntarily limiting the number of hours spent in bed and by adhering to rigid bedtime and rising time. For the success of cognitive therapy, it is important to point out how these procedures put the patient back in control: instead of passively "waiting" for sleep like for a whimsical Prima Donna, the patient now decides when sleep is "allowed" to occur. This is a formidable change in attitude that may take time to achieve, but the effort is rewarded by the patient's sense of "know-how" of sleep.

Similarly, the overwhelming concern about the deleterious daytime consequences of insomnia can first be discussed from the perspective of the vicious cycle of worrying about sleep that prevents sleep from happening, or the overactive arousals system. The underlying belief about the rigid connection between the quality of sleep and daytime performance can then be challenged with the use of diaries that require the patient both to log their sleep at night and to rate several aspects of their daytime functioning. The analysis of several weeks of data helps the patient see how tenuous the connection between nocturnal sleep and daytime performance is once the obvious differences between the best and the worst nights are ignored and the more typical average nights are examined. The prospective nature of logs and diaries thus makes them an excellent tool to challenge the patient's notions that are heavily biased by the memories of the best and the worst nights.

Cognitive therapy is a powerful tool that helps the patient understand the nature of the problem and one's active role in the process of solving it. However, it is rarely used alone. More typically, cognitive and behavioral techniques are used simultaneously to help and reinforce each other. As the beliefs change, the patient becomes more motivated to comply with the demands of behavioral methods, and the improvement gained from the changes in behavior provides evidence and supports for the new and healthier ways to think about one's sleep. Cognitive restructuring also becomes an important part of a behavioral approach as the patient raises questions that are specific to the behavioral change the clinician aims to effect. Below we examine several typical issues that come up in the process of such behavioral techniques as SCT, SRT, and circadian rhythm entrainment techniques.

In the beginning of SCT, the patient may think that once they get out of bed in the middle of the night they will become wide awake, while staying in bed ensures that at least some sleep does occur. As a counterargument, the patient should be asked to consider how much aggravation is created by fruitless tossing and turning, and how unsuccessful attempts to fall asleep make them "dread" the following night, thus undermining their ability to sleep in the long run. The patient may also be concerned that sleep loss, inevitable at the beginning of the treatment, will impact their ability to function during the day. It should be discussed that while daytime deficits may in fact occur at the beginning of treatment, they already comprise a substantial portion of the patient's complaints, and that the quality of sleep they currently get utilizing the strategy of waiting in bed is poor. On the other hand, the treatment aims to improve their sleep quality and continuity, which in turn will lead to improvement in daytime alertness. The long-term nature of the improvements and the active role of the patient in taking control of their sleep pattern should be emphasized. In addition, the patient may detest getting out of the warm comfortable bed, so steps need to be taken ahead of time to prepare a place to sit and read in sufficient comfort in the middle of the night.

Similarly, with SRT the patient may fear sleep loss and the subsequent daytime sleepiness, and dislike the prohibition to indulge in "resting" in bed outside of a restricted time window. The patient may also be alarmed at how few hours of sleep are actually allowed, and express the need for more sleep, not less. These concerns should be countered with the analysis of the maladaptive behavioral cycle that continues to produce light, fragmented, unpredictable and unsatisfying sleep. It also should be pointed out that the first goal of treatment is not to produce more sleep, but to produce more continuous and predictable sleep, which is more satisfying and refreshing. The concept of sleep efficiency can be introduced, and the patient is encouraged to use the SRT methods to make sleep more efficient. As prospective sleep logs are collected, the patient's attention should be directed to shorter sleep latencies and shorter and fewer awakenings, thereby reinforcing the patient's efforts. The complaint of increased daytime sleepiness during the initial phases of SRT can be re-interpreted as the indication that the patient's brain can and does generate sleep need, and now the goal is to direct this sleep propensity to the allocated hours.

A common difficulty patients experience with light therapy is the need to allocate specific time for light exposure. Patients complain that it takes too much time and often wonder if they can do light exposure after getting to work or use a ceiling light or an open window instead. Careful explanations have to be given about the nature of the circadian system's response to light and the need for exact parameters, including length, timing and amount of brightness, for successful treatment. Education is also an important component of chronotherapy in terms of teaching the patient how to prepare for the process of shifting their sleep hours around the clock, organize their activity in a way compatible with the treatment during the active phase, and adhere to the new schedule in the maintenance phase.

Sleep hygiene instructions have face value and may be familiar to the patient to a substantial degree. Most insomnia sufferers would agree that such practices as varying bedtimes, excessive caffeine consumption, daytime napping, and surfing the web in the middle of the night interfere with a good night's sleep. However, patients continue to engage in dysfunctional behaviors as these behaviors have become part of their lifestyle during months and years of trying to cope with immediate demands in the face of sleeplessness. Two arguments against sleep hygiene instructions the patient is likely to bring up in therapy are the inability to perform daily activities without that snooze or cup of coffee, etc., and the failure of previous attempts at better sleep habits to improve sleep quality. The clinician should sensitively but firmly educate the patient about the detrimental effects of maladaptive behaviors and emphasize long-term gains over the inclination to give in to the immediate pressures. Unlike haphazard short-lived attempts the patient may have made in the past, a unified treatment program is laid out that addresses multiple issues simultaneously and therefore has a cumulative effect on sleep.

Other cognitive techniques that do not target sleep-related misconception rather aim to change the patient's overall attitude or produce a state of reduced arousal at night. For example, the patient is frequently instructed to "defer worrying" about difficulty sleeping and to allow oneself to have insomnia for the next couple of months [13]. This instruction is supported by the logic that the patient's insomnia has been going on for many months and often years, and improvement will not happen in one night. Allowing oneself to have insomnia helps the patient reduce the anxiety about a given night and instead concentrate on the overall pattern and long-term gains.

The method of paradoxical intention may also be used with patients who are concerned about having minimal amount of sleep or no sleep at all[47]. Paradoxical intention, initially used for compulsive behaviors, involves, essentially, "prescribing the symptom" and, in case of insomnia, would require the patient to stay in bed in the dark while keeping oneself awake all night using only will power (e.g., excessive fidgeting or self-pinching are not allowed). This approach is not in common usage. This recommendation is presented under the guise of having to collect detailed observations, and hourly phone calls to the clinician's answering machine throughout the night may be incorporated to document wakefulness. Paradoxical intention serves to eliminate the effort of trying to fall asleep, thereby reducing anxiety about not sleeping, which helps sleep come uninvited and provide evidence that the patient's brain may, in fact, generate sleep.

The patient may be instructed to schedule an hour during the early evening, for planning and worrying about different tasks, and to record such plans and worries in a journal [13]. The aim of this technique is to provide the patient with the sense of accomplishment and closure, however temporary, with regard to daily stressors, and to confine worrying to the daytime. The patient should be encouraged to build a "mental wall" between the stressors of the day and the peaceful respite of the night, the symbolic representation of which can be physically closing and putting away the worry journal until the next day.

Another cognitive technique, guided imagery, is similar to meditation and will be described in the section on relaxation techniques.

Relaxation Techniques and Biofeedback

Progressive muscular relaxation, deep breathing and guided imagery are treatment methods that aim at one's inability to achieve physiological relaxation and minimize anxiety to allow sleepiness to take effect and allow for sleep onset. Relaxation has been found to be a useful complement or component of cognitive behavior therapy, and, at least one study has shown that relaxation was found to cause greater change in total sleep time than CBT or placebo at post-treatment and greater improvement in sleep efficiency at follow up [48].

Progressive muscle relaxation starts by asking the patient to sit comfortably in a chair and told to tense a muscle for ten seconds and then relax it and to focus on the experience of shifting tension. An entire series of muscle groups are sequentially targeted. Once the patient learns the technique with a practitioner, he or she is asked to use it at bedtime to help promote sleep [49]. It is important to choose a patient who will be appropriate for this treatment as it may worsen one's ability to sleep in patients who experience no muscular tension [50]. Lichstein *et al* [51] looked at the efficacy of sleep compression (similar to SRT) as well as relaxation when compared to placebo and found that both treatments were more effective than placebo in reducing WASO. Sleep compression and relaxation led to similar results at 6 weeks of treatment, but sleep compression had greater effect at one year follow up [51]. Deep breathing is another method of relaxation that switches patient's attention fully to breathing and targets underlying anxiety. The patient is asked to sit or lie quietly with eyes closed. In one regimen the patient breathes in slowly through the nose, holds his/her breath for 2-3 seconds and exhales slowly and evenly, repeating the sequence 10-15 times before bedtimes. In a randomized controlled trial by Waters *et al* [52] relaxation treatment was shown to have greater effect on sleep onset than sleep restriction and stimulus control while the latter two measures had greater effect on sleep maintenance variables. Guided imagery [53] focuses the patient's thoughts on a sequence of pleasurable and familiar images with a plot. The person must be able to "walk" through the sequence smoothly and without distraction, resulting in minimization of anxiety.

In summary, the cognitive-behavioral approach to insomnia encompasses an array of therapies designed to strengthen homeostatic and circadian sleep drives and to lower arousal during bedtime. Different techniques compliment and reinforce each other, and a multimodal treatment, known as cognitive behavioral therapy for insomnia (CBT-I) is effective [54]. CBT-I involves cognitive therapy and stimulus control in combination with one or more other methods, typically sleep restriction and relaxation training [54]. The cognitive-behavioral approach also motivates the patient to implement life style changes.

Pharmacological Treatment of Insomnia

This chapter will review very briefly the pharmacologic therapy of insomnia and for effects of sleep medications on sleep the reader will be advised to read also Chapter 16 (Medications and Sleep).

The medications used in conjunction with cognitive behavioral therapy or in place of it when the latter is not a viable option should be optimized to target the specific type of insomnia. Sleep onset insomnia may require a different approach from the one used in management of sleep maintenance insomnia or combination of the two kinds. Insomnia co-morbid with medical or psychiatric conditions may call for adjustments based on the underlying symptoms and medications used to manage these symptoms. There are no reliable predictors of response to insomnia medications. In addition to the type of insomnia, the clinician must consider the duration of insomnia as it ranges from intermittent to chronic nightly difficulty with sleep. In the patients with intermittent insomnia, use of pharmacotherapy should be minimized to avoid potential side effects and to take the medication costs into consideration. Studies that assess efficacy suggest the use of zolpidem 10 mg 3-5 times per week for up to 3 months and zolpidem CR 12.5 mg 3-7 times per week for maximum of 6 months [55, 56]. The patients who are best suited for short-term treatment or intermittent use may be those who are able to predict that they may have difficulty falling asleep before they go to bed.

GABA receptor modulators are among the broadest class of agents used in treatment of primary and co-morbid insomnia. Benzodiazepines are agents whose chemical configuration mimics that of GABA. They bind to the alpha subunit of GABA receptor complex with resultant effect of inhibition. Studies in animals have shown that benzodiazepines may bind to the alpha subunits in different parts of the brain. There are 5 types of alpha subunits numbered 1 through 5. Binding to each of these subunits leads to a range of actions, including myorelaxation, anxiolysis, analgesia as well as to the less desirable side effects of gait instability and cognitive impairment. Hence, binding in amygdala to alpha 2 and 3 subunits may lead to relief from anxiety while binding in the cerebellum specifically to alpha 1 subunit may cause ataxia.

There are three unique agents - zolpidem, zaleplon and eszopiclone - that are different from benzodiazepines in structure but bind strongly at the alpha subunit. Zolpidem and zaleplon bind to the alpha 1 subunit while eszopiclone has binding sites on alpha 1, 2 and 3 subunits. Non-benzodiazepines have been studied in double blind, placebo-controlled studies of primary insomnia in the elderly and shown to be efficacious. However, in older individuals use of hypnotics carries a greater risk of adverse effects due to greater sensitivity to cognitive impairment, unsteadiness resulting in falls, interactions with other medications and alterations in metabolism with age.

Other than GABA receptor modulators, agents that block receptors responsible for promoting wakefulness have been used effectively in managing insomnia, often in conjunction with other underlying conditions. Histamine is a neurotransmitter that follows diurnal fluctuations, with rising concentrations in the morning, shortly before awakening. Antihistamine agents such as diphenhydramine, certain anti-depressants such as mirtazapine and antipsychotic medications are most effective in prolonging sleep in the last hour of the sleep period. However, literature supports only the effect of doxepin in 1-6 mg dosage in prolongation of sleep at the end of the night without subsequent cognitive impairment in the hours following awakening [57]. Anti-serotoninergic agents currently in development are aimed at preventing awakenings in the middle of the night but show less success in managing sleep difficulties at sleep onset or close to the time of awakening. Current agents that have blocking effect on serotonin 5H2 receptors are antidepressants trazodone and mirtazapine as well as antipsychotics quietipine and olanzapine. The side effect that may influence compliance with these medications is weight gain due to increased appetite. Antipsychotics that also block dopamine carry a negative side effect profile that includes extrapyramidal symptoms. An array of medication classes block acetylcholine but carry the risk of dangerous side effects like narrow angle glaucoma and less dangerous but significant effects of blurred vision, constipation, urinary retention. Patients may complain of dry mouth. Among these agents are tricyclic antidepressants like doxepin, amitriptyline, trimipramine, antihistaminergic agent diphenhydramine, dopamine antagonists quietiapine and olanzapine. Another type of agent is a melatonin receptor agonist, ramelteon that has demonstrated efficacy in several studies.

Literature suggests that a few studied agents may be helpful in insomnia co-morbid with medical condition. The following double-blind, placebo-controlled studies have pointed to efficacy: in rheumatoid arthritis, eszopiclone 3 mg led to improvement in sleep and pain ratings [58]. An earlier study by Walsh et al [59] described efficacy of triazolam at 0.125-0.250 mg in a small sample of 15 subjects of improving sleep and decreasing joint stiffness upon awakening. Zolpidem and ramelteon have been reported to improve sleep in patients with COPD [60].

In patients with insomnia and psychiatric co-morbidity, eszopiclone 3 mg showed efficacy in improving sleep in patients with major depressive disorder (MDD) [55] as well as anxiety in patients with generalized anxiety disorder (GAD) [61]. Zolpidem extended-release 12.5 mg was found to be efficacious in improving sleep of subjects with GAD [62]. In patients with insomnia following alcohol abstinence, trazodone at 150-200 mg has been found to be effective by subjects' self report [63]. Other medication that may be used in this subset of patients is gabapentin, although no systematic evidence for its efficacy exists. In patients who suffer from post-traumatic stress disorder (PTSD) and in whom insomnia is associated with nightmares, alpha-1 adrenergic antagonist prazosin has been shown to help minimize nightmares and improve symptoms associated with PTSD [64].

In summary, pharmacological treatment of insomnia entails precise assessment of the type of insomnia, duration, existence of other conditions, patient's age and degree of daytime disability as a result of insomnia. It should be used as much as possible in conjunction with other approaches such as cognitive behavioral therapy. Potential side effect profile of each medication must also be considered in optimizing medication management.

RESEARCH OUTLOOK

Research on insomnia encompasses investigation of causes and evaluation of treatment efficacy. These two main lines of inquiry complement each other: studies of causes are necessarily correlative, while studies of treatments targeting the presumed causes can employ various measures of control. See the section below titled "What we don't know" for fruitful directions for future research.

What do we know:

One factor that appears to play a major role in insomnia is arousal. Studies consistently find increased physiologic arousal in insomnia patients in comparison to normal controls on various measures, including respiratory and heart rates, oxygen consumption, muscle tension, body temperature, circulating levels of cortisol and adrenaline, and spectral EEG power [9-12]. Emotional arousal and psychological distress have also been shown to be associated with insomnia in a number of studies [11, 65, 66]. Cognitive patterns and personality qualities, such as coping styles, appraisal of stressful situations, worrying, perfectionism and perception of control, serve to modulate arousal and have also been implicated in insomnia [67-71]. One source of arousal at night has to do with negative expectations about sleep itself and with worrying about the consequences of sleeplessness. The association between these maladaptive cognitions and continuing sleep initiation and maintenance difficulties has been established in a number of studies [13, 14, 46, 72, 73].

Several treatment modalities for insomnia target physiological and cognitive arousal and maladaptive cognitions: relaxation techniques, biofeedback, and cognitive therapy. Relaxation techniques have been shown to improve sleep in insomnia patients in a number of controlled and clinical trial studies, including audio-guided relaxation [48], progressive muscle relaxation [51,74-76], guided imagery [53], and biofeedback [50, 76], although the need for careful patient selection has been stressed [50]. Cognitive therapy targeting maladaptive cognitive patterns and misperceptions about sleep has also been shown to be effective for insomnia treatment [45, 53, 77]. Paradoxical intention as a cognitive technique that aims to reduce subjective distress associated with sleeplessness has also been successful at least in some patients [47, 78].

The importance of homeostatic drive and circadian drive for sleep regulation has been well established [5, 79]. A behavioral therapy that directly aims to increase homeostatic drive to sleep at the appropriate time of night is Sleep

Restriction Therapy (SRT) [21, 22]. The effectiveness of SRT in reducing difficulty falling and staying asleep has been empirically supported [78, 80]. For the adjustment and stabilization of endogenous circadian rhythms, the light therapy has been shown very effective [24, 25, 29-35]. Chronotherapy can also be used successfully for the treatment of the delayed sleep phase type [39].

One of the oldest behavioral treatments of insomnia, Stimulus Control Therapy (SCT), is based on well-established principles of conditioning and has received considerable empirical support [19, 20, 81-84]. The SCT, together with cognitive therapy, has become an important element of the multimodal treatment approach termed cognitive behavior therapy for insomnia (CBT-I) [54]. In addition to the SCT and cognitive therapy, CBT-I also employs other behavioral techniques, most often SRT and some form of relaxation training [54]. Studies investigating the effectiveness of this multimodal treatment found CBT-I effective in patients with both primary insomnia [85, 86] and with insomnia co-morbid with medical [87, 88] or psychiatric [89] conditions, as well as in older patients [90]. The CBT-I has been found to be at least as effective as pharmacological therapy in both young to middle-aged [91] and older [90, 92] insomnia sufferers.

Sleep hygiene instructions as a stand-alone treatment received only limited empirical support; however, it is often used in combination with other treatment modalities or as part of CBT-I [43, 80, 92].

What we don't know:

The current understanding of insomnia rests on the general biological model of sleep regulation as well as on the clinically driven conceptualization of the forces behind the development and progression of insomnia. However, the exact nature of the interplay between biological, psychological and behavioral aspects of insomnia remains to be elucidated. In terms of treatment, a number of specific questions need to be answered. For example:

1) It has been suggested that different components of a cognitive behavioral treatment program may be more appropriate for different types of patients [47, 50, 93]. The interaction between the patient variables and the treatment variables needs to be clarified.

2) One study suggests that four sessions of CBT-I may be the optimal treatment course [94]; however, that may depend on the frequency of sessions. The effect of the frequency and the number of sessions on the effectiveness of treatment deserves further investigation.

3) A recent study tested a novel approach to insomnia treatment termed Intensive Sleep Retraining [95]. A small number of patients with primary insomnia spent a night in the sleep lab and were kept awake except for brief regularly scheduled sleep episodes., Significant improvements in several measures of sleep quality were present immediately after treatment and persisted at a 2-month follow up without any additional interventions. This experimental treatment is intriguing, and its applicability and efficacy merit further research.

4) The idea that behavioral conditioning plays an important role in sleep regulation has long been part of clinical approach to insomnia. One of the most empirically supported behavioral treatments, Stimulus Control Therapy, is based on the principles of conditioning [19, 20]. The effect of the novel Intensive Sleep Retraining treatment [95] described in the preceding paragraph appears to involve conditioning, as the patients are trained to fall asleep quickly with multiple successful trials. The term "conditioned insomnia" has been used interchangeably with psychophysiologic or primary insomnia, implying that sleeplessness can be conditioned. However, there is little empirical evidence to our knowledge that either falling asleep can be conditioned or that a cognitive or physiological arousal can be produced by such a cue as a bed in a person who otherwise feels tired and at a time of night when sleep normally occurs. The role of conditioning in sleep and insomnia needs to be further investigated to bridge the gap between the theoretical understanding of sleep mechanisms and the clinical practice.

5) It has been suggested that in order to adequately meet the need for treatment in the large population of patients with insomnia, a "stepped care" approach should be taken [96]. This approach proposes to deliver non-pharmacological treatment in multiple levels, with the "entry level" self-help materials on the lowest end, an individualized therapy by a trained specialist on the highest end, and such forms of delivery as telephone contacts and a supervised group therapy by mid-level health practitioners in the middle. This approach aims to provide an established treatment to a large number of admittedly underserved insomnia patients in a time and cost effective manner. However, further research is

needed to establish the efficacy of various methods of treatment delivery involved, to evaluate the appropriateness of screening and upstream referral procedures, and to investigate the potential effects of a failure at a lower level on the patient's ability to benefit from a higher level treatment delivery.

REFERENCES

[1] Edinger JD, Bonnet MH, Bootzin RR, *et al*. Derivation of research diagnostic criteria for insomnia: report of an American Academy of Sleep Medicine Work Group. Sleep 2004; 27: 1567-1596.

[2] Buysse DJ, Reynolds CF 3rd, Hauri PJ, *et al*. Diagnostic concordance for DSM-IV sleep disorders: a report from the APA/NIMH DSM-IV field trial. Am J Psychiatry 1994; 151: 1351-1360.

[3] Ohayon MM, Roberts RE. Comparability of sleep disorders diagnoses using DSM-IV and ICSD classifications with adolescents. Sleep 2001; 24: 920-925.

[4] Buysse DJ, Reynolds CF 3rd, Kupfer DJ, *et al*. Clinical diagnoses in 216 insomnia patients using the International Classification of Sleep Disorders (ICSD), DSM-IV and ICD-10 categories: a report from the APA/NIMH DSM-IV Field Trial. Sleep 1994; 17: 630-637.

[5] Borbely AA. A two process model of sleep regulation. Hum Neurobiol 1982; 1: 195-204.

[6] Wager-Smith K, Kay SA. Circadian rhythm genetics: from flies to mice to humans. Nat Genet 2000; 26: 23-27.

[7] Edgar DM, Dement WC, Fuller CA. Effect of SCN lesions on sleep in squirrel monkeys: evidence for opponent processes in sleep-wake regulation. J Neurosci 1993; 13: 1065-1079.

[8] Dijk DJ, Czeisler, CA. Paradoxical timing of the circadian rhythm of sleep propensity serves to consolidate sleep and wakefulness in humans. Neurosci Lett 1994; 166: 63-68.

[9] Bonnet MH, Arand DL. Hyperarousal and insomnia. Sleep Med Rev 1997; 2: 97-108.

[10] Bonnet MH, Arand DL. 24-hour metabolic rate in insomniacs and matched normal sleepers. Sleep 1995; 18: 581-588.

[11] Vgontzas AN, Tsigos C, Bixler EO, *et al*. Chronic insomnia and activity of the stress system: A preliminary study. J Psychosom Res 1998; 45: 21-31.

[12] Perlis ML, Smith MT, Andrews PJ, Orff H, Giles DE. Beta/gamma EEG activity in patients with primary and secondary insomnia and good sleeper controls. Sleep 2001; 24: 110-117.

[13] Morin CM. Insomnia: psychological assessment and management. New York: Guilford; 1993.

[14] Harvey AG, Tang NK, Browning L. Cognitive approaches to insomnia. Clin Psychol Rev 2005; 25: 593-611.

[15] Espie CA. Understanding insomnia through cognitive modeling. Sleep Med 2007; 8(Suppl 4): S3-S8.

[16] Espie CA, Broomfield NM, MacMahon KM, Macphee LM, Taylor LM. The attention-intention-effort pathway in the development of phyyshophysiologic insomnia: A theoretical review. Sleep Med Rev 2006; 10: 215-245.

[17] Spielman AJ. Assessment of insomnia. Clin Psychol Rev 1986; 6: 11-25.

[18] Spielman AJ, Caruso LS, Glovinsky PB. A behavioral perspective on insomnia treatment. Psychiatr Clin North Am 1987;10: 541-553

[19] Bootzin RR. A stimulus control treatment for insomnia. Proceedings of the American Psychological Association 1972; 395-396.

[20] Bootzin RR, Epstein D, Wood JM. Stimulus control instructions. In: Hauri P, editor. *Case studies in insomnia*. New York: Plenum; 1991, pp, 19-28.

[21] Spielman AJ, Saskin P, Thorpy MJ. Treatment of chronic insomnia by restriction of time in bed. Sleep 1987; 10: 45-56.

[22] Glovinsky PB, Spielman AJ. The insomnia answer: breakthrough solutions for getting to sleep, staying asleep, broken sleep. New York: Perigee; 2006.

[23] Czeisler CA, Allan JS, Strogatz SH, Ronda JM, Sanchez R, Rios CD, Freitag WO, Richardson GS, Kronauer RE. Bright light resets the human circadian pacemaker independent of the timing of the sleep-wake cycle. Science 1986; 233: 667-671.

[24] Czeisler CA. The effect of light on the human circadian pacemaker. Ciba Found Symp 1995; 183: 254-302.

[25] Arendt J, Broadway J. Light and melatonin as zeitgebers in man. Chronobiol Int 1987; 4: 273-282.

[26] Gillette MU. Tischkau SA. Suprachiasmatic nucleus: the brain's circadian clock. Recent Prog Horm Res 1999; 54: 33-59.

[27] Murphy PJ, Campbell SS. Physiology of the circadian system in animals and humans. J Clin Neurophysiol 1996; 13: 2-16.

[28] Scheer FA, Pirovano C, Van Someren EJ, Buijs RM. Environmental light and suprachiasmatic nucleus interact in the regulation of body temperature. Neuroscience 2005; 132: 465-477.

[29] Shanahan TL, Zeitzer JM, Czeisler CA. Resetting the melatoning rhythm with light in humans. J Biol Rhythms 1997; 12: 556-567.

[30] Minors DS, Waterhouse JM, Wirz-Justice AA. A human phase-response curve to light. Neurosci Lett 1991; 133: 354-361.

[31]   Kripke DF, Elliott JA, Youngstedt SD, Rex KM. Circadian phase response curves to light in older and young women and men. J Circadian Rhythms 2007; 10: 4.

[32]   Rosenthal NE, Joseph-Vanderpool JR, Levendosky AA, Johnston SH, Allen R, Kelly KA, Souetre E, Schultz PM, Starz KE. Phase-shifting effets of bright morning light as treatment for delayed sleep phase syndrome. Sleep 1990; 13: 354-361.

[33]   Campbell SS, Dawson D, Anderson MW. Alleviation of sleep maintenance insomnia with timed exposure to bright light. J Am Geriatr Soc 1993; 41: 829-836.

[34]   Lack L, Wright H. The effect of evening bright light in delaying the circadian rhythms and lengthening the sleep of early morning awakening insomniacs. Sleep 1993; 16: 436-443.

[35]   Lack L, Wright H, Kemp K, Gibbon S. The treatment of early-morning awakening insomnia with 2 evenings of bright light. Sleep 2005; 28: 616-623.

[36]   Pande AC. Light-induced hypomania. Am J Psychiatry 1985; 142: 1126.

[37]   Lockley SW, Brainard GC, Czeisler CA. High sensitivity of the human circadian melatonin rhythm to resetting by short wavelength light. J Clin Endocrinol Metab 2003; 88: 4502-4505.

[38]   Sasseville A, Paquet N, Sevigny J, Hebert M. Blue blocker glasses impede the capacity of bright light to suppress melatonin production. J Pineal Res 2006; 41: 73-78.

[39]   Czeisler CA, Richardson GS, Coleman RM, Zimmerman JC, Moore-Ede MC, Dement WC, Weitzman ED. Chronotherapy: Resetting the circadian clocks of patients with delayed sleep phase insomnia. Sleep 1981; 4: 1-21.

[40]   Weitzman ED, Czeisler CA, Coleman RM, *et al*. Delayed sleep-phase syndrome. A chronobiological disorder with sleep-onset insomnia. Arch Gen Psychiatry 1981; 38: 737-746.

[41]   Hauri, P. Sleep hygiene, relaxation therapy and cognitive interventions. In P. Hauri, Critical issues in psychiatry: Case studies in insomnia. New York: Plenum Medical Book 1991; 65-84

[42]   Adamson J, Burdick JA. Sleep of dry alcoholics. Arch Gen Psychiatry1973; 28(1): 146-149.

[43]   Pallesen S, Nordhus IH, Kvale G, Nielsen GH, Havik OE, Johnsen BH, Skjotskift S. Behavioral treatment of insomnia in older adults: an open clinical trial comparing two interventions. Behav Res Ther 2003; 41: 31-48

[44]   Harvey L. Inglis SJ, Espie CA. Insomniacs' reported use of CBT components and relationship to long-term clinical outcome. Behav Res Ther 2002; 40: 75-83.

[45]   Morin CM, Stone J, Trinkle D, Mercer J, Remsberg S. Dysfunctional beliefs and attitudes about sleep among older adults with and without insomnia complaints. Psychol Aging 1993; 8: 463-467.

[46]   Edinger JD, Fins AI, Glenn DM, *et al*. Insomnia and the eye of the beholder: are there clinical markers of objective sleep disturbances among adults with and without insomnia complaints? J Consult Clin Psych 2000; 68: 586-593.

[47]   Espie CA, Lindsay WR. Paradoxical intention in the treatment of chronic insomnia: Six case studies illustrating variability in therapeutic response. Behav Res Ther 1985; 23: 703-709.

[48]   Rybarczyk B, Lopez M, Benson R, Alsten C, Stepanski E. Efficacy of two behavioral treatment programs for co-morbid geriatric insomnia. Psychol Aging 2002; 17: 288-298.

[49]   Ebben MR, Spielman AJ. Non-pharmacological treatments for insomnia. J Behav Med 2009; 32: 244-254.

[50]   Hauri P, Percy L, Hellikson C, Russ D. The treatment of psychophysiologic insomnia with biofeedback: A replication study. Biofeedback Self Regul 1982; 7: 223-235.

[51]   Lichstein KL, Riedel BW, Wilson NM, Lester KW, Aguillard RN. Relaxation and sleep compression for late life insomnia: a placebo controlled trial. J Consult Clin Psychol 2001; 69: 227-239.

[52]   Waters WF, Hurry MJ, Binks PG, *et al*. Behavioral and hypnotic treatments for insomnia subtypes. Behav Sleep Med 2003; 1: 81-101.

[53]   Harvey AG, Payne S. The management of unwanted pre-sleep thoughts in insomnia: distraction with imagery versus general distraction. Behav Res Ther 2002; 40: 267-277.

[54]   Schutte-Rodin S, Broch L, Buysse D, Dorsey C, Sateia M. Clinical Guideline for the Evaluation and Management of Chronic Insomnia in Adults. J Clin Sleep Med 2008; 4: 487–504.

[55]   Krystal AD. Treating the health, quality of life, and functional impairments in insomnia. J Clin Sleep Med 2007; 3(1): 63-72.

[56]   Perlis ML, McCall WV, Krystal AD, Walsh JK. Long-term, non-nightly administration of zolpidem in the treatment of patients with primary insomnia. J Clin Psychiatry 2004; 65(8): 1128-37.

[57]   Scharf M, Rogowski R, Hull S, et al. Efficacy and safety of doxepin 1 mg, 3 mg, and 6 mg in elderly patients with primary insomnia: a randomized, double-blind, placebo-controlled crossover study. J Clin Psychiatry 2008; 69(10): 1557-64.

[58]   Roth T, Price JM, Amato DA, Rubens RP, Roach JM, Schnitzer TJ. The effect of eszopiclone in patients with insomnia and coexisting rheumatoid arthritis: a pilot study. Prim Care Companion J Clin Psychiatry 2009; 11(6): 292-301.

[59]   Walsh JK, Muehlbach MJ, Lauter SA, Hilliker NA, Schweitzer PK. Effects of triazolam on sleep, daytime sleepiness, and morning stiffness in patients with rheumatoid arthritis. J Rheumatol 1996; 23(2): 245-52.

[60]   Kryger M, Roth T, Wang-Weigand S, Zhang J. The effects of ramelteon on respiration during sleep in subjects with moderate to severe chronic obstructive pulmonary disease. Sleep Breath 2009; 13(1): 79-84.

[61]   Pollack M, Kinrys G, Krystal A, *et al.*Eszopiclone coadministered with escialopram in patients with insomnia and comorbid generalized anxiety disorder. Arch Gen Psychiatry 2008; 65(5): 551-62.

[62]   Fava M, Asnis GM, Shrivastava R, *et al.* Zolpidem extended-release improves sleep and next-day symptoms in comorbid insomnia and generalized anxiety disorder. J Clin Psychoparmacol 2009; 29(3): 223-30.

[63]   Le Bon O, Murphy JR, Staner L, *et al.* Double-blind, placebo-controlled study of the efficacy of trazodone in alcohol post-withdrawal syndrome: polysomnographic and clinical evaluations. J Clin Psychopnarmacol 2003; 23 (4): 377-83.

[64]   Boynton L, Bentley J, Strachan E, Barbato A, Raskind M. Preliminary findings concerning the use of prazosin for the treatment of posttraumatic nightmares in a refugee population. J Psychiatr Pract 2009; 15(6): 454-9

[65]   Kales A, Caldwell AB, Preston TA, Healey S, Kales JD. Personality patterns in insomnia. Arch Gen Psychiatry 1976; 33(9): 1128-1134

[66]   Drake DL, Richardson G, Roehrs T, Scofield H, Roth T. Vulnerability to stress-related sleep disturbance and hyperarousal. Sleep 2004; 27: 285-291.

[67]   Morin CM, Rodrigue S, Ivers H. Role of stress, arousal, and coping skills in primary insomnia. Psychosom Med 2003; 65(2): 259-267.

[68]   Dorsay CM, Bootzin RR. Subjective and psychophysiologic insomnia: an examinatyion of sleep tendency and personality. Biol Psychiatry 1997; 41: 209-216.

[69]   Vincent NK, Walker JR. Perfectionism and chronic insomnia. J Psychoson Res 2000; 49(5): 349-354.

[70]   Fernández-Mendoza J, Vela-Bueno A, Vgontzas AN, Ramos-Platón MJ, Olavarrieta-Bernardino S, Bixler EO, De la Cruz-Troca JJ. Cognitive-emotional hyperarousal as a premorbid characteristic of individuals vulnerable to insomnia. Psychosom Med 2010; 72(4): 397-403.

[71]   Ottoni GL, Lorenzi TM, Lara DR. Association of temperament with subjective sleep patterns. J Affect Disord 2010; 128(1-2): 120-7.

[72]   Fichten CS, Creti L, Amsel R, Brender W, Weinstein N, Libman E. Poor sleepers who do not complain of insomnia: myths and realities about psychological and lifestyle characteristics of older good and poor sleepers. J Behav Med 1995 Apr; 18(2): 189-223.

[73]   Wicklow A, Espie CA. Intrusive thoughts and their relationship to actigraphic measurement of sleep: towards a cognitive model of insomnia. Behav Res Ther 2000; 38(7): 679-693.

[74]   Reedman R, Papsdorf JD. Biofeedback and progressive relaxation treatment of sleep-onset insomnia: A controlled, all-night investigation. Biofeedback Self Regul 1976; 1(3): 253-271.

[75]   Gustafson R. Treating insomnia with a self-administered muscle relaxation training program: a follow-up. Psychol Rep 1992; 70(1): 124-126.

[76]   Nicassio PM, Boylan MB, McCabe TG. Progressive relaxation, EMG biofeedback and biofeedback placebo in the treatment of sleep-onset insomnia. Br J Med Psychol 1982; 55(pt2): 159-166.

[77]   Harvey AG, Sharpley AL, Ree MJ, Stinson K, Clark DM. An open trial of cognitive therapy for chronic insomnia. Behav Res Ther 2007; 45(10): 2491-2501.

[78]   Morin CM, Bootzin RR, Buysse DJ, Edinger JD, Espie CA, Lichstein KL. Psychological and behavioral treatment of insomnia: update of the recent evidence (1998-2004). Sleep 2006; 29(11): 1398-1414.

[79]   Borbély AA, Achermann P. Sleep homeostasis and models of sleep regulation. J Biol Rhythms 1999; 14(6): 557-568.

[80]   Taylor DJ, Schmidt-Nowara W, Jessop CA, Ahearn J. Sleep restriction therapy and hypnotic withdrawal versus sleep hygiene education in hypnotic using patients with insomnia. J Clin Sleep Med 2010; 6(2): 169-175.

[81]   Morin CM, Azrin NH. Stimulus control and imagery training in treating sleep-maintenance insomnia. J Consult Clin Psychol 1987; 55: 260-262.

[82]   Espie CA. Comparative outcome studies involving relaxation, paradox and stimulus control treatments. In: Espie CA, Ed. The psychological treatment of insomnia. Toronto: Wiley 1991; 178-206.

[83]   Morin CM, Culbert JP, Schwartz SM. Nonpharmacological interventions for insomnia: a meta-analysis of treatment efficacy. Am J Psychiatry 1994; 151: 1172-1180.

[84]   Baillargeon L, Demers M, Ladouceur R. Stimulus-control: nonpharmacologic treatment for insomnia. Can Fam Physician 1998; 44: 73-79.

[85]   Edinger JD, Wohlgemuth WK, Radtke RA, Marsh GR, Quillian RE. Cognitive behavioral therapy for treatment of chronic primary insomnia: a randomized controlled trial. JAMA 2001; 285(14): 1856-1864.

[86]   Edinger JD, Wohlgemuth WK, Radtke RA, Coffman CJ, Carney CE. Dose-response effects of cognitive-behavioral insomnia therapy: a randomized clinical trial. Sleep 2007; 30(2): 203-212.

[87]   Edinger JD, Wohlgemuth WK, Krystal AD, Rice JR. Behavioral insomnia therapy for fibromyalgia patients: a randomized clinical trial. Arch Intern Med 2005; 165(21): 2527-2535.

[88]   Jungquist CR, O'Brien C, Matteson-Rusby S, *et al.* The efficacy of cognitive-behavioral therapy for insomnia in patients with chronic pain. Sleep Med 2010; 11(3): 302-309.

[89]   Edinger JD, Olsen MK, Stechuchak KM, *et al.* Cognitive behavioral therapy for patients with primary insomnia or insomnia associated predominantly with mixed psychiatric disorders: a randomized clinical trial. Sleep 2009; 32(4): 499-510.

[90]   Omvik S, Sivertsen B, Pallesen S, Bjorvatn B, Havik OE, Nordhus IH. Daytime functioning in older patients suffering from chronic insomnia: treatment outcome in a randomized controlled trial comparing CBT with zopiclone. Behav Res Ther 2008; 46(5): 623-641.

[91]   Jacobs GD, Pace-Schott EF, Stickgold R, Otto MW. Cognitive behavior therapy and pharmacotherapy for insomnia: a randomized controlled trial and direct comparison. Arch Intern Med 2004; 164(17): 1888-1896.

[92]   Sivertsen B, Omvik S, Pallesen S, *et al.* Cognitive behavioral therapy vs zopiclone for treatment of chronic primary insomnia in older adults: a randomized controlled trial. JAMA 2006; 295(24): 2851-2858.

[93]   Edinger JD, Carney CE, Wohlgemuth WK. Pretherapy cognitive dispositions and treatment outcome in cognitive behavior therapy for insomnia. Behav Ther 2008; 39(4): 406-416.

[94]   Edinger JD, Wohlgemuth WK, Radtke RA, Coffman CJ, Carney CE. Dose-response effects of cognitive-behavioral insomnia therapy: a randomized clinical trial. Sleep 2007; 30(2): 203-212.

[95]   Harris J, Lack L, Wright H, Gradisar M, Brooks A. Intensive Sleep Retraining treatment for chronic primary insomnia: a preliminary investigation. J Sleep Res 2007; 16(3): 276-284.

[96]   Espie CA. "Stepped care": a health technology solution for delivering cognitive behavioral therapy as a first line insomnia treatment. Sleep 2009; 32(12): 1549-558.

[97]   Harvey A, Spielman A. Insomnia: Diagnosis, Assessment and Outcomes. In: Kryger M, Roth T, Dement W, eds. Principles and practices of sleep medicine, Fifth edition, Saunders.

CHAPTER 10

Circadian Rhythm Sleep Disorders

Saiprakash B. Venkateshiah, M.D.*

Assistant Professor of Medicine - Emory University, Adjunct Clinical Assistant Professor of Medicine – Morehouse School of Medicine, Division of Pulmonary, Critical Care and Sleep Medicine, Emory University School of Medicine, Atlanta Veterans Affairs Medical Center, Atlanta, GA 30033, USA

Abstract: Suprachiasmatic nucleus is the master circadian clock that regulates various endogenous circadian rhythms. Light and social cues are important factors that help align the endogenous circadian rhythms to the 24 hour day. Circadian rhythm sleep disorders can be due to abnormalities in the endogenous circadian clock ("intrinsic disorders") such as delayed sleep phase type, advanced sleep phase type, free running type, and irregular sleep wake rhythm type. Shift work or air travel leads to an artificial mismatch between the endogenous circadian clock and the external environment ("extrinsic disorders") leading to shift work disorder and jet lag disorder. Individuals with circadian rhythm sleep disorders are presented with insomnia or excessive sleepiness or both.

These disorders are under recognized in the general population but they can affect a significant number of people if a the large number of shift workers and air travelers are considered. The symptoms may be misdiagnosed for other common sleep disorders such as sleep apnea or insomnia. Meticulous history and sleep diary data are integral tools in diagnosing CRSD. Actigraphs (activity monitors) may supplement the sleep diary data. In the past two decades major advances have been made in understanding the genetic basis of these disorders. Understanding the circadian principles has led to various therapeutic options such as phototherapy and exogenous melatonin.

TOPIC DISCUSSION (CLINICAL OUTLOOK)

Introduction

Circadian rhythm sleep disorders (CRSD) are a group of disorders that may present with insomnia, excessive sleepiness or both. According to the International Classification of Sleep Disorders, second edition (ICSD-2), the general criteria for CRSDs are: i) there is a persistent or recurrent pattern of sleep disturbance due primarily to alterations in the circadian timekeeping system or a misalignment between the endogenous circadian rhythm and exogenous factors that affect the timing or duration of sleep, ii) the circadian related sleep disruption leads to excessive sleepiness, insomnia or both and iii) sleep disturbance that is associated with impairment of social, occupational or other areas of functioning. The diagnosis also requires that the disorder not be better explained by another current sleep disorder, medical, neurological, mental, medication use or substance use disorder [1]. This criterion is important so that common disorders that cause excessive daytime sleepiness or insomnia should not be overlooked when an individual presents with these nonspecific symptoms.

There are six disorders described by the ICSD-2 and we will be discussing them in the chapter:

1. Delayed sleep phase type

2. Advanced sleep phase type

3. Free- running type

4. Irregular sleep- wake type

5. Jet lag type and

6. Shift work type

Address correspondence to Saiprakash B. Venkateshiah: Assistant Professor of Medicine - Emory University, Adjunct Clinical Assistant Professor of Medicine – Morehouse School of Medicine, Division of Pulmonary, Critical Care and Sleep Medicine, Emory University School of Medicine, Atlanta Veterans Affairs Medical Center, Atlanta, GA 30033, USA; E-mail: svenka8@emory.edu

RESEARCH OUTLOOK:

What do we know:

Circadian Rhythm Physiology

Single cells to humans, all living organisms have circadian rhythms. Circadian [Latin *circa* (about) and *dies* (day)] rhythms are those rhythms that occur in approximately 24-hour cycles. Sleep-wake cycle is the most obvious circadian rhythm in the human body, but there are other biologic processes that also exhibit circadian rhythms. Daily oscillations characterize the release of nearly most hormones such as melatonin, cortisol, growth hormone, thyroid stimulating hormone *etc.* However, the observed hormonal oscillations do not simply reflect the output of this internal circadian pacemaker. Sleep exerts a profound influence on hormone secretion. Moreover, the secretion of hormones such as renin and human growth hormone are strongly influenced by sleep or wakefulness, while melatonin and cortisol levels are relatively unaffected. More likely is the possibility that these daily hormonal profiles are due to a complex interaction between the output of the circadian clock, periodic behavioral changes, light exposure, the timing of sleep and wakefulness, neuroendocrine feedback loop mechanisms, gender, and age [2].

Cardiovascular function (decreased heart rate, blood pressure, sympathetic activity at night), pulmonary function (increased bronchial hyperresponsiveness during early morning), renal function (decreased nocturnal urine output) and cognitive performance are some of the multiple physiological processes that exhibit circadian rhythmicity. It is difficult to distinguish whether these processes are exhibiting circadian or diurnal rhythms. A Circadian rhythm is generated by an endogenous circadian (approximately 24 hour) oscillator. A diurnal rhythm refers to an observed 24-hour pattern which may be caused either by an endogenous circadian pacemaker and/or other events within the 24- hour day such as sleep-wake patterns, light exposure, activity, meals, social contacts, changes in posture etc [3]. Despite the various confounding masking factors, circadian modulation of core body temperature and endogenous melatonin is very strong, thereby leading to the use of these circadian phase markers in research. Melatonin levels in the systemic circulation are very low during the daytime and begin to rise approximately 2 hours before normal bedtime [4]. Melatonin levels tend to peak near the middle of the nocturnal sleep and decline over the rest of the sleep period. Core body temperature is high during daytime and low during nighttime. The core body temperature minimum has been used as a circadian phase marker.

To understand the importance of circadian day-night timekeeping system, we should understand the process that governs the duration and timing of human sleep. "Two-process model" of sleep wake regulation was first described by Borbely [5] (Fig. 1). The two processes are the homeostatic drive and the circadian system. Homeostatic drive for sleep builds up with each hour of wakefulness. Maintaining wakefulness for most of the day, *i.e.*, for 16-18 hours, builds up substantial homeostatic sleep pressure to initiate (nocturnal) sleep. This homeostatic system is not enough to maintain sleep for the entire night as the homeostatic sleep drive is mostly satisfied by the middle of the night. The mechanism by which human beings maintain sleep for the entire night is explained by the effects of the "second process"- the circadian system. Circadian system actively drives sleep during the night, reaching its maximal effect near and just after the normal wake time [6, 7]. Circadian system is also necessary to maintain stable alertness during 16-18 hours of daytime despite the homeostatic sleep drive building up after every hour of wakefulness. The circadian system actively promotes daytime wakefulness and its maximal activity reaches a few hours (1-3 hours) before habitual bedtime [8]. This has been described as a "forbidden zone" for sleep [9].

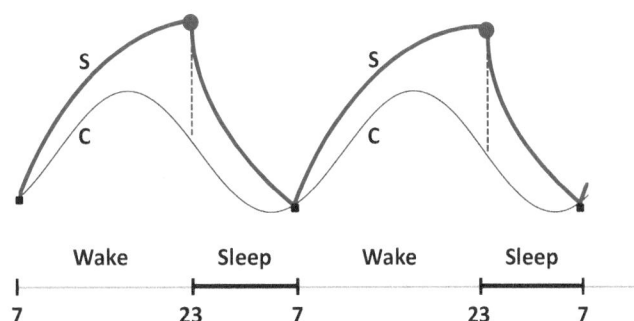

Figure 1: Graph of the Two-process model of sleep regulation. S is the homeostatic sleep drive, which rises during wakefulness and declines during sleep. C is the circadian rhythm cycle as measured by body temperature. The greatest propensity for sleep occurs at the trough of the body temperature. Optimal time for sleep occurs when S is at peak and C is in trough, which coincides

with the usual nighttime sleep period (dark bar). Wake up usually occurs where S and C intersect. With permission: From Borbely AA, Acherman P. Sleep homeostasis and models of sleep regulation. In: Kryger MH, Roth T, Dement WC, (eds.), Principles and practice of sleep medicine (3rd ed). WB Saunders Co., 2000 Fig. **29**-5 A page 384 .

Suprachiasmatic nucleus (SCN) in the hypothalamus is considered the master circadian clock of the body [10]. SCN neurons generate and maintain a self-sustaining rhythm *via* an autoregulatory feedback loop in which oscillating circadian gene products regulate their own expression through a complex system of transcription, translation and posttranslational processes [11-13]. The free-running period of the circadian clock (when human beings are completely isolated from external time cues under carefully controlled lighting conditions) is slightly greater than 24 hours [14]. Precise alignment between the internal circadian rhythms and the 24-hour social and physical environment requires daily adjustments with synchronizing (entraining) agents. Light, melatonin secreted by the pineal gland, and physical activity are the main synchronizing agents for the circadian clock in humans [15]. Light is the the primary synchronizing or entraining agent or *zeitgeber* (time-giver, time cue, in German) [16]. Transduction of this time cue occurs in retinal ganglion cells, which are specialized cells distinct from rods and cones, which are the retinal photoreceptors that mediate vision [17-19]. The light input from the retinal ganglion cells is passed through the retinohypothalamic tract to the suprachiasmatic nucleus (SCN), the master circadian clock [10, 20, 21]. SCN modulates multiple functions such as core body temperature, endogenous melatonin, cortisol and the sleep-wake cycle through its output pathways. Circadian modulation of core body temperature and endogenous melatonin is very strong, thereby leading to the use of these circadian phase markers in research.

The circadian system uses the environmental light-dark cycle as its primary synchronizing cue, so that there is proper orientation to the desired nocturnal sleep schedule [22]. The time of exposure determines the effect of light on the circadian clock. The circadian clock is relatively unresponsive to bright light delivered during the middle of the waking day [22]. Exposure to light near the end of the normal sleep episode or in the early morning hours results in a "phase advance", *i.e.*, shift the clock to an earlier clock time. Exposure to light in the late evening through the middle of the night results in a "phase delay", *i.e.*, shifts the clock to a later clock time [13, 16, 22]. There is emerging literature suggesting that the circadian system is maximally sensitive to visible light in the blue light spectral region [18, 19].

Melatonin, a pineal gland hormone, is also an important synchronizing agent for the circadian system. SCN regulates the nocturnal secretion of melatonin through an indirect pathway, from the superior cervical ganglion to the pineal gland [13, 23, 24]. Melatonin levels in the systemic circulation are very low during the daytime and begin to rise approximately 2 hours before normal bedtime [4]. Melatonin levels tend to peak near the middle of the nocturnal sleep and decline over the rest of the sleep period. Melatonin also resets the phase of the circadian rhythm, but in a direction opposite to that of light exposure- melatonin delays circadian rhythms when administered in the morning and advances them when administered in the afternoon or early evening [25].

Therefore, bright light exposure and melatonin have found a place in the treatment of various CRSD.

Prevalence of CRSD

The exact prevalence of CRSD is unknown. One telephone survey that evaluated the symptoms of excessive sleepiness or insomnia in night and rotating shift work population in the community suggested about a third of shift workers had symptoms suggestive of shift work sleep disorder [26]. There are about 30 million air travelers annually from the USA who travel for destinations that entail flights crossing five or more time zones. The incidence of jet lag disorder is unknown, but it presumably affects a substantial number of people due to the sheer volume of air travel [27]. Obviously, these disorders are of significant public health importance, as they impact a large number of people.

The prevalence of CRSD in a clinic population is generally small [28, 29]. A case series from a clinic in Israel showed that delayed sleep phase disorder was the most common CRSD (83%), followed by free-running circadian disorder (12%). Advanced sleep phase disorder and irregular sleep wake type were rare (less than 2%) [29]. These clinic prevalence estimates are probably an underestimate, as most of the CRSD are under-recognized.

There is normally a delay in adolescents and an advance during middle age and elder subjects in the circadian phase. There is no clear cut demarcation which separates these "normal" delays or advances from pathological states. Moreover shift work and jet lag are due to situations created by mankind wherein there is an artificial mismatch between the endogenous circadian timekeeping mechanism and the 24-hour day but not due to any pathology in the circadian clock. It can be argued that naming these entities as syndromes rather than disorders may be appropriate but we shall adhere to the ICSD-2 definition in this chapter and use the terminology circadian disorders.

Diagnostic Tools

Sleep Logs and Diaries:

Diaries that record the sleep-wake periods (sleep logs) are one of the tools widely used to diagnose CRSD. In a typical sleep diary, there is documentation of the bedtime, sleep onset latency, time spent awake during the night after sleep onset and final wake up time (mention is also made if the alarm was needed or not). Sleep diaries also include the time of consumption of food, alcohol, and caffeine, recorded every evening. Sleep diaries are simple, easy to use and can provide data on both quality and quantity of sleep. Unfortunately there are no standardized sleep logs and each clinics construct their own. Electronic diaries have been used in one study to assess sleepiness in shift workers [30]. This may hold promise for standardization of sleep logs in the future. The practice parameters of the American Academy of Sleep Medicine (AASM) recommend the use of a sleep log or diary in the assessment of patients with a suspected CRSD (strength of recommendation: *guideline, i.e.,* patient-care strategy that reflects a moderate degree of clinical certainty) [31].

Actigraphy

Actigraphs, also known as activity monitors, are devices that detect activity by sensing motion by an internal accelerometer. They are worn on the wrist alike usual watches. They can provide a reasonably accurate estimate of sleep and wakefulness obtained across many days and nights up to 2-3 weeks), hence they may help in the longitudinal assessment of sleep-wake patterns.

There is generally good agreement across studies showing that actigraphy data correlate with polysomnography, sleep logs and markers of circadian phase in patients with CRSD. Furthermore, actigraphy may also be useful as a tool to evaluate treatment response of CRSD. The practice parameters of the AASM recommend the use of actigraphy in the evaluation of patients with a suspected CRSD and also as an outcome measure in evaluating treatment response (strength of recommendation: *guideline, i.e.,* patient-care strategy that reflects a moderate degree of clinical certainty) [31].

Polysomnography

Polysomnography (sleep study) is *not routinely indicated* for the diagnosis of CRSD. It is only indicated to rule out other co-existent sleep disorders in patients with symptoms suggestive of CRSD and possibly another primary sleep disorder [31, 32]. Patients with CRSD can very well have a second sleep disorder, such as sleep apnea, which is very prevalent in the community and hence sleep studies are indicated mainly to rule out other sleep disorders if they have suggestive symptoms rather than to diagnose CRSD *per se.* AASM practice parameters' recommendation is *standard* (patient care strategy that reflects a high degree of clinical certainty) [31].

The Morningness-Eveningness Questionnaire (MEQ)

This questionnaire contains 19 questions aimed at determining when the person's tendency to be active lies during the daily span [33]. This helps to determine whether a person is a "morning lark" or a "night owl" type. These questionnaires have been used in the evaluation of CRSD in some studies but, overall, there is insufficient evidence to recommend the routine use of Morningness-Eveningness Questionnaire for the clinical evaluation of CRSD. AASM practice parameter recommendation is *option* (patient care strategy that reflects uncertain clinical use) [31].

Circadian Phase Markers:

Core body temperature and onset of endogenous melatonin release under dim lighting conditions (Dim Light Melatonin Onset - DLMO) have been used as markers to identify circadian phase [4]. Circadian phase markers are useful to determine circadian phase and confirm the diagnosis of Free Running Disorder in sighted and unsighted patients but there is insufficient evidence to recommend their routine use in the diagnosis of other CRSD. AASM practice parameters' recommendation is *option* (patient care strategy that reflects uncertain clinical use) [31].

Delayed Sleep Phase Disorder (DSPD)

Delayed sleep phase disorder is characterized by a delay of the usual sleep period as much as 2 to 6 hours. The prevalence in the general population has been reported to be 0.17% [34]. Its prevalence in adolescents has been reported to be >7% [35]. Estimated prevalence rates for DSPD have ranged from 0.2 to 10% of the population [34-37]. It is possible that the wide variability in the prevalence estimates is due to using different severity criteria for delayed phase. Nevertheless, it is a condition typically seen in adolescents. There is a normal propensity for small delays of the sleep-wake schedule and circadian phase should during adolescence [38]. There are social-behavioral factors that aggravate the delay in adolescents [39]. Social and behavioral factors (evening social activities, staying late for homework, watching television, surfing the internet, playing videogames *etc.*) also favor the delaying of the sleep-wake schedule. DSPD may be an extreme form of this normal delay phenomenon observed in adolescence. DSPD has been associated with delayed endogenous circadian rhythms such as delayed sleep-timing, core body temperature and melatonin circadian rhythms [36, 40-46].

The cause of the circadian phase delay is unclear. Postulated mechanisms include: a) a longer than normal circadian period [47, 48], b) excessive sensitivity to evening light, which promotes the delay of the circadian clock or diminished sensitivity to morning light, which decreases the phase advancing properties of morning light [49], or c) genetic mutations in the circadian genes (seen in familial forms of DSP) [50-53].

Patients with delayed sleep phase disorder typically have difficulty falling asleep at the desired (conventional) sleep time until a few hours later. Due to the delay in their circadian rhythm, these individuals, when they attempt to sleep at the desired bedtime, are unable to fall asleep, as their circadian clock is in the "wake maintenance zone" at that time. Consequently, they have significant difficulty waking up at the conventional (desired) wake time. This is because they are trying to wake up around the most "sleepy" circadian time. These individuals typically present with complaints of sleep onset insomnia during the night and excessive daytime sleepiness because they have to wake up earlier than the desired time to meet work or social obligations, at least during the weekdays. Hence, their sleep duration is curtailed as they have a delay in their sleep onset. This leads to chronic sleep restriction and accumulation of sleep debt, thereby resulting in daytime sleepiness. The symptoms are typically noted during weekdays, when the patients have to conform to a desired sleep and wake time schedule due to school, social or work obligations. When they do not have any school or work obligations (weekends, vacation) and are left to sleep *ad libitum*, they demonstrate a normal sleep quality and duration. They typically fall asleep between 2-6 AM and wake up between 10 AM -1 PM. Some individuals have their social and work schedules delayed to conform to their delayed sleep wake schedule and they do not suffer any adverse impact from this disorder and they should not be diagnosed as having DSPD. Delayed sleep phase disorder should also be distinguished from the normal, asymptomatic "night owls" or "evening types".

Diagnosis

The diagnosis of a delayed sleep wake schedule is established from a sleep-wake diary of at least 1 or 2 weeks of recording. The diary typically shows a delayed sleep pattern and sleep initiation difficulty. Wrist actigraphy recordings that are used as surrogate markers for sleep and wakefulness are also helpful, if available. Polysomnography is *not* indicated in the routine assessment of DSPD [31, 54].

Treatment

Treatments of delayed sleep phase disorder are aimed at changing the circadian rhythm phase or timing. They are i) morning bright light exposure, ii) exogenous melatonin administration and iii) chronotherapy. The primary goal of therapy is to better align the sleep-wake cycle in relation to desired work and social schedules by advancing the timing of sleep-wake cycle. Occasionally, the same objective can be accomplished by progressively delaying the sleep-wake cycle. Since there is also a social and behavioral component aggravating the phase delay, these should also be addressed so as to optimize and sustain treatment benefits. Lifestyle considerations such as maintaining a regular sleep wake schedule, choosing to pursue any stimulating social or work activities in the morning instead of the evening, and trying to relax in the evening avoiding bright light [36]. We shall discuss here in more detail various strategies to alter the circadian rhythm phase.

Morning Bright Light Therapy

Morning bright light helps phase advance the circadian rhythm. Morning bright light therapy in combination with avoiding bright light in the evening has been shown to be an effective approach to achieve earlier sleep and wake times [43]. One approach would be to administer bright light of 2,000 to 2,500 lux for 1 to 2 hours between 6 and 8 AM [55]. At least one hour of phototherapy is recommended to begin with, following the late habitual rise time. This leads to a small phase advance of the circadian rhythm, so that patients start to fall asleep earlier and wake up earlier. Each successive sleep cycle is moved 30 minutes earlier every day, with the hour of phototherapy being linked to that progressively earlier scheduled wake time. Once the desired sleep-wake time is reached, then patients can be maintained on a shorter 30 minute bout of morning phototherapy. Patients are cautioned to avoid bright light exposure 2 hours prior to bedtime because light exposure at that time leads to phase delay of the circadian rhythm which can counteract the phase advance effects of morning light exposure [22]. In patients who exhibit an extreme delay in the timing of circadian rhythms, the time of light exposure should be given later in the morning in order to avoid exposure at a time that would actually further delay circadian rhythms [13].

Outdoor bright light is a very effective form of light therapy. During winter months when it is generally darker, artificial lights should be considered. Artificial light sources are commercially available. Artificial white light (broad-spectrum) is commonly used to shift the circadian rhythm phase. Wavelengths in the blue end of the visible spectrum (420-500 nm wave length) have been found to have a maximal effect on the circadian phase [18, 56, 57]. Targeted wave length light therapy for phase shifting is not used routinely, but holds promise for the future.

Adherence with bright light therapy may be limited by the inability of many patients to wake up early in the morning, and to schedule their social and professional activities around the light therapy regimen [58, 59]. Sleeping in, even after a late night should be avoided or at least minimized to prevent a relapse. Patients should continue morning bright light exposure and avoid wearing sunglasses in the morning, if possible [36].

The optimal timing, duration and dosing of morning light remain to be determined. Practice parameters of the AASM suggest morning light exposure in the treatment of DSPD (strength of recommendation: *guideline*, *i.e.*, patient care strategy that reflects a moderate degree of clinical certainty) [31].

Melatonin

Melatonin administration is also capable of shifting the circadian rhythm [60]. The phase response curve for melatonin administration shows that melatonin in the early evening leads to phase advances of the circadian rhythm - effect opposite to that of light therapy. Melatonin used in doses of 0.3 mg to 3 mg approximately 5 to 7 hours before sleep time for 4 weeks has been shown to be effective [13, 61]. Melatonin has also been evaluated in various studies on patients with DSPD [44, 62-65]. It is difficult to make comparisons due to the various dosing, time of administration and number of doses. Early evening melatonin has been shown to lead to phase advance [44, 61, 63]. It has also been shown to cause reduced sleepiness during daytime and improve sleep overall [66, 67]. Melatonin commercial production and marketing are largely unregulated and it is available over the counter as a nutritional supplement. Many of the melatonin products purchased from health stores in the US were found to contain unidentified impurities [68]. Melatonin is not approved by the Food and Drug Administration for the treatment of CRSD. The duration of treatment, dosage and time of administration remain yet to be determined. Long-term efficacy and safety of melatonin is still unclear. Adverse effects reported with melatonin administration include nausea, drowsiness, dizziness and headaches [69]. Melatonin in the evening in combination with morning bright light therapy produced an additive phase advance response compared to morning bright light therapy alone in a recent study, suggesting that this treatment strategy holds promise but further studies are awaited [70].

Practice parameters of the AASM suggest properly timed melatonin administration for the treatment of DSPD (strength of recommendation: *guideline* - patient care strategy that reflects a moderate degree of clinical certainty) [31].

Chronotherapy

Chronotherapy is a treatment strategy in which the bedtime and waketime is progressively delayed each day until the desired bedtime for the patient is reached [71]. The circadian rhythm in humans is usually slightly greater than 24 hours, hence there is a natural tendency in individuals for phase delaying relative to the 24-hour clock. Consequently, it should be easier to delay rather than advance the sleep wake cycle. A recommended regimen is 2-hour delays of the sleep period until the target bedtime and waketime are reached. Previously recommended 3-hour delays of bedtime can result, after a few days to inadvertent bright light exposure in the morning, in a counterproductive inhibition of the circadian phase delay [71]'[36].

Chronotherapy can take from 8 to 10 days to complete and it may not be practical and/or acceptable. Social and work activities have to be planned around the chronotherapy treatment schedule which can be challenging. Chronotherapy can be a treatment strategy in some individuals, especially those who have severe delayed sleep phase disorder. As an example, in individuals falling asleep between 4 - 6 AM, it may be a lot easier and quicker to delay the sleep wake cycle each day and reach the desired bedtime and wake time, rather than phase advance. Once the desired bedtime and waketime are reached, then it is necessary to maintain this sleep schedule (consolidation phase). Sleeping in and daytime napping should be strongly discouraged. It is also necessary to obtain bright light exposure in the morning and avoid bright lights in the evening (*i.e.*, encourage exposure to dim lights in the evening).

Practice parameters of the AASM suggest chronotherapy as an *option* (strength of recommendation - patient care strategy that reflects uncertain clinical use) for the treatment of DSPD [31].

What we don't know:

The etiology and mechanisms of causation of DSPD are still not clear. The discovery of various genetic mutations in circadian genes in familial DSPD have given us insight into some of the mechanisms of causation of DSPD but more research is clearly needed. We do not have definite clinical markers to separate the normal phase delay seen in adolescents from DSPD which is truly pathological. Research is also needed to determine the impact of social and behavioral factors in causing or aggravating DSPD. Research is also needed to determine the exact intensity, duration and timing of administration of bright light to advance the sleep phase. If the morning timing of light administration is incorrect, then light administration can paradoxially worsen the phase delay. Studies are needed to determine the efficacy of blue light regarding its phase shifting properties and to determine if it is superior to white light. More research is needed to determine the exact dose of melatonin, and timing of administration in the evening to derive the maximum phase shifting effect. Research is also needed to determine if melatonin receptor agonists have any role in phase shifting for treatment of DSPD. Research to determine the role of combination therapy with melatonin and bright light should be pursued. More studies are needed to evaluate the role and efficacy of chronotherapy.

Advanced Sleep Phase Disorder (ASPD)

Advanced sleep phase disorder (ASPD) is characterized by a sleep pattern that is several hours earlier than the desired time, *i.e.*, patients fall asleep earlier and wake up earlier. On a flip side, patients have a normal sleep quality and duration when they are allowed to choose their own (preferred) sleep schedule. There is no particular standard for how much earlier a sleep schedule should be to qualify as abnormal. If the sleep pattern causes impairment of social or occupational functioning, then it would be termed abnormal. ASPD patients typically complain that they cannot stay awake in the evening until the desired bedtime and fall asleep between 6 and 9 PM. They typically wake up in the early morning (2-5 AM), well in advance of the desired rising time [1]. They can present with either excessive sleepiness (evening), insomnia (early morning) or both. Advanced sleep phase is usually seen in middle-aged and older adults. About 1% of middle-aged adults have ASPD. ASPD is much less prevalent than DSPD [34, 72].

Possible mechanisms for the ASPD that are postulated include:

a) short circadian period of the pacemaker [73]

b) increased sensitivity of retina to morning light exposure [74]

c) circadian phase that appears resistant to delays from evening bright light [75]

d) mutations in the circadian genes [76, 77]

Familial Advanced Sleep Phase Disorder

Familial ASPD was identified in three kindreds of Northern European descent with autosomal dominant transmission. These individuals had markedly advanced sleep onset/offset, core body temperature troughs and endogenous melatonin rhythms. One of the individuals had a significant shortening of circadian period to 23.3 hours (normal period is slightly greater than 24 hours) [73]. Genetic analysis of the affected individuals showed a mis-sense mutation in a casein kinase (CK1c) binding region of a Period gene (hPer2) [76]. A separate mis-sense mutation, in a different casein kinase gene (CK1δ) was reported in a Japanese FASPD cohort [77].

Diagnosis

A careful clinical history is very important in identifying ASPD. A careful history is essential to rule out other disorders that present with sleep complaints such as depression and poor sleep hygiene measures (maintaining irregular sleep wake schedule, evening napping, etc).

Sleep diary and/or actigraphy recordings over 7 days can be helpful to demonstrate stable phase advance of the circadian rhythm. Polysomnography is not routinely indicated for the diagnosis of ASPD but may be useful to exclude other disorders if clinically suspected such as obstructive sleep apnea.

Treatment

There is a paucity of published literature regarding treatment of ASPD. Treatments such as bright light exposure (phototherapy), oral melatonin and chronotherapy have been considered.

Phototherapy

Bright light exposure in the evening causes a phase delay of the circadian clock. There are very few studies which evaluated bright light therapy in this condition and found it to be effective. In one study, bright light at 4,000 lux was administered at home for 2 hours, between 8 PM and 11 PM, for 12 consecutive nights. Significant phase delays were observed in the treatment group, with an average bedtime delay of about 30 minutes [78]. Another study used light of 2,500 lux for 4 hours between 8 PM and 1AM, for two nights [79].

Adherence to phototherapy can be challenging because adequate phototherapy requires proper light device use and placement of the lighting device with respect to patients [75]. Caution should be exercised when using phototherapy in individuals who are on photosensitizing drugs or those with retinal pathology [80]. Furthermore, various light boxes are commercially available (different spectra and light intensity, with probable different safety profiles).

Practice parameters of the AASM suggest timed light exposure for treatment of patients with ASPD as an option (strength of recommendation *option* - patient care strategy that reflects uncertain clinical use) [31].

Melatonin

Oral melatonin in the morning phase delays the circadian clock (effect opposite to that of light). Melatonin administration after awakening in the morning appears to be a physiologically plausible option for patients with ASPD but there are no systematic reports of its use [81]. Moreover, melatonin is a sleep promoting agent (soporific action). Use of hypnotics in the morning in patients who have ASPD, especially in elderly raises safety considerations and hence proper safety precautions should be followed with its use.

Other concerns with melatonin as a drug have been addressed earlier in this chapter (section on therapy for DSPD). Melatonin in total daily doses of 10 mg or less in healthy individuals appears to be safe for short term use, but low-dose melatonin of 0.5 mg may suffice for producing circadian phase shifts.

Practice parameters of the AASM suggest timed oral melatonin for treatment of patients with ASPD as an option (strength of recommendation *option* - patient care strategy that reflects uncertain clinical use) [31].

Chronotherapy

Chronotherapy is a treatment strategy by which the bedtime and wake time of patients is delayed or advanced for several hours each day until the desired times are reached. Once attained, then patients should try to maintain a regular sleep-wake schedule. There is a paucity of literature on the use of chronotherapy for ASPD. One case report of chronotherapy successfully advanced the sleep schedule by 3 hours every other day over a 2-week period [82].

Practice parameters of the AASM suggest prescribed sleep-wake scheduling for treatment of patients with ASPD as an option (strength of recommendation *option* - patient care strategy that reflects uncertain clinical use) [31].

Behavioral Modifications

Behavioral modifications are an integral part of treatment of ASPD. Patients should avoid early morning bright light exposure as it can advance their circadian phase (make them fall asleep and wake up earlier). There are also some studies that have suggested that evening naps can cause phase advance in individuals [83, 84]. Hence, evening naps should be avoided. This requires a major behavioral change in elderly individuals (most patients with ASPD), who are accustomed to taking morning walks and evening naps.

Patients should maintain a regular sleep wake schedule and should consider evening bright light exposure to maintain proper alignment of the circadian clock with the desired bedtime and wakeup time.

What we don't know:

We do not know how far advanced the sleep phase should be to label it as pathological and we do not have any clinical markers to differentiate this from the normal phase advance seen in elderly individuals. More research is needed to elucidate the etiology and mechanisms of causation of advanced sleep phase disorder including the role of the circadian genes. There are limited studies with light therapy for treatment of ASPD and more studies are warranted to determine the efficacy of light therapy, intensity and duration of light exposure, and role of blue light versus white light spectrum.

More studies are also needed to determine the role of chronotherapy as treatment. More studies are needed to determine the efficacy of melatonin for treatment including the dose, timing of administration in the morning and safety of administering a sedating agent in the morning. Studies to evaluate the efficacy of combination therapy (light, chronotherapy and melatonin) are also needed.

Free-Running Type

Free-running disorder (FRD) is also known as non-24-hour sleep-wake syndrome or hypernychthemeral syndrome. The sleep and wake times of patients with FRD vary because their circadian rhythm is not entrained in a stable way to the 24-hour day [13]. Daily light-dark cycle is the most powerful environmental synchronizing agent of the circadian pacemaker to the 24-hour day. When kept in an environment without time cues, human subjects typically have an endogenous circadian rhythm that is slightly longer than 24 hours (24.2) hours [14, 85]. When the circadian rhythm is allowed to run freely, the sleep period will drift later (delay) each day. This leads to progressively later bedtimes and wake up times each day. It is not surprising that most of the patients with FRD are blind, as they are unable to perceive light to synchronize their circadian clock. More than half of those with no light perception have non-entrained circadian rhythms, and many of those have FRD [86-88]. Exact prevalence of FRD is unknown, but is likely to afflict between one thirds and two thirds of the totally blind [89]. Rarely, FRD may also be seen in individuals with preserved vision [90, 91].

As discussed earlier in the chapter, the retinal ganglion cells (different from rods and cones) transmit light to the suprachiasmatic nucleus so that the endogenous circadian rhythm is entrained to the 24-hour light-dark cycle. Lack of light perception in blind individuals is the likely etiology of FRD [88]. Some blind individuals may still able to entrain the light to synchronize the circadian rhythm if they have an intact ganglion cell layer [92-94]. The other completely visually blind individuals who do not exhibit FRD are mostly entrained to the 24-hour social day (not the 24-hour light-dark cycle) through non-photic time cues such as strict scheduling of activities, exercise, mealtime and social interactions [89, 95-97]. The etiology of FRD in sighted individuals is less clear. In one case series of sighted individuals with FRD about 28% of the patients had psychiatric disorders [91]. Etiologies postulated in sighted individuals are either decreased exposure or responsiveness of the circadian clock to light or non photic entraining agents or longer endogenous circadian period that is outside the range of entrainment [13, 89, 98, 99].

Patients typically present with periods of excessive sleepiness, insomnia or both alternating with asymptomatic periods. Most individuals live on a 24 hour social day and attempt a regular sleep wake schedule. The gradual drifting ("free runs") of the circadian pacemaker leads to these symptoms when the circadian phase is out of synchrony with the social sleep episode[90]. There will be asymptomatic periods when the circadian pacemaker is in synchrony with the social sleep period. This happens when the continued circadian drift eventually leads to realignment with the desired social sleep episode.

Diagnosis is established by the clinical history that reveals a gradual delay in the sleep onset and wake every day. A sleep diary or actigraph recorded over ≥ 2 weeks should be able to confirm the free-running type. Circadian phase markers such as core body temperature trough or dim light melatonin onset may be useful to demonstrate the free-running circadian rhythm, but their clinical role is not well established.

Treatment

There are no large controlled trials for treating FRD. Treatment options are mostly based on case studies. Light exposure and melatonin administration have been tried in treating FRD.

Treatment in Sighted Individuals

- **Phototherapy**

There is a typical phase delay of circadian pacemaker each day in FRD. To counteract this delay, the strategy to advance the circadian pacemaker by morning light exposure has been tried [100-102].

Practice parameters of the AASM suggest circadian phase shifting by timed light exposure for treatment in sighted individuals with FRD as an option (strength of recommendation *option* -patient care strategy that reflects uncertain clinical use) [31].

- **Melatonin**

Timed oral melatonin can cause a shift of the phase of the circadian pacemaker and the effects are opposite to that of timed light exposure. Early evening melatonin administration causes a phase advance and this strategy is employed to counteract the phase delays of FRD.

There are reports in which sighted FRD patients were treated with melatonin at bedtime (most common dose used was 3 mg), with successful phase advance [65, 103-105].

Practice parameters of the AASM suggest circadian phase shifting by timed oral melatonin for treatment in sighted individuals with FRD as an option (strength of recommendation *option* -patient care strategy that reflects uncertain clinical use) [31].

Treatment in Blind Individuals

Melatonin offers promise in blind individuals with FRD as there are studies that have successfully entrained free-running rhythms with varying doses, timing and duration. Studies have tried melatonin at 10 mg or 5 mg doses, but there are studies that have shown that circadian phase shifts can be accomplished by lower doses of 0.5 mg [106-114]. Melatonin not only entrains the circadian rhythm, but also has soporific properties.

Practice parameters of the AASM suggest timed melatonin administration for the treatment of FRD in blind individuals (strength of recommendation *guideline* - patient care strategy that reflects a moderate degree of clinical certainty) [31].

What we don't know:

More studies are needed to determine the exact dose, timing and duration of treatment of melatonin in blind individuals with FRD. Large controlled trials for treatment of FRD in sighted individuals are required but may be difficult to accomplish due to the rarity of this condition. More research is needed to evaluate the efficacy of phototherapy in blind and sighted individuals with FRD. Research is also needed to evaluate the role of hypnotics and wake promoting agents to treat insomnia and excessive sleepiness respectively in blind and sighted individuals with FRD.

Irregular Sleep Wake Rhythm Disorder

Irregular sleep wake rhythm disorder is also known as no circadian rhythm, grossly disturbed sleep wake rhythm, low amplitude circadian rhythm or chaotic sleep-wake rhythm. These alternative names accurately describe the sleep abnormality noted in this condition. Irregular sleep wake rhythm disorder (ISWRD) is characterized by the lack of a clearly defined circadian rhythm of sleep and wake. The sleep wake pattern is disorganized temporally and the sleep-wake periods are variable throughout the 24-hour period. Individuals have multiple irregular sleep bouts (at least three) during a 24-hour period, but the total sleep time per 24 -hour period is essentially normal for age [1]. Nighttime sleep is very fragmented and multiple naps are noted during the daytime. Typically, the longest sleep episode occurs between 2 and 6 AM [115, 116]. Patients usually present with insomnia during the night and excessive sleepiness during the day.

The prevalence of ISWRD increases with age. Age itself is not an independent risk factor, but the age-related increased frequency of medical, neurological and psychiatric conditions greatly contribute to the development of ISWRD. It is commonly seen in institutionalized older individuals, particularly in those with Alzheimer's disease [117]. Central nervous system disorders such as traumatic brain injury and mental retardation have also been associated with ISWRD [115, 118, 119].

Dysfunction of the central processes responsible for circadian rhythm generation and decreased exposure to external synchronizing agents such as light and social activities have been postulated to play a role in the development and maintenance of ISWRD [116]. Studies have demonstrated age-related loss of neurons and functional changes in SCN and decrease in neurons within SCN in patients with Alzheimer's disease [120-122]. Neurodegeneration of the SCN (circadian pacemaker) is thought to be responsible for development of ISWRD in older individuals. In addition, older individuals with multiple co-morbid neurological and medical conditions have less exposure to daytime light [123]. Reduced exposure to external synchronizing agents, such as light and social activity is most pronounced in patients with Alzheimer's disease residing in long-term care facilities. Other factors that can lead to impaired nocturnal sleep and daytime sleepiness in these individuals and which need to be taken into consideration in the differential diagnosis are medication effects.

Diagnosis

Sleep logs and actigraphy monitoring for at least 7 days show multiple irregular sleep bouts (at least three) during a 24 hour period, but the total sleep time per 24 hour period is essentially normal for age [1]. Actigraphy may be very useful in individuals who have severe cognitive impairment and cannot complete a sleep log.

Treatment

Treatment goals are to consolidate sleep during the night and wakefulness during the day. Measures aimed at enhancing exposure to the various SCN time cues are also very important [116].

Light Therapy

Patients should be exposed to bright light during the day. They should avoid bright light during the evening and night [116, 124, 125]. In demented patients, morning bright light exposure at 3,000 to 5,000 lux for 2 hours over 4 weeks has led to decreased daytime napping and increased nighttime sleep [126]. Light may decrease agitated behavior and lead to stronger circadian rhythm amplitudes [124-126].

Practice parameters of the AASM suggest daytime bright light exposure for treatment of nursing home residents with dementia and ISWRD as an option (strength of recommendation *option* -patient care strategy that reflects uncertain clinical use) [31].

Melatonin

Studies evaluating melatonin use in ISWRD showed less consistent results. However, small studies revealed some success in using melatonin to treat sleep disturbances in children who have psychomotor retardation and ISWRD [127].

Practice parameters of the AASM suggest that melatonin is not indicated for treatment of ISWRD in older people with dementia and suggest that it may be indicated for children with ISWR and severe psychomotor retardation as an option (strength of recommendation *option* - patient care strategy that reflects uncertain clinical use) [31].

Mixed Modality Therapy

Daytime structured physical and social activities should be encouraged in individuals with ISWRD [128-130]. Use of a multimodal approach including an increase in sunlight exposure and social activity in the day and a decrease in daytime naps and night time noise may be effective [116].

Practice parameters of the AASM suggest mixed modality approaches combining bright light exposure, physical activity, and other behavioral elements in treatment of ISWRD among elderly people with dementia, including nursing home residents with a strength of recommendation *guideline* -patient care strategy that reflects a moderate degree of clinical certainty [31].

What we don't know:

More research is needed in the use of light therapy (timing, intensity and duration) for patients with ISWRD. More research evaluating the use of melatonin in adults and children with ISWRD is needed particularly the dose, timing, duration and safety of melatonin use. Role of melatonin receptor agonists have to be evaluated also. The efficacy of structuring the sleep/wake schedule and activities in these individuals also need further studies. Use of stimulants and hypnotics in these individuals warrant further studies. More research is awaited in evaluating whether using a combination of treatments is more effective than a single treatment modality.

Shift Work Disorder (SWD)

Shift Work Disorder (SWD) is seen in individuals who have misalignment of their endogenous circadian clock with their work schedule. The ICSD-2 diagnostic criteria for SWD state that there is a complaint of insomnia or excessive sleepiness associated with the shift work schedule over the course of at least one month. Sleep logs or actigraphy monitoring for at least 7 days should demonstrate disturbed circadian and sleep-time misalignment [1]. Even though there are a lot of shift workers in the general population, the current definition of SWD requires further validation and the literature specific to SWD is still sparse.

Overall, there is a paucity of epidemiologic data for SWD. As per the US department of labor, bureau of labor statistics (www.bls.gov), there are 22 million shift workers in the US. Of these, there are 3.8 million who work regular night shifts and 3.3 million more who work rotating night shifts [131]. About 20% of the workforce in industrialized countries are shift workers and 40 to 80% of night workers complain of sleep difficulties, but the actual prevalence of clinically significant cases is still unclear [115]. Telephone survey data suggest that approximately a third of shift workers report symptoms suggestive of SWD fulfilling the minimum diagnostic criteria [26]. Since approximately 6% of all US workers are night or rotating shift workers, the overall prevalence of SWD in the general population is approximately 1%, which is probably an underestimate [26]. In a recent study, SWD was reported in 2% of 4,471 US police officers [132]. The difference in the prevalence rates is probably due to non-standardized criteria of SWD used.

Risk Factors

Vulnerability to SWD is dependent on shift type and pattern, age, circadian preference, and susceptibility to sleep disturbance [133]. Night shift workers are more susceptible to SWD than rotating-shift workers (32.1% of night shift workers met the minimum diagnostic criteria for SWD compared to 26.1% of rotating-shift workers) [26]. Since it is easy to delay the sleep time rather than advance it, early morning shift workers are more susceptible to SWD than evening shift workers [134]. Timing of shifts and shift schedule changes have been shown to significantly affect sleep, with rotating shift workers demonstrating the greatest sleep quality impairments. Workers on rotating shifts experienced significantly more difficulty sleeping, with higher proportion demonstrating increased sleep latency, higher number of night time awakenings, excessive sleepiness, higher work absence and work-related accidents than those on fixed daytime or nighttime shifts [134]. Clockwise versus counter-clockwise shift rotations also play a role in adjusting to shift work.Since it is easy to delay sleep rather than advance it, clockwise shift rotations are more beneficial to workers than counterclockwise rotations [135]. Clockwise (forward rotating) shift schedule was found to be particularly beneficial to older workers who showed larger improvements in excessive sleepiness compared with their younger counterparts [136].

Advancing age is a risk factor for shift work intolerance on the basis of the current literature [80, 137-141]. Although older shift workers (ages 53 - 59 years) appear to adapt better to acute sleep deprivation initially compared to younger workers (ages 19 - 29 years), they show a reduced capacity of circadian adaptation when exposed to consecutive night shifts and are more sleepy than younger workers [140].

Lifestyle factors and choices can cause or contribute to excessive sleepiness and insomnia in shift workers. There are represented by: presence of other people at home (who may disrupt the attempted sleep), social obligations during the normal waking day that require the worker to be awake instead of resting, deliberately staying awake in-between transition between shift patterns, and workers attempting to sleep at conventional times during weekends and off days [133]. These sleep hygiene issues need to be carefully addressed in shift workers in order to better control their symptoms.

There is no intrinsic abnormality in the circadian clock in shift workers, but the mismatch is due to their work schedule. They are trying to be awake while working at a time when their circadian clock is trying to promote sleep and they are trying to fall asleep when their circadian clock is maximally alert. Insomnia and excessive sleepiness are the characteristic symptoms of SWD and can lead to fatigue, difficulty concentrating, headache, irritability or depressed mood and diminished work performance [142, 143].

There is usually a shortening of sleep by 1 to 4 hours in night shift workers compared to daytime workers [144-146]. This leads to chronic partial sleep deprivation impairing social and cognitive function, and pathological sleepiness can also lead to safety and health hazards [13]. Although there is no evidence that shift work directly affects longevity, shift work has adverse health effects, even in the absence of SWD [147, 148].

There are various co-morbidities associated with shift work. Shift workers have higher rates of peptic ulcers and gastrointestinal problems such as constipation and diarrhea compared to day workers [26, 149, 150]. Nighttime shift work can be associated with significant metabolic disturbances. *i.e.*, metabolic syndrome, obesity, elevated cholesterol and raised triglyceride levels [151]. Probable explanations for the metabolic disturbances and gastrointestinal symptoms in SWD may be due to sleep deprivation, eating at unusual times of the day leading to gastric secretions at unconventional times, consumption of caffeine and alcohol used as coping strategies by many shift workers [131, 152].

Shift workers compared with daytime workers have an increased risk of developing cardiovascular disease [26, 153]. Multiple mechanisms are posited for the shift work-related cardiovascular morbidity such as changes in hormones, autonomic and sympathetic cardiac control, metabolic rates and chronotropic heart function while working at night along with increased rate of smoking and more frequent rates of obesity in this population [151, 153, 154].

Occupations typically associated with night shift work such as health care workers, firefighters, and law enforcement have been associated with increased rates of breast, prostate and colorectal cancer [155-159]. Women shift workers are more likely than day workers to experience irregular menses, reduced fertility and pregnancy-related problems [160-162]. Also, increased rates of depression have been observed in shift workers, especially in women [26, 163].

Shift workers are more likely to have work-related accidents [134, 164, 165]. Workers commuting home after night shifts report more accidents than day workers [166-168]. There are very few studies published regarding SWD and the rate of accidents. The sheer number of shift workers in the general population suggests that this can be an issue of great public importance when the actual impact of SWD becomes well defined.

Diagnosis

Diagnosis is established when the complaints of excessive sleepiness or insomnia occur in relation to the work schedule and other causes of excessive sleepiness (such as OSA) and insomnia (such as depression-associated insomnia) have been excluded. Sleep logs or actigraphy monitoring for at least 7 days should demonstrate disturbed circadian and sleep-time misalignment [1]. Polysomnography may be indicated to rule out other sleep disorders, if clinical suspicion exists.

TREATMENT

Treatment of SWD Involves a Multimodal Approach

General Measures

Individuals should evaluate if they can make changes to the shift work patterns. They should consider avoiding working more than 4 consecutive 12-hour night shifts. They also should consider avoiding shifts longer than 12 hours [169]. Rotating shift workers should be encouraged to rotate their shifts in a clockwise rather than counter-clockwise direction. Shift workers should also follow proper sleep hygiene measures. They should try to create the proper conditions for sleep if they attempt to sleep during the daytime - dark bedroom by using window curtains and/or blinds, ensure a comfortable temperature in the bedroom, reduce noise exposure, and avoid large meals, caffeine, alcohol or smoking before the sleep period [170]. Whenever possible, they should avoid performing activities perceived as social obligations during the normal wake day which limit resting periods, deliberately staying awake in between transition between shift patterns, and attempting to sleep at conventional times during weekends and off days.

Shift workers should also take adequate precautions to reduce the risk of motor vehicle accidents during the commute home after the shift work. They should consider using public transportation or taxi service, consider taking a nap before driving home, and, if driving, to pull over and take a nap if they become sleepy and try to minimize the commute time by staying close to the work place, if feasible [170].

Planned (Scheduled) Naps

Several studies have shown that napping increases alertness, vigilance, improves reaction times and decreases accidents during night shift work [171-175]. The optimal timing (pre-shift versus on-shift) and duration of naps have yet to be defined. Short naps of less than an hour appear to improve alertness in night shift workers [172]. In another study, a longer nap during the night shift (120 minutes versus 60 minutes) was better in sustaining cognitive performance [176]. Napping before a night shift in combination with caffeine has also been shown to improve performance [171]. There are some practical difficulties in taking naps in the workplace, as there may not be adequate napping space and "napping during work" may be considered conflicting with optimal productivity.

Practice parameters of the AASM suggest planned napping before or during the night shift to improve alertness and performance among night shift workers (strength of recommendation-*standard* - patient care strategy that reflects a high degree of clinical certainty) [31].

Timed Light Exposure

Studies have shown that light therapy can be used to entrain the circadian pacemaker to adapt to night shift work. The optimal dose and duration of bright light exposure has yet to be determined. Studies have utilized light of different intensities (2,350 to 12,000 lux) administered in various schedules (20 minutes during breaks, four 20-minute periods throughout the night shift, 30-minute exposures, at least 50% of the shift, etc with or without restriction of daytime light exposure using goggles). Subjective improvements in work performance, alertness and mood have been shown with timed light exposure compared to ordinary light exposure [177-182].

Practice parameters of the AASM suggest timed light exposure in the work environment and light restriction in the morning, when feasible to decrease sleepiness and improve alertness during night shift work (strength of recommendation *guideline* - patient care strategy that reflects a moderate degree of clinical certainty) [31].

Wakefulness Promoting Agents

FDA has approved Modafinil and Armodafinil (the R-enantiomer of modafinil) for treatment of excessive sleepiness associated with SWD. Modafinil significantly improved wakefulness along with attention, quality of life and self reports of functioning. Additionally, fewer subjects on modafinil reported accidents or near-misses during the commute home compared to placebo [30, 183]. Armodafinil also improved wakefulness, significantly reduced excessive sleepiness at work and during the drive home and did not adversely affect daytime sleep in individuals with SWD [184, 185]. Modafinil in doses of 200 mg to 300 mg or Armodafinil 150mg were used in these studies 30-60 minutes before the start of the work shift for 12 weeks. Headache and nausea were the most common adverse effects with modafinil and armodafinil.

Practice parameters of the AASM suggest modafinil to enhance alertness during the night shift for SWD (strength of recommendation guideline - patient care strategy that reflects a moderate degree of clinical certainty) [31].

Caffeine has also been tried to promote wakefulness during the night shift [186-188]. Appropriate dose and timing of caffeine use have not yet been determined. Tolerance can develop to caffeine with repeated use [189].

Practice parameters of the AASM suggest caffeine to enhance alertness during the night shift for SWD (strength of recommendation: *option* - patient care strategy that reflects uncertain clinical use) [31].

Sleep Promoting Agents (for Help with Daytime Sleep)

Melatonin in doses of 0.5 to 10mg prior to daytime sleep has been evaluated in some studies, with subsequent improvement in daytime sleep quality and duration and also a shift in circadian phase in some subjects. Melatonin failed to enhance alertness during the night [190-195]. The same limitations and caveats of using melatonin as a pharmacologic agent described earlier in this chapter applies.

Practice parameters of the AASM suggest melatonin administration prior to daytime sleep is indicated to promote daytime sleep among night shift workers (strength of recommendation guideline - patient care strategy that reflects a moderate degree of clinical certainty) [31].

Hypnotic medications (triazolam, temazepam, zopiclone, zolpidem) to promote daytime sleep have generally demonstrated improvements in the quality and duration of daytime sleep compared to controls. Effects on nighttime alertness measures were not consistent [196-200]. Only zopiclone has been evaluated among shift workers and the rest of the agents have been evaluated in simulated shift work conditions [200]. Caution should be exercised as there is a possibility of carry-over of sedative effect to the nighttime shift with potential adverse consequences for nighttime safety and work performance. There is also a concern that sedatives may worsen sleep related breathing disorders if co-existent with SWD.

Practice parameters of the AASM suggest hypnotic medications to promote daytime sleep among night shift workers (strength of recommendation *guideline* -patient care strategy that reflects a moderate degree of clinical certainty) [31].

What we don't know:

Research studies need to diagnose subjects according to ICSD-2 diagnostic criteria to test the reliability and validity of these criteria and for comparing treatment results. More research is indicated to evaluate why some individuals are"phase tolerant" and are able to tolerate night shift work better than others. Studies need to elucidate what is normal versus pathologic response to night shift work. Larger controlled studies are necessary to determine the efficacy of naps, their timing in relation to night shift, and duration of naps. Larger controlled studies are needed to determine the efficacy of light, duration and intensity of light exposure during night shift. More research is needed to evaluate the effectiveness of melatonin (and melatonin agonists) to promote daytime sleep, dosage, timing and effect on nighttime alertness. Role of other sedative hypnotics to promote daytime sleep awaits further studies. Modafinil and armodafinil have received FDA approval to improve nighttime alertness but more studies are required to evaluate the role of caffeine to promote nighttime alertness.

Jet Lag

Jet lag is characterized by a temporary mismatch between the sleep wake cycle of the endogenous circadian pacemaker and that of the sleep and wake pattern required by a change in time zone. When the time zones are crossed too rapidly, the circadian clock cannot keep pace, leading to mismatch between the local time and circadian clock. The symptoms are mainly due to the circadian misalignment, but also due to sleep loss. The ICSD-2 defines jet lag disorder as complaints of insomnia and/or excessive daytime sleepiness associated with trans meridian jet travel across at least two time zones, with associated impairment of daytime function, general malaise or somatic symptoms such as gastrointestinal disturbance within one to two days after travel [1].

Jet lag is temporary. Symptoms begin approximately one to two days after air travel. The symptoms are mainly insomnia and daytime sleepiness, but dysphoric mood, cognitive impairment, diminished physical performance and gastrointestinal disturbances have been described. Symptoms of jet lag continue until there is realignment of the circadian system. It is estimated that it takes about one day per time zone travelled for circadian rhythms to adjust to the local time [1]. There are estimates that there is an average resetting of the circadian clock of 92 minutes later each day after westward flight and 57 minutes earlier each day after an eastward flight [201, 202]. Symptoms of jet lag can also be aggravated by non-specific travel fatigue which is a sequel of prolonged immobility in airplane seats, intravascular volume depletion, irregular meal times, irregular sleep leading to sleep deprivation, and other factors linked to long distance travel. Travel fatigue can be reversed within one to two days with adequate diet, volume repletion, rest and sleep [27, 203]. Jet lag is usually self-limited and medically benign, but it may occasionally cause serious misjudgments in business or professional dealings [27].

The incidence of jet lag is unknown but presumably affects a large number of people given the large population of long-distance air travelers. The duration and intensity of jet lag is dependent on multiple factors.: 1) The number of time zones crossed - the larger the number of time zones crossed, the higher the degree of circadian misalignment and more severe the symptoms; 2) The direction of air travel - it is more difficult to travel east than west because it is more difficult to advance the circadian clock versus to delay the circadian clock, as the endogenous period of the circadian clock is longer than 24 hours. Hence, westward travel is more tolerable ("East is a beast, west is best"); 3) Availability of local time cues - most importantly exposure to natural light at the destination facilitates re-entrainment of circadian clock. This depends on the location, time of the year and activity of the traveler; 4) Ability to tolerate circadian misalignment - some individuals are better than others in tolerating phase misalignments. This ability appears to decrease with increasing age [27].

Diagnosis

Diagnosis of jet lag is made on subjective complaints in the context of air travel crossing multiple time zones.

Treatment of Jet Lag

Treatment of jet lag entails resetting of the circadian clock. This can be accomplished by multiple approaches.

Strategic Sleep Scheduling

In case of short duration trips (two days or less), one strategy to minimize jet lag symptoms is to try to maintain home-based sleep hours after arrival at the new destination [204]. In some cases this strategy is not always practical, as it may interfere with desired social or business activities at the destination.

Practice parameters of the AASM suggest that when time at destination is expected to be brief, keeping home-based sleep hours, rather than adopting destination sleep hours, may reduce sleepiness and jet lag symptoms (strength of recommendation *option* - patient care strategy that reflects uncertain clinical use) [31].

Another strategy to minimize jet lag is to try before departure to shift one's sleep schedule by 1 or 2 hours (advance or delay), so that it is in congruence with the destination time zone [27]. In a simulation study, subjects were phase shifted in anticipation of eastward travel with combination of shifting their sleep schedule and bright light exposure to reduce jet leg symptoms [205].

Practice parameters of the AASM suggest the combination of morning exposure to bright light and shifting the sleep schedule one hour earlier each day for three days prior to eastward travel may lessen jet lag symptoms (strength of recommendation *option* - patient care strategy that reflects uncertain clinical use) [31].

Light Exposure

As discussed earlier in this chapter, light is the most important time cue for synchronization of the circadian pacemaker. Exposure to light in the evening shifts the clock to a later time (delays phase) and exposure to light in the morning shifts the clock to an earlier time (advances phase). Travelers can accelerate re-entrainment of the circadian clock by exposure to bright light at the appropriate time. In case of travel up to eight time zones, it is recommended to seek bright light exposure in the morning after eastward travel and evening after westward travel [27].

Travel crossing eight or more time zones presents a different set of circumstances that changes recommendations for light exposure. After eight or more time zones have been crossed, sunlight that would ordinarily be interpreted by the circadian clock as "dawn" may now be interpreted as "dusk" and the other way around. In such situations exposure to light may impede the circadian alignment instead of facilitating it. In such situations avoiding light exposure may be beneficial. Staying indoors for the first few hours of daylight after long eastward travel or for a few hours before dusk after long westward flights may be considered [27, 203, 206, 207]. After few days, such avoidance of light is no longer necessary, as the circadian clock will have shifted substantially. All flights that cross more than 8 to 10 time zones are to be treated as if they were westward according to some experts [203].

Melatonin

Melatonin has its effect on circadian clock resetting but it also works as a hypnotic at higher doses. Melatonin in the evening advances the circadian phase but there is a circadian phase delay when it is given in the morning and hence, the rationale for its use in the treatment of jet lag [208].

Melatonin use is studied extensively for jet lag. Majority of the studies showed significant benefit of melatonin in treatment of jet lag symptoms and improve sleep. Melatonin was administered at bedtime after an eastward flight in most studies [209-215]. Melatonin at bedtime may not be optimal for westward flights since melatonin has the least phase shifting effect when there is overlap with endogenous melatonin secretion [208, 216]. A low, short-acting dose (0.5 mg or less) taken later in the night (second half) is preferable in such circumstances [27].

Doses of melatonin ranged from 0.5 mg to 10 mg have been administered at bedtime but the most common dose used in randomized trials was 5 mg [31]. The efficacy of smaller dose (0.5 mg) of melatonin may be similar to larger doses in relation to phase shifting capabilities [214]. Melatonin is not regulated by the FDA and it is marketed as a nutritional supplement in a 3 mg formulation in the US. Melatonin has been administered up to 3 days prior to departure at a time coinciding with bedtime at the destination. It is not clear at present if treatment with melatonin prior to departure is superior to starting melatonin after reaching the destination [27, 210, 212, 213]. Melatonin has been used up to 5 days upon arrival at the destination [31].

Practice parameters of the AASM suggest melatonin administration at the appropriate time to reduce symptoms of jet lag and improve sleep following travel across multiple time zones (strength of recommendation - *standard* - patient care strategy that reflects a high degree of clinical certainty) [31]. The same caveats and limitations of using melatonin as a pharmacologic agent applies as described earlier in this chapter.

Hypnotics

Hypnotic agents (benzodiazepines and non-benzodiazepenes) have been studied and have been shown to reduce jet lag-induced insomnia [217-226]. Hypnotics are mostly effective in treating the insomnia associated with jet lag, but the benefit for relief of daytime symptoms is unproven [31]. Adverse effects such as confusion, amnesia, etc should be anticipated and adequate precautions followed.

Practice parameters of the AASM suggest short term use of a benzodiazepine receptor agonist hypnotic is indicated for treatment of jet lag-induced insomnia considering potential adverse effects (strength of recommendation *option* - patient care strategy that reflects uncertain clinical use) [31].

Wakefulness Promoting Agents

Caffeine may be used to counteract jet lag-induced sleepiness. Slow-release caffeine 300 mg daily resulted in less daytime sleepiness, but subjects also reported longer sleep onset and more nighttime awakenings [227].

Practice parameters of the AASM suggest caffeine as a way to counteract jet lag induced sleepiness keeping in mind the possibility of nighttime sleep disruption (strength of recommendation *option* - patient care strategy that reflects uncertain clinical use) [31].

There is a paucity of the literature regarding other wakefulness promoting agents being used for jet lag.

What we don't know:

The natural course of jet lag disorder and the exact mechanism by which various factors entrain the circadian clock at the destination remains to be elucidated. The effectiveness of light therapy for JLD has to be established by randomized controlled trials. We do not know the optimal dose of exogenous melatonin and the exact timing of melatonin administration to optimally influence the circadian reentrainment. This is especially relevant for westward travel where in nighttime administration of melatonin would probably not be appropriate as there is already peak endogenous melatonin production. The role for melatonin receptor agonists is not defined yet and trials are warranted to ascertain whether the melatonin receptor agonists have the same efficacy as exogenous melatonin in relation to circadian phase shifting. Studies need to evaluate if other factors such as diet or exercise help to mitigate the symptoms of jet lag disorder.

CONCLUSIONS

Circadian rhythm sleep disorders (CRSD) are those disorders that present with insomnia or excessive sleepiness or both. They can be due to abnormalities in the endogenous circadian clock ("intrinsic disorders") such as delayed sleep phase type, advanced sleep phase type, free running type, and irregular sleep wake rhythm type. Shift work or air travel lead to an artificial mismatch between the endogenous circadian clock and the external environment ("extrinsic disorders") leading to shift work disorder and jet lag disorder.

There disorders are under recognized in the general population but they can affect a significant number of people given the large number of shift workers and air travelers. The symptoms may be misdiagnosed for other common sleep disorders such as sleep apnea or insomnia. Meticulous history and sleep diary data are major tools in diagnosing CRSD. In the past two decades major advances are being made in understanding the genetic basis of these disorders. Understanding the pathophysiologic basis of these disorders has led to various therapeutic options such as phototherapy and exogenous melatonin.

REFERENCES

[1]   American Academy of Sleep Medicine. International classification of sleep disorders 2nd ed.:Diagnostic and coding manual. Westchester: Illinois 2005.
[2]   Czeisler CA, Klerman EB. Circadian and sleep-dependent regulation of hormone release in humans. Recent Prog Horm Res 1999; 54: 97-130; discussion 130-2.
[3]   Klerman EB. Clinical aspects of human circadian rhythms. J Biol Rhythms 2005; 20: 375-86.
[4]   Lewy AJ, Sack RL. The dim light melatonin onset as a marker for circadian phase position. Chronobiol Int 1989; 6: 93-102.
[5]   Borbely AA. A two process model of sleep regulation. Hum Neurobiol 1982; 1: 195-204.
[6]   Stepanski EJ, Wyatt JK. Use of sleep hygiene in the treatment of insomnia. Sleep Med Rev 2003; 7: 215-25.
[7]   Wyatt JK, Cajochen C, Ritz-De Cecco A *et al.* Low-dose repeated caffeine administration for circadian-phase-dependent performance degradation during extended wakefulness. Sleep 2004; 27: 374-81.
[8]   Strogatz SH, Kronauer RE, Czeisler CA. Circadian pacemaker interferes with sleep onset at specific times each day: role in insomnia. Am J Physiol 1987; 253: R172-8.
[9]   Lavie P. Ultrashort sleep-waking schedule. III. 'Gates' and 'forbidden zones' for sleep. Electroencephalogr Clin Neurophysiol 1986; 63: 414-25.
[10]   Moore RY, Eichler VB. Loss of a circadian adrenal corticosterone rhythm following suprachiasmatic lesions in the rat. Brain Res 1972; 42: 201-6.
[11]   Dunlap JC. Molecular bases for circadian clocks. Cell 1999; 96: 271-90.
[12]   Harmer SL, Panda S, Kay SA. Molecular bases of circadian rhythms. Annu Rev Cell Dev Biol 2001; 17: 215-53.

[13]   Lu BS, Zee PC. Circadian rhythm sleep disorders. Chest 2006; 130: 1915-23.

[14]   Czeisler CA, Duffy JF, Shanahan TL *et al.* Stability, precision, and near-24-hour period of the human circadian pacemaker. Science 1999; 284: 2177-81.

[15]   Moore RY. A clock for the ages. Science 1999; 284: 2102-3.

[16]   Czeisler CA, Allan JS, Strogatz SH *et al.* Bright light resets the human circadian pacemaker independent of the timing of the sleep-wake cycle. Science 1986; 233: 667-71.

[17]   Berson DM, Dunn FA, Takao M. Phototransduction by retinal ganglion cells that set the circadian clock. Science 2002; 295: 1070-3.

[18]   Brainard GC, Hanifin JP, Greeson JM *et al.* Action spectrum for melatonin regulation in humans: evidence for a novel circadian photoreceptor. J Neurosci 2001; 21: 6405-12.

[19]   Thapan K, Arendt J, Skene DJ. An action spectrum for melatonin suppression: evidence for a novel non-rod, non-cone photoreceptor system in humans. J Physiol 2001; 535: 261-7.

[20]   Moore RY, Lenn NJ. A retinohypothalamic projection in the rat. J Comp Neurol 1972; 146: 1-14.

[21]   Stephan FK, Zucker I. Circadian rhythms in drinking behavior and locomotor activity of rats are eliminated by hypothalamic lesions. Proc Natl Acad Sci U S A 1972; 69: 1583-6.

[22]   Cvengros JA WJ. Circadian Rhythm Disorders. Sleep Med Clin 2009; 4: 495-505.

[23]   Ebadi M, Govitrapong P. Neural pathways and neurotransmitters affecting melatonin synthesis. J Neural Transm Suppl 1986; 21: 125-55.

[24]   Reppert SM, Perlow MJ, Ungerleider LG *et al.* Effects of damage to the suprachiasmatic area of the anterior hypothalamus on the daily melatonin and cortisol rhythms in the rhesus monkey. J Neurosci 1981; 1: 1414-25.

[25]   Lewy AJ, Ahmed S, Jackson JM, Sack RL. Melatonin shifts human circadian rhythms according to a phase-response curve. Chronobiol Int 1992; 9: 380-92.

[26]   Drake CL, Roehrs T, Richardson G *et al.* Shift work sleep disorder: prevalence and consequences beyond that of symptomatic day workers. Sleep 2004; 27: 1453-62.

[27]   Sack RL. Clinical practice. Jet lag. N Engl J Med 2010; 362: 440-7.

[28]   Kamei Y, Urata J, Uchiyaya M *et al.* Clinical characteristics of circadian rhythm sleep disorders. Psychiatry Clin Neurosci 1998; 52: 234-5.

[29]   Dagan Y, Eisenstein M. Circadian rhythm sleep disorders: toward a more precise definition and diagnosis. Chronobiol Int 1999; 16: 213-22.

[30]   Czeisler CA, Walsh JK, Roth T *et al.* Modafinil for excessive sleepiness associated with shift-work sleep disorder. N Engl J Med 2005; 353: 476-86.

[31]   Morgenthaler TI, Lee-Chiong T, Alessi C *et al.* Practice parameters for the clinical evaluation and treatment of circadian rhythm sleep disorders. An American Academy of Sleep Medicine report. Sleep 2007; 30: 1445-59.

[32]   Kushida CA, Littner MR, Morgenthaler T *et al.* Practice parameters for the indications for polysomnography and related procedures: an update for 2005. Sleep 2005; 28: 499-521.

[33]   Horne JA, Ostberg O. A self-assessment questionnaire to determine morningness-eveningness in human circadian rhythms. Int J Chronobiol 1976; 4: 97-110.

[34]   Schrader H, Bovim G, Sand T. The prevalence of delayed and advanced sleep phase syndromes. J Sleep Res 1993; 2: 51-55.

[35]   Pelayo R TM, Govinski P. Prevalence of delayed sleep phase syndrome among adolescents (abstract). Sleep Res 1988; 17: 392.

[36]   Lack LC WH, Bootzin RR. Delayed Sleep-Phase Disorder. Sleep Med Clin 2009; 4: 229-239.

[37]   Lack LC. Delayed sleep and sleep loss in university students. J Am Coll Health 1986; 35: 105-10.

[38]   Carskadon MA, Wolfson AR, Acebo C *et al.* Adolescent sleep patterns, circadian timing, and sleepiness at a transition to early school days. Sleep 1998; 21: 871-81.

[39]   Hansen M, Janssen I, Schiff A *et al.* The impact of school daily schedule on adolescent sleep. Pediatrics 2005; 115: 1555-61.

[40]   Oren DA, Turner EH, Wehr TA. Abnormal circadian rhythms of plasma melatonin and body temperature in the delayed sleep phase syndrome. J Neurol Neurosurg Psychiatry 1995; 58: 379.

[41]   Shibui K, Uchiyama M, Okawa M. Melatonin rhythms in delayed sleep phase syndrome. J Biol Rhythms 1999; 14:72-6.

[42]   Ozaki S, Uchiyama M, Shirakawa S, Okawa M. Prolonged interval from body temperature nadir to sleep offset in patients with delayed sleep phase syndrome. Sleep 1996; 19: 36-40.

[43]   Rosenthal NE, Joseph-Vanderpool JR, Levendosky AA *et al.* Phase-shifting effects of bright morning light as treatment for delayed sleep phase syndrome. Sleep 1990; 13: 354-61.

[44] Nagtegaal JE, Kerkhof GA, Smits MG, *et al.* Delayed sleep phase syndrome: A placebo-controlled cross-over study on the effects of melatonin administered five hours before the individual dim light melatonin onset. J Sleep Res 1998; 7: 135-43.

[45] Rodenbeck A, Huether G, Ruther E, Hajak G. Altered circadian melatonin secretion patterns in relation to sleep in patients with chronic sleep-wake rhythm disorders. J Pineal Res 1998; 25: 201-10.

[46] Watanabe T, Kajimura N, Kato M, *et al.* Sleep and circadian rhythm disturbances in patients with delayed sleep phase syndrome. Sleep 2003; 26: 657-61.

[47] Reid KJ, Burgess HJ. Circadian rhythm sleep disorders. Prim Care 2005; 32: 449-73.

[48] Regestein QR, Pavlova M. Treatment of delayed sleep phase syndrome. Gen Hosp Psychiatry 1995; 17: 335-45.

[49] Aoki H, Ozeki Y, Yamada N. Hypersensitivity of melatonin suppression in response to light in patients with delayed sleep phase syndrome. Chronobiol Int 2001; 18: 263-71.

[50] Archer SN, Robilliard DL, Skene DJ, *et al.* A length polymorphism in the circadian clock gene Per3 is linked to delayed sleep phase syndrome and extreme diurnal preference. Sleep 2003; 26: 413-5.

[51] Hohjoh H, Takasu M, Shishikura K, *et al.* Significant association of the arylalkylamine N-acetyltransferase (AA-NAT) gene with delayed sleep phase syndrome. Neurogenetics 2003; 4: 151-3.

[52] Iwase T, Kajimura N, Uchiyama M, *et al.* Mutation screening of the human Clock gene in circadian rhythm sleep disorders. Psychiatry Res 2002; 109: 121-8.

[53] Takahashi Y, Hohjoh H, Matsuura K. Predisposing factors in delayed sleep phase syndrome. Psychiatry Clin Neurosci 2000; 54: 356-8.

[54] Littner M, Kushida CA, Anderson WM, *et al.* Practice parameters for the role of actigraphy in the study of sleep and circadian rhythms: an update for 2002. Sleep 2003; 26: 337-41.

[55] Chesson AL, Jr., Littner M, Davila D, *et al.* Practice parameters for the use of light therapy in the treatment of sleep disorders. Standards of Practice Committee, American Academy of Sleep Medicine. Sleep 1999; 22: 641-60.

[56] Wright HR, Lack LC. Effect of light wavelength on suppression and phase delay of the melatonin rhythm. Chronobiol Int 2001; 18: 801-8.

[57] Warman VL, Dijk DJ, Warman GR, *et al.* Phase advancing human circadian rhythms with short wavelength light. Neurosci Lett 2003; 342:37-40.

[58] Regestein QR, Monk TH. Delayed sleep phase syndrome: a review of its clinical aspects. Am J Psychiatry 1995; 152: 602-8.

[59] Thorpy MJ, Korman E, Spielman AJ, Glovinsky PB. Delayed sleep phase syndrome in adolescents. J Adolesc Health Care 1988; 9: 22-7.

[60] Sack RL, Lewy AJ, Hughes RJ. Use of melatonin for sleep and circadian rhythm disorders. Ann Med 1998; 30: 115-21.

[61] Mundey K, Benloucif S, Harsanyi K, *et al.* Phase-dependent treatment of delayed sleep phase syndrome with melatonin. Sleep 2005; 28: 1271-8.

[62] James SP, Sack DA, Rosenthal NE, Mendelson WB. Melatonin administration in insomnia. Neuropsychopharmacology 1990; 3: 19-23.

[63] Dahlitz M, Alvarez B, Vignau J, *et al.* Delayed sleep phase syndrome response to melatonin. Lancet 1991; 337: 1121-4.

[64] Oldani A, Ferini-Strambi L, Zucconi M, *et al.* Melatonin and delayed sleep phase syndrome: ambulatory polygraphic evaluation. Neuroreport 1994; 6: 132-4.

[65] Kamei Y, Hayakawa T, Urata J, *et al.* Melatonin treatment for circadian rhythm sleep disorders. Psychiatry Clin Neurosci 2000; 54: 381-2.

[66] Kayumov L, Brown G, Jindal R, *et al.* A randomized, double-blind, placebo-controlled crossover study of the effect of exogenous melatonin on delayed sleep phase syndrome. Psychosom Med 2001; 63: 40-8.

[67] Dagan Y, Yovel I, Hallis D, *et al.* Evaluating the role of melatonin in the long-term treatment of delayed sleep phase syndrome (DSPS). Chronobiol Int 1998; 15: 181-90.

[68] No authors listed. Melatonin. Med Lett Drugs Ther. 1995; 37(962):111-2.

[69] Buscemi N, Vandermeer B, Hooton N, *et al.* The efficacy and safety of exogenous melatonin for primary sleep disorders. A meta-analysis. J Gen Intern Med 2005; 20: 1151-8.

[70] Revell VL, Burgess HJ, Gazda CJ, *et al.* Advancing human circadian rhythms with afternoon melatonin and morning intermittent bright light. J Clin Endocrinol Metab 2006; 91: 54-9.

[71] Czeisler CA, Richardson GS, Coleman RM, *et al.* Chronotherapy: resetting the circadian clocks of patients with delayed sleep phase insomnia. Sleep 1981; 4: 1-21.

[72] Ando K KD, Ancoli-Israel S. Estimated prevalence of delayed and advanced sleep phase syndromes (abstract). J Sleep Res 1995; 24: 509.

[73] Jones CR, Campbell SS, Zone SE, *et al.* Familial advanced sleep-phase syndrome: A short-period circadian rhythm variant in humans. Nat Med 1999; 5: 1062-5.

[74]   Rufiange M, Dumont M, Lachapelle P. Correlating retinal function with melatonin secretion in subjects with an early or late circadian phase. Invest Ophthalmol Vis Sci 2002; 43: 2491-9.

[75]   Auger R. Advance-Related Sleep Complaints and Advanced Sleep Phase Disorder. Sleep Med Clin 2009; 4: 219-227.

[76]   Toh KL, Jones CR, He Y, *et al.* An hPer2 phosphorylation site mutation in familial advanced sleep phase syndrome. Science 2001; 291: 1040-3.

[77]   Xu Y, Padiath QS, Shapiro RE, *et al.* Functional consequences of a CKIdelta mutation causing familial advanced sleep phase syndrome. Nature 2005; 434: 640-4.

[78]   Campbell SS, Dawson D, Anderson MW. Alleviation of sleep maintenance insomnia with timed exposure to bright light. J Am Geriatr Soc 1993; 41: 829-36.

[79]   Lack L, Wright H, Kemp K, Gibbon S. The treatment of early-morning awakening insomnia with 2 evenings of bright light. Sleep 2005; 28: 616-23.

[80]   Sack RL, Auckley D, Auger RR, *et al.* Circadian rhythm sleep disorders: part I, basic principles, shift work and jet lag disorders. An American Academy of Sleep Medicine review. Sleep 2007; 30: 1460-83.

[81]   Zee PC. Melantonin for the treatment of advanced sleep phase disorder. Sleep 2008; 31: 923; author reply 925.

[82]   Moldofsky H, Musisi S, Phillipson EA. Treatment of a case of advanced sleep phase syndrome by phase advance chronotherapy. Sleep 1986; 9: 61-5.

[83]   Yoon IY, Kripke DF, Elliott JA, *et al.* Age-related changes of circadian rhythms and sleep-wake cycles. J Am Geriatr Soc 2003; 51: 1085-91.

[84]   Buxton OM, L'Hermite-Baleriaux M, Turek FW, van Cauter E. Daytime naps in darkness phase shift the human circadian rhythms of melatonin and thyrotropin secretion. Am J Physiol Regul Integr Comp Physiol 2000; 278: R373-82.

[85]   Moore-Ede MC, Czeisler CA, Richardson GS. Circadian timekeeping in health and disease. Part 1. Basic properties of circadian pacemakers. N Engl J Med 1983; 309: 469-76.

[86]   Lockley SW, Arendt J, Skene DJ. Visual impairment and circadian rhythm disorders. Dialogues Clin Neurosci 2007; 9: 301-14.

[87]   Lockley SW, Skene DJ, Butler LJ, Arendt J. Sleep and activity rhythms are related to circadian phase in the blind. Sleep 1999; 22: 616-23.

[88]   Sack RL, Lewy AJ, Blood ML, *et al.* Circadian rhythm abnormalities in totally blind people: incidence and clinical significance. J Clin Endocrinol Metab 1992; 75: 127-34.

[89]   Uchiyama M, Lockley SW. Non-24-Hour Sleep-Wake Syndrome in Sighted and Blind Patients. Sleep Med Clin 2009; 4: 195-211.

[90]   Okawa M, Uchiyama M. Circadian rhythm sleep disorders: characteristics and entrainment pathology in delayed sleep phase and non-24-h sleep-wake syndrome. Sleep Med Rev 2007; 11: 485-96.

[91]   Hayakawa T, Uchiyama M, Kamei Y, *et al.* Clinical analyses of sighted patients with non-24-hour sleep-wake syndrome: a study of 57 consecutively diagnosed cases. Sleep 2005; 28: 945-52.

[92]   Czeisler CA, Shanahan TL, Klerman EB, *et al.* Suppression of melatonin secretion in some blind patients by exposure to bright light. N Engl J Med 1995; 332: 6-11.

[93]   Klerman EB, Shanahan TL, Brotman DJ, *et al.* Photic resetting of the human circadian pacemaker in the absence of conscious vision. J Biol Rhythms 2002; 17: 548-55.

[94]   Zaidi FH, Hull JT, Peirson SN, *et al.* Short-wavelength light sensitivity of circadian, pupillary, and visual awareness in humans lacking an outer retina. Curr Biol 2007; 17: 2122-8.

[95]   Lockley SW, Skene DJ, Arendt J, *et al.* Relationship between melatonin rhythms and visual loss in the blind. J Clin Endocrinol Metab 1997; 82: 3763-70.

[96]   Klerman EB, Rimmer DW, Dijk DJ, *et al.* Nonphotic entrainment of the human circadian pacemaker. Am J Physiol 1998; 274: R991-6.

[97]   Mistlberger RE, Skene DJ. Nonphotic entrainment in humans? J Biol Rhythms 2005; 20: 339-52.

[98]   Aschoff J, Fatranska M, Giedke H *et al.* Human circadian rhythms in continuous darkness: entrainment by social cues. Science 1971; 171: 213-5.

[99]   Uchiyama M, Shibui K, Hayakawa T *et al.* Larger phase angle between sleep propensity and melatonin rhythms in sighted humans with non-24-hour sleep-wake syndrome. Sleep 2002; 25: 83-8.

[100] Hoban TM, Sack RL, Lewy AJ, *et al.* Entrainment of a free-running human with bright light? Chronobiol Int 1989; 6: 347-53.

[101] Hayakawa T, Kamei Y, Urata J, *et al.* Trials of bright light exposure and melatonin administration in a patient with non-24 hour sleep-wake syndrome. Psychiatry Clin Neurosci 1998; 52: 261-2.

[102] Watanabe T, Kajimura N, Kato M, *et al.* Case of a non-24 h sleep-wake syndrome patient improved by phototherapy. Psychiatry Clin Neurosci 2000; 54: 369-70.

[103] McArthur AJ, Lewy AJ, Sack RL. Non-24-hour sleep-wake syndrome in a sighted man: circadian rhythm studies and efficacy of melatonin treatment. Sleep 1996; 19: 544-53.

[104] Okawa M, Uchiyama M, Ozaki S, *et al.* Melatonin treatment for circadian rhythm sleep disorders. Psychiatry Clin Neurosci 1998; 52: 259-60.

[105] Siebler M, Steinmetz H, Freund HJ. Therapeutic entrainment of circadian rhythm disorder by melatonin in a non-blind patient. J Neurol 1998; 245: 327-8.

[106] Lockley SW, Skene DJ, James K, *et al.* Melatonin administration can entrain the free-running circadian system of blind subjects. J Endocrinol 2000; 164: R1-6.

[107] Sack RL, Brandes RW, Kendall AR, Lewy AJ. Entrainment of free-running circadian rhythms by melatonin in blind people. N Engl J Med 2000; 343: 1070-7.

[108] Hack LM, Lockley SW, Arendt J, Skene DJ. The effects of low-dose 0.5-mg melatonin on the free-running circadian rhythms of blind subjects. J Biol Rhythms 2003; 18: 420-9.

[109] Lewy AJ, Hasler BP, Emens JS, Sack RL. Pretreatment circadian period in free-running blind people may predict the phase angle of entrainment to melatonin. Neurosci Lett 2001; 313: 158-60.

[110] Lewy AJ, Bauer VK, Hasler BP, *et al.* Capturing the circadian rhythms of free-running blind people with 0.5 mg melatonin. Brain Res 2001; 918: 96-100.

[111] Arendt J, Aldhous M, Wright J. Synchronisation of a disturbed sleep-wake cycle in a blind man by melatonin treatment. Lancet 1988; 1: 772-3.

[112] Folkard S, Arendt J, Aldhous M, Kennett H. Melatonin stabilises sleep onset time in a blind man without entrainment of cortisol or temperature rhythms. Neurosci Lett 1990; 113: 193-8.

[113] Lapierre O, Dumont M. Melatonin treatment of a non-24-hour sleep-wake cycle in a blind retarded child. Biol Psychiatry 1995; 38: 119-22.

[114] Tzischinsky O, Pal I, Epstein R *et al.* The importance of timing in melatonin administration in a blind man. J Pineal Res 1992; 12: 105-8.

[115] Wagner DR. Disorders of the circadian sleep-wake cycle. Neurol Clin 1996; 14: 651-70.

[116] Zee PC, Vitiello MV. Circadian Rhythm Sleep Disorder: Irregular Sleep Wake Rhythm. Sleep Med Clin 2009; 2009:213-18.

[117] Sack RL, Auckley D, Auger RR, *et al.* Circadian rhythm sleep disorders: part II, advanced sleep phase disorder, delayed sleep phase disorder, free-running disorder, and irregular sleep-wake rhythm. An American Academy of Sleep Medicine review. Sleep 2007; 30: 1484-501.

[118] Wagner DR. Circadian Rhythm Sleep Disorders. Curr Treat Options Neurol 1999; 1: 299-308.

[119] Witting W, Kwa IH, Eikelenboom P, *et al.* Alterations in the circadian rest-activity rhythm in aging and Alzheimer's disease. Biol Psychiatry 1990; 27: 563-72.

[120] Swaab DF, Fliers E, Partiman TS. The suprachiasmatic nucleus of the human brain in relation to sex, age and senile dementia. Brain Res 1985; 342: 37-44.

[121] Swaab DF. Ageing of the human hypothalamus. Horm Res 1995; 43: 8-11.

[122] Zhou JN, Hofman MA, Swaab DF. VIP neurons in the human SCN in relation to sex, age, and Alzheimer's disease. Neurobiol Aging 1995; 16: 571-6.

[123] Van Someren EJ, Kessler A, Mirmiran M, Swaab DF. Indirect bright light improves circadian rest-activity rhythm disturbances in demented patients. Biol Psychiatry 1997; 41: 955-63.

[124] Ancoli-Israel S, Gehrman P, Martin JL, *et al.* Increased light exposure consolidates sleep and strengthens circadian rhythms in severe Alzheimer's disease patients. Behav Sleep Med 2003; 1: 22-36.

[125] Ancoli-Israel S, Martin JL, Kripke DF, *et al.* Effect of light treatment on sleep and circadian rhythms in demented nursing home patients. J Am Geriatr Soc 2002; 50: 282-9.

[126] Mishima K, Okawa M, Hishikawa Y, *et al.* Morning bright light therapy for sleep and behavior disorders in elderly patients with dementia. Acta Psychiatr Scand 1994; 89: 1-7.

[127] Pillar G, Shahar E, Peled N, *et al.* Melatonin improves sleep-wake patterns in psychomotor retarded children. Pediatr Neurol 2000; 23: 225-8.

[128] Naylor E, Penev PD, Orbeta L, *et al.* Daily social and physical activity increases slow-wave sleep and daytime neuropsychological performance in the elderly. Sleep 2000; 23: 87-95.

[129] Benloucif S, Orbeta L, Ortiz R, *et al.* Morning or evening activity improves neuropsychological performance and subjective sleep quality in older adults. Sleep 2004; 27: 1542-51.

[130] Niggemyer KA, Begley A, Monk T, Buysse DJ. Circadian and homeostatic modulation of sleep in older adults during a 90-minute day study. Sleep 2004; 27: 1535-41.

[131] Culpepper L. The social and economic burden of shift-work disorder. J Fam Pract 2010; 59: S3-S11.

[132] Rajaratnam SMW BL, Lockley SW, et .al. Screeing for Sleep Disorders in North American Police Officers(abstract). Sleep 2007; 30(suppl): A209.

[133] Schwartz JR. Recognition of shift-work disorder in primary care. J Fam Pract 2010; 59: S18-23.

[134] Ohayon MM, Lemoine P, Arnaud-Briant V, Dreyfus M. Prevalence and consequences of sleep disorders in a shift worker population. J Psychosom Res 2002; 53: 577-83.

[135] Czeisler CA, Moore-Ede MC, Coleman RH. Rotating shift work schedules that disrupt sleep are improved by applying circadian principles. Science 1982; 217: 460-3.

[136] Harma M, Tarja H, Irja K, et al. A controlled intervention study on the effects of a very rapidly forward rotating shift system on sleep-wakefulness and well-being among young and elderly shift workers. Int J Psychophysiol 2006; 59: 70-9.

[137] Marquie JC, Foret J. Sleep, age, and shiftwork experience. J Sleep Res 1999; 8: 297-304.

[138] Marquie JC, Foret J, Queinnec Y. Effects of age, working hours, and job content on sleep: a pilot study. Exp Aging Res 1999; 25: 421-7.

[139] Harma M, Knauth P, Ilmarinen J, Ollila H. The relation of age to the adjustment of the circadian rhythms of oral temperature and sleepiness to shift work. Chronobiol Int 1990; 7: 227-33.

[140] Harma MI, Hakola T, Akerstedt T, Laitinen JT. Age and adjustment to night work. Occup Environ Med 1994; 51: 568-73.

[141] Smith L, Mason C. Reducing night shift exposure: a pilot study of rota, night shift and age effects on sleepiness and fatigue. J Hum Ergol (Tokyo) 2001; 30: 83-7.

[142] Schwartz JR, Roth T. Shift work sleep disorder: burden of illness and approaches to management. Drugs 2006; 66: 2357-70.

[143] Shen J, Botly LC, Chung SA, et al. Fatigue and shift work. J Sleep Res 2006; 15: 1-5.

[144] Akerstedt T. [Increased risk of accidents during night shift. An underestimated problem are fatigue-induced accidents]. Lakartidningen 1995; 92: 2103-4.

[145] Akerstedt T. Shift work and disturbed sleep/wakefulness. Occup Med (Lond) 2003; 53: 89-94.

[146] Knauth P, Landau K, Droge C, et al. Duration of sleep depending on the type of shift work. Int Arch Occup Environ Health 1980; 46: 167-77.

[147] Taylor PJ, Pocock SJ. Mortality of shift and day workers 1956-68. Br J Ind Med 1972; 29: 201-7.

[148] Boggild H, Suadicani P, Hein HO, Gyntelberg F. Shift work, social class, and ischaemic heart disease in middle aged and elderly men; a 22 year follow up in the Copenhagen Male Study. Occup Environ Med 1999; 56: 640-5.

[149] Knutsson A. Health disorders of shift workers. Occup Med (Lond) 2003; 53: 103-8.

[150] Segawa K, Nakazawa S, Tsukamoto Y, et al. Peptic ulcer is prevalent among shift workers. Dig Dis Sci 1987; 32: 449-53.

[151] Biggi N, Consonni D, Galluzzo V, et al. Metabolic syndrome in permanent night workers. Chronobiol Int 2008; 25: 443-54.

[152] Garbarino S, Beelke M, Costa G, et al. Brain function and effects of shift work: implications for clinical neuropharmacology. Neuropsychobiology 2002; 45: 50-6.

[153] Boggild H, Knutsson A. Shift work, risk factors and cardiovascular disease. Scand J Work Environ Health 1999; 25: 85-99.

[154] Furlan R, Barbic F, Piazza S, et al. Modifications of cardiac autonomic profile associated with a shift schedule of work. Circulation 2000; 102: 1912-6.

[155] Hansen J. Increased breast cancer risk among women who work predominantly at night. Epidemiology 2001; 12: 74-7.

[156] Davis S, Mirick DK, Stevens RG. Night shift work, light at night, and risk of breast cancer. J Natl Cancer Inst 2001; 93: 1557-62.

[157] Demers PA, Checkoway H, Vaughan TL, et al. Cancer incidence among firefighters in Seattle and Tacoma, Washington (United States). Cancer Causes Control 1994; 5: 129-35.

[158] Schernhammer ES, Laden F, Speizer FE, et al. Rotating night shifts and risk of breast cancer in women participating in the nurses' health study. J Natl Cancer Inst 2001; 93: 1563-8.

[159] Schernhammer ES, Laden F, Speizer FE, et al. Night-shift work and risk of colorectal cancer in the nurses' health study. J Natl Cancer Inst 2003; 95: 825-8.

[160] Nurminen T. Shift work and reproductive health. Scand J Work Environ Health 1998; 24 Suppl 3: 28-34.

[161] Uehata T, Sasakawa N. The fatigue and maternity disturbances of night workwomen. J Hum Ergol (Tokyo) 1982; 11 Suppl: 465-74.

[162] Miyauchi F, Nanjo K, Otsuka K. [Effects of night shift on plasma concentrations of melatonin, LH, FSH and prolactin, and menstrual irregularity]. Sangyo Igaku 1992; 34: 545-50.

[163] Scott AJ, Monk TH, Brink LL. Shiftwork as a Risk Factor for Depression: A Pilot Study. Int J Occup Environ Health 1997; 3: S2-S9.

[164] Ayas NT, Barger LK, Cade BE, *et al.* Extended work duration and the risk of self-reported percutaneous injuries in interns. JAMA 2006; 296: 1055-62.

[165] Garbarino S, De Carli F, Nobili L, *et al.* Sleepiness and sleep disorders in shift workers: a study on a group of italian police officers. Sleep 2002; 25: 648-53.

[166] Akerstedt T, Peters B, Anund A, Kecklund G. Impaired alertness and performance driving home from the night shift: a driving simulator study. J Sleep Res 2005; 14: 17-20.

[167] Steele MT, Ma OJ, Watson WA, *et al.* The occupational risk of motor vehicle collisions for emergency medicine residents. Acad Emerg Med 1999; 6: 1050-3.

[168] Barger LK, Cade BE, Ayas NT, *et al.* Extended work shifts and the risk of motor vehicle crashes among interns. N Engl J Med 2005; 352: 125-34.

[169] Folkard S, Tucker P. Shift work, safety and productivity. Occup Med (Lond) 2003; 53: 95-101.

[170] Thorpy MJ. Managing the patient with shift-work disorder. J Fam Pract 2010; 59: S24-31.

[171] Schweitzer PK, Randazzo AC, Stone K, *et al.* Laboratory and field studies of naps and caffeine as practical countermeasures for sleep-wake problems associated with night work. Sleep 2006; 29: 39-50.

[172] Sallinen M, Harma M, Akerstedt T, *et al.* Promoting alertness with a short nap during a night shift. J Sleep Res 1998; 7: 240-7.

[173] Purnell MT, Feyer AM, Herbison GP. The impact of a nap opportunity during the night shift on the performance and alertness of 12-h shift workers. J Sleep Res 2002; 11: 219-27.

[174] Garbarino S, Mascialino B, Penco MA, *et al.* Professional shift-work drivers who adopt prophylactic naps can reduce the risk of car accidents during night work. Sleep 2004; 27: 1295-302.

[175] Bonnefond A, Muzet A, Winter-Dill AS, *et al.* Innovative working schedule: introducing one short nap during the night shift. Ergonomics 2001; 44: 937-45.

[176] Kubo T, Takeyama H, Matsumoto S, *et al.* Impact of nap length, nap timing and sleep quality on sustaining early morning performance. Ind Health 2007; 45: 552-63.

[177] Yoon IY, Jeong DU, Kwon KB, *et al.* Bright light exposure at night and light attenuation in the morning improve adaptation of night shift workers. Sleep 2002; 25: 351-6.

[178] Boivin DB, James FO. Circadian adaptation to night-shift work by judicious light and darkness exposure. J Biol Rhythms 2002; 17: 556-67.

[179] Budnick LD, Lerman SE, Nicolich MJ. An evaluation of scheduled bright light and darkness on rotating shiftworkers: trial and limitations. Am J Ind Med 1995; 27: 771-82.

[180] Costa G, Ghirlanda G, Minors DS, Waterhouse JM. Effect of bright light on tolerance to night work. Scand J Work Environ Health 1993; 19: 414-20.

[181] Lowden A, Akerstedt T, Wibom R. Suppression of sleepiness and melatonin by bright light exposure during breaks in night work. J Sleep Res 2004; 13: 37-43.

[182] Stewart KT, Hayes BC, Eastman CI. Light treatment for NASA shiftworkers. Chronobiol Int 1995; 12: 141-51.

[183] Erman MK, Rosenberg R, For The USMSWSDSG. Modafinil for excessive sleepiness associated with chronic shift work sleep disorder: effects on patient functioning and health-related quality of life. Prim Care Companion J Clin Psychiatry 2007; 9: 188-94.

[184] Drake C WJ, Roth T. Armodafinil improves sleep latency in patients with shift work disorder. Sleep 2006; 29(suppl): A64.

[185] Roth T CC, Walsh JK, et.al. Randomized, double-blind, placebo-controlled study of armodafinil for the treatment of excessive sleepiness associated with chronic shift work disorder(abstract 161). Neuropsychopharmacology 2005; 30: S140.

[186] Jay SM, Petrilli RM, Ferguson SA, *et al.* The suitability of a caffeinated energy drink for night-shift workers. Physiol Behav 2006; 87: 925-31.

[187] Muehlbach MJ, Walsh JK. The effects of caffeine on simulated night-shift work and subsequent daytime sleep. Sleep 1995; 18: 22-9.

[188] Walsh JK, Muehlbach MJ, Humm TM, *et al.* Effect of caffeine on physiological sleep tendency and ability to sustain wakefulness at night. Psychopharmacology (Berl) 1990; 101: 271-3.

[189] Judelson DA, Armstrong LE, Sokmen B, *et al.* Effect of chronic caffeine intake on choice reaction time, mood, and visual vigilance. Physiol Behav 2005; 85:629-34.

[190] Sharkey KM, Fogg LF, Eastman CI. Effects of melatonin administration on daytime sleep after simulated night shift work. J Sleep Res 2001; 10: 181-92.

[191] Sharkey KM, Eastman CI. Melatonin phase shifts human circadian rhythms in a placebo-controlled simulated night-work study. Am J Physiol Regul Integr Comp Physiol 2002; 282: R454-63.

[192] Sack RL, Lewy AJ. Melatonin as a chronobiotic: treatment of circadian desynchrony in night workers and the blind. J Biol Rhythms 1997; 12: 595-603.

[193] James M, Tremea MO, Jones JS, Krohmer JR. Can melatonin improve adaptation to night shift? Am J Emerg Med 1998; 16: 367-70.

[194] Jorgensen KM, Witting MD. Does exogenous melatonin improve day sleep or night alertness in emergency physicians working night shifts? Ann Emerg Med 1998; 31: 699-704.

[195] Yoon IY, Song BG. Role of morning melatonin administration and attenuation of sunlight exposure in improving adaptation of night-shift workers. Chronobiol Int 2002; 19: 903-13.

[196] Walsh JK, Schweitzer PK, Anch AM, et al. Sleepiness/alertness on a simulated night shift following sleep at home with triazolam. Sleep 1991; 14: 140-6.

[197] Walsh JK, Sugerman JL, Muehlbach MJ, Schweitzer PK. Physiological sleep tendency on a simulated night shift: adaptation and effects of triazolam. Sleep 1988; 11: 251-64.

[198] Porcu S, Bellatreccia A, Ferrara M, Casagrande M. Performance, ability to stay awake, and tendency to fall asleep during the night after a diurnal sleep with temazepam or placebo. Sleep 1997; 20: 535-41.

[199] Monchesky TC, Billings BJ, Phillips R, Bourgouin J. Zopiclone in insomniac shiftworkers. Evaluation of its hypnotic properties and its effects on mood and work performance. Int Arch Occup Environ Health 1989; 61: 255-9.

[200] Moon CA, Hindmarch I, Holland RL. The effect of zopiclone 7.5 mg on the sleep, mood and performance of shift workers. Int Clin Psychopharmacol 1990; 5 Suppl 2: 79-83.

[201] Aschoff J, Hoffmann K, Pohl H, Wever R. Re-entrainment of circadian rhythms after phase-shifts of the Zeitgeber. Chronobiologia 1975; 2: 23-78.

[202] Takahashi T, Sasaki M, Itoh H, et al. Re-entrainment of circadian rhythm of plasma melatonin on an 8-h eastward flight. Psychiatry Clin Neurosci 1999; 53: 257-60.

[203] Waterhouse J, Reilly T, Atkinson G, Edwards B. Jet lag: trends and coping strategies. Lancet 2007; 369:1117-29.

[204] Lowden A, Akerstedt T. Retaining home-base sleep hours to prevent jet lag in connection with a westward flight across nine time zones. Chronobiol Int 1998; 15: 365-76.

[205] Burgess HJ, Crowley SJ, Gazda CJ, et al. Preflight adjustment to eastward travel: 3 days of advancing sleep with and without morning bright light. J Biol Rhythms 2003; 18:318-28.

[206] Daan S, Lewy AJ. Scheduled exposure to daylight: a potential strategy to reduce "jet lag" following transmeridian flight. Psychopharmacol Bull 1984; 20:566-8.

[207] Eastman CI, Burgess HJ. How To Travel the World Without Jet lag. Sleep Med Clin 2009; 4: 241-255.

[208] Lewy AJ, Bauer VK, Ahmed S, et al. The human phase response curve (PRC) to melatonin is about 12 hours out of phase with the PRC to light. Chronobiol Int 1998; 15: 71-83.

[209] Herxheimer A, Petrie KJ. Melatonin for the prevention and treatment of jet lag. Cochrane Database Syst Rev 2002: CD001520.

[210] Arendt J, Aldhous M, Marks V. Alleviation of jet lag by melatonin: preliminary results of controlled double blind trial. Br Med J (Clin Res Ed) 1986; 292: 1170.

[211] Claustrat B, Brun J, David M, et al. Melatonin and jet lag: confirmatory result using a simplified protocol. Biol Psychiatry 1992; 32: 705-11.

[212] Petrie K, Conaglen JV, Thompson L, Chamberlain K. Effect of melatonin on jet lag after long haul flights. BMJ 1989; 298: 705-7.

[213] Petrie K, Dawson AG, Thompson L, Brook R. A double-blind trial of melatonin as a treatment for jet lag in international cabin crew. Biol Psychiatry 1993; 33: 526-30.

[214] Suhner A, Schlagenhauf P, Johnson R et al. Comparative study to determine the optimal melatonin dosage form for the alleviation of jet lag. Chronobiol Int 1998; 15: 655-66.

[215] Edwards BJ, Atkinson G, Waterhouse J, et al. Use of melatonin in recovery from jet-lag following an eastward flight across 10 time-zones. Ergonomics 2000; 43: 1501-13.

[216] Burgess HJ, Revell VL, Eastman CI. A three pulse phase response curve to three milligrams of melatonin in humans. J Physiol 2008; 586: 639-47.

[217] Suhner A, Schlagenhauf P, Hofer I, et al. Effectiveness and tolerability of melatonin and zolpidem for the alleviation of jet lag. Aviat Space Environ Med 2001; 72: 638-46.

[218] Paul MA, Gray G, Sardana TM, Pigeau RA. Melatonin and zopiclone as facilitators of early circadian sleep in operational air transport crews. Aviat Space Environ Med 2004; 75: 439-43.

[219] Jamieson AO, Zammit GK, Rosenberg RS, et al. Zolpidem reduces the sleep disturbance of jet lag. Sleep Med 2001; 2: 423-30.

[220] Buxton OM, Copinschi G, Van Onderbergen A, *et al.* A benzodiazepine hypnotic facilitates adaptation of circadian rhythms and sleep-wake homeostasis to an eight hour delay shift simulating westward jet lag. Sleep 2000; 23: 915-27.

[221] Daurat A, Benoit O, Buguet A. Effects of zopiclone on the rest/activity rhythm after a westward flight across five time zones. Psychopharmacology (Berl) 2000; 149: 241-5.

[222] Donaldson E, Kennaway DJ. Effects of temazepam on sleep, performance, and rhythmic 6-sulphatoxymelatonin and cortisol excretion after transmeridian travel. Aviat Space Environ Med 1991; 62: 654-60.

[223] Hirschfeld U, Moreno-Reyes R, Akseki E, *et al.* Progressive elevation of plasma thyrotropin during adaptation to simulated jet lag: effects of treatment with bright light or zolpidem. J Clin Endocrinol Metab 1996; 81: 3270-7.

[224] Lavie P. Effects of midazolam on sleep disturbances associated with westward and eastward flights: evidence for directional effects. Psychopharmacology (Berl) 1990; 101: 250-4.

[225] Reilly T, Atkinson G, Budgett R. Effect of low-dose temazepam on physiological variables and performance tests following a westerly flight across five time zones. Int J Sports Med 2001; 22: 166-74.

[226] Morris HH, 3rd, Estes ML. Traveler's amnesia. Transient global amnesia secondary to triazolam. JAMA 1987; 258: 945-6.

[227] Beaumont M, Batejat D, Pierard C, *et al.* Caffeine or melatonin effects on sleep and sleepiness after rapid eastward transmeridian travel. J Appl Physiol 2004; 96: 50-8.

CHAPTER 11

Narcolepsy

Emmanuel Mignot, M.D., Ph.D.[*]

Professor of Medicine, Department of Psychiatry and Behavioral Sciences, Stanford University, Stanford University Center for Narcolepsy, 701b Welch Rd, Room 145, Palo Alto, CA, USA

Abstract: Narcolepsy with and without cataplexy has two different nosological entities. Narcolepsy-cataplexy is strongly associated with HLA-DQB1*0602 and usually caused by a selective deficiency in the hypothalamic neuropeptide hypocretin (orexin). The cause of hypocretin deficiency is most likely an autoimmune attack directed against hypocretin cells. Diagnosis is performed clinically, with the additional sleep tests such as the Multiple Sleep Latency Test, or in some cases, by measuring hypocretin-1 levels in the Cerebrospinal fluid (CSF).

To date, therapy is mostly pharmacological and does not act directly on the hypocretin system. Stimulant compounds seem to increase alertness by activating dopaminergic transmission in the brain, while antidepressant therapy reduces cataplexy by increasing adrenergic and serotoninergic transmission. The mode of action of gamma-hydroxybutyrate (sodium oxybate), a treatment for cataplexy and disturbed nocturnal sleep is uncertain, but may involve GABA-B receptors. Narcolepsy without cataplexy is primarily diagnosed using MSLT, with a finding of a short mean sleep latency ($\leq$ 8 min) and at least 2 Sleep Onset REM Periods (SOREMPs). The population-based prevalence of narcolepsy without cataplexy is unknown. It is likely that many cases of narcolepsy without cataplexy have very different pathogenesis, and/or result from false-positive MSLT. A minority of cases without cataplexy have hypocretin deficiency. For cases without cataplexy or hypocretin deficiency, research is needed to better understand the pathophysiology. Therapy is similar to that used for cases with cataplexy, although amphetamine stimulants should be used with more caution.

TOPIC DISCUSSION (CLINICAL OUTLOOK)

Introduction

In the International Classification of Sleep Disorders (ICSD-2) [1], narcolepsy with and without cataplexy are now two distinct disease entities. In most narcolepsy cases with cataplexy and in fewer cases without cataplexy, a deficiency in the hypothalamic neuropeptide called hypocretin, with subsequent low CSF hypocretin-1, is causative [2]. Almost all cases with hypocretin deficiency share a specific Human Leukocyte Antigen (HLA) genetic marker called DQB1*0602 and have a likely autoimmune etiology, as hypocretin-secreting cells in the brain are missing in postmortem studies, as opposed to other neurons in the same parafornical areas of the lateral hypothalamus [3, 4]. In contrast, a diagnosis of narcolepsy without cataplexy (as defined clinically by excessive daytime sleepiness and polysomnographically by a positive MSLT), likely represents a complex constellation of medical conditions and pathologies [5, 6].

Symptoms

Typically, the following pentad is used to characterize clinically the narcoleptic patients:

Sleepiness. The excessive daytime sleepiness seen in narcolepsy can be characterized by a background of chronic sleepiness throughout the day, punctuated by irresistible episodes of sleep. The typical narcoleptic will usually fall asleep in inactive settings (in a lecture, at a movie, etc), sleep for a short duration (typically 10-20 minutes) and awaken feeling refreshed. However, after a few hours of wakefulness, a narcoleptic may begin to feel sleepy once again and the pattern repeats itself. There may also be sudden sleep attacks in situations where one would normally not fall asleep (interactive conversation, while eating, etc).

---

*Address correspondence to Emmanuel Mignot: Professor of Medicine, Department of Psychiatry and Behavioral Sciences, Stanford University, Stanford University Center for Narcolepsy, 701b Welch Rd Room 145, Palo Alto, CA, USA; E-mail: mignot@stanford.edu

Cataplexy is a feature unique to narcolepsy. It is characterized by a sudden loss of muscle tone provoked by strong emotions, typically positive in nature (laughter, elation, etc), although negative emotions can, though less commonly, provoke cataplexy as well. Consciousness remains intact, memory for the event is complete and respiration is undisturbed. Duration is typically a few seconds to several minutes and complete immediate recovery is the norm. The degree of muscle atonia is variable, ranging from a mild sensation of weakness, head droop, facial sagging, jaw drop, slurred speech, to buckling of the knees and collapse to the ground. Patients often learn to avoid conditions that provoke cataplexy.

Hypnagogic hallucinations are vivid sensations occurring at sleep onset. They may be visual, auditory, tactile or kinetic phenomena. They are often described as if someone or something is in the same room and frequently are frightening or anxiogenic in nature. Hypnopompic hallucinations are similar REM-related phenomena and happen at transitions between (REM) sleep and wakefulness, although their diagnostic value may to be inferior to that of the hypnagogic hallucinations.

Sleep paralysis typically presents during the transition from sleep to wakefulness as a transient, generalized inability to move or speak. This can last from one to several minutes and often occur with hypnagogic hallucinations, making for an even more disturbing experience.

Finally, many narcoleptics also experience *disrupted nighttime sleep,* with frequent awakenings, which may, further contribute to their excessive daytime sleepiness. They may also report memory lapses with associated automatic behaviors.

Diagnosis

If cataplexy is present and typical, the diagnosis can be made *on clinical grounds alone*, although it is advisable to conduct an MSLT or a CSF hypocretin-1 level measurement to objectively document the abnormalities before initiating therapy, when the patient is still drug-free.

The *Multiple Sleep Latency Test* (MSLT) is used to provide an objective measure of excessive daytime sleepiness and to document the presence of at least 2 sleep onset REM periods (SOREMPs), which are the hallmark of narcolepsy. For MSLT results to be valid, one must first ensure no other sleep disorder exists that could account for the degree of excessive daytime sleepiness observed. Therefore, one must perform an overnight polysomnogram the night prior to the MSLT (generally to exclude sleep apnea or dramatically reduced nocturnal sleep). Other confounding factors such as medications that can influence sleep (antidepressants reduce REM sleep and must be withdrawn at least 2 weeks prior to MSLT), stimulants, etc must all be controlled prior to polysomnographic investigation for narcolepsy.

During overnight polysomnography, narcoleptics commonly show a short sleep latency (less than 10 minutes) and a SOREMP (REM occurs within 20 minutes of sleep onset). There may also be frequent awakenings. The MSLT in a narcoleptic typically shows sleep latencies of less than 10 minutes (often less than 5 minutes) and 2 or more SOREMPs. As for any diagnostic test, the MSLT is not a perfect test. For example, 5-15% of cases of narcolepsy with cataplexy or hypocretin deficiency do not have a positive MSLT. Similarly, approximately 2-4% of the general population without any obvious narcolepsy complaints has a positive MSLT when population-based samples are tested.

The observation that cerebrospinal fluid (CSF) hypocretin-1 levels are decreased in patients with narcolepsy provides a new test to diagnose this disorder [2, 7]. If positive in an ambulatory patient, the test is highly predictive of narcolepsy/hypocretin deficiency. False positive results are rare, and typically occur in patients with severe brain or metabolic abnormalities, for example comatose patients after a head trauma. The most commonly used cut-off is 110 pg/mL (when performed at Stanford University), or 30% of the mean of multiple control CSF levels (if measurements are conducted elsewhere). If values are below this cut-off, measurement is especially predictive in cases with definite cataplexy (99% specificity, 87% sensitivity). Most of these cases have undetectable CSF hypocretin-1 levels (<40 pg/ml). Almost all subjects with low CSF hypocretin in this context (~99%) are positive for the genetic marker HLA-DQB1*0602, thus HLA typing prior to the lumbar puncture is often advised (however, it is estimated that 25% of the general population in the US is HLA-DQB1*0602-positive by chance) [3]. A good indication to measure the CSF hypocretin-1 levels is for the situation with "negative" MSLT and strong suspicion that cataplexy is present, although not pathognomonic (often at disease onset), or when the MSLT cannot be optimally performed due to inability to discontinue various medications that can affect the predictive value of the test.

Epidemiology Prevalence Studies

Population-based prevalence studies of narcolepsy-cataplexy have been performed in various countries and used different designs. Since cataplexy is a pathognomonic symptom, this allows for a rapid first-screen. In a study performed in Finland, 11,354 individual twin subjects were asked to respond to a questionnaire. Three narcoleptic subjects with cataplexy and abnormal MSLT results were identified, leading to a prevalence of 0.026% [4]. Other studies have led to similar prevalence (0.013 to 0.067%) in Great Britain, France, Hong Kong, Czech Republic, and in the United States [5-7]. Narcolepsy-cataplexy may be less frequent in Israel (0.002%) and more frequent in Japan (0.16-0.18%) [5], but these studies were not adequately designed, so a direct comparison is difficult. It is of interest to note that DQB1*0602 is rare in Israel (4-6%), Japan (8%), Korea (13%), but less so in most Caucasian populations (25%), Chinese (25%) and African American population (38%); thus, a linear relationship between the prevalence of narcolepsy and DQB1*0602 is not expected.

The prevalence of narcolepsy without cataplexy is largely unknown. Narcolepsy without cataplexy represented 20-50% of individuals in a case series [8]. Expectedly, patients without cataplexy are more likely to be under-diagnosed (e.g., cases of co-existent narcolepsy and sleep apnea), undiagnosed (no major complaint) or misdiagnosed (e.g., as depression or sleep apnea) [9]. Some studies have suggested that 1-3% of the adult population may have unexplained sleepiness and multiple SOREMPs during MSLT testing [14, 15]. A recent study identified all diagnosed narcoleptic patients in the Olmsted County (MN, USA) using the medical records-linkage system of the Rochester Epidemiology project [7]. The study identified 0.036% of the population with narcolepsy-cataplexy and 0.021% with narcolepsy without cataplexy, suggesting a significant prevalence for narcolepsy without cataplexy variant [7]. In King County (WA, USA), a similarly designed, recent study found 0.031% of the population with narcolepsy, and only 0.009% with narcolepsy without cataplexy (27% of DQB1*0602 positive) [6]. As mentioned above, however, it is clear that registry-based estimations of diagnosed narcolepsy without cataplexy prevalence probably underestimate, while population-based epidemiological studies that do not exclude other confounding factors, overestimate the true population prevalence.

What percent of narcolepsy without cataplexy cases has hypocretin deficiency is also unknown. In some centers, when all other causes of daytime sleepiness have been excluded, it may reach 30%, while in others may be as low as 5% with a mean of 15% overall and 31% of HLA-positive subjects in a recent metaanalysis of 162 samples tested in our center [10]. This is also reflected by the % DQB1*0602 positivity in such sample, ranging from 27% (slightly above the 23% population frequency in Caucasians), to 40% in a larger, multicenter drug trial [8] and other samples [2, 10].

Twin Studies and Environmental Factors in Narcolepsy

As mentioned above, the only systematic twin study available was performed by Hublin *et al* in Caucasian Finns [4], but the three twin individuals identified with narcolepsy were dizygotic, hence uninformative to establish concordance in monozygotic twins. Approximately twenty monozygotic twin reports are available in literature (see reference by Mignot [5] for review). Five to seven are discordant for narcolepsy, depending how strictly concordance is determined clinically [5]. Most cases of human narcolepsy therefore require the influence of environmental factors for the pathology to develop. This is also substantiated by the fact that onset is generally not at birth, but rather in adolescence [11, 12], suggesting some triggering factors.

The nature of the environmental factor involved is still unknown. Frequently cited factors are head trauma, sudden change in sleep/wake habits [13] or various infections. These factors may be involved, but most studies have used a retrospective design, limiting the value of any reported difference. Interestingly, a recent paper has suggested increased births for narcolepsy in March and decreased frequency in September, suggesting the influence of perinatal factors [14]. A study also found increased passive smoking as a risk factor for the development of narcolepsy in a well designed epidemiological cohort study [15]. Finally, three studies have also found an association with past streptococcus infections [16-18] and, rarely, a possible precipitation by H1N1 vaccination with the adjuvanted Pandremix vaccine [18].

Familial Aspects of Human Narcolepsy

Narcolepsy is occasionally a familial disorder. The risk of a first-degree relative to develop narcolepsy-cataplexy has been shown to be only 1-2% [see [5] for review]. A larger portion of relatives (4-5%) may have isolated daytime sleepiness, when other causes of daytime sleepiness have been excluded [5]. These figures are important to keep in mind, as they are helpful in reassuring patients regarding the risk to their children and relatives. A 1-2% risk is 10- to 40-fold higher than in the general population, but remains manageable. A 4-5% risk for daytime sleepiness is not negligible, although similar values have been reported for excessive daytime sleepiness in the general population, independent of narcolepsy.

Pathogenesis [Narcolepsy, Hypocretin (Orexin) Deficiency and Autoimmunity]

Animal Models

Narcolepsy was first reported in dogs, where it can be either due to hypocretin deficiency [19], or due to a mutation in the hypocretin receptor 2 [20, 21]. Several genetically engineered rodent models of narcolepsy lacking hypocretin or its receptors are also now available [22], [23]. The fact that rodent models without the hypocretin gene, but with intact hypocretin-producing cells have narcolepsy demonstrates causality between narcolepsy and hypocretin pathway deficiency.

Human Data

Concordant with the observation that most cases of human narcolepsy are sporadic and not "fully genetic" like in dogs or mice, an extensive screening study did not identify significant preprohypocretin, hypocretin receptor 1 and 2 (Hcrtr1, Hcrtr2) mutations in human narcolepsy cases [24, 25]. Surprisingly, even familial cases of narcolepsy (some of which were HLA-DQB1*0602 negative) did not have any hypocretin mutations, suggesting further heterogeneity in genetic cases [24]. Furthermore, only one case with a signal peptide mutation of the preprohypocretin gene was identified. This case had very early disease onset (6 months), severe narcolepsy with cataplexy, DQB1*0602 negativity and undetectable Hcrtr-1 cerebrospinal fluid levels [24]. This important observation indicates that hypocretin system gene mutations can cause narcolepsy similar to the animal models.

The observation that narcolepsy is associated with Human Leukocyte Antigen (HLA) DR2 was first reported in Japan in 1983. Because many HLA (also called Major Histocompatibility Complex or MHC) associated diseases are known to be autoimmune, this discovery led to the hypothesis that narcolepsy may result from an autoimmune insult within the Central Nervous System (CNS). The finding of hypocretin cell loss in human narcolepsy [24, 26] suggests that the autoimmune process could target this small population of hypothalamic neurons. Attempts at verifying an autoimmune mediation had been disappointing so far [27]. Human narcolepsy is not associated with any striking pathological changes in the CNS and/or increased frequency in the occurrence of oligoclonal bands in the CSF. Gliosis in human narcolepsy brains has been reported but remains controversial, as are imaging findings suggesting macroscopic hypothalamic changes [28]. Similarly, peripheral immunity does not seem to be altered even around disease onset.

More recently, several new discoveries strongly supported an autoimmune basis for narcolepsy. First, using a genome-wide association study (GWAS) design, we found that narcolepsy/hypocretin deficiency is strongly associated with T-cell receptor (TCR) alpha polymorphisms [29]. Interestingly, the TCR is the natural receptor of HLA class II when presenting antigenic peptides, hence it seems a logical candidate. Furthemore, unlike HLA proteins, the T-cell receptor is only expressed in immune cells, so this finding makes it almost certain that narcolepsy must involve an autoimmune or infectious phenomenon. Second, we found that streptococcal infections are likely to be an infectious trigger for narcolepsy in Caucasians [17]. Third, another group, led by Dr. Tafti in Switzerland, reported that 14% of narcolepsy cases have high titers of antibodies (1/100, >2SD of control sera values) directed against the protein tribbles homolog 2 (TRIB2) (versus 5% of 42 controls), a protein partially co-localized with hypocretin in the hypothalamus [30].

Curiously however, of the many HLA-associated diseases that have undergone GWAS, none have been shown to have predisposing factors in the TCR regions. We believe this may be due to the extreme specificity of the autoimmune process in narcolepsy, involving a single main HLA-DQB1*0602 allele association (>99% of hypocretin deficient cases are HLA-DQB1*0602 positive), a specific infectious trigger (*Streptococcus pyogenes*) and a specific TCR idiotype (which would be marked by our TCR associated polymorphisms). The possibility of determining the trimolecular HLA - streptococcus peptide - TCR idiotype interaction that mediates autoimmunity in narcolepsy would be unprecedented as a model for the study of autoimmune diseases. Indeed, TCR idiotypes have been involved in many animal models of immune response, but never definitively in the context of a human autoimmune disease.

Secondary Narcolepsy

Von Economo was the first to suggest that narcolepsy may have its origins in the posterior hypothalamus and in some cases a secondary etiology [31]. The cause of idiopathic narcolepsy that had been described some 50 years earlier was also speculated to involve this general area. This hypothesis was further refined by many authors who noted that tumors or other lesions located close to the third ventricle were also associated with secondary narcolepsy and hypothesized that the posterior hypothalamic region may be the culprit. A postulated hypothalamic cause of narcolepsy was widespread until the 1940s but was then ignored during the psychoanalytic boom and replaced by brainstem hypothesis [31].

Reports of third ventricle lesions (hypothalamus and upper midbrain) in association with narcolepsy (such as tumors) have been described for over 80 years [31], thus it is clear that these tumors can cause or precipitate narcolepsy. Interestingly, when with cataplexy, a number of these cases have been shown to be HLA-DR2 or DQB1*0602 positive, suggesting that the association could be partially coincidental. In these cases, it is also possible that the emergence of the tumor induced blood brain barrier damage or an inflammatory response in the region that could have favored the development of hypocretin cell loss through an autoimmune attack. In some of these cases, CSF hypocretin may be low or intermediate (110-200 pg/ml), although often the data is difficult to interpret as cataplexy is not clearly present, and in some cases measurement have been made in very ill patients. Such intermediate levels may nonetheless reflect damage to nearby hypocretin projection sites, with sufficient preservation of cell bodies to maintain detectable levels of hypocretin-1. Alternatively (or additionally), other regions in the upper-midbrain may also contribute to the symptomatology, especially sleepiness, as initially proposed by Von Economo.

The complex area of genetic or congenital disorders associated with primary central hypersomnolence is also of great interest. Specific familial syndromes combining HLA negative narcolepsy-cataplexy with ataxia and deafness in one publication [32], obesity - type 1 diabetes in another [33] are especially interesting, as both cataplexy and low to undetectable CSF hypocretin-1 have been documented. Genetic disorders such as Coffin-Lowry Syndrome [34], Moebius syndrome [35], Norrie's Disease [35], Pradder-Willi syndrome [2], Neimann-Pick Type C [2] and myotonic dystrophy [36] have been reported to be associated with daytime sleepiness and/or cataplexy-like symptoms. CSF Hcrt-1 has been measured in cases of Neimann-Pick Type C, a condition where occulomotor symptoms are frequent, and intermediate levels have been found in some cases with cataplexy [2]. This condition is remarkable as cataplexy is often triggered by typical emotions (laughing) and responsive to anti-cataplectic treatment. Some diseases are associated with the development of both narcolepsy and sleep disordered breathing, such as myotonic dystrophy [36] and Prader-Willi Syndrome [2]; in such cases, primary hypersomnia should only be diagnosed if excessive daytime sleepiness does not improve after adequate treatment of sleep-disordered breathing. We have explored CSF hypocretin-1 levels in such cases, and have found that some but not all of these patients have very low CSF Hcrt-1 levels (< 110 pg/mL), suggesting hypocretin deficiency [2]. Similarly, in one case of late-onset Congenital Hypoventilation Syndrome, a disorder with reported hypothalamic abnormalities [37], we found very low CSF Hypocretin-1 levels in an individual with otherwise unexplained sleepiness and cataplexy-like episodes [2]. Excellent response to anti-cataplectic therapy was observed in this case.

Pharmacological Studies: Monoaminergic and Cholinergic Interactions in Hypocretin Deficiency

In the past, the most commonly prescribed anti-cataplectic agents were tricyclic antidepressants (TCAs). These compounds have complex pharmacological profiles which include monoamine (serotonin, norepinephrine, epinephrine and dopamine) re-uptake inhibition, and for older TCAs, cholinergic, histaminic and alpha-adrenergic blocking effects [38]. Using narcoleptic canines, we found that inhibition of adrenergic but not dopaminergic or serotoninergic re-uptake or other properties is critical to explain anti-cataplectic efficacy for antidepressant compounds. This observation fits well with available human pharmacological data [38] as protriptyline, desipramine, viloxazine, and atomoxetine, four adrenergic-specific uptake blockers with no effect on serotonin transmission, are effective and potent anti-cataplectic agents. In contrast, fluoxetine and other specific serotonin reuptake inhibitors (SSRIs) are only active on cataplexy at relatively high doses, an effect likely to be mediated by the weak adrenergic uptake effects of these compounds and their metabolites [39]. A typical and very effective anti-cataplectic compound now commonly used is venlafaxine, a dual serotonin and noreprinephrine re-uptake blocker.

Commonly prescribed stimulants include amphetamine-like drugs, such as dextroamphetamine, methamphetamine, methylphenidate, pemoline and modafinil. Like tricyclic antidepressant compounds, amphetamine-like drugs are very nonspecific pharmacologically. Their main effect is to globally increase monoaminergic transmission by stimulating monoamine release and blocking monoamine re-uptake. Abuse and dose escalation can occur with amphetamine, especially in cases without cataplexy and when using short acting formulations. Less abuse is reported with methylphenidate, while modafinil is believed to have very little addictive potential, if any. Recent studies have demonstrated that the wake-promoting effect of these compounds is secondary to stimulation of dopamine release and re-uptake inhibition [40, 41]. The mode of action of modafinil is still unclear; this compound seems to also selectively inhibit dopamine re-uptake [42]. All these compounds are ineffective in dopamine transporter knock-out mice, suggesting a primary mediation of wake promotion *via* dopaminergic systems [41]. Interestingly, compounds selective for dopaminergic transmission have no effect on cataplexy whereas amphetamine-like compounds with combined dopaminergic and adrenergic effects have some anti-cataplectic properties at high doses [39]. Adrenergic effects of amphetamine-like stimulants also correlate with the respective effects of these compounds on normal REM sleep [38]. Dopaminergic specific uptake blockers have little effect on REM sleep when compared to adrenergic or serotoninergic compounds [38]. The most important effects of dopaminergic re-uptake blockers is to reduce total sleep time and slow wave sleep. This preferential effect of dopaminergic uptake blockers on NREM sleep correlates with electrophysiological data. As opposed to adrenergic or serotoninergic neurons, the firing rate of dopaminergic neurons is known to remain relatively constant during REM sleep [38].

Gamma-hydroxybutyric (GHB) acid, also called sodium oxybate, is a sedative anesthetic compound known to increase slow wave sleep, and to a lesser extent REM sleep [38]. Occasional abuse in the context of rave parties has been reported and the prescription of the compound is highly supervised. Because slow wave sleep is associated with growth hormone (GH) release, GHB also induces GH release and has been abused by athletes. When administered at night, it consolidates sleep and improves daytime functioning. Because of its short half-life, it must be administered twice a night. Interestingly, cataplexy and daytime alertness also improve over time, sometimes producing a full therapeutic effect only after several months of treatment and dose adjustments (see the reference Guilleminault *et al* [43]).

The mode of action of GHB on sleep and narcolepsy is unclear. GHB has a major effect on dopamine transmission, reducing firing rate and raising brain content of dopamine [38]. Other effects on opiod, glutamatergic and acetylcholine transmission have been reported [44]. Specific GHB receptors have been identified, but the compound is also a GABA-B agonist [44]. Most studies to date suggest that the sedative hypnotic effect is mediated *via* GABA-B agonist activity [44, 45]. Whether this effect also mediates the anti-cataplectic effects after long term administration is unknown. Human or animal studies using other GABA-B agonists, for example high-dose baclofen (another GABA-B agonist), would be needed to answer these questions.

The effects of more than 200 compounds with various modes of action have been examined in human patients and narcoleptic canines (see the reference by Nishino *et al* [38] for review). Almost all the effects have been reported for monoaminergic and cholinergic compounds. These systems have been studied more intensively than others because selective pharmacological probes for these systems are generally available. With cataplexy being easier to study than sleep in canines, most studies have also focused on cataplexy rather than sleepiness. For cataplexy, the findings were generally consistent with pharmacological studies of REM sleep. As is the case for REM sleep, the regulation of cataplexy is modulated positively by cholinergic systems and negatively by monoaminergic tone [38]. Muscarinic M2 or M3 receptors are mediating the cholinergic effects, while monoaminergic effects are mostly modulated by postsynaptic adrenergic alpha-1 receptors and presynaptic D2/D3 autoreceptors [38].

A number of studies have shown abnormal cholinergic and monoaminergic receptor density and neurotransmitter levels in human or canine narcolepsy brain and CSF samples [38]. Local injection studies in selected brain areas of narcoleptic canines (basal forebrain and brainstem) have also shown functional relevance for some of these abnormalities. As a result, cholinergic hypersensitivity, dopaminergic abnormalities and decreased histaminergic tone are likely to be critical downstream mediators of the expression of the narcolepsy symptomatology. The cholinergic/monoaminergic imbalances observed in narcolepsy are best illustrated by the finding that in asymptomatic heterozygote animals for the hypocretin receptor-2 mutation, a combination of cholinergic agonists with an alpha-1 blocker or a D2/D3 agonist can trigger cataplexy [46].

RESEARCH OUTLOOK

What do we know:

The cause of most narcolepsy without cataplexy cases is unknown, and there is no clear therapeutic protocol to follow for these patients. There is not a single NIH grant funded to exclusively study narcolepsy without cataplexy or idiopathic hypersomnia and much research is needed in this area. Regarding narcolepsy with hypocretin deficiency, rapid progress is being made, although funding for this pathology is limited to a few researchers. Additional genetic and immunology research is likely to lead to better diagnostic tests and possibly preventive strategies. Treatments to date are mostly pharmacologically based and do not directly act on the hypocretin system. Future therapies based on CNS-penetrating hypocretin agonists in established cases, and immune suppression in recent onset cases, are a logical next step in narcolepsy/hypocretin deficiency.

What we don't know:

What is the clinical spectrum of the hypocretin deficiency syndrome?

In almost all cases with cataplexy, and rare (~5-15%) cases without clear cataplexy, narcolepsy is associated with HLA-DQB1*0602 and a profound deficiency in the hypothalamic neuropeptide system hypocretin (orexin) [10]. The cause of hypocretin deficiency is an autoimmune attack directed against hypocretin cells. It is however still uncertain whether many more cases without cataplexy may have partial hypocretin cell loss, with only sleepiness and SOREMPs as a result. Most probably, only a fraction of narcolepsy/no cataplexy subjects have partial hypocretin cell loss of autoimmune origin, but the percentage of subject is low [10]. The new findings of autoantibodies in narcolepsy may be give new insight into this question [30].

What are the other causes of narcolepsy, especially narcolepsy without cataplexy?

As mentioned above, it is likely that narcolepsy without cataplexy is an artificial construct encompassing a large number of problems. In some cases, the MSLT may have been positive by chance and sleepiness can be due to associated sleep disordered breathing, psychiatric issues (psychiatry, anxiety), circadian disturbances, and sleep deprivation/insufficient or disturbed nocturnal sleep. A combination of multiple issues is not uncommon. Other cases may be postinfectious, and with CNS pathologies of unknown etiologies. A recent study has shown decreased histamine levels in the CSF of such patients, suggesting histamine abnormalities [47]. These cases are often more difficult to treat, and evolution is unpredictable (from chronic drug resistance to spontaneous remission). There is a critical need for studying these cases at the genetic, pathophysiological and therapeutic levels.

What treatments do we want to develop: hypocretin supplementation?

In narcolepsy/hypocretin deficiency, ~80% of patients can recover ~80% functioning with adequate therapy (behavioral, antidepressant, stimulants, sodium oxybate). Developing hypocretin-based therapies would likely be almost curative for these patients. Experiments aimed at studying the effects of hypocretins on sleep after systemic and central (e.g., intracerebroventricular injection and/or local perfusion in selected brain areas) administration have been conducted [48]. Central administration of hypocretin-1, for example in the ventricle of wild type rodents or normal canines, is strongly wake-promoting [48].

Experiments conducted after intravenous (IV) and intracerebroventricular (ICV) administration of hypocretin-1 have been performed in hypocretin deficient narcoleptic dogs and narcoleptic mice [48]. Intravenous administration was not effective, but ICV injection reversed all the symptoms in mice. Unfortunately, injection of hypocretins in human third or lateral ventricles are not a viable option. We attempted intranasal administration in animal models, but results were not encouraging (S. Taheri *et al*, unpublished results). We also examined the possibility of intrathecal administration by implanting a Medtronic pump with catheterization of the cisterna magna in a single hypocretin deficient narcoleptic canine [49]. Our hope was that at high dose, some reverse flow would occur back into deeper brain structure, providing therapeutic relief. A positive result would have had therapeutic application, as these pumps are frequently used in humans for the treatment of pain or spasticity using intrathecal administration. Disappointingly, we did not observe any significant effect on cataplexy [49], probably because the hypocretin did not diffuse in upper ventricular compartments. Overall, these results strongly suggest that in order to be effective, a CNS penetrating hypocretin agonist will have to be developped. To date, most of the pharmaceutical industry's efforts have been focused on hypocretin antagonists for treatment of insomnia.

What treatments do we want to develop: Other symptomatic treatments?

Additionally, new symptomatically -based therapy could help difficult cases, and cases without cataplexy [50]. Most of the current efforts are only improving existing therapies, for example developing a longer half-life derivative of modafinil instead of modafinil. Having additional adrenergic re-uptake inhibitors could be helpful. In addition, there are multiple efforts aiming at developing histamine H3 receptor antagonists as wake promoting agents. H3 receptors are autoreceptors and thus blocking H3 increases histamine release, promoting wakefulness [51]. If made available, it is likely these compounds could be helpful in some cases, especially in cases with narcolepsy without cataplexy or hypersomnia [50].

What treatments do we want to develop: immune therapies?

The proof of an autoimmune basis of narcolepsy pathogenesis raises the possibility that, if narcolepsy is diagnosed close to onset, it could be stopped. In one case, 2 months after an abrupt onset, we tried high-dose prednisone but did not observe significant effects on symptoms and CSF Hcrt-1 levels [52]; however, in this case, very low hypocretin-1 levels were already observed, suggesting the possibility that irreversible damage to cells had already occurred. In another cases with recent onset, intravenous immunoglobulin administration (IVIG) was reported to have positive effects, suggesting the need for further studies [53], [54]. In our experience, IVIG had a marginal effect, and at best delayed the development of the full-blown syndrome. There is a need for a double-blind placebo study to address this therapeutic modality.

More interestingly, the discovery of the TCR association with narcolepsy suggests that a specific TCR idiotype could be involved in triggering the autoimmune attack. It may therefore be possible to use drugs suppressing T cell function, or even eventually an antibody directed against the TCR idiotype, that could block the disease from further developing. All these therapies, if successful, will have to be administered early in the course of the disease, thus most likely effort at early diagnosis and prevention are needed (see below).

How can we better diagnose narcolepsy with hypocretin deficiency?

Measuring blood hypocretin levels has been tried repetitively. To date, preliminary results suggested that very low and variable levels of hypocretin-1 are present in blood, but they do not seem to be decreased in narcolepsy. Nonetheless, it may be possible to design an essay measuring in the blood small amounts of a CNS-derived hypocretin metabolite.

Ongoing genome-wide association studies may reveal additional genetic factors involved in narcolepsy. In the future, using HLA and TCR genotyping, it may be possible to gauge an approximate individual risk to develop narcolepsy. This way, high-risk subjects could be better monitored and possibly treated more aggressively when they develop a specific streptococcal or viral infection.

The discovery of anti-tribbles 2 antibodies in the pathogenesis of narcolepsy is likely only a beginning; more autoantibodies are likely to be discovered. Most of the anti-tribbles 2 positive subjects had onset within 3 years, but only 30% of these subjects had detectable levels[30]; hence, without improving the test's performance, it is not likely to have much diagnostic value. It seems likely that the test will be improved, and that other autoantibodies will be discovered, and some of them may become even more predictive. This will likely improve our diagnostic armamentarium for narcolepsy, especially at disease onset.

The discovery of a TCR association may also have diagnostic consequences if one or a few specific TCR recombinants involved in the pathophysiology of narcolepsy is ever characterized. The presence of these autoreactive clones could then be monitored in susceptible individuals (for example, in HLA-positive cases) and, if present before disease onset, suppressed using immune therapies.

Could narcolepsy be the model for other CNS autoimmune diseases?

Interestingly, whereas there are hundreds of known HLA-associated autoimmune diseases affecting other organs, very few autoimmune diseases are known to affect neurons, the most complex antigenic cells. One likely explanation is the presence of the blood-brain barrier, which may need other co-factors to facilitate penetration, such as infections with fever or head trauma. In the case of narcolepsy, the phenotype of hypocretin deficiency with cataplexy may have the fortune of being very unique, thus allowing its recognition among other conditions presenting with hypersomnia. In many other cases of brain lesions or animal knock-out models, symptoms are non specific or well compensated, thus most autoimmune brain diseases may have been conjoined with or mislabeled as other conditions, such as depression or schizophrenia. In favor of this hypothesis is the recent finding of a signal in the HLA complex in several recent genome wide association studies of schizophrenia [55]. It is also possible that neurons are protected against epitope spreading because of their inability to express HLA class II and regenerate, and thus autoimmune insults typically remain very specific when affecting the respective neurons.

The discovery of a specific HLA molecule DQB1*0602 and possibly a specific TCR idiotype in narcolepsy may finally offer the opportunity for the first time to understand how HLA alleles actually predispose to autoimmune disorders.

REFERENCES

[1]   Medicine AAoS. ICSD-2. International Classification of Sleep Disorders, 2nd Edition: Diagnostic and Coding Manual. Westchester, Illinois: American Academy of Sleep Medicine; 2005.
[2]   Mignot E, Lammers GJ, Ripley B, *et al.* The role of cerebrospinal fluid hypocretin measurement in the diagnosis of narcolepsy and other hypersomnias. Arch Neurol 2002; 59: 1553-62.
[3]   Mignot E, Lin L, Rogers W *et al.* Complex HLA-DR and -DQ interactions confer risk of narcolepsy-cataplexy in three ethnic groups. Am J Hum Genet 2001; 68: 686-99.
[4]   Hublin C, Kaprio J, Partinen M, *et al.* Daytime sleepiness in an adult, Finnish population. J Intern Med 1996; 239:417-23.
[5]   Mignot E. Genetic and familial aspects of narcolepsy. Neurology 1998; 50: S16-22.
[6]   Longstreth WT, Jr. , Ton TG, Koepsell T, *et al.* Prevalence of narcolepsy in King County, Washington, USA. Sleep Med 2008.
[7]   Silber MH, Krahn LE, Olson EJ, Pankratz VS. The epidemiology of narcolepsy in Olmsted County, Minnesota: a population-based study. Sleep 2002; 25: 197-202.
[8]   Mignot E, Hayduk R, Black J *et al.* HLA DQB1*0602 is associated with cataplexy in 509 narcoleptic patients. Sleep 1997; 20: 1012-20.
[9]   Chen W, Mignot E. Narcolepsy and hypersomnia of central origin: Diagnosis, Differential Pearls, and Management. In: Barkoukis T, Avidan A, Eds. Review of Sleep Medicine. 2nd ed. Philadelphia: Butterworth Heinman Elsevier; 2007. pp. 75-94.
[10]   Bourgin P, Zeitzer JM, Mignot E. CSF hypocretin-1 assessment in sleep and neurological disorders. Lancet Neurol 2008; 7: 649-62.
[11]   Dauvilliers Y, Billiard M, Montplaisir J. Clinical aspects and pathophysiology of narcolepsy. Clin Neurophysiol 2003; 114: 2000-17.
[12]   Okun ML, Lin L, Pelin Z, *et al.* Clinical aspects of narcolepsy-cataplexy across ethnic groups. Sleep 2002; 25: 27-35.
[13]   Orellana C, Villemin E, Tafti M, *et al.* Life events in the year preceding the onset of narcolepsy. Sleep 1994; 17: S50-3.
[14]   Dauvilliers Y, Carlander B, Molinari N, *et al.* Month of birth as a risk factor for narcolepsy. Sleep 2003; 26: 663-665.
[15]   Ton TG, Longstreth WT, Jr. , Koepsell T. Active and Passive Smoking and Risk of Narcolepsy in People with HLA DQB1*0602: A Population-Based Case-Control Study. Neuroepidemiology 2008; 32: 114-121.
[16]   Longstreth WT, Jr. , Ton TG, Koepsell TD. Narcolepsy and streptococcal infections. Sleep 2009; 32: 1548.
[17]   Aran A, Lin L, Nevsimalova S, *et al.* Elevated anti-streptococcal antibodies in patients with recent narcolepsy onset. Sleep 2009; 32: 979-83.

[18] Dauvilliers Y, Montplaisir J, Cochen V, *et al.* Post-H1N1 narcolepsy-cataplexy. Sleep 2010; 33: 1428-30.

[19] Ripley B, Fujiki N, Okura M, *et al.* Hypocretin levels in sporadic and familial cases of canine narcolepsy. Neurobiol Dis 2001; 8: 525-34.

[20] Hungs M, Fan J, Lin L, *et al.* Identification and functional analysis of mutations in the hypocretin (orexin) genes of narcoleptic canines. Genome Res 2001; 11: 531-9.

[21] Lin L, Faraco J, Li R, *et al.* The sleep disorder canine narcolepsy is caused by a mutation in the hypocretin (orexin) receptor 2 gene. Cell 1999; 98: 365-76.

[22] Chemelli RM, Willie JT, Sinton CM, *et al.* Narcolepsy in orexin knockout mice: molecular genetics of sleep regulation. Cell 1999; 98: 437-51.

[23] Hara J, Beuckmann CT, Nambu T, *et al.* Genetic ablation of orexin neurons in mice results in narcolepsy, hypophagia, and obesity. Neuron 2001; 30: 345-54.

[24] Peyron C, Faraco J, Rogers W, *et al.* A mutation in a case of early onset narcolepsy and a generalized absence of hypocretin peptides in human narcoleptic brains. Nat Med 2000; 6: 991-7.

[25] Olafsdottir BR, Rye DB, Scammell TE, *et al.* Polymorphisms in hypocretin/orexin pathway genes and narcolepsy. Neurology 2001; 57: 1896-9.

[26] Thannickal TC, Moore RY, Nienhuis R, *et al.* Reduced number of hypocretin neurons in human narcolepsy. Neuron 2000; 27: 469-74.

[27] Scammell TE. The frustrating and mostly fruitless search for an autoimmune cause of narcolepsy. Sleep 2006; 29: 601-2.

[28] Overeem S, Steens SC, Good CD, *et al.* Voxel-based morphometry in hypocretin-deficient narcolepsy. Sleep 2003; 26: 44-6.

[29] Hallmayer J, Faraco J, Lin L, *et al.* Narcolepsy is strongly associated with the T-cell receptor alpha locus. Nat Genet 2009; 41: 708-11.

[30] Cvetkovic-Lopes V, Bayer L, Dorsaz S, *et al.* Elevated Tribbles homolog 2-specific antibody levels in narcolepsy patients. J Clin Invest.

[31] Mignot E. A hundred years of narcolepsy research. Arch Ital Biol 2001; 139: 207-20.

[32] Melberg A, Ripley B, Lin L *et al.* Hypocretin deficiency in familial symptomatic narcolepsy. Ann Neurol 2001; 49: 136-7.

[33] Hor H, Vicário JL, C. P *et al.* Familial narcolepsy, obesity, and type 2 diabetes with hypocretin deficiency. The European Journal of Medical Sciences 2008; 138: 5S.

[34] Nelson GB, Hahn JS. Stimulus-induced drop episodes in Coffin-Lowry syndrome. Pediatrics 2003; 111: 197-202.

[35] Parkes JD. Genetic factors in human sleep disorders with special reference to Norrie disease, Prader-Willi syndrome and Moebius syndrome. J Sleep Res 1999; 8 (Suppl 1): 14-22.

[36] Martinez-Rodriguez JE, Lin L, Iranzo A *et al.* Decreased hypocretin-1 (Orexin-A) levels in the cerebrospinal fluid of patients with myotonic dystrophy and excessive daytime sleepiness. Sleep 2003; 26: 287-90.

[37] Katz ES, McGrath S, Marcus CL. Late-onset central hypoventilation with hypothalamic dysfunction: a distinct clinical syndrome. Pediatr Pulmonol 2000; 29: 62-8.

[38] Nishino S, Mignot E. Pharmacological aspects of human and canine narcolepsy. Prog Neurobiol 1997; 52: 27-78.

[39] Mignot E, Renaud A, Nishino S, *et al.* Canine cataplexy is preferentially controlled by adrenergic mechanisms: evidence using monoamine selective uptake inhibitors and release enhancers. Psychopharmacology (Berl) 1993; 113: 76-82.

[40] Nishino S, Mao J, Sampathkumaran R, Shelton J. Increased dopaminergic transmission mediates the wake-promoting effects of CNS stimulants. Sleep Res Online 1998; 1: 49-61.

[41] Wisor JP, Nishino S, Sora I, *et al.* Dopaminergic role in stimulant-induced wakefulness. J Neurosci 2001; 21: 1787-94.

[42] Mignot E, Nishino S, Guilleminault C, Dement WC. Modafinil binds to the dopamine uptake carrier site with low affinity. Sleep 1994; 17: 436-7.

[43] Guilleminault C. Narcolepsy Syndrome. In: Kryger MH, Roth T, Dement WC, Eds. Principles and Practice of Sleep Medicine. Philadelphia: W. B. Saunders Co. ; 2003.

[44] Castelli MP, Ferraro L, Mocci I *et al.* Selective gamma-hydroxybutyric acid receptor ligands increase extracellular glutamate in the hippocampus, but fail to activate G protein and to produce the sedative/hypnotic effect of gamma-hydroxybutyric acid. J Neurochem 2003; 87: 722-32.

[45] Queva C, Bremner-Danielsen M, Edlund A *et al.* Effects of GABA agonists on body temperature regulation in GABA(B(1))-/- mice. Br J Pharmacol 2003; 140: 315-22.

[46] Mignot E, Nishino S, Sharp LH, *et al.* Heterozygosity at the canarc-1 locus can confer susceptibility for narcolepsy: induction of cataplexy in heterozygous asymptomatic dogs after administration of a combination of drugs acting on monoaminergic and cholinergic systems. J Neurosci 1993; 13: 1057-64.

[47] Nishino S, Sakurai E, Nevsimalova S, *et al.* Decreased CSF histamine in narcolepsy with and without low CSF hypocretin-1 in comparison to healthy controls. Sleep 2009; 32: 175-80.

[48] Nishino S, Fujiki N, Yoshida Y, Mignot E. The effects of hypocretin-1 in hypocretin receptor-2 mutated and hypocretin deficient narcoleptic dogs. Sleep 2003; 26: A287.

[49] Schatzberg SJ, Barrett J, Cutter K, *et al.* The effect of hypocretin replacement therapy in a 3-year-old weimaraner with narcolepsy. J Vet Intern Med 2004; 18: 586-8.

[50] Mignot E, Nishino S. Emerging therapies in narcolepsy-cataplexy. Sleep 2005; 28: 754-63.

[51] Lin JS, Dauvilliers Y, Arnulf I, *et al.* An inverse agonist of the histamine H(3) receptor improves wakefulness in narcolepsy: studies in orexin-/- mice and patients. Neurobiol Dis 2008; 30: 74-83.

[52] Hecht M, Lin L, Kushida CA, *et al.* Report of a case of immunosuppression with prednisone in an 8-year-old boy with an acute onset of hypocretin-deficient narcolepsy. Sleep 2003; 26: 809-810.

[53] Lecendreux M, Maret S, Bassetti C, *et al.* Clinical efficacy of high-dose intravenous immunoglobulins near the onset of narcolepsy in a 10-year-old boy. J Sleep Res 2003; 12: 1-2.

[54] Dauvilliers Y, Abril B, Mas E, *et al.* Normalization of hypocretin-1 in narcolepsy after intravenous immunoglobulin treatment. Neurology 2009; 73: 1333-4.

[55] Stefansson H, Ophoff RA, Steinberg S, *et al.* Common variants conferring risk of schizophrenia. Nature 2009; 460: 744-7.

CHAPTER 12

Idiopathic Hypersomnia

Dan Cohen, M.D.[1,*], Asim Roy, M.D.[2] and Randip Singh, M.D.[3]

[1]*Instructor in Neurology, Harvard Medical School - Beth Israel Deaconess Medical Center, Associate Physician, Brigham and Women's Hospital, Boston, MA, USA;* [2]*Assistant Clinical Professor of Neurology, University of Pittsburgh Medical Center, Pittsburgh, PA, USA and* [3]*Overlake Sleep Disorders Center, Bellevue, WA, USA*

Abstract: Idiopathic hypersomnia is a primary sleep disorder of central nervous system origin. It is an uncommon sleep disorder. However, it impacts patients significantly in their day to day activity. It is seen less frequently than narcolepsy. It is described clinically with excessive daytime sleepiness, often prolonged episodes of non-refreshing sleep, prolonged naps and difficulty in awakening from sleep. The difficulty awakening from sleep is often labeled as "sleep drunkenness". At this time, the pathophysiology of this disorder is not well understood. It is very important to exclude other potential causes and therefore is a diagnosis of exclusion. Treatment for this disorder is in the similar algorithm as patients with narcolepsy; however the response is not consistent. Therefore, this specific disorder is one of the frustrations for most clinicians who treat these patients. This section will review the epidemiology, pathogenesis, clinical features, diagnostic criteria, differential diagnosis, treatment and future outlook of this frustrating disorder.

TOPIC DISCUSSION (CLINICAL OUTLOOK)

Introduction

As the name implies, idiopathic hypersomnia is a sleep disorder of unknown etiology, characterized by excessive sleepiness and yet poorly understood. It was first described by Bedric Roth in the 1950's [1, 2]. He based this description on extensive histories on over 600 patients. Naps and nocturnal sleep periods are often prolonged in duration, usually very efficient and uninterrupted. Sleep inertia and morning awakenings are possible associated symptoms in these individuals. Idiopathic hypersomnia may be considered a heterogenous nosologic category and, therefore, diagnosis, epidemiology, and defining characteristics remain somewhat obscure. The diagnosis of the condition is generally established after exclusion of other causes of excessive daytime sleepiness (EDS) [3]. Several clinical (sub)types have been described. However, the lack of distinct clinical features, pathognomic markers or specific laboratory tests makes the diagnosis difficult. It shares several features with narcolepsy, such as: similar age of onset, chronicity, and short mean sleep latencies. Nevertheless, several features may constitute very distinct differences and will be discussed further in this chapter.

Epidemiology

There have not been any proper studies looking at the prevalence of idiopathic hypersomnia. The difficulty in establishing consistent criteria for diagnosis has clearly been a limiting factor. Therefore, this remains yet undetermined. It was estimated that in a sleep clinic patient population, the condition is at about $1/10^{th}$ as common as narcolepsy [4]. On the other hand, another study suggested that idiopathic hypersomnia occurs at about 40 to 60% as often as narcolepsy [5]. The gender distribution is felt to be equal. While the age of onset of typical symptoms is variable, the usual age of onset is during adolescence to early adulthood. The symptom progression is insidious in nature, typically occurring over weeks to months; afterwards, the symptoms typically remain stable and become chronic. There is a small subset of patients who may have spontaneous resolution of symptoms [6].

Clinical Features

Excessive daytime sleepiness (EDS) represents the salient clinical feature. The hypersomnolence occurs despite a normal overnight sleep architecture, excellent efficiency and fairly normal sleep duration, and often with longer total

---

*Address correspondence to Dan Cohen:** Instructor in Neurology, Harvard Medical School - Beth Israel Deaconess Medical Center, Associate Physician, Brigham and Women's Hospital, Boston, MA, USA; E-mail: dcohen2@bidmc.harvard.edu

sleep times. Patients endorse symptoms related to hypersomnia, in particular having difficulty waking up, non-restorative napping, wanting to go back to sleep, and therefore, "sleep inertia" or "sleep drunkenness" as a prominent complaint. The symptoms are generally experienced daily. Co-morbid depression is not uncommon in this setting and the higher depression and anxiety scores, the more disabling this condition tends to be [7]. Inappropriate "microsleeps" are dangerous and automatic behaviors are often described by patients. Hypnagogic hallucinations and sleep paralysis are more common than in normal individuals. Idiopathic hypersomnia with a long sleep time is more often associated with an evening chronotype. They tend to have delayed sleep phase type circadian pattern. The typical onset is in childhood and generally becomes a lifelong disorder; however, some series suggest improvement may occur in up to 25% [7]. There are two (sub)types, that have been differentiated based on whether the sleep is long (>10 hours) or not [8]. One study suggests that hypersomniacs with long sleep time were younger (29 ± 10 vs. 40 ± 13 years), slimmer (body mass index: 26 ± 5 vs 23 ± 4 kg/m^2), and had lower Horne-Ostberg scores and higher sleep efficiencies than those without long sleep time [9].

Pathophysiology

This has remained highly elusive and currently is still unknown. Daytime sleepiness often occurs after an infection (most likely viral), surgery, mild head trauma or episodes of over-exhaustion [6]. About half of the cases have some familial component [10]. There has been an association with diabetes [6]. A hypothalamic disorder has been proposed by some, but this is still speculative. The hypothalamic areas involved in the control of food intake (hunger and satiety centers) and the areas active in the metabolic regulation are not felt to be affected since being overweight has not been associated with this condition [6].

There have been multiple studies reporting an over-representation of HLA-DQ1, DR5 and DQ3 phenotypes [6, 7]. The HLA DQB1*0602 phenotype, described in narcolepsy, has been found equally represented in hypersomniacs and controls. The observation merits a note that these genetic-based evaluations have been relatively inconsistent [6] Therefore, HLA typing is not currently recommended in the diagnosis of idiopathic hypersomnia.

Cerebrospinal fluid (CSF) analysis has shown normal cell counts, protein and glucose levels. Several studies have also shown abnormal regulation of dopamine and norepinephrine, which suggests abnormal functioning of the arousal system [11]. Furthermore, circadian and homeostatic control abnormalities have been suggested [12]. It has been reported that idiopathic hypersomnia patients have phase delays in their melatonin and cortisol secretion patterns [13]. CSF hypocretin-1 levels have been shown to have utility in the diagnosis of narcolepsy with cataplexy [14]. However, most studies looking at CSF hypocretin-1 levels in idiopathic hypersomnia have found normal levels [15].

Diagnosis

Over the years, there have been many modifications to the diagnostic criteria of idiopathic hypersomnia. Furthermore, there have been very few studies to help with the diagnosis of idiopathic hypersomnia. The International Classification of Sleep Disorders (ICSD-2) has recently established updated guidelines for the diagnosis of idiopathic hypersomnia [8]. According to this classification, there are two (sub)types of idiopathic hypersomnia, one with long sleep time and one with short sleep time. Patients with the long sleep type variant typically sleep more than 10 hours. The short sleep time variant patient sleeps less than 10 hours, but more than 6 hours. Key diagnostic features include: excessive daytime sleepiness (EDS), prolonged naps that are typically not refreshing, difficulty awakening in the morning, usually begins before the age of 30, must last more than 6 months and exclusion of other causes of hypersomnia [8]. The Epworth Sleepiness Scale (ESS) is a useful, well validated scale to help understand the subjective degree of sleepiness in a patient [16]. An overnight polysomnogram is typically required to exclude other causes of hypersomnia.

It is recommended that patients maintain a sleep diary or are studied with actigraphy for 1 to 2 weeks prior to the study [17]. The latter can show the patient's usual sleep-wake schedules (if regular) and possibly point out towards other problems (light exposure, sleep fragmentation, etc). Some studies and authors have advocated the use of 24-hour continuous polysomnography monitoring, although this is not cost-effective [10].

Medication use should also be ascertained thoroughly and the ones that are known to affect nocturnal sleep, sleep onset and/or alertness should be discontinued for at least 2 weeks prior to testing (depending on their pharmacokinetics). It is also often recommended to perform a urine toxicology screen on the day of the testing. Overnight sleep studies are typically normal in this population, except for the long duration, increased stage N3 sleep and (often) high sleep efficiencies [3, 6]. However, these findings are nonspecific and cannot solely be used in diagnosis. Other sleep disorders should be excluded during the sleep study. Not uncommon, the presence of periodic limb movements without restless legs symptoms can be observed [18]. A Multiple Sleep Latency Test (MSLT) is typically performed the next day. The mean sleep latency is usually between 5 to 10 minutes in idiopathic hypersomnia, however there are patients that fall on either side of that range. In one study, only about 4% of patients had sleep-onset REM periods during the MSLTs [6]. Unfortunately, there are multiple inherent limitations to the overnight sleep studies and the MSLTs. The primary limitation is the duration of the study; typically the patient cannot have a prolonged sleep period during the overnight portion, and the nap tests are limited to 20 minutes, which are typically much shorter than the reported longer duration naps these patients take. Therefore, it is possible that these patients can have normal sleep studies.

Differential Diagnosis

Many conditions need to be excluded before establishing a diagnosis of idiopathic hypersomnia (see Tables **1** and **2**).

Table 1. Narcolepsy vs. Idiopathic Hypersomnia – clinical features

Differentiating features	**Narcolepsy**	**Idiopathic Hypersomnia**
EDS	Yes	Yes
Sleep Paralysis	Yes	Not usual
Hypnogogic Hallucinations	Yes	Not usual
Cataplexy	Yes	No
Sleep Drunkenness	Not usual	Often seen
Disrupted Night Sleep	Yes	Not usual
Nap Duration	Short, Brief (20 minutes)	Long (few hours)
Naps refreshing	Often	Not usual
Total Sleep Times	<10 hours	>10 hours (typically)

Table 2. Hypersomnia – differential diagnosis

Narcolepsy with or without cataplexy
Idiopathic Hypersomnia with or without long sleep times
Chronic sleep insufficiency
Long sleeper
Sleep disordered breathing (including UARS)
Hyperomnia associated with psychiatric disorder
Chronic Fatigue Sydrome
Postviral Hypersomnia
Circadian Rhythm Disorders
Hypersomnia associated with neurologic disorders
Periodic or Recurrent Hypersomnia (Kleine-Levin syndrome, hypersomnia associated with menstrual cycle)
Medications/Drugs

Narcolepsy is the most common diagnosis considered on the differential list, especially narcolepsy without cataplexy. However, in the setting of daytime sleepiness, definite cataplexy, at least two sleep-onset REM periods on MSLT and/or decreased CSF hypocretin-1 levels, the diagnosis of narcolepsy is definitive. There are patients with idiopathic hypersomnia that have sleep attacks and also have short refreshing naps, and there are patients with narcolepsy that have long non-refreshing naps and extended nocturnal sleep periods [4, 5, 19]. If cataplexy is not present or it is atypical in description, then sleep-onset REM periods on MSLT and the presence of HLA DQB1*0602 are helpful to differentiate narcolepsy from idiopathic hypersomnia. CSF hypocretin-1 levels are not helpful in distinguishing these two diagnoses, since it is usually normal in both populations [20].

Another diagnosis in the differential is chronic sleep insufficiency in long sleepers. Usually, a careful history is adequate in distinguishing this diagnosis [21]. These individuals typically show on their sleep log a difference of at least 2 hours between their weekday and weekend schedule. Occasionally, actigraphy is necessary to help with the diagnosis [22]. It is important to recognize that these patients improve symptomatically when they are allowed to sleep their desired sleep duration.

Sleep disordered breathing and upper airway resistance syndrome are also to be considered in the differential diagnosis. However, clinically, these patients complain of daytime sleepiness associated with snoring; overnight polysomnography should identify these patients. It has been suggested that in patients with snoring and idiopathic hypersomnia, a trial of positive pressure may be recommended [6].

Several psychiatric disorders may also be associated with hypersomnia, as many symptoms can overlap. These are typically EDS, long unrefreshing naps, long sleep periods, and even sleep inertia. Overnight sleep study findings in patients with psychiatric disorders generally are increased N1 sleep and decreased N3 sleep. The mean sleep latency tends to be normal in most cases. It has been reported however that psychiatric disorders may have abnormal MSLT findings and idiopathic hypersomnia cases can have normal sleep latencies on the nap test [23, 24]. Circadian rhythm disorders are typically differentiated by clinical history, sleep log or actigraphy.

Hypersomnia associated with viral syndromes or neurologic disorders can often demonstrate similar presentation as idiopathic hypersomnia does. They often can have prolonged sleep periods, sleep inertia, excessive sleepiness and even have abnormal MSLTs. History, clinical examination and imaging studies may be important differentiating tools in these cases [25-27].

Treatment

Since significant questions remain about disease pathogenesis (hence no available pathogenic therapy), all treatments available are geared towards relieving symptoms.

A first therapeutic modality is to increase sleep duration; although these patients tend to remain symptomatic despite the sleep elongation [6]. Patients should be advised on proper sleep hygiene and behavioral techniques, although these measures usually have minimal impact on their outcome. Naps are encouraged (similar to narcolepsy), but these patients tend to have already prolonged non-refreshing naps.

In general, the pharmacologic therapy available for idiopathic hypersomnia is similar to the treatment used for narcolepsy. When the response to therapy for idiopathic hypersomnia is compared to the one for narcolepsy, idiopathic hypersomnia patients often have less of a response to these treatments. To date, there have only been a handful of studies evaluating medications in idiopathic hypersomnia. One group evaluated 77 patients with idiopathic hypersomnia. This study initiated therapy with modafinil and 70% remained on monotherapy for a median follow-up of almost 4 years. However, 75% of these patients required higher than recommended doses of modafinil, *i.e.*, more than 400 mg per day. About 15% of patients switched to dexamphetamine. Another 10% either added caffeine or dexamphetamine to modafanil due to lack of monotherapy's efficacy [5]. A more recent study demonstrated a "complete response" to any of the medications in about 65% of patients. In this population, the medication dosages were within the typical recommended doses. This study also demonstrated some discordance between response to treatment and Epworth Sleepiness Scale (ESS) changes. There were a significant number of patients on traditional stimulants which have not been evaluated well before. According to this study, methylphenidate as monotherapy may be more effective than modafinil, however these results did not achieve statistical significance [28]. In 2001, Montplaisir *et al* reported that slow-release melatonin administered at bedtime improved symptoms in ten patients suffering from idiopathic hypersomnia [18]. The use of antidepressants may be recommended in patients with overlapping psychiatric disorders prior to stimulant therapy. The use of activating antidepressants would be preferred in this setting. Some patients may have spontaneous symptomatic improvement or even complete resolution, or a more benign clinical course, without a need for long-term stimulant therapy.

RESEARCH OUTLOOK

What do we know:

Fundamentally, the sleep-wake cycle is determined by a switch-like mechanism that is generated by a network of mutually-inhibitory arousal and sleep-promoting circuits [29]. Sleep homeostatic and circadian processes regulate the activity of the sleep-wake circuitry to ultimately control the brain state. Sleep homeostasis reflects the sleep-wake history, with increasing pressure to sleep in the setting of sleep loss. The circadian process reflects the near 24-hour intrinsic rhythmic activity of the circadian pacemaker located in the hypothalamic suprachiasmatic nucleus. Conceivably, idiopathic hypersomnia may reflect abnormalities in homeostatic or circadian processes, their interactions, or the integrity of the sleep-wake circuitry itself. It is possible that the phenotypic expression of idiopathic hypersomnia may stem from multiple, distinct underlying mechanisms across individuals with this disorder.

While little is known about the causes of idiopathic hypersomnia, there has been some recent attention to possible abnormalities of sleep homeostasis in this disorder. Following waking activity, sleep appears critical for restoring brain energy metabolism, neuronal reorganization and repair [30, 31]. Sleep homeostasis may therefore be conceptualized as an accumulating need for sleep to (teleologically) facilitate brain recovery. A marker of sleep homeostasis is represented by the slow wave activity (SWA) during sleep electroencephalography (EEG). SWA refers to the spectral power in the frequency range of approximately 0.5-4.5Hz, predominantly seen during NREM slow wave sleep (SWS); SWA increases with the duration of prior wakefulness and dissipates during sleep according to a saturating exponential function [32, 33]. Acoustic suppression of SWA without waking participants during the first 3-5 hours of sleep causes an increase or a rebound in SWA during the subsequent hour of sleep [34]. Knock-out mice that lack the adenosine A1 receptor gene do not have a compensatory rise in SWA during recovery sleep following sleep deprivation, leading to impairments in working memory performance [35]. Conversely, pharmacological enhancement of SWA during shortened sleep opportunities in humans can improve waking performance and counteract some of the negative effects of sleep loss [36]. These data suggest not only that SWA is a marker of the homeostatic need for sleep, but also that the ability to generate adequate SWA is a prerequisite for the homeostatic recovery function of sleep. In a case series of 75 patients with idiopathic hypersomnia, 24-hour PSG showed reduced SWS percentage compared to controls, and the last epochs of SWS occurred later in the morning [9]. The total amount of SWS was normal, but patients with idiopathic hypersomnia had to sleep longer to achieve sufficient amounts of SWS. In another study, patients with idiopathic hypersomnia had lower SWA across the night, particularly in the first two NREM-REM cycles compared to controls [12]; the temporal decline in SWA was preserved. These data suggest that the ability to generate sufficient SWA may be impaired in idiopathic hypersomnia, and patients with this disorder therefore have to sleep longer to dissipate homeostatic sleep pressure.

Idiopathic hypersomnia may reflect a fundamental abnormality of the sleep-wake circuitry. In their spectral analysis study cited above [12], the authors report that reductions in faster frequency rhythms (alpha, beta, sigma bands) were also seen, but did not reach statistical significance. They proposed an alternative explanation for their results: the reduction in faster frequency rhythms may reflect a fundamental problem with arousal circuits in this disorder, causing patients with idiopathic hypersomnia to sleep more. The history of excessive sleep time with potentially normal homeostatic mechanisms would lead to a reduction in the amount of SWA recorded during sleep compared to controls. Therefore, the level of homeostatic pressure may actually be low, yet a fundamental failure of arousal circuits may reduce their level of alertness. Similar to narcolepsy (+/-) cataplexy with normal or reduced hypocretin status, patients with idiopathic hypersomnia have lower levels of CSF histamine than controls and hypersomnia from sleep apnea, a non-central cause of hypersomnia [37]. Reduced CSF histamine is believed to reflect the activity of histaminergic arousal circuits [38]. Although the significance of the reduced CSF histamine in idiopathic hypersomnia is not entirely clear, it may be consistent with the hypothesis that idiopathic hypersomnia reflects an abnormality in arousal circuits.

What we don't know:

Is idiopathic Hypersomnia an Extreme form of "Long Sleepers"?

The amount of sleep individuals need on a consistent basis to maintain normal cognitive, mood, cardiovascular, immune, and metabolic function varies along a spectrum. Individuals that are considered long sleepers are considered to be at one extreme of the normal physiological spectrum; long sleepers have normal daytime functioning, provided that they consistently meet their sleep needs. In contrast, patients with idiopathic hypersomnia report feeling sleepy, despite consistent extended sleep durations. It is not clear whether there are any common or overlapping mechanisms in idiopathic hypersomnia and long sleepers. It has been proposed that long sleepers may have a longer biological night than normal, a circadian factor that leads to extended sleep durations [39]. It is currently unknown whether patients with idiopathic hypersomnia have circadian abnormalities, and circadian protocols in idiopathic hypersomnia are necessary. Long sleepers are capable of generating compensatory increases in SWA following sleep deprivation. In fact, following 40 hours of continuous wakefulness, naturally long compared to short sleepers had a 2-fold greater relative increase in the amount of NREM SWA; the time constant for the decline in SWA, which reflects the dissipation of homeostatic sleep pressure across the sleep episode, did not differ between long and short sleepers [40]. Therefore, long sleepers do not appear to have abnormalities in homeostatic mechanisms; the authors concluded also that shorter sleepers live under and tolerate higher homeostatic sleep pressures compared to longer sleepers. Similar experiments in idiopathic hypersomnia could determine whether the SWA increase in response to sleep restriction is blunted in idiopathic hypersomnia, a finding that would suggest that there is a homeostatic regulatory abnormality in idiopathic hypersomnia and a fundamentally distinct physiology from long sleepers.

Does Idiopathic Hypersomnia Share Mechanisms of Chronic Sleep Loss?

Adenosine concentrations in the brain increase with hours of wakefulness, and this product of brain energy metabolism promotes sleepiness in a negative feedback manner [41-45]. In the setting of extended sleep loss, there is an up-regulation of adenosine receptor density [46, 47] and a functional sensitization of the adenosine system. Therefore, there are multiple homeostatic mechanisms acting on different time scales. In humans, extended sleep episodes may allow complete recovery of a short-term homeostatic process, so that performance soon after waking is restored to normal. However, despite this rapid recovery of short-term homeostatic mechanisms, the cumulative effect of chronic sleep loss over the past several weeks causes performance to deteriorate more rapidly for each hour spent awake [48], consistent with a change in the sensitivity or gain of the homeostatic system [49]. Protocols with idiopathic hypersomnia patients that measure performance shortly after waking from extended sleep episodes and the time course of decline in performance *within* extended wake episodes may determine whether the dynamics of the short or long-term homeostatic processes deviate from normal. Additionally, functional imaging of the adenosine system [50] may assess whether there is increased adenosine receptor binding or an exaggerated up-regulation in response to sleep loss.

Is Sleep Drunkenness an Extreme form of Normal Sleep Inertia?

Sleep drunkenness is a fairly specific finding in idiopathic hypersomnia [5, 9] and is characterized by profound difficulty waking, with confusion, automatic behavior, and repeated returns to sleep. Sleep inertia reflects the cognitive impairment seen shortly after waking that dissipates according to an exponential saturating function over approximately two hours [51]. The mechanisms involved in both phenomena are not clear, but likely reflect asymmetries in tendency of the sleep-wake circuitry to transition between states. Comparison of the time constant of dissipation of sleep inertia in idiopathic hypersomnia compared to healthy controls may be a reasonable first step in understanding the potential relationship between these phenomena.

Are New Drug Targets on the Horizon to Improve the Treatment of Idiopathic Hypersomnia?

CSF concentrations of histamine are reduced in idiopathic hypersomnia, suggesting impaired neurotransmission in the histaminergic arousal circuits [37]. The H_3 receptor is located on pre-synaptic neurons and acts as an autoreceptor, serving as a feedback mechanism to prevent excessive histaminergic neurotransmission. H_3 receptor antagonists increase histamine neurotransmission and enhance wakefulness [52], suggesting a possible new therapeutic target to help these patients. Further advances in the neurobiology of idiopathic hypersomnia can determine other pathways, hence targeting other components of the sleep-wake circuitry, enhancing sleep SWA, manipulating the adenosine system or other homeostatic mechanisms, or modulating the circadian system.

REFERENCES

[1]   Shneerson J, John MS. Sleep medicine: a guide to sleep and its disorders. Malden, Mass: Blackwell Pub 2005. ; vi: pp. 325.
[2]   Passouant P, Billiard M. Narcolepsy. Rev Prat 1976; 26: 1917-23.

[3]   Roth B, Nevsimalova S, Rechtschaffen A. Hypersomnia with "sleep drunkenness". Arch Gen Psychiatry 1972; 26: 456-62.

[4]   Aldrich MS. The clinical spectrum of narcolepsy and idiopathic hypersomnia. Neurology 1996; 46: 393-401.

[5]   Anderson KN, Pilsworth S, Sharples LD, *et al*. Idiopathic hypersomnia: a study of 77 cases. Sleep 2007; 30: 1274-81.

[6]   Bassetti C, Aldrich MS. Idiopathic hypersomnia. A series of 42 patients. Brain 1997; 120 (Pt 8): 1423-35.

[7]   Billiard M. Idiopathic hypersomnia. Neurol Clin 1996; 14: 573-82.

[8]   American Academy of Sleep Medicine. The international classification of sleep disorders : diagnostic and coding manual. Westchester, Ill. : American Academy of Sleep Medicine 2005; xviii: 297.

[9]   Vernet C, Arnulf I. Idiopathic hypersomnia with and without long sleep time: a controlled series of 75 patients. Sleep 2009; 32: 753-9.

[10]   Billiard M, Dauvilliers Y. Idiopathic Hypersomnia. Sleep Med Rev 2001; 5: 349-358.

[11]   Faull KF, Guilleminault C, Berger PA, Barchas JD. Cerebrospinal fluid monoamine metabolites in narcolepsy and hypersomnia. Ann Neurol 1983; 13: 258-63.

[12]   Sforza E, Gaudreau H, Petit D, Montplaisir J. Homeostatic sleep regulation in patients with idiopathic hypersomnia. Clin Neurophysiol 2000; 111: 277-82.

[13]   Nevsimalova S, Blazejova K, Illnerova H, *et al*. A contribution to pathophysiology of idiopathic hypersomnia. Suppl Clin Neurophysiol 2000; 53: 366-70.

[14]   Mignot E. Perspectives in narcolepsy and hypocretin (orexin) research. Sleep Med 2000; 1: 87-90.

[15]   Bassetti C, Gugger M, Bischof M, *et al*. The narcoleptic borderland: a multimodal diagnostic approach including cerebrospinal fluid levels of hypocretin-1 (orexin A). Sleep Med 2003; 4: 7-12.

[16]   Johns MW. A new method for measuring daytime sleepiness: the Epworth sleepiness scale. Sleep 1991; 14: 540-5.

[17]   Frenette E, Kushida CA. Primary hypersomnias of central origin. Semin Neurol 2009; 29: 354-67.

[18]   Montplaisir J, Fantini L. Idiopathic hypersomnia: a diagnostic dilemma. A commentary of "Idiopathic hypersomnia" (M. Billiard and Y. Dauvilliers). Sleep Med Rev 2001; 5: 361-362.

[19]   Sturzenegger C, Bassetti CL. The clinical spectrum of narcolepsy with cataplexy: a reappraisal. J Sleep Res 2004; 13: 395-406.

[20]   Ripley B, Overeem S, Fujiki N, *et al*. CSF hypocretin/orexin levels in narcolepsy and other neurological conditions. Neurology 2001; 57: 2253-8.

[21]   Roehrs T, Zorick F, Sicklesteel J, *et al*. Excessive daytime sleepiness associated with insufficient sleep. Sleep 1983; 6: 319-25.

[22]   Roehrs TA, Roth T. Chronic insufficient sleep and its recovery. Sleep Med 2003; 4: 5-6.

[23]   Billiard M, Dolenc L, Aldaz C, *et al*. Hypersomnia associated with mood disorders: a new perspective. J Psychosom Res 1994; 38 Suppl 1: 41-7.

[24]   Nofzinger EA, Thase ME, Reynolds CF, 3rd *et al*. Hypersomnia in bipolar depression: a comparison with narcolepsy using the multiple sleep latency test. Am J Psychiatry 1991; 148: 1177-81.

[25]   Ulivelli M, Rossi S, Lombardi C *et al*. Polysomnographic characterization of pergolide-induced sleep attacks in idiopathic PD. Neurology 2002; 58: 462-5.

[26]   Bassetti C, Mathis J, Gugger M *et al*. Hypersomnia following paramedian thalamic stroke: a report of 12 patients. Ann Neurol 1996; 39: 471-80.

[27]   Guilleminault C, Mondini S. Mononucleosis and chronic daytime sleepiness. A long-term follow-up study. Arch Intern Med 1986; 146: 1333-5.

[28]   Li M, Auger R R. , Slocumb N L. , Morgenthaler T I. Idiopathic Hypersomnia: clinical features and response to treatment. Journal of Clinical Sleep Medicine 2009; 5: 562-568.

[29]   Saper CB, Scammell TE, Lu J. Hypothalamic regulation of sleep and circadian rhythms. Nature 2005; 437: 1257-63.

[30]   Savage VM, West GB. A quantitative, theoretical framework for understanding mammalian sleep. Proc Natl Acad Sci U S A 2007; 104: 1051-6.

[31]   Tononi G, Cirelli C. Sleep and synaptic homeostasis: a hypothesis. Brain Res Bull 2003; 62: 143-50.

[32]   Borbely AA, Baumann F, Brandeis D, *et al*. Sleep deprivation: effect on sleep stages and EEG power density in man. Electroencephalogr Clin Neurophysiol 1981; 51: 483-95.

[33]   Dijk DJ, Brunner DP, Beersma DG, Borbely AA. Electroencephalogram power density and slow wave sleep as a function of prior waking and circadian phase. Sleep 1990; 13: 430-40.

[34]   Dijk DJ, Beersma DG. Effects of SWS deprivation on subsequent EEG power density and spontaneous sleep duration. Electroencephalogr Clin Neurophysiol 1989; 72: 312-20.

[35]   Bjorness TE, Kelly CL, Gao T, *et al*. Control and function of the homeostatic sleep response by adenosine A1 receptors. J Neurosci 2009; 29: 1267-76.

[36]   Walsh JK, Randazzo AC, Stone K, *et al.* Tiagabine is associated with sustained attention during sleep restriction: evidence for the value of slow-wave sleep enhancement? Sleep 2006; 29: 433-43.

[37]   Kanbayashi T, Kodama T, Kondo H, *et al.* CSF histamine contents in narcolepsy, idiopathic hypersomnia and obstructive sleep apnea syndrome. Sleep 2009; 32: 181-7.

[38]   Soya A, Song YH, Kodama T, *et al.* CSF histamine levels in rats reflect the central histamine neurotransmission. Neurosci Lett 2008; 430: 224-9.

[39]   Aeschbach D, Sher L, Postolache TT, *et al.* A longer biological night in long sleepers than in short sleepers. J Clin Endocrinol Metab 2003; 88: 26-30.

[40]   Aeschbach D, Cajochen C, Landolt H, Borbely AA. Homeostatic sleep regulation in habitual short sleepers and long sleepers. Am J Physiol 1996; 270: R41-53.

[41]   Benington JH, Kodali SK, Heller HC. Stimulation of A1 adenosine receptors mimics the electroencephalographic effects of sleep deprivation. Brain Res 1995; 692: 79-85.

[42]   Benington JH, Heller HC. Restoration of brain energy metabolism as the function of sleep. Prog Neurobiol 1995; 45: 347-60.

[43]   Christie MA, Bolortuya Y, Chen LC, *et al.* Microdialysis elevation of adenosine in the basal forebrain produces vigilance impairments in the rat psychomotor vigilance task. Sleep 2008; 31: 1393-8.

[44]   Landolt HP. Sleep homeostasis: a role for adenosine in humans? Biochem Pharmacol 2008; 75: 2070-9.

[45]   Porkka-Heiskanen T. Adenosine in sleep and wakefulness. Ann Med 1999; 31: 125-9.

[46]   Elmenhorst D, Basheer R, McCarley RW, Bauer A. Sleep deprivation increases A(1) adenosine receptor density in the rat brain. Brain Res 2009; 1258: 53-8.

[47]   Basheer R, Bauer A, Elmenhorst D, *et al.* Sleep deprivation upregulates A1 adenosine receptors in the rat basal forebrain. Neuroreport 2007; 18: 1895-9.

[48]   Cohen DA, Wang W, Wyatt JK, *et al.* Uncovering residual effects of chronic sleep loss on human performance. Sci. Transl. Med 2010; 2: 14ra3.

[49]   McCarley RW. Neurobiology of REM and NREM sleep. Sleep Med 2007; 8: 302-30.

[50]   Elmenhorst D, Meyer PT, Winz OH, *et al.* Sleep deprivation increases A1 adenosine receptor binding in the human brain: a positron emission tomography study. J Neurosci 2007; 27: 2410-5.

[51]   Jewett ME, Wyatt JK, Ritz-De Cecco A, *et al.* Time course of sleep inertia dissipation in human performance and alertness. J Sleep Res 1999; 8: 1-8.

[52]   Bonaventure P, Letavic M, Dugovic C, *et al.* Histamine H3 receptor antagonists: from target identification to drug leads. Biochem Pharmacol 2007; 73: 1084-96.

CHAPTER 13

Sleep-Related Movement Disorders

Brian Koo, M.D.[*]

Assistant Professor of Neurology, Case Western Reserve School of Medicine, 11100 Euclid Avenue, Cleveland OH 44106, USA

Abstract: Under normal circumstances, movement is relatively suppressed during sleep. Motor system activity reflects this paucity of movement as it decreases from drowsiness to slow wave sleep (SWS) and then further in rapid eye movement (REM) sleep. Some movement during sleep in fact is adaptive with small shifts in body weight preventing pressure-related injuries such as nerve palsy and skin ulceration. Other movements occurring during sleep serve no obvious purpose and may even fragment sleep, especially when recurrent. This latter constellation of movements constitutes the sleep-related movement disorders. This chapter will focus on the sleep-related movement disorders which are largely characterized by repetitive, non-epileptic, purposeless movement which occurs during sleep. Many of the sleep-related movement disorders are clinically benign or on the severe end of the normal spectrum and as such our discussion will begin with an introduction to normal movement during sleep. The chapter continues with a discussion of benign sleep-related movement then the clinically recognized sleep-related movement disorders. Special attention will be given to restless legs syndrome (RLS) and periodic limb movement disorder (PLMD) as these entities are both common and a major source of morbidity.

TOPIC DISCUSSION (CLINICAL OUTLOOK)

Normal Motor Physiology and Sleep

Movement is a seemingly simple task which occurs almost simultaneously with thought command. The mechanism of movement is, however, far from simple, as it requires that multiple electrical signals interact precisely and rapidly from pre-motor, motor and cerebellar cortices to basal ganglia, spinal cord, root, nerve and, finally, to muscle. Grossly speaking, the motor system can be broken into central (brain and spinal cord) and peripheral (root, nerve, muscle, *etc.*) components. Across different states of normal consciousness, these divisions of the motor system interact uniquely to either facilitate or inhibit movement.

Over the course of a day, the frequency of movement occurrence is governed by two major influences: circadian rhythmicity and sleep-wake cycling. It is no secret that humans, left unstressed, will sleep at night and remain active during the day. This pattern is maintained by the brain's master circadian clock, the suprachiasmatic nucleus. To a smaller degree, there may be an ultradian effect on the motor system even during the day, coincident with a 90-minute basic rest-activity cycle akin to the cycling of sleep [1]. Of course, this ultradian rhythmicity continues on this 90-minute cycle during sleep as one progresses from light, slow wave and then to REM sleep.

By definition, sleep is characterized by relatively little movement, while wakefulness is accompanied by frequent movement. In the waking moments preceding sleep, movement arrest alternates with only brief periods of activity, as the individual assumes a posture suitable for slumber. On polysomnography, this pattern is seen with low chin and leg electromyographic (EMG) signal, interspersed with short periods of increased signal. As drowsiness ensues, the transition from wake to sleep is often accompanied by a sudden myoclonic flexion of an extremity or of the entire body [2,4]. These hypnic jerks or "sleep starts" are normal, unless occurring frequently with sleep interruption [3].

Initially, as non-rapid-eye-movement (NREM) sleep is achieved, chin and leg EMG signal drops further and is interrupted even less frequently by short periods of increased EMG, coincident only with arousal. Postural changes as well as movement in general decrease in frequency from stage N1, stage N2 to Stage N3 as both central and peripheral motor systems are relatively quiescent [5]. Brief small amplitude movements may occur. These movements, termed sleep myoclonus, resemble fasciculation potentials on EMG and emerge from NREM, but even more so from REM sleep [6].

*Address correspondence to Brian Koo:** Assistant Professor of Neurology, Case Western Reserve School of Medicine, 11100 Euclid Avenue, Cleveland OH 44106, USA; E-mail: brian.koo@uhhospitals.org

Octavian C. Ioachimescu (Ed)

The activity of the motor system is completely distinct in rapid-eye-movement (REM) sleep. Bursts of small myoclonic movement often occur during phasic REM, perhaps reflecting sustained activity in the central motor component and movement occurring during dreams. In fact, REM sleep enhances learning of complex motor tasks, while REM deprivation impairs such performance [7,8]. As the central motor component is active, the peripheral motor component is inhibited, to ensure that sleep is kept free of excessive movement which might be dangerous. Normally, in REM sleep there is little movement, reflecting the glycinergic inhibition of spinal α- motor neurons [9]. When REM-associated inhibition of α- motor neurons is interrupted, REM sleep behavior disorder may result, in which dream content is acted out and normal movement of wakefulness escapes into sleep (reviewed in more detail in Chapter 14).

Benign and Normal Variants of Sleep-related Movement

In different circumstances, sleep can be associated with a number of different movements often occurring at sleep onset or in the light stages of NREM sleep. Different types of benign sleep-related movement is listed in Table **1**. These movements are most often innocuous but when they occur frequently, sleep can be disrupted. In addition, these benign movements can be mimicked by other movements which may suggest a pathologic process occurring in the neuraxis.

Hypnic Jerk

The "sleep start" or hypnic jerk (HJ) is perhaps the most commonly experienced normal variant of sleep-related movement, occurring in 60% to 70% of the population [10]. It consists of a sudden myoclonic flexion of an extremity or of the entire body, occurring at the transition between wakefulness and sleep. The movement is often sufficient in amplitude and rigor to startle the once drowsy individual out of slumber. Not uncommonly, the HJ is associated with a sensation of falling, providing further stimulus for alarm. Repetitive or particularly intense hypnic jerks can induce sleep-onset insomnia or even fear of falling asleep. The exact mechanism of the hypnic jerk has not been worked out but, hypothetically, reticular formation instability at sleep onset may result in sudden descending electrical bursts and myoclonus.

Table 1: Benign sleep-related movement.

Benign Sleep-Related Movement
Hypnic jerk
Propriospinal myoclonus
Fragmentary myoclonus
Hypnagogic foot tremor
Alternating leg muscle activation

On EMG, HJs occur as brief isolated events (less than 250 msec) which consist of muscle potentials occurring either simultaneously or in rapid succession [4]. Electroencephalography (EEG) shows stage N1 sleep or drowsiness and the jerk is often coincident with a vertex sharp wave. Hypnic jerks can be confused with fragmentary or propriospinal myoclonus.

Propriospinal Myoclonus

Propriospinal myoclonus (PSM), like the hypnic jerk, occurs at the transition from wakefulness to sleep but, unlike the latter phenomenon, involves several muscle groups in propagation [11]. Movement is most often flexion involving abdominal and trunk muscles initially, then spreading to the neck and proximal extremities. Episodes may be isolated but more frequently occur sporadically or in clusters. Just as with intense hypnic jerks, sleep onset insomnia and anxiety concerning sleep onset may result. Pathophysiologically, propriospinal myoclonus arises most frequently from a myoclonic thoracic spinal generator with microscopic abnormalities visible only by high-resolution diffusion tensor imaging with fiber tracking [12]. EEG shows alpha rhythm, while EMG demonstrates activation of abdominal and truncal muscles with subsequent rostral and caudal propogation into neck and extremity muscles. The myoclonic activity lasts between 200 and 2000 msec.

Care must be taken to rule out any disease in thoracic or cervical spinal cord as myelopathy associated with disc herniation, ischemia and infection have all been reported to cause propriospinal myoclonus [13-15]. Additionally,

PSM occurs more often in persons with restless legs syndrome than in the normal population [16]. If associated with insomnia or psychiatric comorbidity, PSM may be alleviated or lessened with clonazepam.

Fragmentary Myoclonus

Fragmentary myoclonus (FM) is characterized by small fascicular muscle twitches of the fingers, toes or corners of the mouth, which often go unnoticed by the subject. These movements can occur both during wakefulness and sleep, but occur more often during sleep in both REM and NREM stages [17]. The movements resemble muscular twitches of REM sleep, but unlike these latter movements which occur in isolated bursts, FM develops more excessively throughout sleep. As such these movements can occur in compact periods of at least 20 minutes and at least 5 EMG potentials per minute, this can be called *excessive fragmentary myoclonus of sleep*. FM occurs more commonly in men and in up to 10% of persons with excessive daytime sleepiness of different etiology. There is a possible association between FM and excessive daytime sleepiness (EDS); however, causality is not certain, as FM is often found incidentally in persons being undergoing polysomnography for other reasons.

EMG shows very brief potentials, lasting between 75 and 150 msec. Polysomnographically, FM occurs in all sleep stages, but at a somewhat decreased rate during slow wave sleep [18]. Just as in PSM, myelopathy should be ruled out, especially if deep tendon reflexes are brisk. The differential diagnosis includes intense or frequent hypnic jerking, PSM and segmental myoclonus. As it usually goes unnoticed and is often noticed incidentally on PSG, treatment for FM is seldom necessary but, if needed, clonazepam may be helpful.

Hypnagogic Foot Tremor

Hypnagogic foot tremor (HFT) consists of rhythmic movement of the feet and, more specifically, of the toes, which occurs most frequently at sleep onset, but can occur in NREM sleep as well [19]. It is a benign condition lasting seconds to minutes, which is often found incidentally on PSG. Approximately 7.5% of persons undergoing PSG for other reasons have HFT [20]. The movement is often unnoticed and clinically insignificant to the affected person and only brought to their attention by a bed partner. Other times, persons with HFT are aware that they move the feet at night and can voluntarily suppress movement if so requested. Even so, the movements are executed without intention or awareness. Rarely, if the movements are excessive, they may result in insomnia. HFT may also be associated with restless legs syndrome or obstructive sleep apnea. On EMG, the bursts typically last 250-1000 msec, occurring at a frequency of 1-2 Hz with trains of at least 4 bursts, often lasting for about 15 seconds [20].

Alternating Leg Muscle Activation

Alternating leg muscle activation (ALMA) is often considered with HFT, as these two entities share features suggesting that they may not be completely distinct. ALMA consists of brief unilateral anterior tibialis activation (leading to ankle dorsiflexion), which occurs in an alternating (left, right, left, *etc.*) fashion, usually shortly after an arousal [21]. Like HFT, ALMA is often discovered incidentally on PSG where it has been shown to occur in 1.1% of random polygraphic studies. On EMG, individual leg activations usually last between 100 and 500 msec with a frequency between 0.5 and 3 Hz. Trains last between 1 and 30 seconds [20].

Sleep-Related Rhythmic Movement Disorder

Sleep-related rhythmic movement disorder (RMD) is a class of disorder occurring in drowsiness or sleep which is characterized by repetitive, often stereotyped movement of large amplitude in large muscle groups. As the name suggests, the movements are often rhythmic, such as body rocking, head rolling or even head banging (*jactatio capitis*). RMD occurs most frequently in the pediatric population, but may continue or arise in adults. Infants are most commonly affected, with some reports estimating a 59% prevalence of body rocking, head rolling or banging [22]. The prevalence decreases to 5% as children reach the fifth year of life and becomes rarer as age increases as toddlers grow out of the movement [22]. The cause or physiology of RMD is not completely understood, but has been postulated to represent a soothing means to aid in sleep onset. Movement most commonly occurs at sleep onset, but may be found in any stage including REM sleep [23].

When RMD does persist into or beyond toddler years, movements are often disturbing to the caregiver or bed partner and may also be violent, sometimes resulting in bodily harm. Body rocking is most common and involves the entire body or torso. This behavior may occur with the individual seated or on both hands and knees. Head banging is perhaps the most disturbing of the RMDs (at least to the caregiver). It occurs either with the patient seated, repeatedly extending the neck and thus banging the occiput of the head or with the individual prone, flexing the neck and banging the head vertex. The latter movement generally causes less injury as the surface struck is often either pillow or mattress, while in occipital head banging the surface is often a hard headboard or wall. Head rolling is also common and consists of side-to-side head movement with the child often in the supine position. Other less common rhythmic movement include body or leg rolling in which either body or leg is swayed in a rolling fashion.

Movements occur with a frequency between 0.5 and 2 per second. The duration of the entire episode varies greatly, but in general is less than 15 minutes [22]. Care must be taken to ensure that the patient is in a safe environment, as severe head banging may result in injury to the skull, eye or even the brain [24-26]. Injury occurs especially if there is concomitant developmental delay or neuropsychological abnormality (*e.g.*, autism). In these cases, aggressive psychotherapy and head gear may prove useful. Tricyclic antidepressants and benzodiazepines have been used with some success [27,28]. RMD is often confused with seizures, even though movements of body rocking, head banging and head rolling rarely correlate with seizure activity on EEG. Nevertheless, focal activity which occurs unilaterally in a rhythmic fashion should be distinguished from seizure electrographically. The differential diagnosis of RMD includes sleep-related bruxism, hypnagogic foot tremor, seizures - as mentioned above, and rhythmic voluntary sucking.

Nocturnal Leg Cramps

Nocturnal leg cramps consist of painful involuntary contractions of muscles, often in the calf or foot, which either awakens the person from sleep or occurs during relaxed wakefulness. Leg cramps are common in the elderly, as up to 33% of those older than 60 years of age have cramps at least once every two months with daily muscle cramps occurring in approximately 6% of this population [29]. In general, nocturnal muscle cramps are benign, but can be quite painful, causing sleep-onset insomnia or frequent awakenings. Contraction of multiple motor units (often in the gastrocnemius and small foot muscles) results from spontaneous firing of anterior horn cells at a frequency of 300 msec [30]. Episodes last from seconds to minutes and abate spontaneously, but can be relieved by stretching the affected muscle.

Vigorous exercise may potentiate cramps, even in young individuals. In the elderly, as muscles and tendons shorten with disuse and at times become less pliant with intravascular volume depletion, nocturnal leg cramps occur more frequently. Nocturnal cramps have also been associated with diabetes, peripheral vascular disease, thyroid disease, electrolyte abnormalities, pregnancy and a variety of medications such as: diuretics, β-agonists, steroids, morphine, cimetidine and statins [31-33]. Painful muscular cramping can also occur from myelopathy, peripheral neuropathy and myopathy, so care should be taken to distinguish these entities by thorough history and neurologic examination. Restless legs syndrome (RLS), the syndrome of painful feet, moving toes and rheumatologic diseases may also be confused with this entity. Confusion with RLS is quite common, but the two are most easily differentiated as nocturnal cramps are quite painful and are associated with a physically contracted muscle, both these features being absent in RLS.

Conservative treatment should be attempted initially, with maintenance of adequate hydration and assurance that electrolyte levels are normal. Stretching the affected muscles before sleep can prevent or, at the very least, decrease cramp frequency. Quinine has been used in the past with good success, supported by evidence from clinical practice and randomized trials [34-36]. This anti-parasitic drug was used for many years, but more recently has fallen out of favor, mainly because of its toxic effects on the hematologic, renal, neurologic, cardiac, and endocrine systems. In 2007 the FDA banned the prescription of quinine for leg cramps because of adverse effects and cited that design of previously completed controlled trials was flawed. Other medicines which may have efficacy in the treatment of nocturnal leg cramps include diltiazem, gabapentin, naftidrofuryl and vitamin B complex [37].

RESTLESS LEGS SYNDROME

Introduction

Restless legs syndrome (RLS) is a sensorimotor phenomenon characterized by an urge to move which is often associated with a sensory discomfort. By diagnostic necessity, RLS must occur or worsen with inactivity and in evening hours; additionally, there must be temporary relief of symptoms with movement. RLS was likely first recognized in the 17th century, but sentinel work did not occur until the 1940s, when Karl Ekbom popularized the disorder by highlighting its adverse effects on sleep and daytime functioning [38,39]. More recently, main stream medicine has recognized the morbidity associated with RLS, as it can cause significant disturbance in sleep, mood and quality of life.

Epidemiology

RLS occurs commonly in Europe and North America, with prevalence estimates between 4% and 11%, the prevalence being highest in France, lowest in Germany and intermediate in the United States [40]. These prevalence rates are based upon individuals having any frequency of RLS symptoms. The prevalence of clinically significant RLS, defined as RLS symptoms twice per week with at least moderate distress, ranged from 1.3% to 4.2%. Prevalence estimates from natives of South America and Asia are generally under 3%, with the exception of South Korea where the prevalence was found to be 7.5% [41-44]. Prevalence by country can be found in Table **2**.

Table 2: RLS prevalence by country.

Country	RLS Prevalence
United States	7.6%[40]
France	10.8%[40]
Germany	4.1%[40]
Japan	0.6%[41]
South Korea	7.5%[44]

There is some controversy as to whether RLS occurs less commonly in persons of color. Most studies conducted in Asia and South America support this notion, as described above. Unfortunately, there have been no systematic epidemiologic studies carried out in Africa. There seems to be a relative paucity of African-American patients presenting in RLS clinics. A small study looking at African-American versus Caucasian hemodialysis patients found that RLS was more common in Caucasians [45]. The Johns Hopkins group challenged these findings by polling a large population (n = 1071) in East Baltimore. RLS was diagnosed by household interview and was found in 4.7% of African-Americans and 3.8% of Caucasians, the difference being statistically nonsignificant [46].

Classification

RLS can be conveniently classified as primary or secondary. In the secondary form, RLS is due to a pre-existing condition such as: peripheral neuropathy, pregnancy, renal failure, iron deficiency, multiple sclerosis, Parkinson's disease, use of dopamine receptor blocking drugs, myelopathy or stroke (Table **3**). In the primary form, RLS occurs in the absence of a precipitating disorder. Primary RLS, more often than its secondary relative, occurs at a younger age, in women more than men and in persons with a family history of RLS. To the clinician, symptoms of secondary RLS may be indistinguishable from those of primary RLS; however, secondary RLS symptoms can be more painful, more often bilateral and show a less prominent circadian pattern. The caveat here is that when symptoms stray too far from 'typical' RLS, then alternative diagnoses should be considered, as RLS mimics are abundant (see Differential Diagnosis) [47].

Table 3: Secondary RLS and its associated diagnoses.

Secondary RLS
Peripheral neuropathy
Renal failure
Pregnancy
Iron deficiency anemia
Multiple sclerosis
Parkinson's disease
Use of dopamine receptor antagonist Spinal cord disease

Evaluation

Because of the great number of RLS causes and mimics, it is important to be vigilant for secondary causes or alternative diagnoses when seeing patients with RLS symptoms. History should be taken inquiring about weakness, numbness or tingling distinct from RLS symptoms, bowel or bladder incontinence, transient neurologic phenomenon, bradykinesia, gait difficulty, bleeding issues and the possibility of pregnancy. Medications should be checked for dopamine receptor blocking agents, which might include typical or atypical antipsychotics, tricyclic or selective serotonergic antidepressants and, finally, antiemetics such as metoclopromide.

The neurologic exam should focus on looking for clues of secondary causes, which might include hypopmimia (blunted facial expression, increased tone, tremor and festinating gait for Parkinson's disease, muscular weakness in arms or legs with brisk reflexes for myelopoathy and stroke, decreased sensation especially of pain and temperature and diminished reflexes for peripheral neuropathy, and, finally, afferent pupillary defect or other focal findings for multiple sclerosis. Helpful diagnostic testing is contingent on findings on history and exam but may include brain or spine imaging for stroke, multiple sclerosis or spinal cord disease, hemoglobin A1c for neuropathy associated with diabetes, complete blood count with or without iron studies for suspected anemia, blood urea nitrogen and creatinine for renal dysfunction and β-human chorionic gonadotropin for pregnancy. In patients with primary RLS, a serum ferritin level should be checked, as it is often low [48].

Symptoms

RLS is a clinical diagnosis based upon essential diagnostic criteria outlined above. The central tenet of RLS is the *urge to move*; a patient without this complaint absolutely does not have RLS. The urge to move may drive the patient to get up and walk, rub, stretch, shake or even hit the affected body part. The urge to move is often, but not always, associated with a sensory discomfort that patients have difficulty describing. Adjectives used to describe the sensory discomfort may include creepy-crawly, tingling, aching, inner energy, cramping, burning or pulling. Symptoms by definition *worsen or arise with inactivity and in the evening hours*. Patients with severe, and especially longstanding RLS, may describe symptoms without a diurnal pattern. In these cases it is helpful to ask if the nighttime symptoms are worse than the daytime symptoms or if there was once a time when the symptoms were predominantly nocturnal. In our experience, patients with severe RLS not uncommonly deny that movement temporarily relieves symptoms. It is important to ask further if the severity of the symptoms is lessened by movement or if there was once a time when movement alleviated symptoms. If the patient still answers negatively, a tentative diagnosis of RLS can be made in the correct clinical setting, but caution should be exercised.

Other ancillary features of RLS which may support a diagnosis include family history, response to dopaminergic agents, insomnia and the presence of periodic leg movements during sleep (PLMS) [49]. The last of these additional features deserves special attention, as it occurs in up to 88% of patients with RLS [50]. Patients will likely not know if they have PLMS, but they may have been told in the past that they kick in bed frequently if the movements are of large amplitude. Individual leg movements consist of dorsiflexion of the ankle and/or of the toes and less often flexion at the knee and even the hip. The presence of PLMS can be assessed by tibial electromyography which is included in routine PSG monitoring. Movements based upon Coleman criteria adopted by the American Academy of Sleep Medicine (AASM) require that movements last between 0.5 and 10 seconds, as most do [51,52]. In order for movements to be considered periodic, individual leg movements must occur at least four in number with an inter-movement interval between 5 and 90 seconds [52]. Duration between each movement is usually between 15 and 30 seconds, but another frequency peak appears around 8 seconds [53]. As a rule, the total number of periodic leg movements are summed and divided by hours of sleep to yield a periodic leg movement index (PLMI). Further, the number of these periodic leg movements resulting in arousal are summed and divided by total sleep time in hours to generate a periodic leg movement arousal index (PLMAI). Both PLMI and PLMAI have been shown to correlate with RLS severity [54,55]. Generally, in RLS patients, the PLMI runs between 20 and 80 per hour. The movements tend to occur in the first two thirds of the sleeping period and less commonly during REM sleep [56]. Finally, periodic leg movements arise not only in sleep but also in wakefulness, called periodic leg movement during wakefulness (PLMW). PLMW are similar to PLMS, but are helpful in that they have higher diagnostic specificity and sensitivity than PLMS [57]. A two minute polysomnographic epoch shown in Fig. **1** demonstrates PLMS.

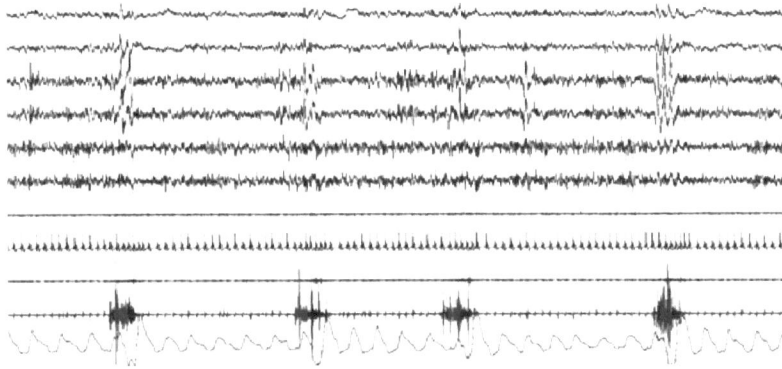

Figure 1: Periodic limb movements during sleep in a patient with RLS on a 2 minute page. Note the occurrence of PLMS between every 20 and 40 seconds. Also note, the increase in heart rate coincident with the movement and relative hyperpnea following movement.

It should be clarified that the diagnosis of RLS is clinical and can be made without PSG. For this reason, in many cases the clinician is unaware if PLMS are present and further how frequently they occur per hour of sleep (PLMI). PSG should be conducted if comorbid sleep-disordered breathing is suspected. With surface leg electromyography PLMS can be quantified in a PLMI; also periodic leg movements during wakefulness (PLMW) can be determined. The presence of PLMW is more specific and sensitive to RLS than is the presence of PLMS [58]. PLMS can also be quantified by using actigraphy. This is best done if actigraphs are placed on both legs to monitor activity [59].

After the diagnosis of RLS has been established, it is important to assess the severity of symptoms. In the research setting, severity scales or even objective testing can be used to assess symptoms severity. The suggested immobilization test (SIT) is a test to measure both motor and sensory symptoms of RLS by provoking symptoms during a one-hour period of inactivity. The patient is fitted with leg surface electromyography (EMG) usually at nighttime and asked to lie awake in bed without moving the legs. This suggested immobilization often provokes both sensory discomfort, an urge to move and motor phenomenon as well. Subjects are asked to rate the degree of sensory discomfort, urge to move and motor activity is monitored by EMG [60]. The International Restless Legs Syndrome Severity Scale (IRLS) is a 40-point, 10-question scale that asks about RLS symptom frequency, severity and the degree of sleep disturbance [61].

In the clinical setting, objective testing and even administering the IRLS is rarely practiced; however, assessing severity is important. Quantifying the frequency of symptoms may be most important, as symptom frequency ranges broadly from rare monthly or bimonthly symptoms to frequent, nightly symptoms. Other significant components in assessing severity includes time of onset, duration of symptoms, degree of relief afforded by movement, intensity of symptoms and degree of sleep disturbance. Severe RLS occurs nightly, manifests as an intense urge to move, inability to relax, causes significant sleep onset and maintenance insomnia and can affect well-being during the day as well. Inability to fall asleep and interrupted sleep are the most troublesome aspects of RLS, followed by inability to get comfortable and sensory discomfort [62]. Sleep-related complaints are also the most common reported symptoms, followed by sensory discomfort [63]. Polysomnography in RLS shows increases in sleep latency and arousal index, but no change in any sleep stage percentages [64]. As other sleep disorders occur more commonly in RLS sufferers, it is vital to take a comprehensive sleep history looking for insomnia, sleep-disordered breathing, excessive sleepiness, parasomnia and circadian rhythm disturbances.

Pathophysiology

Although there are some clues as to mechanism of RLS, there is no pathology which clearly explains the disorder. Theories of dopaminergic system dysfunction and derangement in central iron handling dominate when considering RLS pathophysiology. To a lesser extent, hormonal alterations in the opioid and melanocyte hormone axes have been implicated in RLS physiology.

Much of the evidence supporting a role for *dopaminergic system* dysfunction arises from clinical experience with dopaminergic medications that treat RLS and dopamine receptor blocking agents which cause RLS [65,66]. Despite clinical success with levodopa and dopamine agonists, research trying to elucidate the role of the dopaminergic system in RLS has been conflicting. Early neuropathological studies showed normal levels of substantia nigra tyrosine hydroxylase, but more recent exams from the same group revealed low putaminal dopamine-2-receptor binding and high substantia nigra tyrosine hydroxylase levels [67,68]. Imaging studies have been unrevealing, too. SPECT studies have showed normal presynaptic dopamine transporter binding and normal postsynaptic dopamine receptor binding [69-71]. Positron emission tomography (PET) studies have shown either normal or decreased dopamine uptake in the striatum [72-74]. Finally, vesperal dopamine metabolite levels in cerebrospinal fluid do not differ from control levels [75,76]. However, when looking at diurnal changes in metabolite levels, RLS subjects have significantly greater change when compared to controls [77]. In summary, there is some evidence, although conflicting, for a central role of dopamine in the pathogenesis of RLS.

The evidence implicating *iron* as a player in RLS pathophysiology is more convincing. Ekbom was the first to make the connection between iron deficiency and RLS and along with colleagues successfully treated patients with supplemental iron [78,79]. Peripheral or serum iron is best measured by ferritin, a protein which reflects total body iron stores [80]. In fact, ferritin has been shown to correlate with RLS severity, with low levels reflecting more severe symptoms [81]. Iron stores in the brain are also low in RLS. Using magnetic resonance imaging (MRI), low iron content in substantia nigra was demonstrated in two studies [82,83]. Neuropathologically, low ferritin levels are seen in substantia nigra, verifying imaging findings [84]. Cerebrospinal fluid (CSF) analysis provides another means to determine central iron levels. Low CSF ferritin levels and high CSF transferrin have been confirmed by two separate groups [85,86]. From these findings, it is evident that there is an abnormality in central iron handling in RLS. Animal studies have supplied evidence linking iron deficiency with dopaminergic dysfunction, further validating the roles of both iron and dopamine. In these studies rats were fed an iron poor diet. Pathologically, ferritin levels were low in striatum and correlated with low numbers of D_2-receptors and levels of dopamine transporter protein [87,88].

Hormonal dysfunction in RLS is suggested by its emergence in pregnancy, diurnal variations and successful treatment with opiate medication. Just as with dopamine agonists and iron, *opioids* are effective in treating RLS symptoms, suggesting that the opioid system may be involved in RLS pathogenesis. Using PET imaging, severe RLS was associated with decreased opiate binding in neuronal structures which mediate pain, including medial thalamus and amygdala. These findings suggest that RLS is associated with increased endogenous opioid (endorphin) release and that this system may be dysfunctional in persons with RLS [89]. Alpha-melanocyte stimulating hormone (α-MSH) has also been implicated in RLS physiology. Administration of this hormone to rats results in increased locomotion, fragmented sleep and periodic movements during sleep [90]. Interestingly, α-MSH unifies the opioid, dopamine and iron theories as it shares the same precursor protein with β-endorphin, its release is inhibited by dopamine and it modulates iron binding of CNS neuromelanin [91,92].

Genetics

Familial aggregation of RLS is well known. RLS twin studies approximate the phenotypic variation among individuals attributable to genetic variation at 54% to 83% [93,94]. Formal segregation analysis suggests a difference in the manner of inheritance based upon age of onset. In families with early-onset disease (< 30 year-old), a single gene model with autosomal dominant inheritance and high, but variable penetrance, fits. In late-onset disease, a polygenic pattern of inheritance is more likely [95]. Familial linkage studies have identified five positive linkage regions classified as regions RLS1-5 (12q, 14q, 9p, 2q, and 20p) [96-100]. Although exciting, these findings are somewhat marred as the studies include small family numbers and no putative genes have been associated with the loci.

Genome-wide association (GWA) studies have more recently identified polymorphisms in genes which account for 70% of the RLS population risk [101]. These studies compare entire genomes of patients and controls, looking at hundreds of thousands of single nucleotide polymorphisms (SNPs). In a GWA study conducted in Iceland, a significant association was found between polymorphism in the BTBD9 gene on chromosome 6 and RLS associated with PLMS [102]. The same group verified this relationship in a second Icelandic population and also a North American sample [102]. A separate GWA study conducted in German and French-Canadian populations discovered an association between RLS and the Meis1 gene on chromosome 2p14 and MAP2K5 and LBXCOR1 genes on chromosome 15q23 [103]. These associations are robust; however, little is known regarding the normal function of these genes and furthermore how their dysfunction may be related to the phenotypic expression of RLS.

Comorbidity

Because RLS is based upon subjective discomfort and somewhat odd symptomatology, as a disease entity it has been trivialized even by the medical community [104]. RLS is considered by many physicians as just an annoyance with little consequence. Several lines of evidence run contrary to this line of thinking. RLS is often associated with psychiatric comorbidities. One study showed that for RLS sufferers, the odds ratio for diagnosis of major depression and panic disorder were 4.7 and 12.9, respectively [105]. The relationship between RLS and psychiatric diseases is especially complicated as sleep disturbance may result from both psychiatric disease and RLS. The REST study found that the quality of life, as measured by the SF-36, was significantly reduced in those with RLS as compared to the normal population and those with other chronic disease such as diabetes, osteoarthritis and depression [62].

In large epidemiologic studies, RLS has been associated with increased risk of hypertension [106,107]. The link between RLS and hypertension appears to be PLMS. PLMS occur in the vast majority of persons with RLS. These movements are closely followed by increases in both heart rate and blood pressure, especially if the PLMS are associated with arousal. One study found that individual leg movements were associated with increases in systolic and diastolic blood pressure of 22 and 11 mm Hg, respectively [108]. Large community population studies have suggested that there is increased risk for cardiovascular disease, including myocardial infarction and stroke [109,110]. Review of the Sleep Heart Health data showed that RLS was associated with prevalent coronary artery disease and cardiovascular disease, which included both myocardial infarction and stroke [111]. Interestingly, the association between RLS and prevalent hypertension was dropped after adjusting for other cardiovascular risk factors. Similar conclusions were reached after looking at Wisconsin cohort data. Again, RLS was associated with prevalent coronary artery disease and not hypertension; this study did not consider stroke.

Differential Diagnosis

RLS is an entirely clinical diagnosis and, as such, it can be easily mistaken for other entities. It is important to remember that the diagnosis of RLS is not related to any abnormal involuntary movement. Patients will often describe that their legs jump involuntarily but this has no bearing on RLS diagnosis. Additionally, the habitual voluntary nervous movement of the legs does not represent RLS. For this reason, other entities which manifest with excessive movement, including the tremor of Parkinson's disease, essential tremor, chorea or athetosis are not indicative of RLS. Neuropathy, radicular disease and myelopathy cause shooting or burning pain which can be confused with RLS, especially since the discomfort can be alleviated by movement. RLS may also occur secondarily from each of these entities, but with careful history the patient will explain two distinct symptoms. These entities can be distinguished from RLS, as they are often more painful, do not have a circadian rhythmicity and can also occur with motion.

Claudication, either vascular or neurogenic, may be complicated with RLS. Both of these problems cause discomfort, often in the legs. With careful history taking, the differences should be evident, as symptoms of both vascular and neurogenic claudication occur with movement and are alleviated with rest. Additionally, there is no circadian pattern in claudication. Nocturnal leg cramps are very often confused with RLS and even for the experienced neurologist can be difficult to distinguish. Leg cramps occur at night, are associated with an urge to move, get better with movement or stretching and worse with rest, fulfilling all essential RLS criteria. The major distinguishing features are that leg cramps are invariably quite painful, occur in the calves or in the small foot muscles and are associated with a tense, contracted muscle. The patient will often call the entity a cramp. Not uncommonly, RLS coexists with nocturnal leg cramps, but the patients have no problem distinguishing the two problems symptomatically.

Periodic limb movement disorder (PLMD) will be described in the next section but should be mentioned briefly here, as the non-sleep specialist often equates periodic limb movements during sleep with RLS. PLMS occur in about 80% of persons with RLS; however, PLMS are nonspecific, occurring even in normal persons. PLMD can only be diagnosed when there are PLMS associated with daytime sleepiness in the absence of RLS symptoms. RLS with PLMS and daytime sleepiness is simply RLS.

Finally, the disorder most resembling RLS is akathisia. Akathisia, like RLS, occurs in the setting of dopamine receptor blockade. Both akathisia and RLS are associated with an urge to move and temporary alleviation with movement. The urge to move in akathisia is often of the entire body and at times more severe than that seen in RLS. Additionally, in akathisia the urge to move occurs constantly without circadian rhythmicity. Unlike RLS, akathisia is infrequently accompanied by sensory discomfort.

Treatment

Secondary RLS

In determining proper treatment for RLS, it is important to distinguish primary from secondary RLS. In secondary RLS, treatment of the underlying cause may minimize RLS symptoms and help avoid the addition of another medication. In the case of diabetic neuropathy, for example, tight glycemic control may be helpful to reduce further neuropathic damage and help decrease symptom worsening. In RLS associated with iron deficiency anemia, treatment with iron is essential. And in Parkinson's related RLS, increasing doses of levodopa or nighttime levodopa may be helpful. The most dramatic example of treating the underlying cause occurs in chronic renal disease, where kidney transplantation is often curative of RLS.

At times, even in secondary RLS, treatment of the cause may not necessarily result in better RLS control. This is likely the case in RLS associated with multiple sclerosis, spinal cord disease, various diseases of nerve or nerve root (*e.g.* hereditary neuropathy, Guillain-Barré syndrome) or pregnancy. In these cases RLS should be treated directly, with the choice of agent depending on the primary cause. In neuropathic diseases, patient often describe the burning pain of neuropathy in addition to the urge to move of RLS. In these cases, gabapentin is the best choice as both neuropathic and RLS symptoms may be alleviated. Gabapentin may also be most suitable for RLS associated with multiple sclerosis, as these patients not uncommonly suffer from large fiber demyelinating neuropathy. In the case of pregnancy, the choice of drugs is limited by teratogenicity. The safest medications with the best efficacy in the treatment of RLS in the pregnant female are the opiate medications. Medication should be reserved for severe RLS. Exercise and stretching should be advised. Potential exacerbating factors should be minimized which might include caffeine, alcohol and poor sleep hygiene.

Primary RLS

As mentioned above, treatment of RLS should begin with a thorough history seeking potential RLS symptom exacerbating factors. Poor sleep hygiene and insufficient sleep should be corrected. Caffeine and alcohol intake should be minimized. Medications should be reviewed, looking specifically for dopamine receptor blocking drugs, which could include antipsychotic, antiemetic agents or antidepressant medications. If these medications are found, then the clinician must weigh the benefits of decreasing RLS symptoms against exacerbation of the problem being treated. In the case of psychiatric disorders, this may be especially complicated. Stopping medications in severe depression or psychosis should be done only with great caution and with the collaboration of a psychiatrist, if at all. With the case of antiemetic medications or when antipsychotics are used for sleep in depression, the decision is much easier to discontinue the offending agent. Commonly used medications for the treatment of RLS and appropriate strengths can be found in Table **4**.

Iron Therapy

The initiation of medical therapy for RLS is contingent on symptom severity; hence it is essential to determine symptom frequency, intensity and degree of sleep disturbance. For mild to moderate RLS, behavioral treatments, as mentioned above, may be adequate. Instruction on regular exercise and stretching may also benefit and obviate the need to start a medicine. Serum ferritin should be measured and treatment with iron should be recommended for ferritin levels of 50 ng/mL or lower. Patients should be instructed to take iron on an empty stomach to enhance absorption; however, if gastrointestinal discomfort develops taking iron with food may be necessary. Vitamin C should also be co-administered, as this also enhances iron absorption. Initial treatment of RLS patients with iron was popularized by Ekbom and colleagues. Intravenous iron was shown to decrease RLS symptom severity [79]. More recently, iron sucrose given intravenously has shown some promise, but further study is needed as results have been somewhat inconsistent [111,112]. For oral iron, patients should be forewarned about constipation, which is a frequent reason for noncompliance. Ferritin should be checked every 6 months with goal levels between 80 and 200 ng/mL. The possibility of iron toxicity should be kept in mind as, rarely, hemochromatosis from iron overload may develop.

Table 4: Medical Treatment of RLS.

Medication	Starting dose	Usual dose
Iron	325 mg BID - TID	325 mg TID
Carbidopa/Levodopa*	25/100 mg nighttime	25/100 – 50/200 mg
Ropinorole*	0.25 mg nighttime	1 mg – 2 mg
Pramipexole*	0.125 mg night	0.5 mg – 1 mg
Gabapentin*	100 – 300 mg night	600 – 900 mg nightly

*Can be used two or even three times daily if symptoms occur during the day or early evening.

Dopamine Levodopa

RLS is exquisitely sensitive to dopaminergic agents. In fact, if the diagnosis is in question then a trial of dopamine with response supports the presence of RLS. Early trials focused on the use of levodopa. Levodopa is taken with carbidopa to decrease the peripheral breakdown of levodopa and to maximize levodopa which crosses the blood brain barrier. Doses of 100/25 and 200/50 mg levodopa/carbidopa have been used with good efficacy, decreasing symptoms severity, improving sleep and decreasing PLMS in one study, from 63 to 45 per hour [113]. One major problem with using levodopa is the short half life, which is 1.5 hours even when given with carbidopa. Because of this short half life, RLS symptoms may recur in the latter part of the night, sometimes waking the patient and necessitating a second dose. For this reason, levodopa with carbidopa may be most suitable for mild to moderate RLS or RLS which occurs infrequently. Large doses of levodopa may lead to the development of augmentation, a phenomenon of sudden RLS symptoms worsening. Augmentation occurs in up to 72% of cases in which levodopa is used, but a more likely rate is 26.7% [114,115]. Augmentation will be further described in the subsequent sections. Other side effects which may limit usage include nausea, headache and fatigue.

Dopamine Agonists

More recently, dopamine agonists (DAs) have become the drug of choice for the treatment of RLS. The longer half lives make them a better choice in moderate to severe RLS. Presently, two dopamine agonists are approved by the Food & Drug Administration for the treatment of RLS, these being ropinorole and pramipexole. A third DA, pergolide, formerly had approval but was taken off the market because of cardiac valvular problems. The dopamine agonists are generally well tolerated, especially since doses used to treat RLS are generally lower than what is used in Parkinson's disease. For this reason, impulsive behavior such as pathological gambling, excessive shopping and impulsive sexual behavior is less frequent, but should be still monitored. More common side effects include nausea, fatigue, abdominal pain, diarrhea and dizziness. Augmentation does occur with the DAs, but at a significantly lower rate than with levodopa [117].

Pramipexole

The efficacy of pramipexole in treating RLS has been demonstrated in four large placebo-controlled trials [117-120].Doses between 0.125 and 0.75 mg were used and decreased IRLS scores 12.3 to 17 points from starting points of approximately 25 to 30. Pramipexole has also been shown to decrease PLMI significantly, in one study from 46 to 9 per total hours of sleep, correlating with improved sleep and subjective quality of life [121]. Side effects are outlined above as for all the dopamine agonists. It is important to keep in mind that augmentation does occur, from rates of 8.5% to 39% in open label trials [122-124]. The typical starting dose is 0.125 mg given shortly before the usual onset of symptoms. The dose can be quickly titrated over 3-5 days to 0.25 mg and then to 0.5 mg in another 3-5 days if needed. Dosing for RLS should not exceed 2 mg.

Ropinirole

The efficacy for ropinirole is very similar to that of pramipexole. Ropinirole has also been studied well in placebo-controlled trials, demonstrating efficacy in reducing RLS symptoms with IRLS scores decreasing significantly between 11.0 and 13.5 points [125-128]. The doses ranged somewhat widely even within studies (0.5 to 4 mg), but most subjects were given between 1 and 2 mg. Again, sleep and quality of life improved, as measured by the RLS-6 and CGI.

Ropinirole treatment significantly decreases PLMI between 36.7 and 56.6 per hour of sleep again with doses between 1 and 2 mg. Symptoms of augmentation should be sought, as well as the other common side effects outline above. Typically the starting dose is 0.25 mg which can be increased after 3-5 days to 0.5 mg and then to 1mg after another 3-5 days with the maximum dose being 4 mg per day.

Augmentation

Augmentation is a major complication of long-term dopamine agent usage, occurring most commonly with the use of levodopa. It was first described by the Johns Hopkins group in 1996 and consists of a deterioration of RLS symptoms, often to a degree that is worse than the initial baseline or untreated severity [129]. This increased severity as well as other characteristic features (Table **5**) distinguish augmentation from tolerance to medication. Typically, augmentation includes (in decreasing order of frequency): earlier diurnal onset of symptoms, overall increase in symptom intensity, shorter latency to symptom onset when at rest, decreased duration of medication efficacy and extension of symptoms to the upper limbs or trunk.

Table 5: Symptoms of augmentation.

Augmentation
Earlier onset of RLS symptoms
Increased RLS symptom intensity
Shorter latency to symptoms when at rest
Decreased duration of medication efficacy
Extension of symptoms to other body parts

It has been suggested that augmentation results from chronically heightened nervous system dopamine levels; however, the mechanism underlying augmentation has not been systematically investigated [130]. If augmentation develops, stopping the offending agent may be helpful. Symptom severity then should be reassessed and the medication could be restarted at a lower dose or given in divided doses. If levodopa has been used, then stopping this agent and changing to a dopamine agonist is advisable. If augmentation is severe and RLS symptoms continue to a severe degree after medication holiday, then switching to an alternative medication such as gabapentin or an opiate is advisable. At the same time, conditions which could potentiate augmentation should be sought and addressed; low ferritin should be treated with iron, antidepressant medication should be examined and poor sleep hygiene should be managed. Finally, preventing the development of augmentation is essential. The lowest effective dose in treating symptoms should be provided and high doses exceeding what is recommended should be avoided.

Other Treatments

Gabapentin is also effective in the treatment of RLS, being an especially good choice when RLS is complicated by peripheral neuropathy. Gabapentin can be used once nightly or, if pain occurs, during the day two to three times daily. In one trial, even 300 mg of gabapentin resulted in decreases in IRLS scores of 10 and in PLMI of 17 movements per hour of sleep [131]. Higher doses of around 1,800 mg result in similar decreases in IRLS and PLMI [132]. Gabapentin can be started at 100-300 mg at nighttime. To treat evening symptoms and nighttime PLMS gabapetin can be used twice daily, usually with doses not exceeding 900 mg twice daily. In severe RLS occurring during both day and night, a maximum dose of 3,600 mg may be necessary. Other anti-epileptic agents seem to be less effective than gabapentin, including carbamazepine and valproic acid [133, 134].

Opioid medications also have efficacy in RLS and are a good choice when symptoms of augmentation occur with the use of dopaminergic agents. Opioids are also the medication of choice for severe RLS which arises or worsens during pregnancy. Oxycodone has been studied in subjects with primary RLS and resulted in a reduction of PLMI from 38.8 to 18.4 per hour sleep. A mean dose of 11.4 mg was used in this trial [135].

Finally, benzodiazepines have also been used in the treatment of RLS. These agents have recently fallen out of favor, as the benzodiazepine-receptor agonists are just as effective with a more benign side effect profile.

SUMMARY

The sleep-related movement disorders are more often than not clinically benign disorders. Disorders including propriospinal myoclonus, excessive fragmentary myoclonus and hypnagogic foot tremor may fragment sleep if movements occur repetitively. RLS is the most clinically significant of the sleep-related movement disorders, as it is quite common and causes significant morbidity. RLS must be distinguished from periodic limb movement disorder and nocturnal leg cramps. All patients with sleep complaints should be screened for RLS, as it is very common and readily treatable with medications. It is noteworthy to mention as a final thought that the symptoms of RLS should not be taken lightly. One reason is that severe RLS is related to increased likelihood of having stroke or coronary events. Finally, RLS symptoms can cause significant morbidity including sleep disruption, depression and simply an inability to relax and stay still at the end of the day.

RESEARCH OUTLOOK

Summary

In recent years, research in the field of RLS has grown immensely. Large epidemiologic studies have shown that not only is RLS quite common in many different countries, but that it causes significant comorbidity with sleep and mood disturbance [62,63]. Furthermore, RLS has been associated with increased cardiovascular risk, possibly related to associated hypertension [64]. Genome-wide association studies have identified so far candidate genes on chromosomes 2 and 6 [102,103]. The majority of current RLS research concerns genetics or pathophysiology, as the exact mechanism underlying RLS has not been completely worked out. This lack of knowledge may be in part secondary to a relative absence of reliable RLS animal models. To date, an animal model in which the A11 dopaminergic system is modulated seems most promising [136]. Work which integrates derangements in iron and dopaminergic system is perhaps most needed.

What do we know:

Through clinical and research experience, it is evident that RLS symptoms are quite responsive to treatment [115,118,132]. As stated in previous sections, RLS is perhaps most responsive to dopaminergic medications, but also responds well to gabapentin and opioid medications. Also, epidemiology of RLS has been investigated, mostly in Western countries and unequivocally showed that this disorder is quite common [40]. Furthermore, these large epidemiologic studies show that not only is RLS common, but it is associated with significant impairment of quality of life [40,62]. Perhaps more compelling to the medical mainstream is the recent association of RLS to cardiovascular events, which include stroke and myocardial infarction in two large population-based studies [64,109]. Recent and current research has focused on genetics and RLS pathophysiology. Through genome-wide array studies, several candidate genes have been identified, which include the BTBD9 gene on chromosome 6 [102], the Meis1 gene on chromosome 2 and the MAP2K5 gene on chromosome 15 [103]. Perhaps most disappointing has been so far the lack of evidence showing derangements in the dopaminergic system when concerning RLS pathophysiology. Iron store abnormalities have been more consistently demonstrated [67,82,83].

What we don't know:

Despite much completed research concerning RLS pathophysiology, the mechanism underlying this disorder has not been clearly identified. Questions regarding pathophysiology have been difficult to address, especially since neuropathology has been sparse as the disorder does not lead to death, at least directly [84]. Furthermore, animal models of RLS have been sparse and in many cases imperfect [88,90,136-138]. Perhaps most needed is research that integrates iron and dopamine, the two leading candidates regarding RLS mechanism. A recent neuropathological study, demonstrated decreased dopamine-2 receptor density in putamen in RLS patients as compared to controls, while showing increased tyrosine hydroxylase in substabtia nigra [139]. These areas have been shown in radiologic studies to contain low levels of iron [140]. These results are encouraging; however, additional research linking dopamine and iron are necessary to delineate the mechanics of RLS.

REFERENCES

[1]   Kleitman N. Basic rest-activity cycle-22 years later. Sleep 1982; 5: 311-17.

[2]   Oswald I. Sudden bodily jerks on falling asleep. Brain 1959; 82(1): 92-103.

[3]   Broughton R, Tolentino MA. Fragmentary pathological myoclonus in NREM sleep. Electroencephalogr Clinical Neurophysiology 1984; 57(4): 303-9.

[4]   Dagnino N, Loeb C, Massazza G, Sacco G. Hypnic physiological myoclonias in man: an EEG-EMG study in normals and neurological patients. Eur Neurol 1969; 2(1): 47-58.

[5]   Wilde-Frenz J, Schulz H. Rate and distribution of body movements during sleep in humans. Perceptual Motor Skills 1983; 56(1): 275-83.

[6]   Montagna P, Liguori R, Zucconi M, *et al.* Physiological hypnic myoclonus. Electroencephalography Clin Neurophysiol 1988; 70(2): 172-6.

[7]   Born J, Rasch B, Gais S. Sleep to remember. Neuroscientist 2006; 12: 410-24.

[8]   Buchegger J, Fritsch R, Meier-Koll A, Riehle H. Does trampolining and anaerobic physical fitness affect sleep? Percept Mot Skills 1991; 73: 243–52.

[9]   Curtis, DR, Johnston GAR. Amino acid transmitters in the mammalian central nervous system. Ergeb Physiol 1974; 69: 97-188.

[10]   Montagna P, Liguori R, Zucconi M, Sforza E, Lugaresi A, Cirignotta F, Lugaresi E. Physiological hypnic myoclonus. Electroencephalogr Clin Neurophysiol 1988; 70(2): 172-6.

[11]   Brown P, Thompson PD, Rothwell JC, Day BL, Marsden CD. Axial myoclonus of propriospinal origin. Brain 1991; 114 (1A): 197-214.

[12]   Roze E, Bounolleau P, Ducreux D, *et al.* Propriospinal myoclonus revisited: Clinical, neurophysiologic, and neuroradiologic findings. Neurology 2009; 72(15): 1301-9.

[13]   Capelle HH, Wöhrle JC, Weigel R, Grips E, Bäzner HJ, Krauss JK. Propriospinal myoclonus due to cervical disc herniation. Case report. J Neurosurg Spine 2005; 2(5): 608-11.

[14]   Nogués M, Cammarota A, Solá C, Brown P. Propriospinal myoclonus in ischemic myelopathy secondary to a spinal dural arteriovenous fistula. Mov Disord 2000; 15(2): 355-8.

[15]   de la Sayette V, Schaeffer S, Queruel C, *et al.* Lyme neuroborreliosis presenting with propriospinal myoclonus. J Neurol Neurosurg Psychiatry 1996; 61(4): 420.

[16]   Vetrugno R, Provini F, Plazzi G, Cortelli P, Montagna P. Propriospinal myoclonus: a motor phenomenon found in restless legs syndrome different from periodic limb movements during sleep. Mov Disord 2005; 20(10): 1323-9.

[17]   Broughton R, Tolentino MA, Krelina M. Excessive fragmentary myoclonus in NREM sleep: a report of 38 cases. Electroencephalogr Clin Neurophysiol 1985;61(2): 123-33.

[18]   Lins O, Castonguay M, Dunham W, Nevsimalova S, Broughton R. Excessive fragmentary myoclonus: time of night and sleep stage distributions. Can J Neurol Sci 1993;20(2): 142-6.

[19]   Wichniak A, Tracik F, Geisler P, Ebersbach G, Morrissey SP, Zulley J. Rhythmic feet movements while falling asleep. Mov Disord 2001; 16(6): 1164-70.

[20]   American Academy of Sleep Medicine. Hypnagogic foot tremor and alternating leg muscle activation. In: Sateia MJ, Ed. The international classification of sleep disorders: diagnostic and coding manual. 2nd ed. Westchester, IL: American Academy of Sleep Medicine, 2005; 213–5.

[21]   Chervin RD, Consens FB, Kutluay E. Alternating leg muscle activation during sleep and arousals: a new sleep-related motor phenomenon. Mov Disord 2003; 18: 551–9.

[22]   Sallustro F, Atwell CW. Body rocking, head banging, and head rolling in normal children. J Pediatr 978; 93(4): 704-8.

[23]   Kohyama J, Matsukura F, Kimura K, Tachibana N. Rhythmic movement disorder: polysomnographic study and summary of reported cases. Brain Dev 2002; 24: 33-8.

[24]   Bemporad JR. Cataracts following chronic head banging: A report of two cases. Am J Psychiatry 1968; 125: 245-9.

[25]   Stuck KJ, Hernandez RJ. Large skull defect in a head banger. Pediatr Radiol 1979; 8: 257-8.

[26]   Mackenzie JM. Headbanging and fatal subdural haemorrhage. Lancet 1991; 338: 1457.

[27]   Chisholm T, Morehouse RL. Adult headbanging: sleep studies and treatment. Sleep 1996; 19(4): 343-6.

[28]   Alves RS, Alóe F, Silva AB, Tavares SM. Jactatio capitis nocturna with persistence in adulthood. Case report. Arq Neuropsiquiatr 1998; 56(3B): 655-7.

[29]   Naylor RJ, Young JB. A general population survey of leg cramps. Age Ageing 1994; 23: 418–20.

[30]   Norris FH, Gasteiger EL, Chatfield EO. An electromyographic study of induced and spontaneous muscle cramp. Electroencephalogr Clin Neurophysiol 1957; 9: 139-47.

[31]   Eaton JM. Is this really a muscle cramp? Postgrad Med J 1989; 86: 227-32.

[32]   McGee SR. Muscle cramps. Arch Intern Med 1990; 150: 511–8.

[33]   Haskell SG, Fiebach NH. Clinical epidemiology of nocturnal leg cramps in male veterans. Am J Med Sci 1997; 313: 210-4.

[34]   Jansen PHP, Veenhuizen KCW, Wesseling ALM, de Boo T, Verbeek AL. Randomised controlled trial of hydroxyquinine in muscle cramps. Lancet 1997; 349: 528–32.

[35]   Diener HC, Dethlefsen U, Dethlefsen-Gruber S, Verbeek P. Effectiveness of quinine in treating muscle cramps: a double-blind, placebo-controlled, parallel-group, multicentre trial. Int J Clin Pract 2002; 56(4): 243-6.

[36]   Warburton A, Royston JP, O'Neill CJA, *et al.* A quinine a day keeps the leg cramps away? Br J Clin Pharmacol 1987; 23: 459–65.

[37]   Katzberg HD, Khan AH, So YT. Assessment: symptomatic treatment for muscle cramps (an evidence-based review): report of the therapeutics and technology assessment subcommittee of the American academy of neurology. Neurology 2010; 74(8): 691-6.

[38]   Willis T. De Animae Brutorum. London, England: Wells and Scott 1672.

[39]   Ekbom KA. Restless legs: a clinical study. Acta Med Scand Supp 1945; 158: 1-122.

[40]   Allen RP, Walters AS, MD; Montplaisir J, *et al.* Restless Legs Syndrome Prevalence and Impact REST General Population Study. Arch Intern Med 2005; 165: 1286-92.

[41]   Kageyama T, Kabuto M, Nitta H, *et al.* Prevalence of periodic limb movement-like and restless legs-like symptoms among Japanese adults. Psychiatry Clin Neurosci 2000; 54: 296–8.

[42]   Rangarajan S, Rangarajan S, D'Souza GA. Restless legs syndrome in an Indian urban population. Sleep Med 2007; 9(1): 88-93.

[43]   Castillo PR, Kaplan J, Lin SC, Fredrickson PA, Mahowald MW. Prevalence of restless legs syndrome among native South Americans residing in coastal and mountainous areas. Mayo Clin Proc 2006; 81(10): 1345-7.

[44]   Cho YW, Shin WC, Yun CH, *et al.* Epidemiology of restless legs syndrome in Korean adults. Sleep 2008; 31(2): 219-23.

[45]   Kutner NG, Bliwise DL. Restless legs complaint in African-American and Caucasian hemodialysis patients. Sleep Med 2002; 3: 497–500.

[46]   Lee HB, Hening WA, Allen RP, Earley CJ, Eaton WW, Lyketsos CG. Race and restless legs syndrome symptoms in an adult community sample in east Baltimore. Sleep Med 2006; 7(8): 642-5.

[47]   Benes H, Walters AS, Allen RP, Hening WA, Kohnen R. Definition of restless legs syndrome, how to diagnose it, and how to differentiate it from RLS mimics. Mov Disord 2007; 22: S401-8.

[48]   O'Keeffe ST, Gavin K, Lavan JN. Iron status and restless legs syndrome in the elderly. Age Ageing 1994; 23(3): 200-3.

[49]   Lugaresi E, Coccagna C, Berti-Ceroni G, Ambrosetto C. Restless legs syndrome and nocturnal myoclonus. In: Gastaut H, Lugaresi E, Berti_Ceroni G, Eds. The abnormalities of sleep in man. Bologna, Italy: Aulo Gaggi 1968; 285-94.

[50]   Montplaisir J, Boucher S, Poirier G, Lavigne G, Lapierre O, Lesperance P. Clinical, polysomnographic, and genetic characteristics of restless legs syndrome: a study of 133 patients diagnosed with new standard criteria. Mov Disord 1997; 12: 61–5.

[51]   Coleman RM. Periodic movements in sleep (nocturnal myoclonus) and restless legs syndrome. In: Guilleminault C, Ed. Sleep and waking disorders: indications and techniques. Menlo Park, CA: Addison-Wesley, 1982; 265–95.

[52]   American Sleep Disorder Association (ASDA). Atlas Task Force of the American Sleep Disorders Association. Recording and scoring leg movements. Sleep 1993; 16: 748–59.

[53]   Ferri R, Zucconi M, Manconi M, Plazzi G, Bruni O, Ferini-Strambi L. New approaches to the study of periodic leg movements during sleep in restless legs syndrome. Sleep 2006; 29(6): 759-69.

[54]   Garcia-Borreguero D, Larrosa O, de la Llave Y, Granizo JJ, Allen RR. Correlation between rating scales and sleep laboratory measurements in restless legs syndrome. Sleep Med 2004; 5(6): 561–5.

[55]   Hornyak M, Hundemer HP, Quail D, Riemann D, Voderholzer U, Trenkwalder C. Relationship of periodic leg movements and severity of restless legs syndrome: a study in unmedicated and medicated patients. Clin Neurophysiol 2007; 118(7): 1532-7.

[56]   Pollmacher T, Schulz H. Periodic leg movements: their relationship to sleep stages. Sleep 1993; 16: 572–7.

[57]   Michaud M, Soucy JP, Chabli A, Lavigne G, Montplasir J. SPECT imaging of striatal pre- and postsynaptic dopaminergic status in restless legs syndrome with periodic leg movements in sleep. J Neurol 2002; 249: 164–70.

[58]   Pollmächer T, Schulz H. Periodic leg movements (PLM): their relationship to sleep stages Sleep. 1993; 16(6): 572-7.

[59]   Sforza E, Johannes M, Claudio B. The PAM-RL ambulatory device for detection of periodic leg movements: a validation study. Sleep Med 2005; 6(5): 407-13.

[60]   Montplaisir J, Boucher S, Nicolas A, *et al.* Immobilization tests and periodic leg movements in sleep for the diagnosis of restless leg syndrome. Movement Disorders 1998; 13(2): 324-9.

[61]   Walters AS, LeBrocq C, Dhar A, *et al.* International Restless Legs Syndrome Study Group. Validation of the International Restless Legs Syndrome Study Group rating scale for restless legs syndrome. Sleep Med 2003; 4(2): 121-32.

[62]   Allen RP, Walters AS, Montplaisir J, *et al.* Restless legs syndrome prevalence and impact: REST general population study. Arch Intern Med 2005; 165(11): 1286-92.

[63]   Hening W, Walters AS, Allen RP, Montplaisir J, Myers A, Ferini-Strambi L. Impact, diagnosis and treatment of restless legs syndrome (RLS) in a primary care population: the REST (RLS epidemiology, symptoms, and treatment) primary care study. Sleep Med 2004; 5(3): 237-46.

[64]   Winkelman JW, Redline S, Baldwin CM, Resnick HE, Newman AB, Gottlieb DJ. Polysomnographic and health-related quality of life correlates of restless legs syndrome in the Sleep Heart Health Study. Sleep 2009; 32(6): 772-8.

[65]   Akpinar S. Treatment of restless legs syndrome with levodopa plus benserazide. Arch Neurol 1982; 39: 739.

[66]   Walters AS, Hening W, Rubinstein M, Chokroverty S. A clinical and polysomnographic comparison of neuroleptic-induced akathisia and the idiopathic restless legs syndrome. Sleep 1991; 14(4): 339-45.

[67]   Connor JR, Boyer P.J, Menzies SL, BS, *et al.* Neuropathological examination suggests impaired brain iron acquisition in restless legs syndrome. Neurology 2003; 61: 304–9.

[68]   Connor JR, Wang XS, Allen RP, *et al.*Altered dopaminergic profile in the putamen and substantia nigra in restless leg syndrome. Brain 2009; 132(9): 2403-12.

[69]   Eisensehr I, Wetter TC, Linke R, *et al.* Normal IPT and IBZM SPECT in drug-naive and levodopa-treated idiopathic restless legs syndrome. Neurology 2001; 57: 1307–9.

[70]   Michaud M, Soucy JP, Chabli A, Lavigne G, Montplaisir J. SPECT imaging of striatal preand postsynaptic dopaminergic status in restless legs syndrome with periodic leg movements in sleep. J Neurol 2002; 249: 164–70.

[71]   Tribl GG, Asenbaum S, Happe S, Bonelli RM, Zeitlhofer J, Auff E. Normal striatal D2 receptor binding in idiopathic restless legs syndrome with periodic leg movements in sleep. Nucl Med Commun 2004; 25(1): 55-60.

[72]   Trenkwalder C, Walters AS, Hening WA, Chokroverty S, Antonini A, Dhawan V, Eidelberg D. Positron emission tomographic studies in restless legs syndrome. Mov Disord 1999; 14: 141–5.

[73]   Turjanski N, Lees AJ, Brooks DJ. Striatal dopaminergic function in restless legs syndrome. 18F-dopa and 11C-raclopride PET studies. Neurology 1999; 52: 932–7.

[74]   Ruottinen HM, Partinen M, Hublin C, *et al.* An FDOPA PET study in patients with periodic limb movement disorder and restless legs syndrome. Neurology 2000; 54: 502–4.

[75]   Earley CJ, Hyland K, Allen RP. CSF dopamine, serotonin, and biopterin metabolites in patients with restless legs syndrome. Mov Disord 2001; 16(1): 144-9.

[76]   Stiasny-Kolster K, Möller JC, Zschocke J, Bandmann O, Cassel W, Oertel WH, Hoffmann GF. Normal dopaminergic and serotonergic metabolites in cerebrospinal fluid and blood of restless legs syndrome patients. Mov Disord 2004; 19(2): 192-6.

[77]   Earley CJ, Hyland K, Allen RP. Circadian changes in CSF dopaminergic measures in restless legs syndrome. Sleep Med 2006; 7(3): 263-8.

[78]   Ekbom KA. Restless legs. Stockholm: Ivar Haeggstroms 1945.

[79]   Nordlander NB. Therapy in restless legs. Acta Med Scand 1953; 145: 453– 7.

[80]   Alvarez-Ossorio L, Kirchner H, Kluter H, Schlenke P. Low ferritin levels indicate the need for iron supplementation: strategy to minimize iron-depletion in regular blood donors. Transfus Med 2000; 10: 107–12.

[81]   O'Keeffe ST, Gavin K, Lavan JN. Iron status and restless legs syndrome in the elderly. Age Ageing 1994; 23: 200 –3.

[82]   Earley CJ, Barker PB, Horska A, Allen RP. MRI-determined regional brain iron concentrations in early- and late-onset restless legs syndrome. Sleep Med 2006; 7: 459–61.

[83]   Allen RP, Barker PB, Wehrl F, Song HK, Earley CJ. MRI measurement of brain iron in patients with restless legs syndrome. Neurology 2001; 56: 263–5.

[84]   Connor JR, Boyer PJ, Menzies SL, Dellinger B, Allen RP, Earley CJ. Neuropathological examination suggests impaired brain iron acquisition in restless legs syndrome. Neurology 2003; 61: 304–9.

[85]   Mizuno S, Mihara T, Miyaoka T, Inagaki T, Horiguchi J. CSF iron, ferritin and transferrin levels in restless legs syndrome. J Sleep Res 2005; 14: 43– 7.

[86]   Earley CJ, Connor JR, Beard JL, Malecki EA, Epstein DK, Allen RP. Abnormalities in CSF concentrations of ferritin and transferring in restless legs syndrome. Neurology 2000; 54: 1698 –700.

[87]   Erikson KM, Jones BC, Hess EJ, Zhang Q, Beard JL. Iron deficiency decreases dopamine D1 and D2 receptors in rat brain. Pharmacol Biochem Behav 2001; 69: 409–18.

[88]   Erikson KM, Jones BC, Beard JL. Iron deficiency alters dopamine transporter functioning in rat striatum. J Nutr 2000; 130: 2831–7.

[89]   Von Spiczak S, Whone A, Hammers A, *et al.* The Role of opioids in Restless Legs Syndrome: an [11C] diprenorphine PET study. Brain 2005; 128: 906-17.

[90]   Koo BB, Feng P, Dostal J, Strohl KP. α-Melanocyte Stimulating Hormone and Adrenocorticotropic Hormone: An Alternative Approach When Thinking About Restless Legs Syndrome? Movement Disorders 2008; 23(9): 1234–42.

[91]   Gonzalez de Aguilar JL, Malagon MM, Vazquez-Martinez RM, Martínez-Fuentes AJ, Tonon MC, Vaudry H, Gracia-Navarro F. Differential effects of dopamine on two frog melanotrope cell subpopulations. Endocrinology 1999; 140: 159–64.

[92]   Nicolaus BJ. A critical review of the function of neuromelanin and an attempt to provide a unified theory. Med Hypotheses 2005; 65: 791–6.

[93]   Desai AV, Cherkas LF, Spector TD, Williams AJ. Genetic influences in self-reported symptoms of obstructive sleep apnoea and restless legs: a twin study. Twin Res 2004, 7: 589– 95.

[94]   Ondo WG, Vuong KD, Wang Q. Restless legs syndrome in monozygotic twins: clinical correlates. Neurology 2000; 55: 1404–6.

[95]   Winkelmann J, Muller-Myhsok B, Wittchen HU, *et al.* Complex segregation analysis of restless legs syndrome provides evidence for an autosomal dominant mode of inheritance in early age at onset families. Ann Neurol 2002; 52: 297–302.

[96]   Desautels A, Turecki G, Montplaisir J, Sequeira A, Verner A, Rouleau GA. Identification of a major susceptibility locus for restless legs syndrome on chromosome 12q. Am J Hum Genet 2001: 69: 1266–70.

[97]   Bonati MT, Ferini-Strambi L, Aridon P, Oldani A, Zucconi M, Casari G. Autosomal dominant restless legs syndrome maps on chromosome 14q. Brain 2003; 126: 1485–92.

[98]   Chen S, Ondo WG, Rao S, Li L, Chen Q, Wang Q. Genomewide linkage scan identifies a novel susceptibility locus for restless legs syndrome on chromosome 9p. Am J Hum Genet 2004; 74: 876–85.

[99]   Pichler I, Marroni F, Volpato CB, *et al.* Linkage analysis identifies a novel locus for restless legs syndrome on chromosome 2q in a South Tyrolean population isolate. Am J Hum Genet 2006; 79: 716–23.

[100] Levchenko A, Provost S, Montplaisir J, *et al.* A novel autosomal dominant restless legs syndrome locus maps to chromosome 20p13. Neurology 2006; 67: 900–1.

[101] Trotti LM, Bhadriraju S, Rye DB. An update on the pathophysiology and genetics of restless legs syndrome. Curr Neurol Neurosci Rep 2008; 8(4): 281-7.

[102] Stefansson H, Rye DB, Hicks A, *et al.* A genetic risk factor for periodic limb movements in sleep. N Engl J Med 2007; 357(7): 639-47.

[103] Winkelmann J, Schormair B, Lichtner P, *et al.* Genomewide association study of restless legs syndrome identifies common variants in three genomic regions. Nat Genet 2007; 39: 1000–6.

[104] Woloshin S, Schwartz LM. Giving legs to restless legs: a case study of how the media helps make people sick. PLoS Med 2006; 3: e170.

[105] Lee HB, Hening WA, Allen RP, *et al.* Restless legs syndrome is associated with DSM-IV major depressive disorder and panic disorder in the community. J Neuropsychiatry Clin Neurosci 2008; 20(1): 101-5.

[106] Ulfberg J, Nystrom B, Carter N, Edling C. Prevalence of restless legs syndrome among men aged 18 to 64 years: an association with somatic disease and neuropsychiatric symptoms. Mov Disord 2001; 16: 1159-63.

[107] Ohayon MM, Roth T. Prevalence of restless legs syndrome and periodic limb movement disorder in the general population. J Psychosom Res 2002; 53: 547-54.

[108] Pennestri MH, Montplaisir J, Colombo R, Lavigne G, Lanfranchi PA. Nocturnal blood pressure changes in patients with restless legs syndrome. Neurology 2007; 68(15): 1213-18.

[109] Winkelman JW, Shahar E, Sharief I, Gottlieb DJ. Polysomnographic and health-related quality of life correlates of restless legs syndrome in the Sleep Heart Health Study. Sleep 2009; 32(6): 772-78.

[110] Winkelman JW, Finn L, Young T. Prevalence and correlates of restless legs syndrome symptoms in the Wisconsin Sleep Cohort. Sleep Med 2006; 7(7): 545-52.

[111] Grote L, Leissner L, Hedner J, Ulfberg J. A randomized, double-blind, placebo controlled, multi-center study of intravenous iron sucrose and placebo in the treatment of restless legs syndrome. Mov Disord 2009; 24(10): 1445-1452.

[112] Earley CJ, Horská A, Mohamed MA, Barker PB, Beard JL, Allen RP. A randomized, double-blind, placebo-controlled trial of intravenous iron sucrose in restless legs syndrome. Sleep Med 2009; 10(2): 206-11.

[113] Trenkwalder C, Stiasny K, Pollmacher T, *et al.* L-DOPA therapy of uremic and idiopathic restless legs syndrome: a double-blind crossover trial. Sleep 1995; 18: 681-8.

[114] Allen RP, Earley CJ. Augmentation of the restless legs syndrome with carbidopa/levodopa. Sleep 1996; 19: 205-213.

[115] Collado-Seidel V, Kazenwadel J, Wetter TC, *et al.* A controlled study of additional SR-L-DOPA in L-DOPA responsive RLS with late night symptoms. Neurology 1999; 52: 285-90.

[116] García-Borreguero D, Allen RP, Kohnen R, et al. International Restless Legs Syndrome Study Group. Diagnostic standards for dopaminergic augmentation of restless legs syndrome: report from a World Association of Sleep Medicine-International Restless Legs Syndrome Study Group consensus conference at the Max Planck Institute. Sleep Med. 2007; 8(5): 520-30.

[117] Trenkwalder C, Stiasny-Kolster K, Kupsch A, Oertel WH, Koester J, Reess J. Controlled withdrawal of Pramipexole after 6 months of open-label treatment in patients with Restless Legs Syndrome. Mov Disord 2006; 21: 1404-10.

[118] Partinen M, Hirvonen K, Jama L, *et al.* Efficacy and safety of pramipexole in idiopathic restless legs syndrome: a polysomnographic dose-finding study—the PRELUDE study. Sleep Med 2006; 7: 407-17.

[119] Oertel WH, Stiasny-Kolster K, Bergthold B, *et al..* Efficacy of pramipexole in restless legs syndrome: a 6-week, multi-center, randomized, double-blind study (Effect-RLS Study). Mov Disord 2007; 22: 213-9.

[120] Winkelman JW, Sethi K, Kushida C, *et al.* Efficacy and safety of pramipexole in restless legs syndrome. Neurology 2006; 67: 1034-9.

[121] Manconi M, Ferri R, Zucconi M, *et al.* First night efficacy of pramipexole in restless legs syndrome and periodic leg movements. Sleep Med 2007; 8(5): 491-7.

[122] Ferini-Strambi L, Oldani A, Castronovo V, Zucconi M. RLS augmentation and pramipexole longterm treatment. Neurology 2001; 56(8, Suppl 3): A20.

[123] Stiasny-Kolster K, Oertel WH. Low-dose pramipexole in the management of restless legs syndrome—an open label trial. Neuropsychobiol 2004; 50: 65-70.

[124] Winkelman JW, Bennet S. Augmentation and tolerance with longterm pramipexole treatment of restless legs syndrome. Sleep Med 2004; 5: 9-14.

[125] Trenkwalder C, Garcia-Borreguero D, Montagna P, *et al.* Therapy with Ropiunirole; Efficacy and Tolerability in RLS 1 Study Group. Ropinirole in the treatment of restless legs syndrome: results from the TREAT RLS 1 study, a 12 week, randomised, placebo controlled study in 10 European countries. J Neurol Neurosurg Psychiatry 2004; 75: 92-97.

[126] Walters AS, Ondo W, Dreykluft T, Grunstein R, Lee D, Sethi K. Ropinirole is effective in the treatment of restless legs syndrome: TREAT RLS 2: A12-week double-blind, randomized, parallelgroup,placebo-controlled study. Mov Disord 2004; 19: 1414-23.

[127] Bogan RK, Fry JM, Schmidt MH, Carson SW, Ritchie SY, for the TREAT RLS US (Therapy with Ropinirole Efficacy and Tolerability in RLS US) Study Group. Ropinirole in the treatment of patients with restless legs syndrome: a US-based randomized, double-blind, placebo-controlled clinical trial. Mayo Clin Proc 2006; 81: 17-27.

[128] Allen R, Becker PM, Bogan R, *et al.* Ropinirole decreases periodic leg movements and improves sleep parameters in patients with restless legs syndrome. Sleep 2004; 27: 907-14.

[129] Allen RP, Earley CJ. Augmentation of the restless legs syndrome with carbidopa/levodopa. Sleep 1996; 19: 205-213.

[130] Paulus W, Trenkwalder C. Less is more: therapy-related augmentation of symptoms in Restless legs syndrome caused by dopaminergic overstimulation. Lancet Neurol 2006; 5: 878–86.

[131] Happe S, Sauter C, Klosch G, Saletu B, Zeitlhofer J. Gabapentin versus ropinirole in the treatment of idiopathic restless legs syndrome. Neuropsychobiology 2003; 48: 82–6.

[132] Garcia-Borreguero D, Larrosa O, de la Llave Y, Verger K, Masramon X, Hernandez G. Treatment of restless legs syndrome with gabapentin: a double-blind, cross-over study. Neurology 2002; 59: 1573–9.

[133] Telstad W, Sorensen O, Larsen S, Lillevold PE, Stensrud P, Nyberg-Hansen R. Treatment of the restless legs syndrome with carbamazepine: a double blind study. Br Med J (Clin Res Ed) 1984; 288: 444-6.

[134] Eisensehr I, Ehrenberg BL, Solti SR, Noachtar S. Treatment of idiopathic restless legs syndrome (RLS) with slow-release valproic acid compared with slow release levodopa/benserazide. J Neurol 2004; 251: 579-83

[135] Walters AS, Winkelmann J, Trenkwalder C, *et al.* Long-term follow-up on restless legs syndrome patients treated with opioids. Mov Disord 2001; 16: 1105-9.

[136] Qu S, Le W, Zhang X, Xie W, Zhang A, Ondo WG. Locomotion is increased in a11-lesioned mice with iron deprivation: a possible animal model for restless legs syndrome. J Neuropathol Exp Neurol 2007; 66(5): 383-8.

[137] Glover J, Jacobs A. Activity pattern of iron-deficient rats. Br Med J 1972; 2: 627–8.

[138] Baier PC, Winkelmann J, Hohne A, Lancel M, Trenkwalder C. Assessment of spontaneously occurring periodic limb movements in sleep in the rat. J Neurol Sci 2002; 198: 71–7.

[139] Connor JR, Wang XS, Allen RP, *et al.* Altered dopaminergic profile in the putamen and substantia nigra in restless leg syndrome. Brain. 2009; 132(Pt 9): 2403-12.

[140] Allen RP, Barker PB, Wehrl F, Song HK, Earley CJ. MRI measurement of brain iron in patients with restless legs syndrome. Neurology. 2001; 56(2): 263-5.

CHAPTER 14

Parasomnias

Kumar S. Budur, M.D., M.S.*

Associate Medical Director: Clinical Science – Neuroscience, Takeda Global Research and Development Inc., 675 North Field Drive, Lake Forest, IL 60045, USA

Abstract: Parasomnias are any undesirable physical events or experiences that happen during falling asleep, staying asleep or during arousals from sleep. Parasomnias are classified primarily based on the stage of sleep from which they originate *i.e.* NREM or REM sleep and by the nature of symptoms, *i.e.* sleep terrors, sleep walking, sleep eating, *etc.* These disorders vary both in frequency and severity and range from relatively benign events such as occasional episode of sleep paralysis to potentially serious and sometimes life-threatening events such as REM sleep behavior disorder. Parasomnias are also considered to be automatisms since the subjects sometimes do not have conscious awareness during these episodes resulting in some medico-legal consequences. Parasomnias can significantly affect the quality of sleep resulting in daytime impairments and they can also affect sleep and safety of the bed-partners. However, a thorough clinical assessment, appropriate tests where indicated, and judicious use of medications can help a vast majority of patients with parasomnia disorders.

TOPIC DISCUSSION (CLINICAL OUTLOOK)

Summary

The prevalence of various parasomnias varies widely and depending on the nature of the clinical practice, it is not uncommon to encounter patients with sleep enuresis, sleep-related eating disorder, REM sleep behavior disorder (RBD), *etc.* Patient with parasomnias usually present with complaints of unusual behaviors or experiences during sleep that results in disturbed sleep, daytime impairment and/or potentially dangerous behaviors that are sometimes associated with injuries to self or others.

Over the years, our understanding of the pathophysiology of parasomnias has advanced significantly and now the association between disorders such as RBD and certain neurodegenerative disorders is well established. A thorough clinical evaluation, including a detailed sleep history and collateral information and physical examination is sufficient to diagnose majority of the patients. However, polysomnography (PSG) is mandatory in certain disorders such as REM sleep behavior disorder. Patient education and, where appropriate, judicious use of medications can help the majority of the patients with parasomnias.

Discussion

The prevalence of various parasomnias varies with age and gender and some disorders are more common and clinically more important than others.

The prevalence and sexual predilection of some of the commonly encountered and clinically important parasomnias are depicted succinctly in Table **1**:

PARASOMNIAS USUALLY ASSOCIATED WITH NREM SLEEP

The disorders of arousal from NREM sleep are characterized by abnormal behaviors associated with sudden partial arousal from slow-wave sleep. Disorders of arousals typically occur during the first third of the night, when slow-wave sleep is prominent. Disorders of arousals are commonly precipitated by sleep deprivation, fever, stress (physical or psychological), psychiatric/neurological disorders and some medications [1].

*Address correspondence to **Kumar S. Budur:** Associate Medical Director: Clinical Science – Neuroscience, Takeda Global Research and Development Inc., 675 North Field Drive, Lake Forest, IL 60045, USA; E-mail: ksbudur@yahoo.com

Table 1: Parasomnia categories and main characteristics. (SSRIs = selective serotonin re-uptake inhibitors, SNRIs = serotonin & norepinephrine re-uptake inhibitors)

Disorder	Prevalence	Sex predilection	Unique features/comments
Confusional arousals	Children aged 3 to 13 years: 17.3%; Children > 15 years and adults: 2.9 to 4.2%;	No sex difference.	- Most of the children "out grow" this disorder - Scheduled awakenings sometimes help.
Sleep walking	17% in children with a peak between the age of 8 to 12 years. Adults: 4%.	No sex difference but sleep walking related injuries are more common in men than women.	- safety is of paramount importance as sleep walking can sometimes result in serious injuries
Sleep terrors	Children: 1 to 6.5%; Adults: 2.2%; greater than 65 years old: 1%.	No sex difference.	- In most cases, sleep terrors tend to resolve spontaneously during adolescence. - Sleep terrors should be distinguished from nocturnal panic attacks which are characterized by full awareness of the surroundings on awakening from sleep.
REM sleep behavior disorder (RBD)	0.38% in the general population and 0.5% in subjects older than 50 years.	Predominantly seen in men > 50 year-old;	- Ensuring safety of the patient and the bed partners is extremely important. - Some medications (mainly SSRIs, SNRIs) can precipitate RBD. - Can have medico-legal consequences
Nightmare disorder	2 to 8% of the general population.	No sex difference during childhood. However, in adolescents and adults, it is more common in females.	- Nightmares are often seen in patients with posttraumatic stress disorder (PTSD) and sometimes persist long after the resolution of other PTSD symptoms.
Sleep enuresis	10% of 6 year olds; 5% of 10 year olds and 1-2% in 18-year old children.	Primary enuresis is more common in men than in women with a ratio of 3:2.	- Behavioral therapy is effective in some patients.
Sleep-related eating disorder	The exact prevalence is unknown but 4.6% in an university setting.	Predominantly affects females.	- Sleep-related eating disorder should be differentiated from nocturnal eating syndrome (NES), that is characterized by over-eating between the evening meal and sleep onset; eating during awakenings at night with no altered consciousness and full recall; and absence of eating any bizarre/uncooked foods that is sometimes seen in patients with sleep-related eating disorder - Behavioral therapy is effective in some patients. - Topiramate and fluoxetine have been found to e effective in some patients.
Sleep related sexual behavior	Exact prevalence is unknown	No information available but men appear to be involved in many of the reported cases	- Also known as "sexsomnia" - It is considered as a variant of confusional arousal but can occur as part of sleep walking, as well. - Behaviors described include: masturbation, sexual molestation/assault, loud sexual vocalizations, etc followed by amnesia to these events - These behaviors can result in significant personal, medical and legal implications

The following is a brief description of some of the important aspects of commonly observed parasomnias:

Confusional Arousals

Confusional arousals are recurrent episodes of mental confusion or confusional behavior which occur during an arousal or awakening from night time sleep or a daytime nap. Confusional arousals are typically seen in children in the age group of 3 to 13 years and majority of the children tend to "outgrow" this disorder.

Some of the common precipitants for confusional disorder include: sleep deprivation, primary sleep disorders (sleep apnea, restless legs syndrome), physical/emotional stress, febrile illness, environmental stimuli such as noise, alcohol/illicit drug use and psychiatry conditions such as depression, anxiety, *etc.*

Sleep Walking

Sleep walking is characterized by ambulation in sleep, during which the subject is completely asleep, has altered state of consciousness or impaired judgment. It is often difficult to wake up a person during an episode of sleep walking; if awakened, sleep-walkers tend to have either mental confusion or lack of memory (either partial or complete) about the episode. During an episode of sleep walking, some patient's exhibit routine behaviors but these occur at inappropriate times and sometimes they may engage in inappropriate or non-goal directed behaviors. Sleep walking can be potentially dangerous to self or others.

Sleepwalking is a common disorder, affecting approximately 15 % of children and 4 % of adults, with peak prevalence between ages 8 and 12. In the majority of cases, sleepwalking begins in the first decade of life and remit spontaneously by adolescence. However, onset in adulthood can also occur. Childhood-onset sleepwalking continues into adulthood in about 20 % of cases. Sleepwalking has a strong genetic predisposition, increasing in relation to the number of affected parents. Although there is no sex difference, sleep walking associated injuries are more common in men than in women.

Common precipitants for sleep walking include: sleep deprivation, primary sleep disorders (sleep apnea, restless legs syndrome), physical/emotional stress, febrile illness, environmental stimuli such as noise, alcohol/illicit drug use and psychiatry conditions such as depression, anxiety, *etc.*

Sleep Terror

Sleep terror is characterized by sudden episode of terror in sleep, usually commencing with a loud scream or a cry associated with intense fear. It is often difficult to wake up a person during an episode of sleep terror and, if awakened, they have either mental confusion or lack of memory (partial or complete) for the episode. Sometimes, sleep terrors can be accompanied by potentially dangerous behaviors towards self or others.

Sleep terrors often occur in children and some of the common precipitants for sleep terrors include: sleep deprivation, primary sleep disorders (sleep apnea, restless legs syndrome), physical/emotional stress, febrile illness, environmental stimuli such as noise, *etc.* Sleep terrors, although benign and usually not need any pharmacological therapy, can be very distressing to the family, especially the parents who often feel helpless [2].

PARASOMNIAS USUALLY ASSOCIATED WITH REM SLEEP

The three disorders that are recognized under this category include REM sleep behavior disorder, recurrent isolated sleep paralysis and nightmare disorder.

REM Sleep Behavior Disorder (RBD)

RBD is characterized by abnormal behaviors that occur during REM sleep, that can cause injury to self or others, or cause sleep disruption. It is a relatively rare disorder with a prevalence of 0.38% in subjects under the age of 50 years and the prevalence is slightly higher (0.5%) in subjects older than 50 years. Although rare, RBD is an important parasomnia since about a third of the patients with RBD may have injurious behaviors for self or others, which may have also medico-legal implications.

The typical presentation in RBD is that of a recurrent dream-enactment behavior in men over the age of 50 years. These episodes occur about two hours after the onset of sleep, coinciding with the onset of the first episode of REM sleep but also commonly occur during the last one-third of the sleep, where REM sleep is predominantly observed. After awakening from an episode, the patients become alert quickly and typically describe unpleasant dream content (violent dreams, chasing, etc). The observed actions during these episodes usually correspond to the dream content. A history of injury to self or the bed partner is not uncommon in patients with RBD. For reasons not known, RBD is more common in men than in women.

Some of the common precipitants of RBD include: medications (mainly psychotropics such as selective serotonin reuptake inhibitors, serotonin and norepinephrine reuptake inhibitors), alcohol/drug abuse, sleep apnea (pseudo-RBD [see below]), *etc*. RBD is frequently associated with neurodegenerative disorders, such as Parkinson's disease, dementia with Lewy bodies, and multiple system atrophy [3, 4]. These disorders share a common pathologic lesion composed of abnormal aggregates of alpha-synuclein protein in the brain. RBD may precede the diagnosis of the underlying neurodegenerative disorder by several decades and may serve as an indicator of an evolving synucleinopathy.

A polysomnogram (PSG) in these patients typically shows excessive muscle tone during REM sleep. PSG is essential to establishing the diagnosis. In fact, RBD is the only parasomnia for which a sleep study is required for confirmation.

One of the important differential diagnoses for RBD is pseudo-RBD. It is a phenomenon characterized by sleep apnea presenting with abnormal behaviors in sleep, mimicking RBD. These patients, typically have severe sleep apnea with significant oxygen desaturations, muscle atonia in REM on PSG, and clinical features including snoring, witnessed apneas, excessive daytime sleepiness, *etc*. Pseudo-RBD is perhaps best classified as a parasomnia due to a medical condition (sleep apnea). It is important to differentiate RBD from pseudo-RBD since it has clinical implications [5]. Treatment of the underlying cause (here sleep apnea), will usually result in resolution of RBD-like symptoms [6].

Recurrent, Isolated Sleep Paralysis

Recurrent isolated sleep paralysis is characterized by episodes of lack of ability to move the trunk or all limbs either during sleep initiation or waking up in the morning. These episodes are usually brief, lasting for seconds, but sometimes it may last up to a few minutes.

Nightmare Disorder

Nightmare disorder is characterized by repeated episodes of awakenings from sleep (usually REM sleep, and therefore, seen more commonly during the second half of the sleep period), associated with recall of dreams that are disturbing with feelings of fear, anxiety and other unpleasant emotions. The patients experience difficulty in returning to sleep.

Other Parasomnias

The most common disorders in this category are sleep enuresis and sleep-related eating disorder.

Sleep Enuresis

Sleep enuresis is characterized by repeated, involuntary voiding of urine during sleep for at least two times per week in children who are at least five-year old [7]. In addition, depending on whether these children were or were not consistently "dry" before, they are categorized to have secondary or primary sleep enuresis, respectively. Primary enuresis presents with a history of involuntary voiding during sleep since infancy. However, for secondary enuresis, a period of dryness lasting at least 6 months before bedwetting returns is required. Many causes and associations for secondary enuresis are identified including psychosocial stress, sleep apnea, urinary tract infections, diabetes mellitus, diabetes insipidus, constipation, *etc*. In fact, sleep apnea is increasingly diagnosed in children with sleep enuresis and it is now one of the common causes of secondary enuresis [8]. The enuresis during sleep should occur at least twice a week to be considered clinically problematic and sleep enuresis, as a diagnosis, should not be considered in children under the age of 5 years.

Sleep-Related Eating Disorder (SRED)

Sleep-related eating disorder (SRED) is characterized by repeated episodes of involuntary eating and/or drinking during arousal from sleep. During these episodes, the patients have variable levels of consciousness, with partial or complete recall of the episode. In addition, patients with SRED often consume inedible substances such as uncooked food, raw meat, detergents, etc and realize about it only in the morning [9, 10]. Other features include morning anorexia, unrefreshing sleep and adverse health consequences related to consumption of high-calorie foods, inedible substances, *etc*. SRED is predominantly seen in females and the usual age of onset is in the third decade of life.

SRED is sometimes associated with other sleep disorders such as sleep apnea, periodic limb movement disorder, etc that can cause a partial arousal in NREM sleep. A related condition, called Nocturnal Eating Syndrome (NES), however, is characterized by over-eating between the evening meal and nocturnal sleep onset and sometimes eating again after awakening from sleep with full recall. An association between the use of sedative/hypnotic medications and sleep-related eating disorder has been described [11, 12].

Various parasomnias, *i.e.* different disorders of arousals can occur in the same patient and, occasionally, REM parasomnias can also be observed in the same patient. It is important to note that other disorders such as seizures, sleep apnea, sleep-related dissociative disorders can also cause sleep-related behaviors without awareness, or with partial awareness.

In the majority of patients with parasomnias, the diagnosis is accomplished by a detailed clinical history, while a polysomnogram (PSG) is not typically indicated. However, PSG should be considered in patients with potentially injurious behaviors or behaviors that disrupt others during sleep; atypical features including those suggestive of other disorders such as sleep apnea or seizures; if the patient has daytime impairments such as excessive daytime sleepiness, fatigue; and also in patients who do not respond to appropriate therapy. Patients with parasomnias do not necessarily show abnormalities during a PSG. They may have slow-wave sleep arousals on a PSG in the absence of abnormal behaviors or they may have REM sleep with much reduced muscle tone but not associated with any abnormal motor behaviors.

Managing patients with parasomnias consists primarily of educating the patient and family members about the disorder, maintaining a safe sleeping environment that is free of any objects that are potentially dangerous to the patient or others. Securing doors, windows and other exits is essential. The patients should avoid stimuli that could precipitate an episode of parasomnia, such as sleep deprivation, and maintain a regular sleep-wake cycle. Treatment of co-morbid sleep and psychiatric disorders and, if possible, avoidance of any medications that could potentially precipitate parasomnias are also important. Stress reduction, psychotherapy and hypnosis have been found to be helpful in some patients. Sometimes the frequency or the severity of the disorder necessitates treatment with medications such as benzodiazepines or tricyclic antidepressants.

Treatment with benzodiazepines is effective in RBD and clonazepam is often considered the first-line therapy. However, prior to starting benzodiazepines, all patients must be evaluated for sleep apnea and, if present, should be treated appropriately since benzodiazepines can worsen sleep apnea by suppressing upper airway tone and/or respiratory centers. Other agents such as melatonin, dopamine agonists and some antiepileptic drugs are also found to be effective in the treatment of RBD. Patients should be educated about the association between RBD and synucleinopathies, which are a group of neurodegenerative disorders characterized by fibrillary aggregates of alpha-synuclein protein in selective populations of neurons and glial cells (Parkinson disease, dementia with Lewy bodies, multiple system atrophy, pure autonomic failure, neurodegeneration with brain iron accumulation type I, or Hallervorden-Spatz disease) [3, 4].

RESEARCH OUTLOOK

Summary

Parasomnias are unique sleep disorders that provide us an insight into both the normal and abnormal physiological processes that happen during sleep. Disorders such as confusional arousals, sleep walking, RBD and sleep-related eating disorders have helped us understand the complex interaction of the various neurological pathways and neurotransmitters that lead to sleep initiation and maintenance and presumably help function during the wake period. However, a vast majority of the research findings are the result of experiments in animals, which may or may not correspond to the pathophysiology that occurs in humans with parasomnias.

What do we know:

REM sleep behavior disorders are associated with certain neurodegenerative disorders like Parkinson's Disease (PD), Dementia with Lewy Bodies (DLB), Multiple System Atrophy (MSA), Pure Autonomic Failure (PAF), neurodegeneration with brain iron accumulation type I, or Hallervorden-Spatz disease.

About 45% of patients with idiopathic RBD develop neurodegenerative disorder, on average 12 years after the initial onset of RBD. The most common neurodegenerative disorder observed in these patients is Parkinson's disease.

Sleep related eating disorder has features of both sleep and eating disorders *i.e.* somnambulism and daytime eating disorder; over 90% of patients report some form of amnesia and more than one-third of the subjects have a lifetime diagnosis of eating disorder.

The interaction between sleep apnea and parasomnia disorders is complex: sleep apnea can predispose or induce both disorders of arousal during NREM and REM sleep. Sleep related eating disorder can cause or worsen sleep apnea by inducing obesity.

What we don't know:

Many of the non-REM parasomnias such as confusional arousals, sleep terrors, and sleep walking are limited to pediatric age group and most of the children tend to "outgrow" these disorders. However, the reasons for this seem to be unknown. Further research in this area might not only help to understand the pathophysiology and help develop targets for effective treatments, but also help to understand the relationship between pediatric and adult parasomnias.

The current understanding of the pathophysiology of RBD stems mainly from animal models. It is presumed to generally apply to the disease pathophysiology in humans. However, better understanding of the illness in humans will enable us to further understand some of the complex relationship between RBD and synucleinopathies.

Treating RBD with benzodiazepines is associated with an improvement in symptoms. However, persistence of high muscle tone during REM sleep is still noted on PSG in these patients. Further understanding of the mechanism by which drugs like benzodiazepines and tricyclic antidepressants affect RBD will help in better understanding of the pathophysiology of not just RBD, but also other neurodegenerative disorders.

Although dopaminergic agents have been found to be helpful in the treatment of some patients with RBD, and PET or SPECT brain scans have shown decreased binding to presynaptic dopamine receptors in the nigrostriatal system, it is yet to be determined if dopaminergic dysfunction is the cause of RBD or if it is an epiphenomenon.

REFERENCES

[1]   Schenck CH, Pareja JA, Patterson AL, *et al.* Analysis of polysomnographic events surrounding 252 slow-wave sleep arousals in thirty-eight adults with injurious sleepwalking and sleep terrors. J Clin Neurophysiol 1998; 15(2): 159-166.
[2]   Mason TB, Pack AI. Pediatric parasomnias. Sleep 2007; 30(2): 141-51.
[3]   Iranzo A, Molinuevo JL, Santamaria J, *et al.* Rapid-eye-movement sleep behaviour disorder as an early marker for a neurodegenerative disorder: a descriptive study. Lancet Neurol 2006; 5(7): 572-7.
[4]   Boeve BF, Silber MH, Parisi JE, *et al.* Synucleinopathy pathology and REM sleep behavior disorder plus dementia or parkinsonism. Neurology 2003; 61(1): 40-5.
[5]   Schenck CH, Boyd JL, Mahowald MW. A parasomnia overlap disorder involving sleepwalking, sleep terrors, and REM sleep behavior disorder in 33 polysomnographically confirmed cases. Sleep 1997; 20(11): 972-81.
[6]   Iranzo A, Santamaria J. Severe obstructive sleep apnea/hypopnea mimicking REM sleep behavior disorder. Sleep 2005; 28(2): 203-6.
[7]   Fritz G, Rockney R. Summary of the practice parameter for the assessment and treatment of children and adolescents with enuresis. J Am Acad Child Adolesc Psychiatry 2004; 43(1): 123-5.
[8]   Brooks LJ, Topol HI. Enuresis in children with sleep apnea. J Pediatr 2003; 142(5): 515-8.
[9]   Winkelman JW. Clinical and polysomnographic features of sleep-related eating disorder. J Clin Psychiatry 1998; 59(1): 14-9.
[10]   Eveloff SE, Millman RP. Sleep-related eating disorder as a cause of obstructive sleep apnea. Chest 1993; 104(2): 629-30.
[11]   Morgenthaler TI, Silber MH. Amnestic sleep-related eating disorder associated with zolpidem. Sleep Med 2002; 3(4): 323-7.
[12]   Vetrugno R, Manconi M, Ferini-Strambi L, *et al.* Nocturnal eating: sleep-related eating disorder or night eating syndrome? A videopolysomnographic study. Sleep 2006; 29(7): 949-54.

CHAPTER 15

Sleep and Aging

Yohannes Endeshaw, M.D., M.P.H.[*]

Associate Professor, Department of Aging and Geriatric Research, College of Medicine, University of Florida, Gainesville, FL, USA

Abstract: Advances in science and technology over the last century have resulted in a steady increase in the average life expectancy of human beings, especially in developed countries. This trend implies a gradual increase in the proportion of older adults in the general population and that this group of the population will account for an increasing and significant proportion of patients seen by physicians in most clinical disciplines in the near future. For this reason, understanding the aging process and associated changes that occur in the different organs and systems is of paramount importance. Accordingly, age-related changes occur in sleep and wake system and these are described below.

TOPIC DISCUSSION (CLINICAL OUTLOOK)

THE AGING PROCESS

Advances in science and technology have resulted in a steady increase in the average life expectancy of human beings in general, especially in developed countries. In the United States, the current average life expectancy at birth is 80.4 years and 75.2 years for females and males, respectively; at age 65, average life expectancy is 20.0 years and 17.2 years for females and males, respectively [1]. This trend implies a gradual increase in the proportion of older adults in the general population (Table 1) and that this group of the population will account for an increasing and significant proportion of patients seen by physicians in most clinical disciplines. For this reason, understanding the aging process and age-related changes that occur in different organs and systems, is of paramount importance.

Table 1: United States Population Projection by Age Groups.

Calendar Year	Age Groups						
	0 – 4 years	5 to 19 years	20 to 44 years	45 to 64 years	65 to 84 years	85 years and over	
2000	6.81	21.74	36.89	22.13	10.92	1.51	100.00
2010	6.94	20.01	33.81	26.22	11.04	1.98	100.00
2020	6.83	19.64	32.35	24.91	14.10	2.16	100.00
2030	6.68	19.48	31.56	22.63	17.01	2.64	100.00
2040	6.71	19.22	31.04	22.61	16.49	3.93	100.00
2050	6.69	19.31	31.18	22.18	15.68	4.97	100.00

Source: U.S. Census Bureau, 2004, U.S. Interim Projections by Age -http://www.census.gov/ipc/www/usinterimproj/

The changes related to aging occur in all physiological systems and are associated with a gradual decline in function. However, these changes occur at variable rates in different individuals, depending on both intrinsic and extrinsic factors. "Successful aging" is a term that has been used to describe the impact of aging on the global functional status of the individual. In general, the term implies absence of disease-related disability, high functional capacity (physical and mental) and active engagement in daily life activities. Associations between sleep related

***Address correspondence to Yohannes Endeshaw:** Associate Professor, Department of Aging and Geriatric Research, College of Medicine, University of Florida, Gainesville, FL, USA; E-mail: yendeshaw@aging.ufl.edu

Octavian C. Ioachimescu (Ed)

characteristics and increased morbidity status have been reported, suggesting that sleep-related factors could have some roles in determining aging status of older adults.

Changes in sleep architecture and sleep stage distribution, as well as alterations in the activities of the circadian timing system have been described to occur in association with aging. However, the clinical significance of these changes, especially in otherwise health older adults is not clearly understood. In addition, sleep related complaints, daytime sleepiness and primary sleep disorders are reported to be common among older adults. Although some studies have indicated adverse impact of these sleep disorders on the functional status of older adults, this issue still remains controversial.

RESEARCH OUTLOOK

What do we know:

Aging-related changes occur in all physiological systems and are associated with a gradual decline in function [2]. However, these changes occur at a different rate in different individuals, depending on both intrinsic and extrinsic factors [3]. For this reason, chronological age may not reflect the extent of aging in an individual, and instead biological age (also referred to as physiological age or functional age) would be preferred for this purpose [4-6]. However, the quest to identify a universal biomarker (a biochemical, physiological or physical measure the can be used to determine biological age) has not been successful so far [7]. Given the importance of sleep for normal bodily functions, it would be important to investigate if sleep-related measures can be used for this purpose. For example, one recent study has reported that regularity of electroencephalographic (EEG) arousals (entropy-based measures of EEG arousals) associated with sleep disorders such as sleep disordered breathing may be a useful biomarker for co-existent hypertension [8]. Similar studies would have to be performed in order to identify sleep-related measures that could serve as biomarker(s) of biological aging.

"Successful aging" is another term used to describe the impact of aging on global functional status. In general, the term indicates absence of disease-related disability, high functional capacity (physical and mental) and active engagement in daily life activities [9]. Previous reports have indicated biological, personal and environmental factors as significant predictors of successful aging [9]. Sleep-related factors have also been shown to be significantly associated with measures that indicate successful aging, as defined above. For example, among community dwelling women, lower insomnia rating scale (less sleep disturbance) was significantly associated with less disability, higher life satisfaction score and positive psychological adaptation [10]. In another study, older adults (age $\geq$ 75 years) with no significant co-morbidity reported good sleep quality (based on sleep diary measures), suggesting that good sleep quality may be indicative of good physical health (or successful aging) [11]. This finding is in agreement with a previous report that showed that sleep-related complaints among older adults are associated with increased morbidity [12]. Furthermore, objective sleep measures of sleep such as actigraphy-derived short sleep time, reduced sleep efficiency and increased wake period after sleep onset were reported to be associated with poor physical [13, 14] and cognitive function [15]. Although cause-and-effect relationship cannot be inferred from cross-sectional studies, these studies suggest the possibility that co-morbid conditions are potential causes of associated insomnia. However, there is also the possibility that chronic insomnia could contribute to the pathogenesis or worsening of these conditions. Studies involving younger individuals have reported that sleep deprivation may result in metabolic abnormalities that could result in significant morbidity [16]. It is possible that optimal physical health and good quality and quantity of sleep would have reciprocal effects on each other. For a more extensive review, the reader is recommend to refer to a review article by Bliwise DL [17]. Future studies should focus on studies that would examine the direction of the association between physical / mental health and sleep, or on a sleep related measures(s) that would predict "successful aging".

In the following sections, we will describe changes in sleep and wakefulness associated with age, and sleep-disorders that are commonly encountered among older adults. It should be noted that: (1) older adults are a heterogeneous group of people, with varying functional and cognitive status, and (2) participants of most of the studies referred in this chapter were community-dwelling older adults who are independent in their activities of daily living and with no significant cognitive impairment. Hence, these factors should be taken into consideration when one interprets the results of such studies. Furthermore, each section is discussed in relation to aging or as it relates to older adults; and it would not be a comprehensive review of the sleep related subject or disorder. For this reason, the reader is advised to refer to the specific sleep related topic for a complete review of the subject.

What we don't know:

Several tasks still await answer(s) and could represent center points for future research:

- Identify sleep related biomarker(s) that would help determine the actual biological age.

- Determine objective sleep measures or sleep characteristics (sleep quality and quantity) which could predict successful aging.

- The impact of quality and quantity of sleep at mid-life on the aging process or the occurrence of disability and institutionalization later in life?

AGE-RELATED CHANGES IN SLEEP ARCHITECTURE

Sleep Continuity and Sleep Stage Distribution

TOPIC DISCUSSION (CLINICAL OUTLOOK)

Previous studies have revealed age-related changes in sleep architecture and sleep stage distribution, and these included: increase in stages N1 and N2, decrease in stages N3 and R (REM) sleep, increase in wake time after sleep onset (WASO) and decrease in sleep efficiency [18-24]. However, most of these studies were limited by small sample size and other methodological issues, such as confounding by co-morbidity and medications. More recently, a meta-analysis of studies that reported sleep architecture in healthy (non-clinical) individuals ranging in age between 5 years and 102 years was published [25]. Included in the analysis were 47 studies, (with a total of 2,391 participants; 1,474 men and 917 women) which measured sleep using polysomnography or actigraphy in "nonclinical" study participants. Results indicated that there were significant age-related changes in most indices of sleep measures and sleep architecture, with large effect size for total sleep time, sleep efficiency and slow wave sleep (all decreased with age) and WASO (increased with age); medium effect size for REM sleep percent (decreased with age) and small effect size for stage N1 percent and REM latency (both increased with age) [25].

These findings corroborate (more or less) previous reports on this issue [17-23]. In addition, this meta-analysis also reported several other notable findings. For example, when participants with mental illness, physical illness and sleep apnea were excluded, the effect size for total sleep time and sleep efficiency increased, suggesting a stronger association between aging and these sleep measures. Other findings of interest that were reported include, significant decline in REM sleep were observed only after age 60 years, and absence of significant difference in sleep latency between middle-aged and older adults. With regards to stage N3 of sleep (slow wave sleep, SWS), there was no significant association with age when studies that included only elderly participants were analyzed, suggesting that the changes may have occurred at an earlier age. This finding is in agreement with previous studies that have reported decline in SWS starting at an earlier age (as early as early adulthood) [26]. Of note, the decrease in SWS is intimately associated with reduction in the levels of growth hormone, which starts during early adulthood [26].

Similar results were reported in another cross-sectional study, in which association between age and polysomnographic sleep measures were described among 2,685 community dwelling older adults (age range between 37 and 92 years, 49.6% female) who participated in the Sleep Heart Health Study (SHHS) [27]. Findings of interest in this analysis included an increase in stage N1 and N2 sleep among participants 61 years or older in comparison to those less than 54 years old, significantly lower SWS among participants 54 years or older as compared to those less than 54 years old, significantly reduced REM sleep in those ≥ 61 years old in relation to those < 61 years old and increase in arousal index and sleep efficiency associated with increasing age [27]. Again, the results of this study are in agreement with previous reports on this issue [17-23]. A remarkable finding in this report was the differential effect of age on sleep continuity and sleep stage distributions among men and women. The effect of age on all indices of sleep architecture was significantly worse among men, in comparison to women. Male study participants had significantly lower SWS in comparison to female study participants, and a significant increase in stages N1 and N2. Similar findings were previously reported among older adults [28-30]. The significance of this gender difference in sleep architecture is not clearly understood. Whether the favorable sleep architecture observed among women explains, at least in part, the 'gender longevity gap'[1] that is described in most countries has not been investigated. Despite this favorable sleep architecture, sleep related complaints are more common among older women in comparison to older men (see below), a finding that is contrary to what one would expect to observe.

RESEARCH OUTLOOK

What do we know:

The aforementioned studies should be viewed in conjunction with their limitations. Ideally, in order to assess changes in sleep measures across time, one would like to look at a random sample of individuals without co-morbidity or medication effects, followed for a long period of time, and hence to be able to develop normative data for different age and gender groups. However, we do not live in an ideal world, and consequently we would have to make best use of the information that is available, understanding its limitations. As described by the authors, the cross-sectional study from SHHS [27] has many strengths, which include: large sample size, exclusion of individuals such as those: on medications known to impact sleep, with history of alcohol consumption (> 14 drinks per week), and those with history of awakenings due to leg cramps, leg jerks, cough or wheezing, and pain. In addition, adjustments for potential confounding factors such as gender, body mass index, respiratory disturbance index, smoking status and history of stroke were made during the analysis. However, as the authors state in the manuscript, sleep measures were derived from a single night study, and whether this could be considered representative of the participants' normal sleep pattern may be questioned. In addition, other potential confounding factors such as periodic leg movements in sleep, undiagnosed depression, effect of non-CNS active medications on sleep (for example beta-blockers) has not been accounted for.

What we don't know:

One question that is frequently raised when describing age-related changes pertains to referential values or normative data for sleep measures in older adults. Should reference values derived from mostly "healthy" young and middle-aged adults be used for older adults? Or is it important to develop normative data based on a reference group of "healthy" older adults? Each approach may have its own advantages and disadvantages. For example, normative data derived from "healthy" older adults provides information about changes that are expected or more than expected for age and this may have important clinical implications. However, it would not provide information about changes that may have occurred at younger age, for example changes in SWS distribution. Last but not least, given the differences in sleep architecture among older men and women, should there be different reference values for the two genders? These issues have important clinical implications and future studies should aim to provide answers to these questions.

Circadian Timing System

Topic Discussion (Clinical Outlook)

In humans, most cellular functions follow a close-to-24-hour circadian rhythm which is highly controlled and coordinated by the master circadian clock located in suprachiasmatic nucleus (SCN) of the anterior hypothalamus [31]. The SCN is entrained by various environmental cues (also known as *zeitgebers,* or time giver, synchronizer), such that activities of the different organs or systems and general individual behaviours coincide with appropriate environmental conditions during the 24-hour light-dark cycle. Light is the primary *zeitgeber,* with projections from the optic nerve (retino-hypothlammic tract) playing a crucial role in synchronization of the SCN to the environment [32], but social signals may also have roles serving as *zeitgebers* [33]. Activities that disrupt the harmony between the circadian rhythm and the environment on a long-term basis (for example, shift work, frequent travel across time zones) would result in disruption of sleep-wake system [34], and may predispose to increased morbidity [35, 36]; and these adverse effects are reported to be worse with aging [34]. In addition, change in pattern of exposure to light and social activities may also adversely affect the activities of the circadian timing system and this would have important clinical implications for older adults. For example, institutionalized older adults stay indoors most of the time, hence get no or limited exposure to light of adequate intensity required for stimulation of the circadian system. Furthermore, the presence of diseases of the eye, such as cataract of the lens or macular degeneration, would limit transmission of light required for activation of the circadian timing system. This implies circadian rhythm related disorders may be more common among this group of the population.

RESEARCH OUTLOOK

What do we know:

Age-related changes in the activity of circadian timing system, including physiological activities and behaviour, have been well described in animals [37-39], and improvements in circadian rhythm functions have been described after transplantation of fetal SCN to old rats [40]. Similar psychological and behavioural changes have been reported among humans as well. For example, in a constant routine procedure involving 27 young men (age range 18–31 years) and 21 older adults (age range 65–80 years), it was noted that the mean circadian temperature amplitude (swing) was significantly lower among older adults in comparison to younger men, that the nadir temperature occurred at an earlier time of the day (phase advance) among older adults when compared to younger men [41]; and these changes were more pronounced in men in comparison to women [41]. These findings may explain the increased wake time during sleep period (night-time) and increased sleep time during wake period (daytime) observed among older adults. However, conflicting results have also been reported on this issue, in which no significant difference in the amplitude and time of the temperature rhythm was observed between older and young adults [42].

One possible explanation for the phase advance in the circadian rhythm observed among older adults is the possibility that the circadian rhythm may get shorter with age. This issue was addressed in a study that determined the period of endogenous circadian rhythm of body temperature, melatonin and cortisol levels [43]. Results indicated that there was no significant difference between younger and older participants in the intrinsic circadian rhythm of these measures; however, there was advance in the circadian phase observed among older adults. As stated by the authors, this implies that the circadian phase advance observed among older adults is not the result of shortening of the intrinsic circadian rhythm.

What we don't know:

Although unequivocal changes in sleep architecture associated with aging have been reported, there are mixed reports about their clinical relevance. Recent epidemiologic studies have shown that healthy older adults with no significant medical or sleep related morbidity do not have increased sleep complaints (see below), regardless of age-related changes in sleep architecture described above. Another issue is related to the significance of gender differences in polysomnographic sleep architecture observed among older men and women? Although older women are described to have favourable sleep architecture and sleep stage distribution, they also are reported to have increased sleep related complaints. These findings suggest that polysomonographically derived measures commonly used to determine sleep quantity and quality may not be good indicators of subjective sleep complaints among older adults.

SLEEP-RELATED COMPLAINTS AMONG OLDER ADULTS

Difficulty Initiating and Maintaining Sleep

Topic Discussion (Clinical Outlook)

Several studies have reported increased prevalence of sleep complaints among older adults, including difficulty initiating, maintaining sleep, early morning awakenings and non-restorative sleep.

RESEARCH OUTLOOK

What do we know:

An epidemiologic study that included community-dwelling older adults from 3 communities in the United States [12] evaluated the occurrence of sleep-related complaints among 9,282 participants aged 65 years or older (average age = 72 years). Trouble falling asleep, waking up from sleep, waking up too early and feeling not rested in the morning were reported by 19%, 30%, 19% and 13% of participants, respectively [12], indicating the common occurrence of these complaints in this group. However, when the prevalence of these complaints was assessed among study participants without significant medical or psychiatric conditions (by self report), the proportion of participants with trouble falling asleep, waking up from sleep, waking up too early and feeling not rested in the morning decreased to 4%, 14%, 4%, 8%, 2% respectively, suggesting that the occurrence of these complaints is influenced by co-morbid conditions.

Another notable report on sleep complaints comes from the National Sleep Foundation in 2002 Sleep in America Polls [44]. This was a telephone interview in which close to 1,000 randomly selected young, middle-aged and older adults participated; results of the survey indicated that the prevalence of sleep-related complaints were not higher among older adults in comparison to young and middle-aged adults (Table **2**). These findings imply that sleep complaints among older adults are not a result of normal aging *per se*, but may be due to associated co-morbidity.

Table 2: Sleep related complaints by Age Group (Source: Sleep Foundation 2002 Sleep in America Poll).

	Age Groups		
	18 – 29 years (N=184) (%)	**30 – 64years (N=650) (%)**	**65 and above (N=161) (%)**
Trouble falling asleep	33	24	19
Waking up from sleep	32	38	32
Waking up too early	20	26	25
Feeling not rested in the morning	49	41	25

It is noteworthy that in both reports the sleep complaints were more common among women in comparison to men. This finding was despite a more "favorable" sleep architecture and sleep stage distribution reported among older women in relation to older men (see above). These findings indicate a mismatch between polysomnography (PSG)-derived measures of sleep quality and quantity and sleep-related complaints.

What we don't know:

- Is this a result of differences in symptom reporting among older men and older women?

- Is it possible that the current visual scoring of EEG recordings on PSG may not be adequate to identify factors that are responsible for sleep related complaints, and are other methods such as EEG spectral analysis better indicators of subjective sleep complaints? [45].

Daytime Sleepiness and Napping

Topic Discussion (Clinical Outlook)

Another common and important sleep complaint among older adults is daytime sleepiness. Previous epidemiological studies have reported variable prevalence rates, ranging from 7% [46], 8% [47], 14% [48], 15% [49], 17% [50] to 19% [51]. Most of these studies used different questionnaires to assess daytime sleepiness. And some of the studies utilized telephone interviews, while others used data that were obtained from questionnaires completed by patients. Furthermore, some of the questionnaires used Likert scale, while others used "Yes"/"No" dichotomy. The different methods used in these studies may explain the different prevalence rates reported. One large epidemiologic study reported a 20% overall prevalence rate of daytime sleepiness using Epworth Sleepiness Scale as a measure of sleepiness (ESS > 11 for male and > 9 for females) [52]. However, despite the differences in the methods used and prevalence rates reported, almost all of these studies reported a significant association between daytime sleepiness and increased morbidity. Daytime sleepiness was significantly associated with cardiovascular morbidity, psychiatric morbidity, sleep related complaints, functional impairment, cognitive impairment and mortality in these studies; indicating that daytime sleepiness could be a potential marker of increased co-morbidity and mortality.

Napping is a common behavior among older adults. While napping has been described to be beneficial in situations of sleep deprivation and shift work [53, 54], the significance of napping among older adults has not been clearly established; and conflicting results have been reported regarding this issue. For example, among healthy older adults, short naps taken at or before 15:00 hours for less than one hour (usually 30 minutes) resulted in improvement in sleepiness, performance, and did not have any adverse effect on nighttime sleep [55]. In another study that compared sleep patterns of healthy older adults while taking naps versus not taking naps, statistically significant decreases in PSG-derived total sleep time and sleep efficiency during periods of napping (mean (standard deviation: 318 (45) minutes vs. 366 (31) minutes; and 74.5 (6.1)% vs. 76.9 (6.4)%, respectively) were reported. However, there were no significant differences in other sleep measures [56]. While the latter study suggests that longer naps may have some adverse consequences, whether these differences have clinical significance or not is a debatable issue. In another more recent study, which monitored sleep patterns with 14-day wrist actigraphy and sleep diary, participants who napped during daytime and evening hours (2 hours before bedtime) were found to have increased sleep efficiency and reduced wake time after sleep onset [57], a finding that is not consistent with traditional teaching and practice [58]. On the other hand, several epidemiological studies have reported a significant association between napping and poor night time sleep, increased morbidity (medical and psychiatric) and increased mortality [46, 59-65]. One of the postulated explanations of the adverse effects of napping relates to an increased risk of adverse cardiovascular events associated with the surge in the sympathetic activity upon awakening from sleep [64, 65].

RESEARCH OUTLOOK

What do we know:

Several factors could explain the conflicting results regarding the consequences of napping. For example, what the study participants understand by the term napping could be very different. For some, it could mean a scheduled sleep during the day which usually occurs at the same time, while for others it may mean dozing off (unintended sleep) during the day, while watching TV or reading. Furthermore, napping is considered as one variable in some studies, and while in other studies, components of napping such as frequency of naps, timing and duration of naps are included in the analysis. For these reasons, the significance of napping among older adults is not clearly established.

In general, daytime sleepiness could occur as a result of altered function of the sleep-wake regulation system [66], which results in inappropriate increase in propensity to sleep (increased activity of sleep promoting centers), or decreased ability to stay awake (decreased activity of wake promoting centers). An increased propensity to sleep could occur in situations in which the individual is not getting adequate sleep during the night (*e.g.*, due to "primary" or "secondary" sleep disorders) or adverse effects of medications with sleep promoting effect. On the other hand, decreased ability to stay awake could occur in situations in which circadian wake drive is impaired (*e.g.* associated with neurodegeneration of SCN) or problems related to decreased activity of the wake-promoting neurotransmitters (*e.g.*, decreased hypocretin activity in narcolepsy). And in some individuals, napping may be a lifelong habit and may not be associated with significant morbidity.

What we don't know:

As stated above, one factor that could contribute for the conflicting results related to effect of napping is different methods of measurement used in these studies. Future studies should focus on developing a standardized measurement that can be used to determine the impact of napping on health status.

Nocturia

Topic Discussion (Clinical Outlook)

Nocturia is a prevalent and bothersome symptom among older adults, with two or more episodes of nocturia reported by more than a third of older adults [67, 68]. Nocturia is an important complaint among older adults because, in addition to sleep disruption, it is reported to be associated with decreased quality of life [67-69], falls [70-72] and even increased mortality [73]. Etiological factors associated with nocturia are multiple and include bladder-related factors (*e.g.*, age-related decreased bladder capacity, bladder outflow obstruction as in benign prostatic hyperplasia), increased urine production during sleep or nocturnal polyuria (age-related decrease in arginin vasopressin levels [74]), medications, diabetes mellitus and cardiovascular morbidity.

RESEARCH OUTLOOK

What do we know:

Of particular interest to this chapter is the relationship between nocturia and sleep disorders. Previous studies have indicated significant associations between increased nocturia and obstructive sleep apnea [75-77]. Increased serum levels of atrial natriuretic peptide resulting in nocturnal polyuria has been described in individuals with obstructive sleep apnea [78, 79]. Another mechanism by which sleep disorders (including sleep apnea, restless legs syndrome and periodic limb movement of sleep) could be related to nocturia is awakening from sleep. Individuals who have increased frequency of nocturia may be awakened from sleep by these primary sleep disorders, but these individuals may report 'urination' as the reason for waking up [76]. Independent association between nocturia and snoring, as well as nocturia and symptoms of restless legs syndrome has been previously reported [71], indicating that nocturia could be caused by underlying "primary" sleep disorders. This implies that sleep disorders should be considered in the differential diagnosis of nocturia.

What we don't know:

Multiple approaches (different questionnaires) have been used to measure daytime sleepiness among older adults previously, and none of them have been validated for use in this group of the population. Hence, developing a validated questionnaire that can be used among different groups of older adults would be essential.

Factors that determine the beneficial effects and / or adverse consequences of napping would also be important.

SLEEP DISORDERS

In the next section, sleep disorders that are commonly encountered among older adults are discussed in brief. The discussion is focused on issues that are particularly relevant to older adults, and the reader is advised to refer to specific chapters on these disorders for detailed discussion on the topic.

Sleep Disordered Breathing (SDB)

Topic Discussion (Clinical Outlook)

Sleep disordered breathing (SDB) in the form of obstructive sleep apnea-hypopnea is a common disorder among older adults. In a recent population-based survey, the prevalence of SDB with an apnea-hypopnea index (AHI) ≥ 5 episodes per hour of sleep was 52.8% among participants ≥ 60 years old. Of these, 32.8% had an AHI between 5 and 14, while 19.9% had an AHI of 15 or more per hour of sleep [80]. This was significantly higher than the rate for subjects less than 60 year-old in the same study. However, when the rate of increase was examined by age, the linear relationship between increasing age and SDB seemed to level off after age 60, and then show a sharp rise after age 80 years (Fig. **1**). The significance of these findings has not been clearly established. Previous reports have speculated that SDB among older adults could show both age-related and age-dependent pattern [81], and this could explain the pattern shown in the Fig. **1**. The male to female ratio in this study was reported to be 2-3 to 1, a value lower than reported among typical sleep clinic populations [82]. This phenomenon has been reported previously and may very well reflect the observed increase in prevalence of SDB among women after menopause [83].

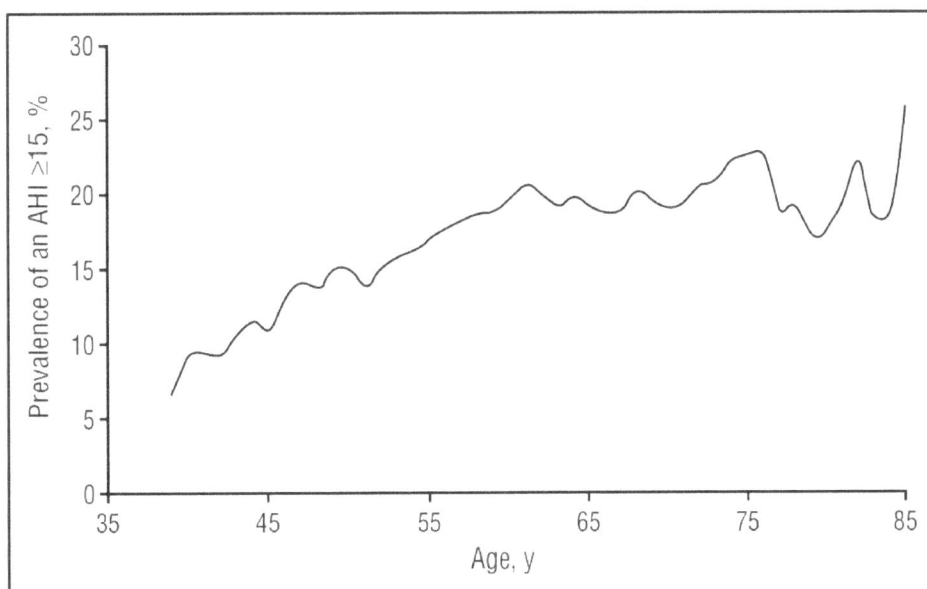

Figure 1: Sleep apnea prevalence versus age (Source: adapted from Young, T. *et al.* Arch Intern Med 2002; 162: 893-900)

This study also reports a decrease in the strength of association between SDB in older adults and traditional risk factors for SDB, such as snoring, obesity, increased neck circumference and hip-to-waist ratio. Several other studies have reported similar findings [80, 84, 85]. Older adults who live alone may not know whether they snore or stop breathing during their sleep, and this may explain, at least in part, the reduced frequency of these symptoms among those with SDB. However, this could also indicate the role of other predisposing factors for SDB among older adults. For example, a decrease in the tone of the upper airway muscles has been described as a possible predisposing factor for SDB in non-obese elderly [86-88]. Another common condition that may change the anatomy of the upper airway and adversely impact its function is edentulism, and previous studies have reported significant association between SDB and edentulism [89, 90]. Edentulism leads to a decrease in the vertical dimension of occlusion, which may result in a reduction of upper airway anatomy (size) and altered activity of upper-airway-dilating muscles; and these changes would predispose subjects to partial or complete obstruction of the upper airway during sleep. And more recently, a significant association has been reported between age-related decline in forced vital capacity and sleep disordered breathing, suggesting that decline in lung function associated with aging could predispose older adults to SDB [16].

RESEARCH OUTLOOK

What do we know:

Despite the common occurrence of SDB among older adults, its significance is not clearly established. For example, significant association between SDB and hypertension (based on casual blood pressure recordings) was reported among participants of SHHS less than 60 years of age, but not among those older than 60 [91, 92]. Similar findings were reported regarding the association between SDB and cardiovascular morbidity [93]. A more recent population-based prospective study reported increased cardiovascular mortality among male participants with severe SDB (RDI >30/hour) less than 70 years of age, but not among men over the age of 70 and women of all ages [94]. Another study that examined the relationship between SDB and mortality reported no significant increase in mortality in men with severe SDB who are between 50 and 79 years old in comparison to mortality of the general population; although in the same study an increase in mortality among participants > 80 year-old with SDB was observed [95]. Based on these and similar reports, opinion that suggests that elderly individuals with SDB may have developed resistance to hypoxia-related tissue injury (ischemic preconditioning) [95, 96] have been proposed. Furthermore, whether SDB among older adults is a different disorder than SDB seen among middle-aged adults has also been raised [97, 98].

On the other hand, several studies have reported significant associations between SDB and biological or functional measures that are relevant to older adults. For example, significant associations between SDB and nocturia [84], non-dipping of blood pressure during sleep [99], slow waking speed [100], disability in performing one or more activities of daily living [100], and falls [101] have been reported. In addition, reports of significant associations between SDB and stroke [102], increased blood pressure, diabetes and low high-density lipoprotein (LDL) [103] have been published. These reports indicate that SDB among older adults is not a benign condition. Future studies, aiming to investigate the significance of SDB among older adults should identify outcome measures that have relevance to functional status and quality of life of older adults. Relevant outcome measures for older adults include performance measures, mobility limitations, falls, quality of life and health care utilization (for example emergency room visits, hospitalizations). Another unresolved issue is if the impact of SDB is different among older men and older women, and future studies should examine if there are gender differences in the adverse effects of SDB.

Published reports examining the efficacy of treatment of SDB among older adults are relatively scarce and remain controversial. Non-surgical treatment options for SDB include oral appliance devices and continuous positive airway pressure (CPAP), but experience with the use of both modalities of treatment among older adults is limited. Loss of teeth and sub-optimal dentition status, common conditions among older adults, would be limiting factors to the use of oral appliance therapy in this group of the population [104, 105]. With regard to CPAP, adherence to CPAP treatment is reported to be 40% t0 50% among sleep clinic population (mostly middle-aged), and there are no reports describing adherence to CPAP exclusively among older adults [106, 107]. In controlled clinical trials, the general compliance of older adults to CPAP was reported to be comparable to that observed in middle-aged adults [106, 107]. Furthermore, CPAP therapy of older adults with obstructive sleep apnea was reported to improve night-time sleep [108], daytime sleepiness [109] and functional status [110], indicating that older adults not only tolerate CPAP use, but would also benefit from its use. However, these studies should be interpreted with caution as they are limited by small sample size (or case report publication), and controlled trials that lasted only a few weeks. Future well designed studies would be required to examine the impact of CPAP therapy on outcomes that are relevant to older adults, including daytime sleepiness, functional status, quality of life and health care utilization.

What we don't know:

What is the impact of treatment of SDB with CPAP among older adults? Does it improve functional status and quality of life; does it reduce health care utilization and mortality?

Restless Legs Syndrome (RLS) and Periodic Limb Movement of Sleep (PLMS)

Topic Discussion (Clinical Outlook)

RLS is a common disorder among older adults, with prevalence rates for the presence of symptoms of RLS ranging between 9% and 24% reported in studies from Europe [111-113], and about 4% in a study from Japan [114]. However, the prevalence of clinically significant RLS (based on frequency and severity of symptoms) is reported to range between 2% and 3% [115-117]. In most studies, the disease is reported to be more common among women, with female-to-male ratios of at least 2:1. Conflicting results are reported on the issue of whether prevalence of RLS increases with age, with some studies showing no significant difference among different age groups [113, 118], while others reported an increase with age [119-121]. However, the diagnostic criteria for RLS were not exactly the same in these studies, and this may partly explain the different results reported. In addition to sleep-related problems, older adults with RLS were more likely to report use of hypnotics [112], anxiety and depression symptoms [112], suggesting that RLS among the elderly may adversely impact health status and their quality of life. Of note, previous studies have reported significant association between use of hypnotics among older adults and adverse outcomes such as falls and cognitive impairment [122, 123].

RESEARCH OUTLOOK

What do we know:

RLS is described to occur in two forms, early onset and late onset disease, and the late onset form, generally characterized by absence of family history and low ferritin levels, is reported more commonly among the elderly [124].

Diagnosis of RLS is based on the international RLS study group diagnostic criteria [115, 125] and RLS rating scale [126]. While these criteria work well for most older adults, the diagnosis of RLS among elderly with cognitive impairment remains a challenge. Although RLS diagnostic criteria for cognitively impaired individuals [115] have been described, they have not been validated among older adults with dementia. The relationship between RLS and abnormal behaviors among older adults with dementia has also not been examined. For example, exacerbation of abnormal behaviors during the evening hours has been described in nursing home residents with cognitive impairment, a phenomenon termed "sun-downing" [127, 128]. Although circadian rhythm disturbances have been thought to explain this phenomenon [129, 130], it is also plausible that these behaviors could be a manifestation of RLS in these individuals who are not able to voice their complaints. Pacing, a common behavior among nursing home residents (NHRs) with dementia, could also be a manifestation of RLS in this group. Given the common occurrence of iron deficiency among NHRs [131], the prevalence of RLS in this group of the population would be expected to be high.

Periodic limb movement disorder of sleep (PLMS), a condition characterized by repetitive movement of the lower extremities (rhythmic extension of the big toe and dorsiflexion of the ankle and flexion at the knee and hip) [132, 133] is also a common condition among older adults [134-136], and these limb movements are independently associated with increased arousals from sleep [136]. RLS and PLMS share a common pathophysiology and a significant proportion of individuals with RLS would also have PLMS [137] (see Chapter 13). Several factors could contribute for the increase in prevalence of RLS/PLMS among older adults. As stated above, iron deficiency state is a common problem among older adults [138]. In addition, the rate of use of psychotropic agents such as serotonin re-uptake inhibitors and anti-psychotic agents is high in this group of the population [139], and these group of medications have been described to precipitate or exacerbate these disorders [140-142]

Management of RLS/PLMS among older adults is similar to management of these conditions among the general population. However, given the increased prevalence of "secondary" RLS or PLMS in this group of the population, emphasis should be given to management of underlying risk factors such as iron deficiency and medication use. The lowest effective dose of dopamine agonists should be used, even if the dose is less than recommended by the drug manufacturer. Doses recommended by manufacturers of these medications are generally based on the results of clinical trials in which healthy, mostly young and middle-aged adults are involved. Given the age-related changes in drug metabolism and the potential drug-drug interactions that could occur among older adults that take multiple medications, these recommended doses may not be optimal for older adults.

What we don't know:

- What are the criteria for the diagnosis of RLS among older adults with cognitive impairment?

- Do RLS /PLMS have adverse impact on functional status and cognitive status of older adults?

- Are abnormal behaviors among older adults with dementia associated with RLS and /or PLMS?

Rapid Eye Movement Sleep Behavior Disorder (RBD)

Topic Discussion (Clinical Outlook)

Rapid eye movement sleep behavior disorder (RBD) is characterized by abnormal behavior during rapid eye movement (REM, R) sleep [143], with a potential for sleep related injuries. It was initially described in adults between the ages of 60 and 72 years [144, 145], but more recently, the disorder has been reported even among younger patients (< 50 years of age) [146]. In one case series in which 39 young (age range 15 – 49 years) and 52 older (age range between 50 and 88) participants were included, idiopathic form of RBD was the predominant diagnosis in both age groups, with 51% and 63% of participants in the young and older groups, respectively [146]. However, etiological factors for secondary form of the disease were significantly different in the two groups. In the younger group, secondary RBD was diagnosed in 19 participants, and associated conditions included narcolepsy in 15, anti-depressant medications in 2 and Parkinson's disease in one person. Among those in the older age groups, conditions associated with secondary RBD were mostly neurodegenerative diseases related to alpha-synuclein deposition (synucleinopathy). Parkinson's disease, multiple system atrophy, Lewy body dementia were associated with RBD in 12, 2 and 1 participant, respectively. The diagnostic criteria for RBD requires both the presence of REM sleep without atonia (RSWA) during PSG recording and history of associated abnormal motor behavior [143]. In situations where RSWA is associated with no behavioral abnormalities (or no complex behavioral abnormalities), a clinical diagnosis of sub-clinical RBD is entertained [143]. Although the natural course of subclinical RBD remains yet to be established, these individuals should be followed up for possible development of RBD or associated conditions.

RESEARCH OUTLOOK

What do we know:

Idiopathic RBD is diagnosed when the disorder is identified in individuals with no neurological or sleep-related disorders. However, at least in one study, patients with idiopathic RBD were reported to have lower scores on neurological tests in comparison to controls [147]; suggesting that the idiopathic form of the disorder may represent earlier stage of neuropathology. In general, 25% to 50% of individuals with idiopathic RBD at the time of initial diagnosis are reported to develop a neurodegenerative disorder (commonly Parkinson's disease and dementia) on follow up, which could range from one year to many years [148-150]. For this reason, it would be prudent to perform a detailed baseline neurological examination and neuropsychological testing in individuals diagnosed with idiopathic RBD. Although the pathophysiology of RBD is understood in general terms, the specific neural circuit or neurotransmitter that is involved in each case is not clearly known [151]. For example, the association of RBD with different disorders (narcolepsy in young adults, neurodegenerative diseases in older adults) suggests that the pathogenesis of the disorder may be different in different groups of individuals with the disorder.

Management of RBD includes both conservative measures and pharmacological interventions. Conservative measures include making the home environment safe, in order to avoid or minimize injuries during the episodes. In homes were firearms are available, they should be kept secure, so they would not be accessed easily during RBD episodes. Ideally, pharmacological treatment of a condition should follow a clear understanding of the pathophysiology involved in the disorder. In situations where this is not clearly established, empirical use of medications is practiced. With regard to RBD, several medications with different mechanism of actions have been used with some degree of success.

In clinical practice, the most commonly used medication is clonazepam, a long-acting benzodiazepine agent. This medication is reported to decrease "phasic" REM activity and there are reports that it may also modify dream content [152, 153]. Supporting data for use of this medication is derived from published case series and case reports, and not randomized controlled clinical trials [153]. The use of benzodiazepine agents among older adults is not without consequences; for this reason, caution is recommended while prescribing this medication. A recent case series of 39 patients with RBD who were treated with Clonazepam reported side effects in up to 58% of the participants, and side effects included daytime sleepiness, confusion and cognitive impairment [154]. Use of melatonin has also been reported to improve symptoms of RBD, and reported mechanism for its favorable effect includes restoration of REM sleep atonia [155-158]. Because these two medications work through different mechanisms, the possibility that their action may be additive when used together has been reported. Other medications reported to be effective for treatment of RBD include Pramipexole [159, 160] and Zopiclone [154]. Future clinical trial with focus on the impact of treatment on REM atonia and motor behavior during sleep are needed to improve management of individuals with RBD.

What we don't know:

- Development of safe and effective medication for treatment of RBD among older adults.

Chronic Insomnia

Topic Discussion (Clinical Outlook):

Insomnia related sleep complaints [161] are common among older adults. An epidemiological study which reported sleep complaints among older adults in the United States indicated that 42% of 9,282 participants complained of difficulty initiating or maintaining sleep most of the time [12] and similar high prevalence rates for insomnia has been reported in other studies as well [162-164]. One of the consistent findings that is reported in all these studies is that complaints related to insomnia are much more common among older adults with co-morbid medical, neurological and psychiatric conditions, in comparison to older adults with no significant co-morbidities, suggesting that these co-morbid conditions may predispose to insomnia [165]. The relationship between insomnia and co-morbidities may be bidirectional, with co-morbidities giving rise to insomnia, and insomnia in turn worsening the status of co-morbidities. For example, insomnia has been reported to lower pain threshold, and successful treatment of insomnia with cognitive behavioral therapy has been reported to improve chronic pain [166, 167]. Another consequence of insomnia among older adults is increased use of sedative hypnotics, and this group of medications is associated with multiple adverse effects as stated below. Furthermore, independent associations between insomnia and increased risk of falls [168-171] and reduced quality of life [172] have been reported. These reports have several implications and these include: insomnia is not a result of normal aging; insomnia is associated with significant adverse effects in this group of the population, and management of insomnia in this group of the population should include optimal treatment of co-morbid conditions (in addition to treatment of insomnia with cognitive behavioral therapy).

RESEARCH OUTLOOK

What do we know:

Use of sedative hypnotics are indicated for short-term treatment of insomnia and data for this recommendation is derived from short-term randomized controlled trials, mostly performed on healthy young and middle-aged adults. Except for one recent study that reported safety profile for 12-months use of a short-acting non-benzodiazepine agent (zaleplon) [173], there is no data on the efficacy and safety of long-term sedative-hypnotics among older adults. However, long-term use of sedative-hypnotics among older adults is common [174, 175] and associated with significant adverse effects related to cognition, gait, balance and daytime fatigue [176-178]. For these reasons, caution should be exercised when prescribing sedative hypnotics for older adults.

Cognitive Behavioral therapy (CBT) for the treatment of chronic insomnia has been used more widely in research and clinical practice in the last decades [58, 179]. This form of therapy aims to correct dysfunctional beliefs and practices that perpetuate insomnia [180]; and more recently has been successfully used among different groups of older adults with chronic insomnia, including community-dwelling older adults [181-183], care givers of dementia patients [184], older adults with co-morbid insomnia [166, 185] and older adults using sedative hypnotics [186]. This indicates that the principles of CBT can be successfully applied for treatment of insomnia among older adults. However, the age cut-off used to define older adults in these studies is variable, with some studies including adults in their 50s as participants, and the number of participants above 75 years of age may be under-represented in most of these studies. In addition, older adults are not a homogenous group, and within each age-group, functional and cognitive status of individuals would vary. For these reasons, future research should focus on the effectiveness of CBT among the oldest old and older adults with functional and cognitive impairment. Previous studies have indicated improvement in anxiety and depression after CBT among older adults with mild to moderate dementia of Alzheimer's type [187, 188], suggesting that this form of therapy can be effective in individuals with dementia. Of particular interest related to this is a report in which CBT along with physical exercise and light therapy resulted in reduction in the number and duration of nighttime awakenings among patients with Alzheimer's disease [189], suggesting that the principles of CBT can be modified and applied for treatment of chronic co-morbid insomnia among older adults with varying functional and cognitive status.

In summary, chronic insomnia is a common problem among older adults and successful management of this condition should include optimal treatment of underlying conditions and CBT. Future research should aim at modifying the principles of CBT for application to older adults with functional and cognitive impairment. The efficacy of long-term treatment of chronic insomnia with sedative hypnotics in this group of the population has not been demonstrated, may be associated with significant adverse effects, and should be used with caution.

Consolidation of wakefulness during the day is one of the functions of the circadian timing system [190]. Previous reports have implicated age-related changes in the circadian timing system, such as reduction in the amplitude of circadian pacemaker outputs, to contribute to sleep and wake consolidation observed among older adults (manifested by increased sleepiness during the day and awakenings during the night). Based on this, bright light therapy has been used for treatment of sleep maintenance insomnia among community-dwelling older adults, as well as institutionalized elderly. Unfortunately, in these studies, use of bright light did not show a consistently favorable result [191-196]. A more recent well designed study did not find significant improvement in objective sleep measures among older adults with primary insomnia (age range 54–78 years, mean age 64 years) after treatment with bright light (4000 Lux) for 12 weeks [197]. Reasons for these conflicting results include dose, timing and duration of light therapy and possibly the heterogeneity of the health status of study participants in different studies. These conflicting results may also suggest the possibility that bright light therapy may be effective in selected group of older adults with certain characteristics. For example, institutionalized older adults with limited light exposure and activities during the day and with no significant pathology in the retina may be a group in whom light exposure may be beneficial. Future studies should aim at identifying older adults with insomnia for whom light therapy would be a treatment option.

What we don't know:

- The efficacy of CBT in older adults with functional impairment.
- The efficacy of CBT in older adults with cognitive impairment.

Advanced Sleep Phase Syndrome

Topic Discussion (Clinical Outlook)

Entrainment of the circadian system to the outside environment results in synchronization of sleep-wake schedule to the dark-light cycle of the environment and appropriate social activities of the individual. When this alignment is lost, sleep-wake schedules may not be fully synchronized with the environment. Earlier bed and wake times are reported among older adults, and this is explained, at least in part, by age-related phase advances in the circadian timing system [198]. However, in some older adults, this phase advance is exaggerated resulting in much earlier bed time and wake time (up to 3 hours before the desired bed time) than what is desired by the individual. These individuals complain of difficulty keeping awake until their desired sleep time and difficulty sleeping until their desired wake time; although their sleep quality and duration may be normal [199].

RESEARCH OUTLOOK

What do we know:

Bright light therapy (≥ 2500 lux) administered during the evening hours has been reported to delay sleep phase among older adults [200, 201]. However, tolerance and adherence to long term use of this amount of light has been reported to be a limitation to use of this form of treatment on a long term basis. Attempts to decrease the intensity of the light to a level that would be more tolerable have not been successful yet. For example, a recent study examined the effect of enhanced evening light (265 lux) in older adults (age range between 60 and 80 years) with advanced sleep phase syndrome, but no significant change was observed in improving objective measures of advance sleep phase [202].

What we don't know:

- Identification of dose, duration and related factors that determine effectiveness of light therapy among older adults.

REFERENCES

[1]   http://www.cdc.gov/nchs/data/hus/hus08.pdf#026.
[2]   Murphy MP, Partridge L. Toward a control theory analysis of aging. [Review]   [139 refs]. Annu Rev Biochem 2008; 77: 777-98.
[3]   Kirkwood TB, Austad SN. Why do we age?. [Review] [75 refs]. Nature 6809; 408:233-8.
[4]   Edwards AS. The myth of chronological age. J Appl Psychol 1950; 34:316-8.
[5]   Nakamura E, Moritani T, Kanetaka A. Effects of habitual physical exercise on physiological age in men aged 20-85 years as estimated using principal component analysis. Eur J Appl Physiol Occup Physiol 1996; 73:410-8.
[6]   Karasik D, Demissie S, Cupples LA, Kiel DP. Disentangling the genetic determinants of human aging: biological age as an alternative to the use of survival measures. J Gerontol A Biol Sci Med Sci 2005; 60:574-87.
[7]   Butler RN, Sprott R, Warner H *et al.* Biomarkers of aging: from primitive organisms to humans. J Gerontol A Biol Sci Med Sci 2004; 59.
[8]   Jamasebi R, Redline S, Patel SR, Loparo KA. Entropy-based measures of EEG arousals as biomarkers for sleep dynamics: applications to hypertension. Sleep 2008; 31:935-43.
[9]   Rowe JW, Kahn RL. Successful aging. [Review]   [62 refs]. Gerontologist 1997; 37:433-40.
[10]   Jeste N, Meeks TW, Fellow I *et al.* Sleep and Successful Aging in Women Over Age 60. Sleep 2008; 31 (Suppl):A100 (0305).
[11]   Driscoll HC, Serody L, Patrick S *et al.* Sleeping well, aging well: a descriptive and cross-sectional study of sleep in "successful agers" 75 and older. Am J Geriatr Psychiatry 2008; 16:74-82.
[12]   Foley DJ, Monjan AA, Brown SL *et al.* Sleep complaints among elderly persons: an epidemiologic study of three communities. Sleep 1995; 18:425-32.
[13]   Goldman SE, Stone KL, Ancoli-Israel S *et al.* Poor sleep is associated with poorer physical performance and greater functional limitations in older women. Sleep 1317; 30:1317-24.
[14]   Dam TT, Ewing S, Ancoli-Israel S *et al.* Association between sleep and physical function in older men: the osteoporotic fractures in men sleep study. J Am Geriatr Soc 1665; 56:1665-73.
[15]   Blackwell T, Yaffe K, Ancoli-Israel S *et al.* Poor sleep is associated with impaired cognitive function in older women: the study of osteoporotic fractures. J Gerontol A Biol Sci Med Sci 2006; 61:405-10.
[16]   Bliwise D. EPIDEMIOLOGY OF AGE-DEPENDENCE IN SLEEP DISORDERED BREATHING (SDB) IN OLD AGE: THE BAY AREA SLEEP COHORT (BASC). Sleep Med Clin. 2009; 4:57-64.
[17]   Bliwise DL. Sleep in normal aging and dementia. Sleep 1993; 16:40-81.
[18]   Feinberg I, Koresko RL, Heller N. EEG sleep patterns as a function of normal and pathological aging in man. J Psychiatr Res 1967; 5:107-44.
[19]   Bonnet MH, Arand DL. EEG arousal norms by age. J Clin Sleep Med 2007; 3:271-4.
[20]   Boselli M, Parrino L, Smerieri A, Terzano MG. Effect of age on EEG arousals in normal sleep. Sleep 1998; 21:351-7.
[21]   Dijk DJ, Duffy JF, Czeisler CA. Age-related increase in awakenings: impaired consolidation of nonREM sleep at all circadian phases. Sleep 2001; 24:565-77.
[22]   Klerman EB, Davis JB, Duffy JF *et al.* Older people awaken more frequently but fall back asleep at the same rate as younger people. Sleep 2004; 27:793-8.
[23]   Hoch CC, Dew MA, Reynolds CF, 3rd *et al.* A longitudinal study of laboratory- and diary-based sleep measures in healthy "old old" and "young old" volunteers. Sleep 1994; 17:489-96.
[24]   Reynolds CF, 3rd, Monk TH, Hoch CC *et al.* Electroencephalographic sleep in the healthy "old old": a comparison with the "young old" in visually scored and automated measures. J Gerontol 1991; 46:M39-46.

[25] Ohayon MM, Carskadon MA, Guilleminault C, Vitiello MV. Meta-analysis of quantitative sleep parameters from childhood to old age in healthy individuals: developing normative sleep values across the human lifespan. Sleep 2004; 27:1255-73.

[26] Van Cauter E, Leproult R, Plat L. Age-related changes in slow wave sleep and REM sleep and relationship with growth hormone and cortisol levels in healthy men. JAMA 2000; 284:861-8.

[27] Redline S, Kirchner HL, Quan SF et al. The effects of age, sex, ethnicity, and sleep-disordered breathing on sleep architecture. Arch Intern Med 2004; 164:406-18.

[28] Reynolds CF, 3rd, Kupfer DJ, Taska LS et al. Sleep of healthy seniors: a revisit. Sleep 1985; 8:20-9.

[29] Fukuda N, Honma H, Kohsaka M et al. Gender difference of slow wave sleep in middle aged and elderly subjects. Psychiatry Clin Neurosci 1999; 53:151-3.

[30] Rediehs MH, Reis JS, Creason NS. Sleep in old age: focus on gender differences. [Review] [56 refs]. Sleep 1990; 13:410-24.

[31] Moore RY, Eichler VB. Loss of a circadian adrenal corticosterone rhythm following suprachiasmatic lesions in the rat. Brain Res 1972; 42:201-6.

[32] Klein DC, Moore RY. Pineal N-acetyltransferase and hydroxyindole-O-methyltransferase: control by the retinohypothalamic tract and the suprachiasmatic nucleus. Brain Res 1979; 174:245-62.

[33] Davidson AJ, Menaker M. Birds of a feather clock together--sometimes: social synchronization of circadian rhythms. [Review] [46 refs]. Curr Opin Neurobiol 2003; 13:765-9.

[34] Sack RL, Auckley D, Auger RR et al. Circadian rhythm sleep disorders: part I, basic principles, shift work and jet lag disorders. An American Academy of Sleep Medicine review. [Review] [197 refs]. Sleep 1460; 30:1460-83.

[35] Sahar S, Sassone-Corsi P. Metabolism and cancer: the circadian clock connection. [Review] [139 refs]. Nat Rev Cancer 2009; 9:886-96.

[36] Kawachi I, Colditz GA, Stampfer MJ et al. Prospective study of shift work and risk of coronary heart disease in women. Circulation 3178; 92:3178-82.

[37] Ingram DK, London ED, Reynolds MA. Circadian rhythmicity and sleep: effects of aging in laboratory animals. Neurobiol Aging 1982; 3:287-97.

[38] Weinert D. Age-dependent changes of the circadian system. [Review] [150 refs]. Chronobiol Int 2000; 17:261-83.

[39] Weinert H, Weinert D, Schurov I et al. Impaired expression of the mPer2 circadian clock gene in the suprachiasmatic nuclei of aging mice. Chronobiol Int 2001; 18:559-65.

[40] Cai A, Scarbrough K, Hinkle DA, Wise PM. Fetal grafts containing suprachiasmatic nuclei restore the diurnal rhythm of CRH and POMC mRNA in aging rats. Am J Physiol 1764; 273.

[41] Czeisler CA, Dumont M, Duffy JF et al. Association of sleep-wake habits in older people with changes in output of circadian pacemaker. Lancet 8825; 340:933-6.

[42] Monk TH, Buysse DJ, Reynolds CF, 3rd et al. Circadian temperature rhythms of older people. Exp Gerontol 1995; 30:455-74.

[43] Czeisler CA, Duffy JF, Shanahan TL et al. Stability, precision, and near-24-hour period of the human circadian pacemaker. Science 5423; 284:2177-81.

[44] Foundation NS. "Sleep in America" Poll. 2002.

[45] Latta F, Leproult R, Tasali E et al. Sex differences in delta and alpha EEG activities in healthy older adults. Sleep 1525; 28:1525-34.

[46] Foley DJ, Vitiello MV, Bliwise DL et al. Frequent napping is associated with excessive daytime sleepiness, depression, pain, and nocturia in older adults: findings from the National Sleep Foundation '2003 Sleep in America' Poll. Am J Geriatr Psychiatry 2007; 15:344-50.

[47] Foley D, Monjan A, Masaki K et al. Daytime sleepiness is associated with 3-year incident dementia and cognitive decline in older Japanese-American men. J Am Geriatr Soc 1628; 49:1628-32.

[48] Ohayon MM, Vecchierini MF. Daytime sleepiness and cognitive impairment in the elderly population. Arch Intern Med 2002; 162:201-8.

[49] Chasens ER, Sereika SM, Weaver TE, Umlauf MG. Daytime sleepiness, exercise, and physical function in older adults. J Sleep Res 2007; 16:60-5.

[50] Newman AB, Spiekerman CF, Enright P et al. Daytime sleepiness predicts mortality and cardiovascular disease in older adults. The Cardiovascular Health Study Research Group. J Am Geriatr Soc 2000; 48:115-23.

[51] Empana JP, Dauvilliers Y, Dartigues JF et al. Excessive daytime sleepiness is an independent risk indicator for cardiovascular mortality in community-dwelling elderly: the three city study. Stroke 1219; 40:1219-24.

[52]   Whitney CW, Enright PL, Newman AB *et al.* Correlates of daytime sleepiness in 4578 elderly persons: the Cardiovascular Health Study. Sleep 1998; 21:27-36.

[53]   Milner CE, Cote KA. Benefits of napping in healthy adults: impact of nap length, time of day, age, and experience with napping. [Review]   [95 refs]. J Sleep Res 2009; 18:272-81.

[54]   Takahashi M. The role of prescribed napping in sleep medicine. [Review]   [60 refs]. Sleep Med Rev 2003; 7:227-35.

[55]   Tamaki M, Shirota A, Hayashi M, Hori T. Restorative effects of a short afternoon nap (<30 min) in the elderly on subjective mood, performance and eeg activity. Sleep Res Online 2000; 3:131-9.

[56]   Monk TH, Buysse DJ, Carrier J *et al.* Effects of afternoon "siesta" naps on sleep, alertness, performance, and circadian rhythms in the elderly. Sleep 2001; 24:680-7.

[57]   Dautovich ND, McCrae CS, Rowe M. Subjective and objective napping and sleep in older adults: are evening naps "bad" for nighttime sleep? J Am Geriatr Soc 1681; 56:1681-6.

[58]   Morin CM, Bootzin RR, Buysse DJ *et al.* Psychological and behavioral treatment of insomnia:update of the recent evidence (1998-2004). [Review] [82 refs]. Sleep 1398; 29:1398-414.

[59]   Picarsic JL, Glynn NW, Taylor CA *et al.* Self-reported napping and duration and quality of sleep in the lifestyle interventions and independence for elders pilot study. J Am Geriatr Soc 1674; 56:1674-80.

[60]   Goldman SE, Hall M, Boudreau R *et al.* Association between nighttime sleep and napping in older adults. Sleep 2008; 31:733-40.

[61]   Yoon IY, Kripke DF, Youngstedt SD, Elliott JA. Actigraphy suggests age-related differences in napping and nocturnal sleep. J Sleep Res 2003; 12:87-93.

[62]   Frisoni GB, De Leo D, Rozzini R, Trabucchi M. Napping in the elderly and its association with night sleep and psychological status. Int Psychogeriatr 1996; 8:477-87.

[63]   Hays JC, Blazer DG, Foley DJ. Risk of napping: excessive daytime sleepiness and mortality in an older community population. J Am Geriatr Soc 1996; 44:693-8.

[64]   Bursztyn M, Ginsberg G, Hammerman-Rozenberg R, Stessman J. The siesta in the elderly: risk factor for mortality? Arch Intern Med 1582; 159:1582-6.

[65]   Campos H, Siles X. Siesta and the risk of coronary heart disease: results from a population-based, case-control study in Costa Rica. Int J Epidemiol 2000; 29:429-37.

[66]   Saper CB, Scammell TE, Lu J. Hypothalamic regulation of sleep and circadian rhythms. [Review]   [100 refs]. Nature 7063; 437:1257-63.

[67]   Bing MH, Moller LA, Jennum P *et al.* Prevalence and bother of nocturia, and causes of sleep interruption in a Danish population of men and women aged 60-80 years. BJU Int 2006; 98:599-604.

[68]   Coyne KS, Zhou Z, Bhattacharyya SK *et al.* The prevalence of nocturia and its effect on health-related quality of life and sleep in a community sample in the USA. BJU Int 2003; 92:948-54.

[69]   Tikkinen KA, Johnson TM, 2nd, Tammela TL *et al.* Nocturia frequency, bother, and quality of life: how often is too often? A population-based study in Finland. Eur Urol 2010; 57:488-96.

[70]   Stewart RB, Moore MT, May FE *et al.* Nocturia: a risk factor for falls in the elderly. J Am Geriatr Soc 1217; 40:1217-20.

[71]   Endeshaw Y. Correlates of self-reported nocturia among community-dwelling older adults. J Gerontol A Biol Sci Med Sci 2009; 64:142-8.

[72]   Temml C, Ponholzer A, Gutjahr G *et al.* Nocturia is an age-independent risk factor for hip-fractures in men. Neurourol Urodyn 2009; 28:949-52.

[73]   Bursztyn M, Jacob J, Stessman J. Usefulness of nocturia as a mortality risk factor for coronary heart disease among persons born in 1920 or 1921. Am J Cardiol 1311; 98:1311-5.

[74]   Asplund R, Aberg H. Diurnal variation in the levels of antidiuretic hormone in the elderly. J Intern Med 1991; 229:131-4.

[75]   Endeshaw YW, Johnson TM, Kutner MH *et al.* Sleep-disordered breathing and nocturia in older adults. J Am Geriatr Soc 2004; 52:957-60.

[76]   Pressman MR, Figueroa WG, Kendrick-Mohamed J *et al.* Nocturia. A rarely recognized symptom of sleep apnea and other occult sleep disorders. Arch Intern Med 1996; 156:545-50.

[77]   Ulfberg J, Thuman R. A non-urologic cause of nocturia and enuresis--obstructive sleep apnea syndrome (OSAS). Scand J Urol Nephrol 1996; 30:135-7.

[78]   Baruzzi A, Riva R, Cirignotta F *et al.* Atrial natriuretic peptide and catecholamines in obstructive sleep apnea syndrome. Sleep 1991; 14:83-6.

[79]   Lin CC, Tsan KW, Lin CY. Plasma levels of atrial natriuretic factor in moderate to severe obstructive sleep apnea syndrome. Sleep 1993; 16:37-9.

[80]   Young T, Shahar E, Nieto FJ *et al.* Predictors of sleep-disordered breathing in community-dwelling adults: the Sleep Heart Health Study. Arch Intern Med 2002; 162:893-900.

[81]   Bliwise DL. Principles and Practice of Sleep Medicine. In: Normal Aging. 4th. Kryger MH, Roth T, WC. D (Editors). Philadelphia: Elsevier Saunders; 2005.

[82]   Guilleminault C, Quera-Salva MA, Partinen M, Jamieson A. Women and the obstructive sleep apnea syndrome. Chest 1988; 93:104-9.

[83]   Bixler EO, Vgontzas AN, Lin HM *et al.* Prevalence of sleep-disordered breathing in women: effects of gender. Am J Respir Crit Care Med 2001; 163:608-13.

[84]   Endeshaw Y. Clinical characteristics of obstructive sleep apnea in community-dwelling older adults. J Am Geriatr Soc 1740; 54:1740-4.

[85]   Enright PL, Newman AB, Wahl PW *et al.* Prevalence and correlates of snoring and observed apneas in 5,201 older adults. Sleep 1996; 19:531-8.

[86]   Fogel RB, White DP, Pierce RJ *et al.* Control of upper airway muscle activity in younger versus older men during sleep onset. J Physiol 2003; 553:533-44.

[87]   Ray AD, Ogasa T, Magalang UJ *et al.* Aging increases upper airway collapsibility in Fischer 344 rats. J Appl Physiol 1471; 105:1471-6.

[88]   Malhotra A, Huang Y, Fogel R *et al.* Aging influences on pharyngeal anatomy and physiology: the predisposition to pharyngeal collapse. Am J Med 2006; 119.

[89]   Bucca C, Carossa S, Pivetti S *et al.* Edentulism and worsening of obstructive sleep apnoea. Lancet 9147; 353:121-2.

[90]   Endeshaw YW, Katz S, Ouslander JG, Bliwise DL. Association of denture use with sleep-disordered breathing among older adults. J Public Health Dent 2004; 64:181-3.

[91]   Haas DC, Foster GL, Nieto FJ *et al.* Age-dependent associations between sleep-disordered breathing and hypertension: importance of discriminating between systolic/diastolic hypertension and isolated systolic hypertension in the Sleep Heart Health Study. Circulation 2005; 111:614-21.

[92]   Nieto FJ, Young TB, Lind BK *et al.* Association of sleep-disordered breathing, sleep apnea, and hypertension in a large community-based study. Sleep Heart Health Study.[Erratum appears in JAMA 2002 Oct 23-30;288(16):1985]. JAMA 2000; 283:1829-36.

[93]   Shahar E, Whitney CW, Redline S *et al.* Sleep-disordered breathing and cardiovascular disease: cross-sectional results of the Sleep Heart Health Study. Am J Respir Crit Care Med 2001; 163:19-25.

[94]   Punjabi NM, Caffo BS, Goodwin JL *et al.* Sleep-disordered breathing and mortality: a prospective cohort study. PLoS Medicine / Public Library of Science 2009; 6.

[95]   Lavie P, Lavie L, Herer P. All-cause mortality in males with sleep apnoea syndrome: declining mortality rates with age. Eur Respir J 2005; 25:514-20.

[96]   Lavie L, Lavie P. Ischemic preconditioning as a possible explanation for the age decline relative mortality in sleep apnea. Med Hypotheses 1069; 66:1069-73.

[97]   Ancoli-Israel S, Coy T. Are breathing disturbances in elderly equivalent to sleep apnea syndrome? Sleep 1994; 17:77-83.

[98]   Young T. Sleep-disordered breathing in older adults: is it a condition distinct from that in middle-aged adults? Sleep 1996; 19:529-30.

[99]   Endeshaw YW, White WB, Kutner M *et al.* Sleep-disordered breathing and 24-hour blood pressure pattern among older adults. J Gerontol A Biol Sci Med Sci 2009; 64:280-5.

[100]   Endeshaw YW, Unruh ML, Kutner M *et al.* Sleep-disordered breathing and frailty in the Cardiovascular Health Study Cohort. Am J Epidemiol 2009; 170:193-202.

[101]   Kaushik S, Wang JJ, Mitchell P. Sleep apnea and falls in older people. J Am Geriatr Soc 1149; 55:1149-50.

[102]   Munoz R, Duran-Cantolla J, Martinez-Vila E *et al.* Severe sleep apnea and risk of ischemic stroke in the elderly. Stroke 2317; 37:2317-21.

[103]   Newman AB, Nieto FJ, Guidry U *et al.* Relation of sleep-disordered breathing to cardiovascular disease risk factors: the Sleep Heart Health Study. Am J Epidemiol 2001; 154:50-9.

[104]   Petit FX, Pepin JL, Bettega G *et al.* Mandibular advancement devices: rate of contraindications in 100 consecutive obstructive sleep apnea patients. Am J Respir Crit Care Med 2002; 166:274-8.

[105]   Chan AS, Lee RW, Cistulli PA. Non-positive airway pressure modalities: mandibular advancement devices/positional therapy. [Review]   [73 refs]. Proc Am Thorac Soc 2008; 5:179-84.

[106]   Weaver TE, Chasens ER. Continuous positive airway pressure treatment for sleep apnea in older adults. [Review] [55 refs]. Sleep Medicine Reviews 2007; 11:99-111.

[107] Ayalon L, Ancoli-Israel S, Stepnowsky C *et al.* Adherence to continuous positive airway pressure treatment in patients with Alzheimer's disease and obstructive sleep apnea. Am J Geriatr Psychiatry 2006; 14:176-80.

[108] Cooke JR, Ancoli-Israel S, Liu L *et al.* Continuous positive airway pressure deepens sleep in patients with Alzheimer's disease and obstructive sleep apnea. Sleep Med 1101; 10:1101-6.

[109] Chong MS, Ayalon L, Marler M *et al.* Continuous positive airway pressure reduces subjective daytime sleepiness in patients with mild to moderate Alzheimer's disease with sleep disordered breathing. J Am Geriatr Soc 2006; 54:777-81.

[110] Endeshaw YW. Successful treatment of obstructive sleep apnea in a nonagenarian. J Am Geriatr Soc 2377; 57:2377-8.

[111] Berger K, von Eckardstein A, Trenkwalder C *et al.* Iron metabolism and the risk of restless legs syndrome in an elderly general population--the MEMO-Study. J Neurol 1195; 249:1195-9.

[112] Celle S, Roche F, Kerleroux J *et al.* Prevalence and clinical correlates of restless legs syndrome in an elderly French population: the synapse study. J Gerontol A Biol Sci Med Sci 2010; 65:167-73.

[113] Rothdach AJ, Trenkwalder C, Haberstock J *et al.* Prevalence and risk factors of RLS in an elderly population: the MEMO study. Memory and Morbidity in Augsburg Elderly. Neurology 1064; 54:1064-8.

[114] Mizuno S, Miyaoka T, Inagaki T, Horiguchi J. Prevalence of restless legs syndrome in non-institutionalized Japanese elderly. Psychiatry Clin Neurosci 2005; 59:461-5.

[115] Allen RP, Picchietti D, Hening WA *et al.* Restless legs syndrome: diagnostic criteria, special considerations, and epidemiology. A report from the restless legs syndrome diagnosis and epidemiology workshop at the National Institutes of Health. [Review]   [140 refs]. Sleep Med 2003; 4:101-19.

[116] Allen RP, Bharmal M, Calloway M. Prevalence and disease burden of primary restless legs syndrome: Results of a general population survey in the United States. Mov Disord 2010.

[117] Allen RP, Stillman P, Myers AJ. Physician-diagnosed restless legs syndrome in a large sample of primary medical care patients in western Europe: Prevalence and characteristics. Sleep Med 2010; 11:31-7.

[118] Hogl B, Kiechl S, Willeit J *et al.* Restless legs syndrome: a community-based study of prevalence, severity, and risk factors. Neurology 1920; 64:1920-4.

[119] Rijsman R, Neven AK, Graffelman W *et al.* Epidemiology of restless legs in The Netherlands. Eur J Neurol 2004; 11:607-11.

[120] Phillips B, Young T, Finn L *et al.* Epidemiology of restless legs symptoms in adults. Arch Intern Med 2137; 160:2137-41.

[121] Allen RP, Walters AS, Montplaisir J *et al.* Restless legs syndrome prevalence and impact: REST general population study. Arch Intern Med 1286; 165:1286-92.

[122] Leipzig RM, Cumming RG, Tinetti ME. Drugs and falls in older people: a systematic review and meta-analysis: I. Psychotropic drugs. J Am Geriatr Soc 1999; 47:30-9.

[123] Peri K. Review: sedative hypnotics may improve sleep quality but increase adverse effects in elderly people with insomnia. Evid Based Nurs 2006; 9:87.

[124] O'Keeffe ST, Gavin K, Lavan JN. Iron status and restless legs syndrome in the elderly. Age Ageing 1994; 23:200-3.

[125] Walters AS. Toward a better definition of the restless legs syndrome. The International Restless Legs Syndrome Study Group. [Review]   [142 refs]. Movement Disorders 1995; 10:634-42.

[126] Walters AS, LeBrocq C, Dhar A *et al.* Validation of the International Restless Legs Syndrome Study Group rating scale for restless legs syndrome. Sleep Med 2003; 4:121-32.

[127] Bliwise DL. What is sundowning?. [Review]   [47 refs]. J Am Geriatr Soc 1009; 42:1009-11.

[128] Bliwise DL, Carroll JS, Lee KA *et al.* Sleep and "sundowning" in nursing home patients with dementia. [Review]   [65 refs]. Psychiatry Res 1993; 48:277-92.

[129] Mahlberg R, Kunz D, Sutej I *et al.* Melatonin treatment of day-night rhythm disturbances and sundowning in Alzheimer disease: an open-label pilot study using actigraphy. J Clin Psychopharmacol 2004; 24:456-9.

[130] Volicer L, Harper DG, Manning BC *et al.* Sundowning and circadian rhythms in Alzheimer's disease. Am J Psychiatry 2001; 158:704-11.

[131] Artz AS, Fergusson D, Drinka PJ *et al.* Mechanisms of unexplained anemia in the nursing home. J Am Geriatr Soc 2004; 52:423-7.

[132] Montplaisir J, Allen RP, Walters AS, Ferini-Strambi L. Restless Legs Syndrome and Perioidic Limb Movments durign Sleep. In: Principles and Practice of Sleep Medicine. Kryger MH, Roth T, WC D (Editors). Philadelphia: Elsevier Saunders; 2005. p. 842.

[133] Hornyak M, Feige B, Riemann D, Voderholzer U. Periodic leg movements in sleep and periodic limb movement disorder: prevalence, clinical significance and treatment. [Review]   [96 refs]. Sleep Medicine Reviews 2006; 10:169-77.

[134] Kripke DF, Ancoli-Israel S, Okudaira N. Sleep apnea and nocturnal myoclonus in the elderly. Neurobiol Aging 1982; 3:329-36.

[135] Ancoli-Israel S, Kripke DF, Klauber MR *et al.* Periodic limb movements in sleep in community-dwelling elderly. Sleep 1991; 14:496-500.

[136] Claman DM, Redline S, Blackwell T *et al.* Prevalence and correlates of periodic limb movements in older women. J Clin Sleep Med 2006; 2:438-45.

[137] Stefansson H, Rye DB, Hicks A *et al.* A genetic risk factor for periodic limb movements in sleep. N Engl J Med 2007; 357:639-47.

[138] Coban E, Timuragaoglu A, Meric M. Iron deficiency anemia in the elderly: prevalence and endoscopic evaluation of the gastrointestinal tract in outpatients. Acta Haematol 2003; 110:25-8.

[139] Furniss L, Craig SK, Burns A. Medication use in nursing homes for elderly people. [Review][61   refs].   Int   J   Geriatr Psychiatry 1998; 13:433-9.

[140] Bakshi R. Fluoxetine and restless legs syndrome. J Neurol Sci 1996; 142:151-2.

[141] Pinninti NR, Mago R, Townsend J, Doghramji K. Periodic restless legs syndrome associated with quetiapine use: a case report. J Clin Psychopharmacol 2005; 25:617-8.

[142] Urbano MR, Ware JC. Restless legs syndrome caused by quetiapine successfully treated with ropinirole in 2 patients with bipolar disorder. J Clin Psychopharmacol 2008; 28:704-5.

[143] American Academy of Sleep Medicine. Rapid Eye Movement Sleep Behavior Disorder. In: The International Classification of Sleep Disorders Diagnostic and Coding Manual. Second. Medicine AAoS (Editor) Westchester, IL: 2005. pp. 148 - 152.

[144] Schenck CH, Bundlie SR, Ettinger MG, Mahowald MW. Chronic behavioral disorders of human REM sleep: a new category of parasomnia. Sleep 1986; 9:293-308.

[145] Schenck CH, Bundlie SR, Patterson AL, Mahowald MW. Rapid eye movement sleep behavior disorder. A treatable parasomnia affecting older adults. JAMA 1786; 257:1786-9.

[146] Bonakis A, Howard RS, Ebrahim IO *et al.* REM sleep behaviour disorder (RBD) and its associations in young patients. Sleep Med 2009; 10:641-5.

[147] Ferini-Strambi L, Di Gioia MR, Castronovo V *et al.* Neuropsychological assessment in idiopathic REM sleep behavior disorder (RBD): does the idiopathic form of RBD really exist? Neurology 2004; 62:41-5.

[148] Postuma RB, Gagnon JF, Vendette M, Montplaisir JY. Idiopathic REM sleep behavior disorder in the transition to degenerative disease. Mov Disord 2225; 24:2225-32.

[149] Iranzo A, Molinuevo JL, Santamaria J *et al.* Rapid-eye-movement sleep behaviour disorder as an early marker for a neurodegenerative disorder: a descriptive study. Lancet Neurol 2006; 5:572-7.

[150] Schenck CH, Bundlie SR, Mahowald MW. Delayed emergence of a parkinsonian disorder in 38% of 29 older men initially diagnosed with idiopathic rapid eye movement sleep behaviour disorder.[Erratum appears in Neurology 1996 Jun;46(6):1787]. Neurology 1996; 46:388-93.

[151] Boeve BF, Silber MH, Saper CB *et al.* Pathophysiology of REM sleep behaviour disorder and relevance to neurodegenerative disease. [Review] [138 refs]. Brain 2007; 130:2770-88.

[152] Lapierre O, Montplaisir J. Polysomnographic features of REM sleep behavior disorder: development of a scoring method. Neurology 1371; 42:1371-4.

[153] Aurora RN, Zak RS, Maganti RK *et al.* Best Practic Guide for the Treatment of REM Sleep Behavior Disorder (RBD). J Clin Sleep Med 2010; 6:85-95.

[154] Anderson KN, Shneerson JM. Drug treatment of REM sleep behavior disorder: the use of drug therapies other than clonazepam. J Clin Sleep Med 2009; 5:235-9.

[155] Boeve BF, Silber MH, Ferman TJ. Melatonin for treatment of REM sleep behavior disorder in neurologic disorders: results in 14 patients. Sleep Med 2003; 4:281-4.

[156] Kunz D, Bes F. Melatonin effects in a patient with severe REM sleep behavior disorder: case report and theoretical considerations. Neuropsychobiology 1997; 36:211-4.

[157] Kunz D, Bes F. Melatonin as a therapy in REM sleep behavior disorder patients: an open-labeled pilot study on the possible influence of melatonin on REM-sleep regulation. Mov Disord 1999; 14:507-11.

[158] Takeuchi N, Uchimura N, Hashizume Y *et al.* Melatonin therapy for REM sleep behavior disorder. Psychiatry Clin Neurosci 2001; 55:267-9.

[159] Fantini ML, Gagnon JF, Filipini D, Montplaisir J. The effects of pramipexole in REM sleep behavior disorder. Neurology 1418; 61:1418-20.

[160] Schmidt MH, Koshal VB, Schmidt HS. Use of pramipexole in REM sleep behavior disorder: results from a case series. Sleep Med 2006; 7:418-23.

[161]   American Academy of Sleep Medicine. Insomnia. In: The International Classification of Sleep Disorders - Diagnostic and Coding Manual. Second. Medicine AAoS (Editor) Westchester, IL: 2005.

[162]   Henderson S, Jorm AF, Scott LR *et al.* Insomnia in the elderly: its prevalence and correlates in the general population. Med J Aust 1995; 162:22-4.

[163]   Morgan K, Dallosso H, Ebrahim S *et al.* Characteristics of subjective insomnia in the elderly living at home. Age Ageing 1988; 17:1-7.

[164]   Quan SF, Katz R, Olson J *et al.* Factors associated with incidence and persistence of symptoms of disturbed sleep in an elderly cohort: the Cardiovascular Health Study. Am J Med Sci 2005; 329:163-72.

[165]   Vitiello MV, Moe KE, Prinz PN. Sleep complaints cosegregate with illness in older adults: clinical research informed by and informing epidemiological studies of sleep. J Psychosom Res 2002; 53:555-9.

[166]   Vitiello MV, Rybarczyk B, Von Korff M, Stepanski EJ. Cognitive behavioral therapy for insomnia improves sleep and decreases pain in older adults with co-morbid insomnia and osteoarthritis. J Clin Sleep Med 2009; 5:355-62.

[167]   Roehrs T, Hyde M, Blaisdell B *et al.* Sleep loss and REM sleep loss are hyperalgesic. Sleep 2006; 29:145-51.

[168]   Brassington GS, King AC, Bliwise DL. Sleep problems as a risk factor for falls in a sample of community-dwelling adults aged 64-99 years. J Am Geriatr Soc 1234; 48:1234-40.

[169]   Latimer Hill E, Cumming RG, Lewis R *et al.* Sleep disturbances and falls in older people. J Gerontol A Biol Sci Med Sci 2007; 62:62-6.

[170]   Stone KL, Ensrud KE, Ancoli-Israel S. Sleep, insomnia and falls in elderly patients. Sleep Med 2008; 9.

[171]   Avidan AY, Fries BE, James ML *et al.* Insomnia and hypnotic use, recorded in the minimum data set, as predictors of falls and hip fractures in Michigan nursing homes. J Am Geriatr Soc 2005; 53:955-62.

[172]   Stein MB, Barrett-Connor E. Quality of life in older adults receiving medications for anxiety, depression, or insomnia: findings from a community-based study. Am J Geriatr Psychiatry 2002; 10:568-74.

[173]   Ancoli-Israel S, Richardson GS, Mangano RM *et al.* Long-term use of sedative hypnotics in older patients with insomnia. Sleep Med 2005; 6:107-13.

[174]   Aparasu RR, Mort JR, Brandt H. Psychotropic prescription use by community-dwelling elderly in the United States. J Am Geriatr Soc 2003; 51:671-7.

[175]   Craig D, Passmore AP, Fullerton KJ *et al.* Factors influencing prescription of CNS medications in different elderly populations. Pharmacoepidemiol Drug Saf 2003; 12:383-7.

[176]   Glass J, Lanctot KL, Herrmann N *et al.* Sedative hypnotics in older people with insomnia: meta-analysis of risks and benefits. BMJ 2005; 331:1169.

[177]   Curran HV, Collins R, Fletcher S *et al.* Older adults and withdrawal from benzodiazepine hypnotics in general practice: effects on cognitive function, sleep, mood and quality of life. Psychol Med 2003; 33:1223-37.

[178]   Schneeweiss S, Wang PS. Claims data studies of sedative-hypnotics and hip fractures in older people: exploring residual confounding using survey information. J Am Geriatr Soc 2005; 53:948-54.

[179]   Morgenthaler T, Kramer M, Alessi C *et al.* Practice parameters for the psychological and behavioral treatment of insomnia: an update. An american academy of sleep medicine report. Sleep 1415; 29:1415-9.

[180]   Edinger JD, Means MK. Cognitive-behavioral therapy for primary insomnia. [Review] [82 refs]. Clin Psychol Rev 2005; 25:539-58.

[181]   Edinger JD, Hoelscher TJ, Marsh GR *et al.* A cognitive-behavioral therapy for sleep-maintenance insomnia in older adults. Psychol Aging 1992; 7:282-9.

[182]   Pallesen S, Nordhus IH, Kvale G *et al.* Behavioral treatment of insomnia in older adults: an open clinical trial comparing two interventions. Behav Res Ther 2003; 41:31-48.

[183]   Sivertsen B, Omvik S, Pallesen S *et al.* Cognitive behavioral therapy vs zopiclone for treatment of chronic primary insomnia in older adults: a randomized controlled trial. JAMA 2851; 295:2851-8.

[184]   McCurry SM, Logsdon RG, Vitiello MV, Teri L. Successful behavioral treatment for reported sleep problems in elderly caregivers of dementia patients: a controlled study. J Gerontol B Psychol Sci Soc Sci 1998; 53:122-9.

[185]   Rybarczyk B, Stepanski E, Fogg L *et al.* A placebo-controlled test of cognitive-behavioral therapy for comorbid insomnia in older adults. J Consult Clin Psychol 1164; 73:1164-74.

[186]   Soeffing JP, Lichstein KL, Nau SD *et al.* Psychological treatment of insomnia in hypnotic-dependant older adults. Sleep Med 2008; 9:165-71.

[187]   Kraus CA, Seignourel P, Balasubramanyam V *et al.* Cognitive-behavioral treatment for anxiety in patients with dementia: two case studies. J Psychiatr Pract 2008; 14:186-92.

[188]   Teri L, Logsdon RG, Uomoto J, McCurry SM. Behavioral treatment of depression in dementia patients: a controlled clinical trial. J Gerontol B Psychol Sci Soc Sci 1997; 52:159-66.

[189] McCurry SM, Gibbons LE, Logsdon RG *et al.* Nighttime insomnia treatment and education for Alzheimer's disease: a randomized, controlled trial. J Am Geriatr Soc 2005; 53:793-802.

[190] Dijk DJ, Duffy JF, Czeisler CA. Contribution of circadian physiology and sleep homeostasis to age-related changes in human sleep. [Review][107 refs]. Chronobiol Int 2000; 17:285-311.

[191] Ancoli-Israel S, Martin JL, Kripke DF *et al.* Effect of light treatment on sleep and circadian rhythms in demented nursing home patients. J Am Geriatr Soc 2002; 50:282-9.

[192] Chesson AL, Jr., Littner M, Davila D *et al.* Practice parameters for the use of light therapy in the treatment of sleep disorders. Standards of Practice Committee, American Academy of Sleep Medicine. Sleep 1999; 22:641-60.

[193] Fetveit A, Bjorvatn B. Bright-light treatment reduces actigraphic-measured daytime sleep in nursing home patients with dementia: a pilot study. Am J Geriatr Psychiatry 2005; 13:420-3.

[194] Forbes D, Morgan DG, Bangma J, Peacock S, Pelletier N, Adamson J. Light therapy for managing sleep, behaviour, and mood disturbances in dementia. Cochrane Database Syst Rev 2004; (2): CD003946. [Review update in: Cochrane Database Syst Rev 2009; (4): CD003946].

[195] Gammack JK. Light therapy for insomnia in older adults. [Review] [37 refs]. Clin Geriatr Med 2008; 24:139-49.

[196] Montgomery P, Dennis J. Bright light therapy for sleep problems in adults aged 60+. [Review] [67 refs]. Cochrane Database of Syst Rev 2002; 2.

[197] Friedman L, Zeitzer JM, Kushida C *et al.* Scheduled bright light for treatment of insomnia in older adults. J Am Geriatr Soc 2009; 57:441-52.

[198] Duffy JF, Dijk DJ, Klerman EB, Czeisler CA. Later endogenous circadian temperature nadir relative to an earlier wake time in older people. Am J Physiol 1478; 275.

[199] American Academy of Sleep Medicine. Circadian Rhythm Sleep Disorder Advance Sleep Phase Type. In: The International Classification of Sleep Disorders Diagnostic and Coding Manual. Medicine AAoS (Editor) Westchester, IL: 2005.

[200] Campbell SS, Dawson D, Anderson MW. Alleviation of sleep maintenance insomnia with timed exposure to bright light. J Am Geriatr Soc 1993; 41:829-36.

[201] Lack L, Wright H. The effect of evening bright light in delaying the circadian rhythms and lengthening the sleep of early morning awakening insomniacs. Sleep 1993; 16:436-43.

[202] Palmer CR, Kripke DF, Savage HC, Jr. *et al.* Efficacy of enhanced evening light for advanced sleep phase syndrome. Behav Sleep Med 2003; 1:213-26

CHAPTER 16

Medications and Sleep

Francoise J. Roux, M.D., Ph.D.[1,*] and Meir H. Kryger, M.D.[2]

[1]*Assistant Professor of Medicine, Section of Pulmonary and Critical Care Medicine Yale University School of Medicine, 333 Cedar Street, Post Office Box 208057, New Haven, CT 06520-8057, USA and [2]Clinical Professor of Medicine, University of Connecticut School of Medicine and Director of Research and Education, Gaylord Sleep Medicine, Wallingford CT., Gaylord Sleep Medicine, 400 Gaylord Farm Road, Wallingford CT 06492, USA*

Abstract: Sleep is essential for optimal mental, physical and social wellbeing (or, generically, health). Sleep disruption and/or deprivation can have adverse health consequences, promoting or worsening cardiovascular disease and diabetes. The sleep-wake cycle is a very tightly regulated process that involves multiple neuro-pharmacological reciprocal interactions. It was recently shown that sleep deprivation and sleep disorders can have adverse metabolic consequences. Multiple medications have a direct or indirect impact on sleep and the waking state. In this article, we review the effects of commonly prescribed medications on the sleep-wake cycle.

TOPIC DISCUSSION (CLINICAL OUTLOOK)

Introduction

A very complex interaction of neuronal networks involving multiple neurotransmitters is necessary to allow the transition from the awake to the sleep state and vice versa. Medications can directly alter this delicate balance and promote either insomnia of hypersomnia, or act indirectly to disturb sleep. It is now appreciated that good-quality sleep is essential to maintain general good health and adequate well-being. In this article we will review the different neurological networks and the neurotransmitters involved in the wake and sleep state and how commonly used medications can impact these pathways.

Neuropharmacology of Wakefulness and Sleep

Wakefulness

The mesopontine ascending reticular activating system in the brainstem is the major contributor to wakefulness. The ascending arousal system projects from the brainstem to hypothalamus and to thalamus, which in turn lead to diffuse cortical activation, with wakefulness as an end-result. Norepinephrine is one of the major neurotransmitter promoting arousal. Dopamine is also a significant contributor to arousal through the activation of Dopamine-1 and Dopamine-2 receptors [1]. The major wakefulness-promoting nuclei are the histaminergic and orexinergic-containing neurons in the hypothalamus and the noradrenergic locus coerulus, the serotoninergic dorsal and median raphe nuclei in the brainstem. The hypocretinergic neurons help maintain and stabilize wakefulness by increasing the activity of the aminergic neurons in the ascending arousal system. These hypocretinergic neurons send projections to the cortex to contribute to wakefulness. The locus coerulus can also promote wakefulness by inhibiting the sleep promoting area such as the ventrolateral preoptic (VLPO). In fact, acetylcholine, noradrenaline and serotonin can all inhibit the neuronal activity of the VLPO, promoting arousal.

Sleep

The complex arousal system described above needs to be suppressed to allow sleep induction. The anterior hypothalamus is the main area responsible for the induction of sleep. The ventrolateral preoptic (VLPO) area in the anterior hypothalamus is the main sleep-promoting nucleus. The VLPO contains gamma-aminobutyric acid (GABA) and galanin neurons which project to and inhibit the wake-promoting areas. The cholinergic neurons of the pedonculopontine nuclei and the laterodorsal tegmental nuclei promote REM sleep. Ablation of the VLPO area results in a state of prolonged wakefulness. Adenosine is also involved in the sleep-wake regulation. During wakefulness

Address correspondence to Francoise J. Roux: Assistant Professor of Medicine, Section of Pulmonary and Critical Care Medicine, Yale, University School of Medicine, 333 Cedar Street, Post Office Box 208057, New Haven, CT 06520-8057, USA; Tel: (203) 785 4163; Fax: (203) 785 3634, USA; E-mail: francoise.roux@yale.edu

Octavian C. Ioachimescu (Ed)

there is also a progressive increase in adenosine which accumulates in the forebrain and promotes NREM sleep by inhibiting the cholinergic centers in the brainstem and decreasing the cortical arousal. The circadian clock of the brain is the suprachiasmatic nucleus (SCN) of the hypothalamus, which regulates the timing of the sleep-wake cycle [2]. The SCN regulates the production of melatonin in a circadian pattern, with high levels secreted at night and low levels during the daytime. As the day progresses, the onset of melatonin production favors sleep initiation.

Sleep is divided into non-rapid eye movement sleep (NREM) and rapid eye movement (REM) sleep. NREM sleep is further subdivided into N1, N2 and N3. Stages N1 and N2 (formerly called stages 1 and 2) represent light sleep, whereas stages N3 (formerly called stages 3 and 4) are considered deep sleep or delta sleep. During the night there are three to four cycles of NREM sleep with episodes of REM sleep about every ninety minutes between the cycles.

In summary, the sleep wake interaction is made of reciprocal groups of neurons, one promoting arousal and inhibiting sleep and the other one inhibiting arousal and promoting sleep, creating a delicate and complex relationship. Medications can affect these homeostatic control systems and lead to symptoms of either hypersomnolence or insomnia.

DRUGS INDUCING EXCESSIVE DAYTIME SOMNOLENCE

Hypnotics

Benzodiazepines

Worldwide, benzodiazepines are very frequently prescribed as hypnotics. The benzodiazepines bind non-selectively to the various sub-units of the gamma aminobutyric acic (GABA)-A receptor in the brain. The GABA is the predominant central nervous system inhibitory neurotransmitter and seems to have also an inhibitory effect on norepinephrine transmission, increasing sedation [3]. This non-selective binding to the GABA-A receptor is responsible not only for the hypnotic effect of the benzodiazepines, but also for their various side effects, such as daytime sedation, cognitive impairment, anterograde amnesia, ataxia, muscle relaxation and dependency. Hypnotic benzodiazepinic medications include temazepam, estazolam, flurazepam, quazepam and triazolam. They differ from each other in term of onset and duration of action, but exert the same effect on sleep architecture. Short-acting benzodiazepines are more likely to cause anterograde amnesia, rebound insomnia and benzodiazepine withdrawal. Temazepam is one of the commonly used benzodiazepines. In healthy subjects, temazepam decreases the sleep latency and the time awake after sleep onset, but also decreases delta sleep [4]. In insomniacs patients, temazepam consolidates sleep, decreases sleep latency and suppresses delta sleep (slow wave sleep or N3) in a sustained fashion [5]. Benzodiazepines alter sleep architecture; in addition to delta suppression they can also slightly decrease REM sleep and prolong its latency. Chronic use of benzodiazepines leads to a slight decrease in effectiveness. Benzodiazepines should be tapered slowly to allow a gradual decline in plasma concentration, avoiding rebound insomnia or withdrawal symptoms. Since benzodiazepines are sedative and muscle relaxant, they can also affect nighttime breathing among susceptible hosts [6]. They have been shown to worsen sleep-disordered breathing and cause hypoventilation in patients with underlying lung impairment, with resulting nocturnal sleep disruption [7].

Non-Benzodiazepinic Agents

The non-benzodiazepines are more selective agents; they promote sleep primarily by the activation of the alpha-1 subunit of the GABA-A receptor in the brain [8]. The non-benzodiazepines include zolpidem, zopiclone, zaleplon and eszopiclone. Their hypnotic effect is comparable to the benzodiazepines, but due to their selectivity, they have no anti-anxiety, myorelaxant or anti-convulsive properties. The duration of action varies from ultra-short, to short, and intermediate for zaleplon, zolpidem and eszopiclone, respectively. Zolpidem is the most commonly prescribed agent amongst the non-benzodiazepine group and is indicated for the short-term treatment of insomnia. Zolpidem can reduce sleep latency and increase sleep duration in healthy volunteers [9]. In patients with chronic primary insomnia, polysomnographic data showed that zolpidem increased total sleep time and did not alter delta or REM sleep. In that study, tolerance did not develop and interruption of zolpidem did not lead to rebound insomnia [10]. In contrast to the benzodiazepines, the non-benzodiazepines preserve the sleep architecture, including delta sleep. The repeated administration of zolpidem during eight days did not alter nocturnal ventilation and oxygenation in patients with chronic obstructive lung disease [11].

Zolpidem had no significant drug interaction with sertraline or fluoxetine in studies involving healthy subjects [12]. However, chlorpromazine and imipramine can increase the sedative effect of zolpidem. Fewer clinically significant interactions with other medications have been reported with the non-benzodiazepines compared to the benzodiazepines, likely due to differences in hepatic metabolism (CYP system polymorphisms) [13].

Antidepressants

In the last two decades the number of antidepressants prescribed for the treatment of insomnia has increased steadily and are used generally off-label. The usage of antidepressants in this setting has not been as well studied compared to the one of the benzodiazepines, especially in non-depressed patients.

Tricyclic Antidepressants (TCAs)

The TCAs can inhibit the reuptake of serotonin and norepinephrine, block histamine H1 receptors, muscarinic cholinergic receptors and, most of them, also block alpha1-adrenoceptors. However, their effects on sleep can be diverse, despite belonging to the same class of medications. They are all associated with daytime somnolence, especially those with greater effect on serotonin than norepinephrine reuptake such as clomipramine, amitriptyline and doxepin [14-16]. Doxepin is one of the most selective and potent H1 antihistaminic agents, known to have significant sedative effects [16]. Low-dose doxepin has been shown to significantly improve sleep maintenance and to be well tolerated in the elderly population [17]. Doxepin has been recently approved as a hypnotic by the US Food and Drug Administration (FDA). In general, tricyclics reduce REM (R) sleep and prolong REM (R) latency, especially clomipramine, a very potent REM (stage R) suppressor. The REM suppressant effects tend to lessen over time but do not return to baseline values. In contrast, trimipramine does not have the same effect on REM sleep than other TCAs and it does not have a serotonin reuptake inhibitory effect. The sedating TCAs, such as amitriptyline, nortriptyline, doxepine and clomipramine, tend to reduce sleep onset latency, improve total sleep time and sleep efficiency. Trimipramine, desipramine and protriptyline are less sedating and can in fact decrease total sleep time. Trimipramine can also increase sleep latency. Of note, TCAs can exacerbate the frequency of periodic leg movements during sleep and may worsen REM sleep behavior disorder.

Selective Serotonin Reuptake Inhibitors (SSRIs)

The SSRI are currently the most commonly prescribed medications to treat depression, since they exhibit significantly fewer side effects than the TCAs. They also have other indications, such as generalized anxiety disorder, social phobia and obsessive-compulsive disorder. SSRIs block primarily the reuptake of serotonin, but can also affect several other receptors. As a result, individual SSRIs may be associated with daytime sedation or insomnia, which may be due to effects on different serotonin (5-HT) receptor subtypes [14]. The SSRIs tend to increase sleep and REM latency, while decreasing REM sleep time and increasing the number of awakenings. Once the SSRIs are discontinued, REM sleep time can initially show a rebound before returning to normal levels [17]. Among the SSRIs, fluoxetine and citalopram are more alerting. In healthy volunteers, fluoxetine increase REM latency and decrease REM sleep [18]. Feige *et al* [19] examined the effect of three-week administration of fluoxetine on sleep parameters in healthy subjects. They found that fluoxetine worsened total sleep time and sleep efficiency and decreased REM sleep. However, discontinuation of fluoxetine restored those indices within two to four days and led to a rebound in REM sleep. SSRIs can also induce prominent eye movement during NREM sleep, which was present in 36% of patients chronically on SSRI in one study [20]. In depressed patients, paroxetine was also found to increase REM latency and decrease REM sleep time [21]. Serotonergic antidepressants can also induce REM sleep behavior disorder [22] and increase the number of periodic leg movements during sleep [23].

Serotonin-Norepinephrine Reuptake Inhibitors (SNRI)

Venlafaxine is an antidepressant introduced in the United States in the 1990's. It is a potent inhibitor of serotonin reuptake but a mild inhibitor of dopamine reuptake. It is also a norepinephrine reuptake inhibitor. The antidepressant activity is mainly due to the increased neurotransmission capacity of the serotonin and norepinephrine, leading to better efficacy of the SNRI compared to the SSRI for severe depression. Venlafaxine has more selective pharmacological characteristics than the TCA's and thus has fewer side effects. The effect of 4-day venlafaxine treatment on sleep architecture was investigated in young normal volunteers by using polysomnography. There was an increase in wake after sleep onset with venlafaxine. REM sleep was initially reduced at the onset of treatment and then totally abolished after 4 days of venlafaxine. An increase in periodic leg movement during sleep was also noted with venlafaxine [24]. The same sleep disturbances were noted in a double-blind, placebo controlled study of the effect of venlafaxine in patients with major depression. The venlafaxine group exhibited a decrease in sleep continuity with increased wake time and a decrease in REM sleep duration with a prolongation of its latency compared with placebo [25]. Duloxetine is a new antidepressant belonging to the SNRI class. Duloxetine was also associated with decreased sleep continuity and total REM sleep duration in healthy volunteers after 7 days of treatment [26].

Norepinephrine Reuptake Inhibitors (NRI)

Reboxetine is a new antidepressant with selective norepinephrine reuptake inhibitor effect. Reboxetine was shown to be as effective as fluoxetine in the treatment of depression [27]. Kuenzel *et al.* examined the effect of short term treatment with reboxetine on sleep parameters in depressed patients [28]. A decrease in total sleep time, sleep efficiency and in the amount of REM sleep were noted after 2 weeks of reboxetine treatment. There has been some concern that reboxetine could have some detrimental cardiovascular effects due to a sympathomimetic effect. Ferrini-Strambi *et al* studied the acute, intermediate and long-term effect of reboxetine on sleep architecture and on sympathetic activity using spectral analysis of heart rate variability in dysthymic patients [29]. The authors found that acute administration of reboxetine led to an increased time awake after sleep onset, number of awakenings and a trend toward an increase in sympathetic activity compared to the placebo group, however these effects disappeared by continuing reboxetine for 4 months. In contrast, the significant decrease in the total amount of REM (R) sleep persisted throughout the acute, short-term and long-term administration of reboxetine. The long-term intake of reboxetine up to 4 months did not cause any significant changes in cardiac autonomic function.

Atypical Antidepressants

Trazodone is very commonly prescribed for insomnia off-label, even in non-depressed patients; unfortunately there is a paucity of studies looking at the effect of trazadone in this patient population. Trazodone and nefazadone are weak serotonin reuptake inhibitors. They are also 5-HT2 receptor antagonists and block alpha1- adrenoceptor activity. Trazodone also blocks histamine H1 receptor. A review of some studies using polysomnography showed that trazodone decreased the number of awakenings during the night, but evidence for its efficacy is overall very limited [30]. Trazodone can increase deep sleep and decrease REM (R) sleep. A large review of the literature showed that trazodone can improve total sleep in patients with major depressive disorder, but there are few data to suggest efficacy in non-depressed patients [31]. Trazodone caused drowsiness and next day sedation, even at low doses. Furthermore, trazodone can induce significant side effects such as syncope, ventricular arrhythmias, QTc prolongation, exacerbation of ischemic attacks, and orthostatic hypotension. In contrast to most other antidepressants, nefazodone has been shown either to have no effect on REM (R) sleep [32] or to increase REM (R) sleep [33], in healthy and depressed subjects. Nefazadone can cause drowsiness, but in some studies does not improve sleep continuity in healthy subjects [34].

Mirtazapine, another antidepressant used off-label for insomnia, blocks alpha2 adrenergic, H1 histaminergic, 5-HT2 and 5-HT3 serotonergic receptors. Mirtazapine can be associated with daytime somnolence and significant weight gain. Aslan *et al.* found that mirtazapine improved sleep efficiency, increased deep sleep, decreased the number of awakenings but, in contrast to other antidepressants, did not decrease REM sleep in healthy subjects [35]. Another recent study in depressed patients confirmed its sedative properties, with improvement in sleep continuity and total sleep time with increased delta sleep, which were maintained even after twenty-eight days of treatment [36].

Agomelatine is a novel antidepressant with melatoninergic receptor agonist and 5-HT2 antagonist effects. A randomized, double-blind trial was conducted in 2 centers in Europe comparing the effect of agomelatine to venlafaxine for 6 week-period on subjective sleep using the Leeds Sleep Evaluation questionnaire (LSEQ) in depressive patients. The authors found that the ease to fall asleep and daytime alertness were superior with agomelatine than with venlafaxine [37]. These results were confirmed in an objective fashion using polysomnography in depressed patients [38]. Six weeks of Agomelatine improved sleep efficiency, increased the duration of N3 and N4 sleep and had no significant effect on REM sleep. There was also an improvement in daytime alertness and in the sleep-wake cycle possibly through the agomelatine's chronobiotic effect on the suprachiasmatic nucleus. The normalization of the sleep-wake cycle may have some impact on the depressive symptoms.

Antipsychotics

Sleep disturbances such as insomnia and circadian rhythm shift are common among psychotic patients [39]. Schizophrenic patients might have normal or decreased delta sleep, and the latter may correlate well with negative symptoms. The antipsychotic medications exert their antipsychotic effect mainly through dopamine receptor blockade. These medications can improve sleep quality by decreasing psychotic symptomatology. All the traditional and newest antipsychotics exhibit sedative properties through their antagonism of histaminergic, serotonergic and alpha-1 adrenergic receptors; among them, aripiprazole seems to be the least sedating agent. Schizophrenic patients experienced subjective better sleep quality with shortened sleep latency and higher sleep efficiency when switched from conventional to atypical antipsychotic medications such as risperidone, olanzapine, quetiapine [40]. This benefit might be attributable to a more potent serotonin receptor blockade effect, which in rats and normal subjects has been shown to increase delta sleep. Indeed, acute and chronic administration of olanzapine in schizophrenics has been shown to significantly improve sleep efficiency, total sleep time and delta sleep [41, 42]. Ziprasidone and risperidone have also been shown to increase delta sleep, whereas clozapine may reduce delta sleep. Among the antipsychotics, risperidone and ziprasidone seem to be the most REM suppressant agents. Antipsychotics can also elicit akathisia, due to their potential extrapyramidal side effects. An increased number of periodic leg movements and the onset of restless leg syndrome due to dopamine antagonism can also be induced by these medications. Quetiapine has been associated with respiratory failure in patients with underlying lung disease or sleep-disordered breathing, even when used at conventional dosage [43]. Conversely, these antipsychotic medications can eventually promote sleep-disordered breathing through weight gain.

Lithium

Lithium is used mainly to treat manic-depressive disease and is associated with excessive daytime somnolence. It has been shown to decrease REM sleep in both depressed and normal subjects. Lithium was also shown to increase delta sleep in healthy subjects, likely through a decrease in 5-HT2 receptor function [44]. Lithium can also decrease vigilance and worsen restless leg syndrome impacting sleep quality.

Antiepileptic Drugs (AEDs)

Epileptic patients often complain of hypersomnia or nocturnal sleep disruption, especially those with partial seizures. Poorly controlled epilepsy can directly disrupt sleep, with decreased sleep time and REM sleep, increased wake after sleep onset and increased number of arousals. Those sleep architecture changes are also found to a lesser degree in patients with controlled epilepsy, suggesting some inherent degree of sleep instability among epileptic patients [45]. Poor sleep quality or sleep deprivation can further worsen epilepsy, leading to a vicious cycle. Most AEDs lead to daytime sedation and some patients may need multiple medications to adequately control seizures further impacting daytime alertness. Anticonvulsants should be carefully selected, since some AEDs can independently affect sleep quality and have various effects on daytime somnolence. Daytime somnolence is a common side effect of barbiturates and benzodiazepines (see above). The older AEDs, namely the barbiturates, carbamazepine and phenytoin, will decrease REM (R) sleep, while benzodiazepines can decrease both REM (R) and delta sleep. Valproate can lead to mild sleep disruption in epileptic patients. Barbiturates, benzodiazepines and possibly phenytoin can decrease upper airway tone, thus promoting sleep-disordered breathing, which can further worsen seizure control. Obstructive sleep apnea has been the most common sleep disorder found in epileptic patients complaining of hypersomnia [46].

Newer AEDs incude gabapentin, lamotrigine, tiagabine, felbamate, zonisamide, topiramate and levetiracetam. Gabapentin and tiagabine increase GABA concentrations [14] and delta sleep. Gabapentin and lamotrigine seem to increase REM sleep and decrease arousals when they were added to other AEDs [46]. Gabapentin is effective for the treatment of restless leg syndrome and periodic leg movements, which can improve sleep quality. The effect of lamotrigine was studied in patients with focal epilepsy who had incomplete seizure control despite treatment with other AEDs. The addition of lamotrigine did not lead to excessive daytime somnolence [47] as shown by the Epworth Sleepiness Scale. Bonanni *et al* [48] evaluated daytime sleep latencies using multiple sleep latency tests in drug-naïve epileptic patients receiving topiramate for two months. The authors found that topiramate did not impair daytime alertness in epileptic patients. Felbamate, lamotrigine and zonisamide can have an alerting effect and should be administered early in the day [49]. In conclusion, the identification, treatment of primary sleep disorders and the selection of AEDs are important in epileptic patients to optimize adequate seizure control and daytime function.

Antiparkinsonian Drugs

Nocturnal sleep disruption is very common in Parkinson disease, affecting up to 60 - 90% of patients and can worsen with disease progression. This patient population is more prone to various primary sleep disorders, such as sleep-disordered breathing, REM sleep behavior disorder, restless legs syndrome and periodic leg movement disorder. Excessive daytime somnolence affects many patients and might be a primary feature in Parkinson disease, but can also be related to a co-existent sleep disorder or to dopaminergic treatment [50].

The antiparkinsonian drugs include the dopamine (D) precursors such as levodopa, the ergot derivative dopamine agonist such as pergolide and the non-ergot dopamine agonists such as pramipexole and ropirinole acting at the D2 -D3 receptors. Dopaminergic agents at low-dose can increase delta and REM (R) sleep and induce hypersomnia. Ergot and non-ergot based dopaminergic agents can cause daytime hypersomnia, however sleep attacks have been linked more often to the latter medication. Decreased sleep latencies have been demonstrated in parkinsonian patients treated with pramipexole which normalized after withdrawal of pramipexole. Frucht and colleagues [51] reported sleep "attacks" among patients with Parkinson disease treated with pramipexole or ropirinole. In contrast, a large study in Germany, of about 3,000 patients with Parkinson disease, examined the occurrence of sleep "attacks" using questionnaires and the Epworth Sleepiness Scale while on dopaminergic treatment. The authors concluded that sleep "attacks" could be demonstrated with all dopaminergic agents, regardless whether ergot or non-ergot based medications were used [52]. Ramzy and colleagues suggested that the total dose of dopaminergic agent was a better predictor of hypersomnia than the use of ergot versus non-ergot based dopaminergic agent (based on polysomnographic recordings) [53]. Anticholinergic drugs used in Parkinson disease such as benztropine can also be sedating.

Opiates

Pain can be a major contributor to sleep disruption. Opioid use, whether acute or chronic, has dramatically increased over the last decade, especially methadone and oxycodone prescription. Opioid receptors are present in the brain and the peripheral nervous system. Opioid medications, morphine and methadone for example, are relatively selective and activate the mu-opioid receptors present in the brainstem respiratory centers and on pain neurons. Acute administration of morphine in healthy subjects disrupts sleep, with increased arousals, wake after sleep onset, N2 sleep [54] and reduced delta and REM (R) sleep [55]. The acute morphine administration led to an increase in lighter stages of sleep without any increase in total sleep time. Acute opioid administration can also lead to respiratory depression in case of overdose or underlying pulmonary compromise, since opioids act as direct depressants on the brainstem respiratory centers. With chronic morphine use, REM (R) sleep is still decreased and many wake episodes during the night can be seen, but these changes are attenuated compared to the ones seen after acute morphine administration. In contrast, chronic methadone administration is more sedative than chronic morphine administration and does not affect much sleep architecture, with the exception of a decrease in waking state [56]. Fatigue and excessive daytime somnolence are frequently observed during chronic opioid use. It has been recently appreciated that up to 30% of patients chronically on methadone therapy could develop central apneas. Chronic opioid use has been associated with the development of central apneas with a significant dose response effect [57]. Opiates can be also useful to treat restless leg syndrome.

Antihistamines

Histamine (H) is one of the major wake–promoting neurotransmitter. Anti-histamines will block the post-synaptic H1 receptor and cause sedation.

The first generation of antihistaminic agents readily penetrates the blood brain barrier due to their high lipophilic properties, with subsequent daytime sedation. They tend to decrease sleep latency and improve sleep continuity. They include hydroxyzine, diphenhydramine, doxylamine, chlorpheniramine, clemastine, promethazine. They are mainly useful to treat symptoms of allergy, but diphenhydramine is often self-prescribed as an OTC (over the counter) hypnotic medication due to its sedative properties, although diphenhydramine is not FDA approved for that indication. However, tolerance to the sedative effect of diphenhydramine develops over time [58]. To date, hydroxyzine is among the most sedating antihistaminic agents.

The second generation of antihistamines are more selective and do not block the cholinergic and adrenergic receptors. They include cetirizine, loratidine, mizolastin, are highly hydrophilic and as such, penetrate less the brain-blood barrier; however, at high doses, they can still be sedative.

The most recently developed antihistaminic agents are levocetirizine, fexofenadine and desloratidine, which reportedly have no anticholinergic properties and are not sedative [59]. The effect of fexofenadine and cetirizine on cognitive performance and sedation was studied in aviators compared to placebo. There was no significant increase in drowsiness with fexofenadine or cetirizine compared to placebo, but the latter was found to impair cognition, which might affect pilots' performance [60]. Since there is some degree of variation in sedation among the new generation of antihistamines, the lowest dose should always be attempted to avoid side effects [61].

DRUGS INDUCING ALERTNESS OR INSOMNIA

Multiple neurotransmitters, such as acetylcholine, serotonin, norepinephrine, histamine, hypocretin, dopamine and glutamate are involved into the promotion of wakefulness.

Amphetamines

The recognition of attention-deficit hyperactivity disorders has dramatically increased over the last decade and, as a result, the prescription of amphetamine derivatives. Furthemore, these agents are used at times to also treat narcolepsy or other hypersomnia syndromes. They include amphetamine, methylphenidate and dextroamphetamine. They promote wakefulness by blocking the reuptake and increasing the release of dopamine, norepinephrine and serotonin in the central nervous system [3]. These neurotransmitters will stimulate the ascending arousal pathway and increase wakefulness. Dopamine has recently been discovered to also contribute to the wakefulness state [62]. Amphetamines increase sleep latency, reduce total sleep time and decrease delta and REM sleep. When given chronically, the sleep efficiency can improve over time. Unfortunately, over a long period of time, amphetamine intake can lead to significant increase in blood pressure and heart rate, limiting their usefulness despite their great effects on wakefulness. Insomnia is also a possible side effect and, more rarely, hallucinations and paranoid ideation. Amphetamines became a second line treatment for narcolepsy due to reports of abuse, tolerance and dependence in patients using these medications.

Modafinil and Armodafinil

This new class of medications is now considered first line treatment for narcolepsy due to less side effects and less abuse potential compared to amphetamines. Modafinil and armodafinil are non-amphetamine stimulants which are FDA-approved for the treatment of narcolepsy, shift-work disorder and sleep-disordered breathing with residual hypersomnia. This increased use is due to their minor side effects and their low potential for abuse in comparison to the amphetamines. The exact mechanism of action of modafinil or armodafinil is still unclear, but might result from some effect at the dopamine and noradrenergic transporter in the central nervous system. Dopaminergic D-1 and D-2 receptors are essential for the wakefulness effect of modafinil [63]. An animal study showed that the potency of modafinil on wake correlated with its affinity to the dopamine transporter [64]. Armodafinil is the R-enantiomer of modafinil and as such, has a much longer half-life. Maintenance wakefulness tests have shown that both modafinil and armodafinil promote wakefulness compared to placebo in narcoleptic patients [65] . Armodafinil has been shown to be effective in treating the sleepiness of shift workers [66]. Modafinil and armodafinil have very few side effects; while headache is one of the most common, anxiety, depression and rash (including Stevens Johnson syndrome) have been reported.

Theophylline

In individuals following normal circadian schedules, adenosine extracellular concentrations in the basal forebrain and other CNS areas tend to increase throughout the day, so that in the evening, it may help promote sleep. Theophylline can antagonize adenosine receptors and thus induce alertness. Theophylline is a bronchodilator used only occasionally in patients with chronic obstructive lung disease and rarely in asthmatics due to its possible toxicity. The effect of theophylline on sleep and wakefulness was assessed in healthy subjects using multiple sleep latency test (MSLT) and polysomnography [67]. Nighttime administration of theophylline, at therapeutic level, delayed sleep latency, increased the number of arousals and wake time, decreasing the total sleep time by approximately one hour. Theophylline also increased alertness during the daytime, with prolonged latency during the MSLT compared to placebo. Sleep quality among asthmatics was shown to improve with salmeterol treatment, but not with theophylline. A large propective study in asthmatics, using questionnaires, showed that 6-month treatment at low dose theophylline did not affect sleep quality [68]. Those results were confirmed by using polysomnography in asthmatics with nocturnal symptoms who were treated with theophylline; specifically, there was no difference in terms of sleep efficiency, sleep latency or number of arousals compared to placebo and salmeterol, even at higher doses of theophylline [69].

Cardiovascular Drugs

Beta-Blockers

Beta-blockers are increasingly prescribed for congestive heart failure since they can decrease mortality. Beta-blockers are well known for their sleep side effects such as nightmares, hallucinations and insomnia, especially with lipophilic agents such as propanolol, metoprolol, oxprenolol, acebutolol, timolol and pindolol, which penetrate the central nervous system more readily. Furthermore, beta-blockers may also decrease melatonin synthesis, which could lead to insomnia; carvedilol seems to be to date the only beta-blocker that does not impair melatonin secretion [70].

HMG CoA Reductase Inhibitors

HMG CoA reductase inhibitors are the most commonly prescribed hypolipemic agents. Pravastatin is a hydrophilic agent, whereas lovastatin is lipophilic. Their effects on sleep architecture were compared to placebo using polysomnography. Neither pravastatin, nor lovastatin had any significant effect on daytime function or nighttime sleep latency, efficiency, number of arousals, and REM density compared to placebo [71]. Another large, placebo-controlled, randomized study reported no significant effect of 3-month therapy with lovastatin and pravastatin on nocturnal sleep [72].

Steroids

Corticosteroids are potent anti-inflammatory medications, which can have significant sleep side effects, including insomnia. In healthy volunteers, dexamethasone increased the wake time after sleep onset and reduced REM sleep compared to placebo [73]. Dexamethasone can increase daytime alertness after nocturnal administration. In some reports, dexamethasone has been shown to decrease delta sleep which seems to be important in memory formation. Indeed, administration of dexamethasone resulted in impaired sleep-facilitating declarative memory in healthy subjects [74]. Anabolic androgenic steroid users had decreased sleep efficiency with higher percentage of wake after sleep onset compared to controls in a study using polysomnography [75].

In summary, sleep and wake cycles are tightly regulated by numerous anatomical pathways involving many neurotransmitters which can be adversely affected by multiple medications. The development of more selective medications is warranted to minimize side effects and disruption of the sleep-wake cycle with possible detrimental health consequences.

Research Outlook

Insomnia is very prevalent, affecting more than half of the population. Since the early 19th century the search for medications to treat insomnia or hypersomnia has evolved from herbal therapy, to the relatively more selective compounds of the 21st century. Most medications are considered relatively safe, with fewer side effects than in the past. Nonetheless, medications used to treat insomnia or excessive daytime somnolence should be still used with caution in certain clinical conditions, since their mechanisms of action and their possible long-term effects have still not been completely elucidated.

What do we know:

- Sleep seems to play an important role in the learning process and memory formation. The biochemical events involved in that process are complex and contribute to promote synapse plasticity. Molecular studies could demonstrate the limitation of the commonly used hypnotics, which are still unable to reproduce a good night of natural sleep [76].

- Most hypnotics act on the GABA-A receptors, which seem to play a major role in memory formation. Anterograde amnesia and impaired daytime function are well known side effects of the hypnotics.

- Studies in animals reported that zolpidem did impair cortical plasticity involved in consolidation of new learning during sleep despite no significant change in sleep architecture, whereas triazolam and ramelteon had no significant impact on that process [77]. Using the same model to trigger synaptic remodeling, another study in animals showed that trazadone could also impair synaptic remodeling during sleep [78].

- In humans, prolonged use of benzodiazepines could lead to long-term cognitive impairment, even after 6 months of benzodiazepinic abstinence [79].

- Conversely, amphetamines seem to increase re-learning potential after traumatic brain injury or stroke.

What we don't know:

- It is still unclear which effects medications could have in different patient populations. The era of personalized medicine may already be here and this is a hot area of research and further developments.

- Benzodiazepines and non-benzodiazepinic agents should be used with extreme caution in patients with traumatic brain injury, since they may impede neural plasticity and prevent full recovery. In contrast, ramelteon might be beneficial since patients with traumatic brain injury have decreased level of melatonin but further research is needed [80].

- It is also unclear to which degree individual variability might also affect the efficacy, half-life and side effects of various pharmacological therapies for sleep disorders [81].

REFERENCES

[1]   Isaac SO, Berridge CW. Wake-promoting actions of dopamine D1 and D2 receptor stimulation. J Pharmacol Exp Ther 2003; 307: 386-94.

[2]   Moore RY. Suprachiasmatic nucleus in sleep-wake regulation. Sleep Med 2007; 8 (Suppl 3): 27-33.

[3]   Mitchell HA, Weinshenker D. Good night and good luck: norepinephrine in sleep pharmacology. Biochem Pharmacol 2010; 79: 801-9.

[4]   Wright NA, Belyavin A, Borland RG, Nicholson AN. Modulation of delta activity by hypnotics in middle-aged subjects: studies with a benzodiazepine (flurazepam) and a cyclopyrrolone (zopiclone). Sleep 1986; 9: 348-52.

[5]   Kripke DF, Hauri P, Ancoli-Israel S, Roth T. Sleep evaluation in chronic insomniacs during 14-day use of flurazepam and midazolam. J Clin Psychopharmacol 1990; 10: 32S-43S.

[6]   Roth T. Hypnotic use for insomnia management in chronic obstructive pulmonary disease. Sleep Med 2009; 10:19-25.

[7]   Guilleminault C. Benzodiazepines, breathing, and sleep. Am J Med 1990; 88: 25S-28S.

[8]   Rudolph U, Crestani F, Benke D, *et al.* Benzodiazepine actions mediated by specific gamma-aminobutyric acid(A) receptor subtypes. Nature 1999; 401: 796-800.

[9]   Walsh JK, Schweitzer PK, Sugerman JL, Muehlbach MJ. Transient insomnia associated with a 3-hour phase advance of sleep time and treatment with zolpidem. J Clin Psychopharmacol 1990; 10: 184-9.

[10]   Monti JM, Monti D, Estevez F, Giusti M. Sleep in patients with chronic primary insomnia during long-term zolpidem administration and after its withdrawal. Int Clin Psychopharmacol 1996; 11: 255-63.

[11]   Girault C, Muir JF, Mihaltan F, *et al.* Effects of repeated administration of zolpidem on sleep, diurnal and nocturnal respiratory function, vigilance, and physical performance in patients with COPD. Chest 1996; 110: 1203-11.

[12]   Holm KJ, Goa KL. Zolpidem: an update of its pharmacology, therapeutic efficacy and tolerability in the treatment of insomnia. Drugs 2000; 59: 865-89.

[13]   Hesse LM, von Moltke LL, Greenblatt DJ. Clinically important drug interactions with zopiclone, zolpidem and zaleplon. CNS Drugs 2003; 17: 513-32.

[14]   DeMartinis NA, Winokur A. Effects of psychiatric medications on sleep and sleep disorders. CNS Neurol Disord Drug Targets 2007; 6: 17-29.

[15]   Goforth HW. Low-dose doxepin for the treatment of insomnia: emerging data. Expert Opin Pharmacother 2009; 10: 1649-55.

[16]   Scharf M, Rogowski R, Hull S, *et al.* Efficacy and safety of doxepin 1 mg, 3 mg, and 6 mg in elderly patients with primary insomnia: a randomized, double-blind, placebo-controlled crossover study. J Clin Psychiatry 2008; 69: 1557-64.

[17]   Winokur A, Gary KA, Rodner S, *et al.* Depression, sleep physiology, and antidepressant drugs. Depress Anxiety 2001; 14: 19-28.

[18]   Vasar V, Appelberg B. The effect of flouoxetine on sleep: a longitudinal, double-blind polysomnographic study of healthy volunteers. J Sleep Research 1992; 1: 240.

[19] Feige B, Voderholzer U, Riemann D, *et al.* Fluoxetine and sleep EEG: effects of a single dose, subchronic treatment, and discontinuation in healthy subjects. Neuropsychopharmacology 2002; 26: 246-58.

[20] Geyer JD, Carney PR, Dillard SC, *et al.* Antidepressant medications, neuroleptics, and prominent eye movements during NREM sleep. J Clin Neurophysiol 2009; 26: 39-44.

[21] Staner L, Kerkhofs M. A double-blind comparison of the effects of paroxetine and amitriptylline on sleep EEG patients with major depression. J Sleep Research 1992; 1: 218.

[22] Schenck CH, Mahowald MW, Kim SW, *et al.* Prominent eye movements during NREM sleep and REM sleep behavior disorder associated with fluoxetine treatment of depression and obsessive-compulsive disorder. Sleep 1992; 15: 226-35.

[23] Yang C, White DP, Winkelman JW. Antidepressants and periodic leg movements of sleep. Biol Psychiatry 2005; 58: 510-4.

[24] Salin-Pascual RJ, Galicia-Polo L, Drucker-Colin R. Sleep changes after 4 consecutive days of venlafaxine administration in normal volunteers. J Clin Psychiatry 1997; 58: 348-50.

[25] Luthringer R, Toussaint M, Schaltenbrand N, *et al.* A double-blind, placebo-controlled evaluation of the effects of orally administered venlafaxine on sleep in inpatients with major depression. Psychopharmacol Bull 1996; 32: 637-46.

[26] Chalon S, Pereira A, Lainey E, *et al.* Comparative effects of duloxetine and desipramine on sleep EEG in healthy subjects. Psychopharmacology (Berl) 2005; 177: 357-65.

[27] Andreoli V, Caillard V, Deo RS, *et al.* Reboxetine, a new noradrenaline selective antidepressant, is at least as effective as fluoxetine in the treatment of depression. J Clin Psychopharmacol 2002; 22: 393-9.

[28] Kuenzel HE, Murck H, Held K, *et al.* Reboxetine induces similar sleep-EEG changes like SSRI's in patients with depression. Pharmacopsychiatry 2004; 37: 193-5.

[29] Ferini-Strambi L, Manconi M, Castronovo V, *et al.* Effects of reboxetine on sleep and nocturnal cardiac autonomic activity in patients with dysthymia. J Psychopharmacol 2004; 18: 417-22.

[30] Mendelson WB. A review of the evidence for the efficacy and safety of trazodone in insomnia. J Clin Psychiatry 2005; 66: 469-76.

[31] James SP, Mendelson WB. The use of trazodone as a hypnotic: a critical review. J Clin Psychiatry 2004; 65: 752-5.

[32] Vogel G, Cohen J, Mullis D, *et al.* Nefazodone and REM sleep: how do antidepressant drugs decrease REM sleep? Sleep 1998; 21: 70-7.

[33] Ware JC, McBrayer RH. REM sleep and nefazodone. Sleep 1998; 21: 795-6.

[34] Sharpley AL, Williamson DJ, Attenburrow ME, *et al.* The effects of paroxetine and nefazodone on sleep: a placebo controlled trial. Psychopharmacology (Berl) 1996; 126: 50-4.

[35] Aslan S, Isik E, Cosar B. The effects of mirtazapine on sleep: a placebo controlled, double-blind study in young healthy volunteers. Sleep 2002; 25: 677-9.

[36] Schmid DA, Wichniak A, Uhr M, *et al.* Changes of sleep architecture, spectral composition of sleep EEG, the nocturnal secretion of cortisol, ACTH, GH, prolactin, melatonin, ghrelin, and leptin, and the DEX-CRH test in depressed patients during treatment with mirtazapine. Neuropsychopharmacology 2006; 31: 832-44.

[37] Lemoine P, Guilleminault C, Alvarez E. Improvement in subjective sleep in major depressive disorder with a novel antidepressant, agomelatine: randomized, double-blind comparison with venlafaxine. J Clin Psychiatry 2007; 68: 1723-32.

[38] Quera-Salva MA, Lemoine P, Guilleminault C. Impact of the novel antidepressant agomelatine on disturbed sleep-wake cycles in depressed patients. Hum Psychopharmacol 2010; 25: 222-9.

[39] Cohrs S. Sleep disturbances in patients with schizophrenia : impact and effect of antipsychotics. CNS Drugs 2008; 22: 939-62.

[40] Yamashita H, Mori K, Nagao M, *et al.* Effects of changing from typical to atypical antipsychotic drugs on subjective sleep quality in patients with schizophrenia in a Japanese population. J Clin Psychiatry 2004; 65: 1525-30.

[41] Muller MJ, Rossbach W, Mann K, *et al.* Subchronic effects of olanzapine on sleep EEG in schizophrenic patients with predominantly negative symptoms. Pharmacopsychiatry 2004; 37: 157-62.

[42] Salin-Pascual RJ, Herrera-Estrella M, Galicia-Polo L, Laurrabaquio MR. Olanzapine acute administration in schizophrenic patients increases delta sleep and sleep efficiency. Biol Psychiatry 1999; 46: 141-3.

[43] Freudenmann RW, Sussmuth SD, Wolf RC, *et al.* Respiratory dysfunction in sleep apnea associated with quetiapine. Pharmacopsychiatry 2008; 41: 119-21.

[44] Friston KJ, Sharpley AL, Solomon RA, Cowen PJ. Lithium increases slow wave sleep: possible mediation by brain 5-HT2 receptors? Psychopharmacology (Berl) 1989; 98: 139-40.

[45] Foldvary-Schaefer N, Grigg-Damberger M. Sleep and epilepsy. Semin Neurol 2009; 29: 419-28.

[46] Foldvary-Schaefer N. Sleep complaints and epilepsy: the role of seizures, antiepileptic drugs and sleep disorders. J Clin Neurophysiol 2002; 19:514-21.

[47] Foldvary N, Perry M, Lee J, *et al.* The effects of lamotrigine on sleep in patients with epilepsy. Epilepsia 2001; 42: 1569-73.

[48] Bonanni E, Galli R, Maestri M, *et al.* Daytime sleepiness in epilepsy patients receiving topiramate monotherapy. Epilepsia 2004; 45: 333-7.

[49]   Bazil CW. Effects of antiepileptic drugs on sleep structure : are all drugs equal? CNS Drugs 2003; 17: 719-28.

[50]   Comella CL. Sleep disorders in Parkinson's disease: an overview. Mov Disord 2007; 22 Suppl 17: S367-73.

[51]   Frucht S, Rogers JD, Greene PE, *et al.* Falling asleep at the wheel: motor vehicle mishaps in persons taking pramipexole and ropinirole. Neurology 1999; 52: 1908-10.

[52]   Paus S, Brecht HM, Koster J, *et al.* Sleep attacks, daytime sleepiness, and dopamine agonists in Parkinson's disease. Mov Disord 2003; 18: 659-67.

[53]   Razmy A, Lang AE, Shapiro CM. Predictors of impaired daytime sleep and wakefulness in patients with Parkinson disease treated with older (ergot) vs newer (nonergot) dopamine agonists. Arch Neurol 2004; 61: 97-102.

[54]   Wang D, Teichtahl H. Opioids, sleep architecture and sleep-disordered breathing. Sleep Med Rev 2007; 11: 35-46.

[55]   Shaw IR, Lavigne G, Mayer P, Choiniere M. Acute intravenous administration of morphine perturbs sleep architecture in healthy pain-free young adults: a preliminary study. Sleep 2005; 28: 677-82.

[56]   Kay DC. Human sleep during chronic morphine intoxication. Psychopharmacologia 1975; 44: 117-24.

[57]   Walker JM, Farney RJ, Rhondeau SM *et al.* Chronic opioid use is a risk factor for the development of central sleep apnea and ataxic breathing. J Clin Sleep Med 2007; 3: 455-61.

[58]   Richardson GS, Roehrs TA, Rosenthal L *et al.* Tolerance to daytime sedative effects of H1 antihistamines. J Clin Psychopharmacol 2002; 22: 511-5.

[59]   McDonald K, Trick L, Boyle J. Sedation and antihistamines: an update. Review of inter-drug differences using proportional impairment ratios. Hum Psychopharmacol 2008; 23: 555-70.

[60]   Vacchiano C, Moore J, Rice GM, Crawley G. Fexofenadine effects on cognitive performance in aviators at ground level and simulated altitude. Aviat Space Environ Med 2008; 79: 754-60.

[61]   Mattila MJ, Paakkari I. Variations among non-sedating antihistamines: are there real differences? Eur J Clin Pharmacol 1999; 55: 85-93.

[62]   Boutrel B, Koob GF. What keeps us awake: the neuropharmacology of stimulants and wakefulness-promoting medications. Sleep 2004; 27: 1181-94.

[63]   Qu WM, Huang ZL, Xu XH, *et al.* Dopaminergic D1 and D2 receptors are essential for the arousal effect of modafinil. J Neurosci 2008; 28: 8462-9.

[64]   Nishino S, Mao J, Sampathkumaran R, Shelton J. Increased dopaminergic transmission mediates the wake-promoting effects of CNS stimulants. Sleep Res Online 1998; 1: 49-61.

[65]   Lankford DA. Armodafinil: a new treatment for excessive sleepiness. Expert Opin Investig Drugs 2008; 17: 565-73.

[66]   Czeisler CA, Walsh JK, Wesnes KA, *et al.* Armodafinil for treatment of excessive sleepiness associated with shift work disorder: a randomized controlled study. Mayo Clin Proc 2009; 84: 958-72.

[67]   Roehrs T, Merlotti L, Halpin D, et al. Effects of theophylline on nocturnal sleep and daytime sleepiness/alertness. Chest 1995; 108: 382-7.

[68]   Mastronarde JG, Wise RA, Shade DM, et al. Sleep quality in asthma: results of a large prospective clinical trial. J Asthma 2008; 45: 183-9.

[69]   Wiegand L, Mende CN, Zaidel G, *et al.* Salmeterol vs theophylline: sleep and efficacy outcomes in patients with nocturnal asthma. Chest 1999; 115: 1525-32.

[70]   Stoschitzky K, Sakotnik A, Lercher P, et al. Influence of beta-blockers on melatonin release. Eur J Clin Pharmacol 1999; 55: 111-5.

[71]   Kostis JB, Rosen RC, Wilson AC. Central nervous system effects of HMG CoA reductase inhibitors: lovastatin and pravastatin on sleep and cognitive performance in patients with hypercholesterolemia. J Clin Pharmacol 1994; 34: 989-96.

[72]   Keech AC, Armitage JM, Wallendszus KR, *et al.* Absence of effects of prolonged simvastatin therapy on nocturnal sleep in a large randomized placebo-controlled study. Oxford Cholesterol Study Group. Br J Clin Pharmacol 1996; 42: 483-90.

[73]   Moser NJ, Phillips BA, Guthrie G, Barnett G. Effects of dexamethasone on sleep. Pharmacol Toxicol 1996; 79: 100-2.

[74]   Plihal W, Pietrowsky R, Born J. Dexamethasone blocks sleep induced improvement of declarative memory. Psychoneuroendocrinology 1999; 24: 313-31.

[75]   Venancio DP, Tufik S, Garbuio SA, *et al.* Effects of anabolic androgenic steroids on sleep patterns of individuals practicing resistance exercise. Eur J Appl Physiol 2008; 102: 555-60.

[76]   Wisor JP, Morairty SR, Huynh NT, *et al.* Gene expression in the rat cerebral cortex: comparison of recovery sleep and hypnotic-induced sleep. Neuroscience 2006; 141: 371-8.

[77]   Seibt J, Aton SJ, Jha SK, *et al.* The non-benzodiazepine hypnotic zolpidem impairs sleep-dependent cortical plasticity. Sleep 2008; 31: 1381-91.

[78]   Aton SJ, Seibt J, Dumoulin MC, *et al.* The sedating antidepressant trazodone impairs sleep-dependent cortical plasticity. PLoS One 2009; 4: e6078.

[79]   Tata PR, Rollings J, Collins M, *et al.* Lack of cognitive recovery following withdrawal from long-term benzodiazepine use. Psychol Med 1994; 24: 203-13.

[80]   Paparrigopoulos T, Melissaki A, Tsekou H, *et al.* Melatonin secretion after head injury: a pilot study. Brain Inj 2006; 20: 873-8.

[81]   Van Dongen HP, Vitellaro KM, Dinges DF. Individual differences in adult human sleep and wakefulness: Leitmotif for a research agenda. Sleep 2005; 28: 479-96.

CHAPTER 17

Sleep and Cardiovascular Disorders

J. Shirine Allam, M.D.[*]

Assistant Professor of Medicine - Emory University, Adjunct Clinical Assistant Professor of Medicine – Morehouse School of Medicine, Division of Pulmonary, Critical Care and Sleep Medicine, Emory University School of Medicine, Atlanta Veterans Affairs Medical Center, Atlanta, GA 30033, USA

Abstract: Sleep has always been associated with the overall concept of health. Over the past decades, the association between sleep and cardiovascular diseases has been emerging. Several sleep disorders are now known to be associated with cardiovascular disease. One of the most notorious associations is with obstructive sleep apnea (OSA). OSA has been linked to a higher incidence of hypertension, with up to 50% of patients with OSA having an elevated blood pressure. Continuous Positive Airway Pressure (CPAP) treatment has been shown to improve blood pressure. The pathogenesis of hypertension in OSA is related to the sympathetic nervous system activation (SNA) that occurs following each apneic episode and that requires the presence of intermittent hypoxia. OSA is similarly linked to an increased risk of cardiac ischemia as well as congestive heart failure.

Treatment with CPAP can improve cardiovascular mortality and left ventricular ejection fraction. OSA is also associated with arrhythmias and strokes. Central sleep apnea and Cheyne Stokes respiration have been described in patients with congestive heart failure and their presence could lead to a worse prognosis. CPAP treatment improves ejection fraction but the effect on mortality has not been proven. Other sleep disorders are linked to increased cardiovascular risk. These include insomnia, short and long sleep duration, circadian rhythm disorders and possibly restless leg syndrome. Sympathetic activation in the form of elevated norepinephrine levels has been documented in patients with OSA. Other markers studied include inflammatory markers and markers of oxidative stress. Although a lot of progress has been made, a specific molecular signature for OSA is yet to be found.

TOPIC DISCUSSION (CLINICAL OUTLOOK)

Introduction

That good sleep is equivalent with good health has been a matter-of-fact knowledge passed on through generations. Disrupted sleep has well known consequences on human beings, starting from fatigue and deterioration of skills, up to complete exhaustion. In the past decade, long term observational studies identified a link between certain sleep disorders and the risk for cardiovascular disease. In this chapter, we will examine this relationship in detail.

Obstructive Sleep Apnea and Cardiovascular Diseases

Obstructive sleep apnea (OSA) is estimated to affect 1 in 5 adults in the United States of America, of which 1 in 15 have a severe form of the disorder defined as more than 30 events per hour. It is only over the past 2 decades that large population-based studies have started to clarify the health care burden and adverse consequences associated with sleep disordered breathing (SDB). One such study, the Wisconsin Sleep Cohort, followed 1,522 individuals with SDB over 18 years and established a higher all-cause mortality risk for untreated patients with severe SDB vs. controls [HR (95% CI)=3.8 (1.6-9.0)], as well as a higher cardiovascular mortality [HR= 5.2 (1.4-19.2)] [1] We will examine below the known associations between OSA and several cardiovascular diseases.

OSA and Hypertension

The first description of OSA in the North American Literature was in 1976 in a report by Guilleminault *et al* [2]. They reported 62 individuals who were diagnosed with OSA and noted that 60% of the adults and 62% of the children had elevated systolic and diastolic blood pressure [2]. Since then, the association between OSA and

---

***Address correspondence to J. Shirine Allam:** Assistant Professor of Medicine - Emory University, Adjunct Clinical Assistant Professor of Medicine – Morehouse School of Medicine, Division of Pulmonary, Critical Care and Sleep Medicine, Emory University School of Medicine, Atlanta Veterans Affairs Medical Center, Atlanta, GA 30033, USA; E-mail: shirine.allam@emory.edu

hypertension (HTN) has been consistently described in observational studies. Roughly, fifty percent of patient with OSA are hypertensive and 30% of hypertensive individuals have diagnosed or non-diagnosed OSA [3-7].

Two prospective studies examined the risk of developing hypertension relative to a baseline apnea hypopnea index (AHI). One was a study of the Wisconsin Sleep Cohort, published in 2000 that followed 709 participants over 4 years [8]. The odds ratios for developing hypertension were adjusted for age, sex, body mass index (BMI), neck and waist circumference, weekly alcohol and cigarette use. The odds ratio to develop hypertension were 1.42 (95%CI 1.13-1.78), 2.03 (1.29-3.17) and 2.89 (1.46-5.64) for participants with minimal (AHI 0.1-4.9), mild (AHI 5.0-14.9) and at least moderate (AHI>15.0) OSA, respectively, when compared with those with AHI of 0 [8]. In a more recent analysis of the Sleep Heart Health study, followed 2,470 participants with baseline in-home polysomnography over 5 years [9]. The risk of developing hypertension was proportional to the baseline AHI, but did not reach statistical significance after adjustment for body mass index (BMI). There was a trend between future hypertension and a baseline AHI>30 that did not reach statistical significance (Odds ratio: 1.53; 95% CI: 0.93-2.47), but did not exclude the possibility of a modest association [9].

The two largest population studies looking into the relationship between OSA and hypertension were published in 2000. They included 6,132 individuals (52.8% of them women) [10] and 2,277 individuals [11] respectively. Both studies showed a strong association between SDB and hypertension. Although the first study found body mass index to explain part of the association [10], the second study concluded that the link was independent of all other relevant risk factors [11].

The interaction between OSA and hypertension is also important in drug resistant hypertension: 83% of patients with drug resistant hypertension have OSA with an AHI>10 [12], and OSA was an independent predictor of uncontrolled hypertension in patients <50 years of age [13].

OSA is now considered by the National Committee on the Detection and Management of Hypertension to be an identifiable cause of hypertension [14]. Additional data has also linked OSA severity with a reduction in nocturnal BP "dipping" [15], which in turn is associated with higher all-cause mortality [16].

The mechanism that links OSA to the development of hypertension has been extensively studied. Alterations in the autonomic nervous system activated inflammatory responses and endothelial dysfunction have all been implicated. However, it is the intermittent hypoxia that occurs in OSA that appears to be the critical element that accounts for most of its immediate and long term cardiovascular consequences [17-19]. It was indeed confirmed that the hypoxic events, and not the increased respiratory efforts, were responsible for the sympathetic nervous system activation that takes place after each respiratory event in OSA [20, 21]. The activation of the nervous system tends to persist after the hypoxia has resolved and is thought to eventually lead to daytime hypertension [22, 23]. The exact mechanism for this is still not well understood.

OSA-related hypertension is often difficult to treat and raises the question of whether treatment with continuous positive airway pressure (CPAP) can result in improved blood pressure control. A myriad of open label studies, controlled trials, systematic reviews and meta-analyses have addressed this issue and have found a mean reduction in blood pressure of 2 mm Hg with CPAP [24]. Despite its doubtful clinical significance, this reduction seemed to be significant in terms of improving cardiovascular outcomes. Blood pressure reduction with CPAP was more pronounced in hypertensive patients and in those with more severe OSA. Response of hypertension to CPAP therapy has not been uniform in all patients. Patients who were not sleepy were not found in initial studies to have a significant blood pressure response to CPAP. However, a recent trial found that CPAP, if used more than 5.6 hours a night for a year, can result in a blood pressure reduction in non sleepy patients with moderate to severe OSA [25]. It is important to note that the majority of subjects (85%) enrolled in these studies have been men and therefore, the response in women is not well studied [24].

OSA and Coronary Artery Disease:

Patients with sleep disordered breathing have been noted to have up to a two-fold increased risk of having coronary artery disease (myocardial ischemia and/or infarction) in observational studies [26-29]. Furthermore, longitudinal studies have described an increased risk of mortality from cardiovascular events in untreated patients with OSA [30, 31]. Even mild to moderate OSA (AHI>10) can result in a 4-fold increased risk of cardiovascular death over a 5-year period in patients with existing coronary artery disease (CAD) [32]. Subclinical coronary atherosclerosis is also independently linked to OSA according to a recent report [33]. Several studies have shown an increase in the rate of in-stent restenosis and adverse cardiovascular events in patients with OSA undergoing angioplasty compared to controls [33, 34].

The pathophysiologic mechanism linking OSA and CAD are similar to those discussed for hypertension. The repetitive hypoxia and reoxygenation episodes are implicated in generating oxidative stress and leading to atherosclerosis [35, 36]. There is also evidence of endothelial dysfunction, abnormal inflammatory responses and lipid dysfunction in patients with OSA, all known to be associated with coronary artery disease [37-39]. The repetitive nocturnal sympathetic activation will therefore be the catalyst that can precipitate ischemic events in an already at risk cardiovascular system. Treatment with CPAP has been shown to improve cardiovascular mortality, reduce atherosclerotic burden and various inflammatory makers [33, 37-42].

OSA and Congestive Heart Failure

Given the association between OSA and HTN, as well as CAD, it is not surprising that OSA is also associated with congestive heart failure, both systolic and diastolic subtypes. Overall, it is estimated that 11-53% of patients with heart failure have OSA [43-47]. The fluid redistribution from the edematous lower extremities to other tissues when recumbent is thought to lead to increased pharyngeal wall edema and therefore predispose to OSA in patients with heart failure [48, 49]. On the other hand, OSA itself is thought to lead to worsening left ventricular function. Significant negative intrathoracic pressures are produced during each obstructive event, generated by respiratory effort against an obstructed airway. The pressures can be up to 5 times more negative than those occurring during normal respiration. This leads to acute changes in the pressure gradient between the left ventricle and the extrathoracic compartment, and therefore an acute elevation in afterload, which leads to a decreased cardiac output [50-53]. In addition, on the right side of the heart, the venous return is increased, distending the right ventricle and displacing the ventricular septum to the left, leading to further impairment of the left ventricular filling and therefore the cardiac output. These changes occur in all individuals with OSA during apneic episodes, but they understandably have a more pronounced effect on an already failing heart, and could lead to further cardiac injury [54].

Treatment of OSA with CPAP in patients with heart failure improves sympathetic activity and reduces the risk of death and hospitalization [55-57]. CPAP also improves ejection fraction and quality of life and reduces urinary norepinephrine levels[58]. A recent study has found that identification and treatment of OSA during a hospital admission for heart failure decompensation results in improvement in the systolic function [59].

OSA and Pulmonary Hypertension

The association between OSA and pulmonary hypertension (PH) is less well established than the one with systemic hypertension. Several observational studies have described a 20 to 41% prevalence of pulmonary hypertension in patients with OSA. However, many of the patients studied may have had co-existent pulmonary or cardiac disease as confounding factors of their pulmonary vascular pressures [60-62]. Overall, the pulmonary pressure elevation associated with OSA was found to be in the mild range [63]. One of the risk factors associated with the pulmonary hypertension include the presence of intrinsic pulmonary parenchymal disorders. CPAP therapy is associated in moderate reductions in the pulmonary artery pressures in both normal controls and patients with pulmonary hypertension.

The current guidelines recommend assessment for sleep-disordered breathing in patients with pulmonary hypertension. However, routine screening for PH in patients with OSA is not recommended [63]. In patients with OSA and PH, treatment with CPAP is recommended with a goal to reduce the pulmonary pressures [63].

OSA and Arrhythmias

During sleep, a normal heart rate is considered to be between 40 and 90 beats per minute. Bradycardia is scored for a heart rate less than 40 and tachycardia for a heart rate more than 90 beats per minute [64].

In a recent large cross sectional study, part of the Sleep Heart Health Study, patients with OSA were found to have 2 to 4-fold increased risk of complex arrhythmias, even after adjustment for possible confounding factors [65]. The most common arrhythmias reported are atrial fibrillation, non-sustained ventricular tachycardia, sinus pauses, second-degree atrioventricular conduction block, and frequent premature ventricular contractions (more than 2 per minute) [65-69].

Although early studies reported a high prevalence of bradyarrhythmias in patients with OSA [66, 68, 69] more recent studies have found a lower prevalence [65, 67, 70, 71]. Nevertheless, bradyarrhythmias are known to occur in patients with OSA. They have been shown to occur even in an electrophysiologically intact conduction system and are thought to result from a surge in vagal output during apneic episodes [72]. The first line of treatment in such cases is CPAP treatment rather than implantation of a cardiac pacemaker [72-74].

The association between OSA and atrial fibrillation has been recently validated [65]. In patients under 65 years of age, obesity and nocturnal desaturations were both independent predictors of incident atrial fibrillation [75]. Treatment with CPAP reduces the recurrence of atrial fibrillation after cardioversion by almost 50% in patients with OSA [76].

OSA and Stroke

There is a high prevalence of sleep disordered breathing in patients with acute stroke, estimated between 44% and 72% [77, 78]. Interestingly, obstructive more often than central events are generally seen in this setting. Furthermore, central events and not obstructive ones tend to improve during the recovery period after an acute stroke [79]. This suggests that obstructive events might have preceded the onset of the stroke. The association of OSA with atherosclerosis, increased thrombotic risk and hypertension, all risk factors for stroke, poses the question of whether OSA itself could be a risk factor for stroke. Although an attractive hypothesis, evidence for a causal relationship is only inferential. In Japanese men with moderate to severe OSA, 25% had evidence of silent infarcts on brain magnetic resonance imaging (MRI) versus 6% of controls [80]. Cerebral blood flow in response to hypoxia is significantly impaired in patients with OSA and reverts back to normal after 4-6 weeks of CPAP therapy [81]. Furthermore, OSA is associated with a significantly increased risk of stroke and death [82, 83]. Patients with OSA have a higher risk of mortality 1 year after a stroke and have more disabilities at discharge and at 3 and 12 months after a stroke [84].

CPAP therapy in patients with acute stroke has been studied and the results are conflicting. Some studies showed good initial compliance but poorer long-term adherence to therapy [85-88]. Compared to those not treated with CPAP, patients on CPAP therapy after a stroke showed improved depression score, wellbeing and lower BP readings at night [85, 86]. However, more recent studies showed a very low compliance with CPAP after stroke and the benefits have not been confirmed [89]. Another consideration is that positional therapy for stroke patients not compliant with CPAP could also be useful [90].

Central Sleep Apnea and Cardiovascular Diseases

Central sleep apnea (CSA) and Cheyne Stokes respiration (CSR) are commonly observed in patients with congestive heart failure [43, 44]. CSA is defined as a cessation of breathing for 10 seconds or more, with no accompanying respiratory effort. Cheyne Stokes respiration is a pattern of cyclic breathing characterized by crescendo-decrescendo tidal volumes followed by a central apnea or central hypopnea. The cycle length is longer than 45 seconds, most commonly close to 60 seconds in duration.

The reported prevalence of CSA/CSR in heart failure is between 15% and 37% [43-45]. The pathophysiology of this phenomenon is linked to a state of chronic hypocapnea [91, 92]. The hypocapnea is induced by a persistent hyperventilation in response to the stimulation of pulmonary vagal afferent C-fibers in the congested lungs of patient with heart failure [93-96], as well as a state of increased central and peripheral chemo-responsiveness [97, 98]. One theory is that at sleep onset, the apnea threshold (or CO_2 value below which the central drive for breathing stops) increases and therefore the circulating CO_2 levels are suddenly below the apnea threshold, leading to a cessation of breathing. As the CO_2 builds back up, the breathing resumes and CO_2 levels start going down. However, because of the circulation delay due to a depressed cardiac output, there is a time lapse before the lower levels of CO_2 are sensed by the central receptors. The respiratory efforts therefore continue for a longer time and the CO_2 value is "overshot" down to below the apnea level again, and the cycle starts once more.

The risk factors for the development of CSA/CSR in patients with heart failure are: older age, male gender, elevated left ventricular filling pressures, increased chemosensitivity, and the presence of hypocapnea [47]. Interestingly, cardiac output and ejection fraction were not predictors of CSA/CSR [47].

Many studies have looked at the significance of CSA/CSR in heart failure and its effect on mortality. The results have been variable but overall, a majority seems to point towards CSA/CSR being an independent predictor of mortality [99-106]. The main question remains whether CSA/CSR is only a reflection of a severely diseased heart or if in itself contributes to the progression of the disease. There is evidence that, much like OSA, CSA/CSR leads to nocturnal surges in sympathetic nervous activity (SNA) that peaks during hyperpneas and dips during apneas [107, 108]. This leads to an overall increase in sympathetic output at night but also during the day, as evidenced by higher measured nocturnal norepinephrine urinary levels and daytime plasma levels in patients with heart failure and CSA/CSR compared to those without CSA/CSR [109]. The higher SNA could lead to more cardiac damage over time and contribute to the overall increased mortality [99].

If CSA/CSR can plausibly contribute to increased mortality in heart failure, the question that naturally follows is whether treatment of CSA/CSR can improve outcomes. Several treatment modalities have been shown to improve CSA/CSR. These include: optimization of the medical management of heart failure [94,110-112], which should be the primary therapy; cardiac resynchronization [113-115]; cardiac transplantation [116], and valve replacement when heart failure is due to valvular heart disorders [117].

Treatment with positive airway pressure has generated a lot of interest. It has been shown to improve some hemodynamic parameters, but its impact on survival is still not well established. The largest randomized control trial to address the effect of CPAP on survival when treating CSA/CSR in heart failure was CANPAP, published in 2001 [118]. Two hundred and fifty eight patients with CSA were followed over a mean duration of 2 years and randomized to a CPAP arm and a control arm. The CPAP arm had an improvement in the apnea hypopnea index, the six-minute walk distance, the ejection fraction and the nocturnal oxygenation. However, there was no difference in transplant-free survival, death, hospitalization rates or quality of life. There was an early divergence in survival favoring the control group over the first 18 months of CPAP treatment. This may have been related to acute changes in hemodynamics, in particular a decrease in cardiac output in a certain population of patients who were preload dependent. In a post-hoc analysis of the CANPAP trial, a subgroup analysis was performed and compared patients who had achieved a good control of their CSA, with an AHI less than 15 events per hour, to the control group [119]. This analysis showed a significant improvement in ejection fraction and transplant-free survival between the 2 groups, favoring the treatment arm. This analysis raised the question of whether therapies that succeed in controlling the AHI may improve survival. Alternatively, the lower AHI may have been a marker of a population with less disease burden and therefore who inherently had a better prognosis, unrelated to CPAP therapy. Several other papers studied the effect of other positive pressure therapies such bilevel positive airway pressure and adaptive servo-ventilation [120-121]. Although hemodynamic parameters were improved in these studies, no long-term data exist yet to comment on overall survival.

Other Sleep Disorders and CVD

Sleep Duration, Insomnia and CVD

Sleep has always been considered to have a restorative function on the organism and the question of how much sleep is needed for health has interested lay people and scientists alike. Several studies have looked in particular at the relationship between sleep duration and cardiovascular mortality and morbidity. Self-reported short sleep duration and sleep complaints have been associated with increased cardiovascular morbidity [122-125]. Shorter sleep duration has also been found to be independently associated with incident coronary artery calcifications and higher blood pressure [126, 127]. Interestingly, both shorter and longer sleep durations have been associated with increased all cause mortality in middle aged adults [128-136]. In the elderly (65 to 85 years), however, a recent population-based study found that only longer sleep durations (>10 hours) were associated with a 1.95 increased risk of cardiovascular mortality in patients with reported poor sleep quality, compared to those who slept 7 hours [137]. Another recent large community-based cohort followed 3,430 Chinese adults for 15.9 years and found a U-shaped association between sleep duration and all cause mortality, with both short and long sleep durations being associated with higher all cause mortality. However, the risk of cardiovascular disease was found to have a linear relationship with sleep duration. The presence of frequent insomnia along with long sleep duration was associated with an increased risk of both cardiovascular and all cause mortality [138]. These results are consistent with other studies that found that sleep duration and quality (insomnia complaints) are both important predictors of cardiovascular disease risk [139-142]. Chronic insomnia has been shown to be associated with increased blood pressure, lack of nocturnal blood pressure dipping and increased risk of diabetes [143-145]

Circadian Rhythm Disorders and CVD

There is a higher incidence of obesity, diabetes and cardiovascular diseases in shift workers [146-150]. This is thought to result from a chronic circadian misalignment [151, 152]. A recent study looked at metabolic and cardiovascular consequences of circadian misalignment in 10 experimental subjects. When these subjects ate and slept about 12 hours out of phase from their habitual times, serum leptin decreased, glucose increased, insulin levels increased, mean blood pressure was elevated and there was a total reversal in serum cortisol circadian rhythm [153]. These findings demonstrated the possible adverse cardiovascular and metabolic effects of circadian rhythm misalignment.

Restless Leg Syndrome and CVD

The relationship between RLS and CVD has been the subject of multiple epidemiologic studies. In these studies, RLS diagnosis was mostly dependent on self-reported RLS symptoms. The incidence of hypertension was found to be disproportionately elevated in RLS patients [154-156]. The risk of self-reported cardiovascular disease was also increased in RLS patients, including coronary artery disease that had adjusted odds ratio of 2.22 (95% CI 1.40-3.53) in one study [157]. The relationship between cardiovascular disease and RLS was only apparent in patients with symptoms more than 16 times a month, and was stronger with more severe disease [157]. The putative mechanism behind this association is thought to be related to the sympathetic nervous system over-activity that is present in RLS [158].

RESEARCH OUTLOOK

What do we know:

As discussed previously, the pathophysiological mechanisms linking OSA and cardiovascular diseases have been extensively studied. Some of the main proposed mechanisms include increased sympathetic activity, oxidative stress from recurrent intermittent hypoxia, increased inflammatory activation, and endothelial dysfunction [159]. We will briefly review some of the evidence behind each of these.

The sympathetic activity in OSA has been measured by direct recording of muscle sympathetic nerve activity (microneurography) and has been found to be elevated in OSA patients compared to controls during the daytime [160, 161], and to decrease with CPAP treatment [162-164]. Norepinephrine levels measured in plasma and urine are also elevated in OSA patients compared to controls [165, 166], but this finding has not been universally reproduced in all studies [161]. In the great majority of studies evaluating this association, CPAP use reduces levels of norepinephrine [36, 58, 164, 167-169].

Studying oxidative stress is more challenging, as many of the studied markers are non-specific and have not been validated to be reliable indicators [159]. Keeping this limitation in mind, several studies have shown increases in possible markers of oxidative stress, including 8-isoprostane [170-172], malondialdehyde [173], thiobarbituric acid reactive substances [39, 174] and reactive oxygen species in white blood cells [38, 175]. Other studies have found no evidence of oxidative stress in OSA [176-178].

Markers of inflammation have also been studied in OSA, mainly Tumor Necrosis Factor α (TNF-α), Interleukin 6 (IL-6) and C-reactive protein (CRP). Most studies show an increase in these markers in OSA compared to BMI-matched controls [42, 171, 179-185], as well as a reduction in these markers with CPAP therapy [170, 181, 184, 185]. Other studies, though, do not demonstrate any difference in inflammatory markers between OSA patients and controls [186-191]. Some of these negative results can be explained by the presence of obesity as a confounding factor, knowing that pro-inflammatory cytokines can be produced by visceral fat cells [159, 192, 193].

Endothelial dysfunction is usually demonstrated by abnormal (reduced) production or activity of nitric oxide (NO) pathway in endothelial cells, as well as abnormal flow-mediated dilatation. Moderate and severe OSA have been associated with endothelial dysfunction which reverses with CPAP use [37]. A recent study has also found evidence of endothelial dysfunction in patients with minimally symptomatic OSA [194]. Another recent study showed that endothelial dysfunction in SDB was due to OSA itself and not to obesity as, unlike subjects with OSA and obesity, those with obesity and no SDB did not demonstrate any decrease in flow-mediated vasodilation or decrease in endothelial nitric oxide synthase production. Furthermore, in the OSA group, these changes were reversed after CPAP treatment [195]. Many more pathways and molecular markers have been studied and proposed to play a role in the pathogenesis of cardiovascular disease in obstructive sleep apnea. A comprehensive review of the subject has been recently published [159]. More studies are needed to identify molecular signatures of OSA that could help in identifying patients at risk for complications and help in early intervention and prevention.

What we don't know:

Although the relationship between OSA and cardiovascular diseases appears to be in the strong associations category, a lot of confounding factors exist, the most important of which is body mass index (BMI). It would be important to know how much risk is attributable to obesity alone, as opposed to the sleep-disordered breathing. Many epidemiological studies have tried to correct their results for obesity (and BMI as a specific metric for this matter), although it is quite debatable if the correct analysis should in fact make the adjustments for confounding factors that are not independent of each other.

The effect of CPAP on risk reduction has not been strongly established for all of the cardiovascular comorbidities associated with OSA and long term studies are still needed to assess the impact of therapy on long term prognosis in patients with hypertension, stroke and congestive heart failure. Furthermore, the optimal number of hours of CPAP use needed to achieve meaningful risk reduction is still a matter of debate.

The exact mechanism(s) behind the increased cardiovascular morbidity in various sleep disorders has yet to be elucidated. It is likely that more than one mechanism is in place, as it was discussed above.

Although our knowledge of the relationship between sleep and cardiovascular health has significantly expanded in the last decade, some interesting and crucial questions remain unanswered. Future long-term studies will be paramount in shedding more light on this important and potential pathogenic association.

REFERENCES

[1]   Young T, Finn L, Peppard PE, *et al.* Sleep disordered breathing and mortality: eighteen-year follow-up of the Wisconsin sleep cohort. Sleep 2008; 31: 1071-8.

[2]   Guilleminault C, Tilkian A, Dement WC. The sleep apnea syndromes. Annu Rev Med 1976; 27: 465-84.

[3]   Fletcher EC, DeBehnke RD, Lovoi MS, Gorin AB. Undiagnosed sleep apnea in patients with essential hypertension. Ann Intern Med 1985; 103: 190-5.

[4]   Kales A, Bixler EO, Cadieux RJ, *et al.* Sleep apnoea in a hypertensive population. Lancet 1984; 2: 1005-8.

[5]   Lavie P, Ben-Yosef R, Rubin AE. Prevalence of sleep apnea syndrome among patients with essential hypertension. Am Heart J 1984; 108: 373-6.

[6]   Silverberg DS, Oksenberg A, Iaina A. Sleep-related breathing disorders as a major cause of essential hypertension: fact or fiction? Curr Opin Nephrol Hypertens 1998; 7: 353-7.

[7]   Williams AJ, Houston D, Finberg S, *et al.* Sleep apnea syndrome and essential hypertension. Am J Cardiol 1985; 55: 1019-22.

[8]   Peppard PE, Young T, Palta M, Skatrud J. Prospective study of the association between sleep-disordered breathing and hypertension. N Engl J Med 2000; 342: 1378-84.

[9]   O'Connor GT, Caffo B, Newman AB, *et al.* Prospective study of sleep-disordered breathing and hypertension: the Sleep Heart Health Study. Am J Respir Crit Care Med 2009; 179: 1159-64.

[10]   Nieto FJ, Young TB, Lind BK, *et al.* Association of sleep-disordered breathing, sleep apnea, and hypertension in a large community-based study. Sleep Heart Health Study. JAMA 2000; 283: 1829-36.

[11]   Lavie P, Herer P, Hoffstein V. Obstructive sleep apnoea syndrome as a risk factor for hypertension: population study. BMJ 2000; 320: 479-82.

[12]   Logan AG, Perlikowski SM, Mente A, *et al.* High prevalence of unrecognized sleep apnoea in drug-resistant hypertension. J Hypertens 2001; 19: 2271-7.

[13]   Grote L, Hedner J, Peter JH. Sleep-related breathing disorder is an independent risk factor for uncontrolled hypertension. J Hypertens 2000; 18: 679-85.

[14]   Chobanian AV, Bakris GL, Black HR, *et al.* The Seventh Report of the Joint National Committee on Prevention, Detection, Evaluation, and Treatment of High Blood Pressure: the JNC 7 report. JAMA 2003; 289: 2560-72.

[15]   Hla KM, Young T, Finn L, *et al.* Longitudinal association of sleep-disordered breathing and nondipping of nocturnal blood pressure in the Wisconsin Sleep Cohort Study. Sleep 2008; 31: 795-800.

[16]   Ben-Dov IZ, Kark JD, Ben-Ishay D, *et al.* Predictors of all-cause mortality in clinical ambulatory monitoring: unique aspects of blood pressure during sleep. Hypertension 2007; 49: 1235-41.

[17]   Brooks D, Horner RL, Kozar LF, *et al.* Obstructive sleep apnea as a cause of systemic hypertension. Evidence from a canine model. J Clin Invest 1997; 99: 106-9.

[18]   Fletcher EC. Invited review: Physiological consequences of intermittent hypoxia: systemic blood pressure. J Appl Physiol 2001; 90: 1600-5.

[19]   Lesske J, Fletcher EC, Bao G, Unger T. Hypertension caused by chronic intermittent hypoxia--influence of chemoreceptors and sympathetic nervous system. J Hypertens 1997; 15: 1593-603.

[20]   Morgan BJ, Denahan T, Ebert TJ. Neurocirculatory consequences of negative intrathoracic pressure vs. asphyxia during voluntary apnea. J Appl Physiol 1993; 74: 2969-75.

[21]   Cutler MJ, Swift NM, Keller DM, *et al.* Hypoxia-mediated prolonged elevation of sympathetic nerve activity after periods of intermittent hypoxic apnea. J Appl Physiol 2004; 96: 754-61.

[22]   Xie A, Skatrud JB, Crabtree DC, *et al.* Neurocirculatory consequences of intermittent asphyxia in humans. J Appl Physiol 2000; 89: 1333-9.

[23]   Prabhakar NR, Peng YJ, Jacono FJ, *et al.* Cardiovascular alterations by chronic intermittent hypoxia: importance of carotid body chemoreflexes. Clin Exp Pharmacol Physiol 2005; 32: 447-9.

[24]   Duran-Cantolla J, Aizpuru F, Martinez-Null C, Barbe-Illa F. Obstructive sleep apnea/hypopnea and systemic hypertension. Sleep Med Rev 2009; 13: 323-31.

[25]   Barbe F, Duran-Cantolla J, Capote F, *et al.* Long-term effect of continuous positive airway pressure in hypertensive patients with sleep apnea. Am J Respir Crit Care Med 2010; 181: 718-26.

[26]   Mooe T, Rabben T, Wiklund U, *et al.* Sleep-disordered breathing in men with coronary artery disease. Chest 1996; 109: 659-63.

[27]   Peker Y, Kraiczi H, Hedner J, *et al.* An independent association between obstructive sleep apnoea and coronary artery disease. Eur Respir J 1999; 14: 179-84.

[28]   Sanner BM, Konermann M, Doberauer C, *et al.* Sleep-Disordered breathing in patients referred for angina evaluation--association with left ventricular dysfunction. Clin Cardiol 2001; 24: 146-50.

[29]   Schafer H, Koehler U, Ewig S, *et al.* Obstructive sleep apnea as a risk marker in coronary artery disease. Cardiology 1999; 92: 79-84.

[30]   Mooe T, Franklin KA, Holmstrom K, *et al.* Sleep-disordered breathing and coronary artery disease: long-term prognosis. Am J Respir Crit Care Med 2001; 164: 1910-3.

[31]   Takama N, Kurabayashi M. Influence of untreated sleep-disordered breathing on the long-term prognosis of patients with cardiovascular disease. Am J Cardiol 2009; 103: 730-4.

[32]   Peker Y, Hedner J, Kraiczi H, Loth S. Respiratory disturbance index: an independent predictor of mortality in coronary artery disease. Am J Respir Crit Care Med 2000; 162: 81-6.

[33]   Sorajja D, Gami AS, Somers VK, *et al.* Independent association between obstructive sleep apnea and subclinical coronary artery disease. Chest 2008; 133: 927-33.

[34]   Steiner S, Schueller PO, Hennersdorf MG, *et al.* Impact of obstructive sleep apnea on the occurrence of restenosis after elective percutaneous coronary intervention in ischemic heart disease. Respir Res 2008; 9: 50.

[35]   Dean RT, Wilcox I. Possible atherogenic effects of hypoxia during obstructive sleep apnea. Sleep 1993; 16: S15-21; discussion S21-2.

[36]   Drager LF, Bortolotto LA, Figueiredo AC, *et al.* Effects of continuous positive airway pressure on early signs of atherosclerosis in obstructive sleep apnea. Am J Respir Crit Care Med 2007; 176: 706-12.

[37]   Ip MS, Tse HF, Lam B, *et al.* Endothelial function in obstructive sleep apnea and response to treatment. Am J Respir Crit Care Med 2004; 169: 348-53.

[38]   Schulz R, Mahmoudi S, Hattar K, *et al.* Enhanced release of superoxide from polymorphonuclear neutrophils in obstructive sleep apnea. Impact of continuous positive airway pressure therapy. Am J Respir Crit Care Med 2000; 162: 566-70.

[39]   Barcelo A, Miralles C, Barbe F, *et al.* Abnormal lipid peroxidation in patients with sleep apnoea. Eur Respir J 2000; 16: 644-7.

[40]   Marin JM, Carrizo SJ, Vicente E, Agusti AG. Long-term cardiovascular outcomes in men with obstructive sleep apnoea-hypopnoea with or without treatment with continuous positive airway pressure: an observational study. Lancet 2005; 365: 1046-53.

[41]   Milleron O, Pilliere R, Foucher A, *et al.* Benefits of obstructive sleep apnoea treatment in coronary artery disease: a long-term follow-up study. Eur Heart J 2004; 25: 728-34.

[42]   Minoguchi K, Yokoe T, Tazaki T, *et al.* Increased carotid intima-media thickness and serum inflammatory markers in obstructive sleep apnea. Am J Respir Crit Care Med 2005; 172: 625-30.

[43]   Ferrier K, Campbell A, Yee B, *et al.* Sleep-disordered breathing occurs frequently in stable outpatients with congestive heart failure. Chest 2005; 128: 2116-22.

[44]   Javaheri S. Sleep disorders in systolic heart failure: a prospective study of 100 male patients. The final report. Int J Cardiol 2006; 106: 21-8.

[45]   Wang H, Parker JD, Newton GE, *et al.* Influence of obstructive sleep apnea on mortality in patients with heart failure. J Am Coll Cardiol 2007; 49: 1625-31.

[46]   Chan J, Sanderson J, Chan W, *et al.* Prevalence of sleep-disordered breathing in diastolic heart failure. Chest 1997; 111: 1488-93.

[47]   Sin DD, Fitzgerald F, Parker JD, *et al.* Risk factors for central and obstructive sleep apnea in 450 men and women with congestive heart failure. Am J Respir Crit Care Med 1999; 160: 1101-6.

[48]   Chiu KL, Ryan CM, Shiota S, *et al.* Fluid shift by lower body positive pressure increases pharyngeal resistance in healthy subjects. Am J Respir Crit Care Med 2006; 174: 1378-83.

[49]   Shiota S, Ryan CM, Chiu KL, *et al.* Alterations in upper airway cross-sectional area in response to lower body positive pressure in healthy subjects. Thorax 2007; 62: 868-72.

[50]   Shivalkar B, Van de Heyning C, Kerremans M, *et al.* Obstructive sleep apnea syndrome: more insights on structural and functional cardiac alterations, and the effects of treatment with continuous positive airway pressure. J Am Coll Cardiol 2006; 47: 1433-9.

[51]   Romero-Corral A, Somers VK, Pellikka PA, *et al.* Decreased right and left ventricular myocardial performance in obstructive sleep apnea. Chest 2007; 132: 1863-70.

[52]   Bordier P. Sleep apnoea in patients with heart failure. Part I: diagnosis, definitions, prevalence, pathophysiology and haemodynamic consequences. Arch Cardiovasc Dis 2009; 102: 651-61.

[53]   Orban M, Bruce CJ, Pressman GS, *et al.* Dynamic changes of left ventricular performance and left atrial volume induced by the mueller maneuver in healthy young adults and implications for obstructive sleep apnea, atrial fibrillation, and heart failure. Am J Cardiol 2008; 102: 1557-61.

[54]   Bradley TD, Hall MJ, Ando S, Floras JS. Hemodynamic effects of simulated obstructive apneas in humans with and without heart failure. Chest 2001; 119: 1827-35.

[55]   Kaneko Y, Floras JS, Usui K, *et al.* Cardiovascular effects of continuous positive airway pressure in patients with heart failure and obstructive sleep apnea. N Engl J Med 2003; 348: 1233-41.

[56]   Kasai T, Narui K, Dohi T, *et al.* Prognosis of patients with heart failure and obstructive sleep apnea treated with continuous positive airway pressure. Chest 2008; 133: 690-6.

[57]   Usui K, Bradley TD, Spaak J, *et al.* Inhibition of awake sympathetic nerve activity of heart failure patients with obstructive sleep apnea by nocturnal continuous positive airway pressure. J Am Coll Cardiol 2005; 45: 2008-11.

[58]   Mansfield DR, Gollogly NC, Kaye DM, *et al.* Controlled trial of continuous positive airway pressure in obstructive sleep apnea and heart failure. Am J Respir Crit Care Med 2004; 169: 361-6.

[59]   Khayat RN, Abraham WT, Patt B, *et al.* In-hospital treatment of obstructive sleep apnea during decompensation of heart failure. Chest 2009; 136: 991-7.

[60]   Bady E, Achkar A, Pascal S, *et al.* Pulmonary arterial hypertension in patients with sleep apnoea syndrome. Thorax 2000; 55: 934-9.

[61]   Sajkov D, Cowie RJ, Thornton AT, *et al.* Pulmonary hypertension and hypoxemia in obstructive sleep apnea syndrome. Am J Respir Crit Care Med 1994; 149: 416-22.

[62]   Sanner BM, Doberauer C, Konermann M, *et al.* Pulmonary hypertension in patients with obstructive sleep apnea syndrome. Arch Intern Med 1997; 157: 2483-7.

[63]   Atwood CW, Jr., McCrory D, Garcia JG, *et al.* Pulmonary artery hypertension and sleep-disordered breathing: ACCP evidence-based clinical practice guidelines. Chest 2004; 126: 72S-77S.

[64]   Iber C, Ancoli-Israel S, Chesson A, Quan S. The AASM Manual for the Scoring of Sleep and Associated Events: Rules, Terminology and Technical Specifications. In: 2007.

[65]   Mehra R, Benjamin EJ, Shahar E, *et al.* Association of nocturnal arrhythmias with sleep-disordered breathing: The Sleep Heart Health Study. Am J Respir Crit Care Med 2006; 173: 910-6.

[66]   Guilleminault C, Connolly SJ, Winkle RA. Cardiac arrhythmia and conduction disturbances during sleep in 400 patients with sleep apnea syndrome. Am J Cardiol 1983; 52: 490-4.

[67]   Hoffstein V, Mateika S. Cardiac arrhythmias, snoring, and sleep apnea. Chest 1994; 106: 466-71.

[68]   Miller WP. Cardiac arrhythmias and conduction disturbances in the sleep apnea syndrome. Prevalence and significance. Am J Med 1982; 73: 317-21.

[69]   Tilkian AG, Guilleminault C, Schroeder JS, *et al.* Sleep-induced apnea syndrome. Prevalence of cardiac arrhythmias and their reversal after tracheostomy. Am J Med 1977; 63: 348-58.

[70]   Flemons WW, Remmers JE, Gillis AM. Sleep apnea and cardiac arrhythmias. Is there a relationship? Am Rev Respir Dis 1993; 148: 618-21.

[71]   Roche F, Xuong AN, Court-Fortune I, *et al.* Relationship among the severity of sleep apnea syndrome, cardiac arrhythmias, and autonomic imbalance. Pacing Clin Electrophysiol 2003; 26: 669-77.

[72]   Grimm W, Hoffmann J, Menz V, *et al.* Electrophysiologic evaluation of sinus node function and atrioventricular conduction in patients with prolonged ventricular asystole during obstructive sleep apnea. Am J Cardiol 1996; 77: 1310-4.

[73]   Becker H, Brandenburg U, Peter JH, Von Wichert P. Reversal of sinus arrest and atrioventricular conduction block in patients with sleep apnea during nasal continuous positive airway pressure. Am J Respir Crit Care Med 1995; 151: 215-8.

[74]   Zwillich C, Devlin T, White D, *et al.* Bradycardia during sleep apnea. Characteristics and mechanism. J Clin Invest 1982; 69: 1286-92.

[75]   Gami AS, Hodge DO, Herges RM, *et al.* Obstructive sleep apnea, obesity, and the risk of incident atrial fibrillation. J Am Coll Cardiol 2007; 49: 565-71.

[76]   Kanagala R, Murali NS, Friedman PA, *et al.* Obstructive sleep apnea and the recurrence of atrial fibrillation. Circulation 2003; 107: 2589-94.

[77]   Turkington PM, Elliott MW. Sleep disordered breathing following stroke. Monaldi Arch Chest Dis 2004; 61: 157-61.

[78]   Yaggi H, Mohsenin V. Obstructive sleep apnoea and stroke. Lancet Neurol 2004; 3: 333-42.

[79]   Parra O, Arboix A, Bechich S, *et al.* Time course of sleep-related breathing disorders in first-ever stroke or transient ischemic attack. Am J Respir Crit Care Med 2000; 161: 375-80.

[80]   Minoguchi K, Yokoe T, Tazaki T, *et al.* Silent brain infarction and platelet activation in obstructive sleep apnea. Am J Respir Crit Care Med 2007; 175: 612-7.

[81]   Foster GE, Hanly PJ, Ostrowski M, Poulin MJ. Effects of continuous positive airway pressure on cerebral vascular response to hypoxia in patients with obstructive sleep apnea. Am J Respir Crit Care Med 2007; 175: 720-5.

[82]   Yaggi HK, Concato J, Kernan WN, *et al.* Obstructive sleep apnea as a risk factor for stroke and death. N Engl J Med 2005; 353: 2034-41.

[83]   Valham F, Mooe T, Rabben T, *et al.* Increased risk of stroke in patients with coronary artery disease and sleep apnea: a 10-year follow-up. Circulation 2008; 118: 955-60.

[84]   Good DC, Henkle JQ, Gelber D, *et al.* Sleep-disordered breathing and poor functional outcome after stroke. Stroke 1996; 27: 252-9.

[85]   Wessendorf TE, Wang YM, Thilmann AF, *et al.* Treatment of obstructive sleep apnoea with nasal continuous positive airway pressure in stroke. Eur Respir J 2001; 18: 623-9.

[86]   Palombini L, Guilleminault C. Stroke and treatment with nasal CPAP. Eur J Neurol 2006; 13: 198-200.

[87]   Sandberg O, Franklin KA, Bucht G, *et al.* Nasal continuous positive airway pressure in stroke patients with sleep apnoea: a randomized treatment study. Eur Respir J 2001; 18: 630-4.

[88]   Scala R, Turkington PM, Wanklyn P, *et al.* Acceptance, effectiveness and safety of continuous positive airway pressure in acute stroke: a pilot study. Respir Med 2009; 103: 59-66.

[89]   Hsu CY, Vennelle M, Li HY, *et al.* Sleep-disordered breathing after stroke: a randomised controlled trial of continuous positive airway pressure. J Neurol Neurosurg Psychiatry 2006; 77: 1143-9.

[90]   Brown DL, Lisabeth LD, Zupancic MJ, *et al.* High prevalence of supine sleep in ischemic stroke patients. Stroke 2008; 39: 2511-4.

[91]   Hanly P, Zuberi N, Gray R. Pathogenesis of Cheyne-Stokes respiration in patients with congestive heart failure. Relationship to arterial PCO2. Chest 1993; 104: 1079-84.

[92]   Naughton M, Benard D, Tam A, *et al.* Role of hyperventilation in the pathogenesis of central sleep apneas in patients with congestive heart failure. Am Rev Respir Dis 1993; 148: 330-8.

[93]   Yu J, Zhang JF, Fletcher EC. Stimulation of breathing by activation of pulmonary peripheral afferents in rabbits. J Appl Physiol 1998; 85: 1485-92.

[94]   Solin P, Bergin P, Richardson M, *et al.* Influence of pulmonary capillary wedge pressure on central apnea in heart failure. Circulation 1999; 99: 1574-9.

[95]   Lorenzi-Filho G, Azevedo ER, Parker JD, Bradley TD. Relationship of carbon dioxide tension in arterial blood to pulmonary wedge pressure in heart failure. Eur Respir J 2002; 19: 37-40.

[96]   Paintal AS. Vagal sensory receptors and their reflex effects. Physiol Rev 1973; 53: 159-227.

[97]   Javaheri S. A mechanism of central sleep apnea in patients with heart failure. N Engl J Med 1999; 341: 949-54.

[98]   Solin P, Roebuck T, Johns DP, *et al.* Peripheral and central ventilatory responses in central sleep apnea with and without congestive heart failure. Am J Respir Crit Care Med 2000; 162: 2194-200.

[99]   Yumino D, Bradley TD. Central sleep apnea and Cheyne-Stokes respiration. Proc Am Thorac Soc 2008; 5: 226-36.

[100]   Sin DD, Logan AG, Fitzgerald FS, *et al.* Effects of continuous positive airway pressure on cardiovascular outcomes in heart failure patients with and without Cheyne-Stokes respiration. Circulation 2000; 102: 61-6.

[101]   Corra U, Pistono M, Mezzani A, *et al.* Sleep and exertional periodic breathing in chronic heart failure: prognostic importance and interdependence. Circulation 2006; 113: 44-50.

[102]   Javaheri S, Shukla R, Zeigler H, Wexler L. Central sleep apnea, right ventricular dysfunction, and low diastolic blood pressure are predictors of mortality in systolic heart failure. J Am Coll Cardiol 2007; 49: 2028-34.

[103]   Lanfranchi PA, Braghiroli A, Bosimini E, *et al.* Prognostic value of nocturnal Cheyne-Stokes respiration in chronic heart failure. Circulation 1999; 99: 1435-40.

[104]   Hanly PJ, Zuberi-Khokhar NS. Increased mortality associated with Cheyne-Stokes respiration in patients with congestive heart failure. Am J Respir Crit Care Med 1996; 153: 272-6.

[105]   Roebuck T, Solin P, Kaye DM, *et al.* Increased long-term mortality in heart failure due to sleep apnoea is not yet proven. Eur Respir J 2004; 23: 735-40.

[106]   Andreas S, Hagenah G, Moller C, *et al.* Cheyne-Stokes respiration and prognosis in congestive heart failure. Am J Cardiol 1996; 78: 1260-4.

[107]   Franklin KA, Sandstrom E, Johansson G, Balfors EM. Hemodynamics, cerebral circulation, and oxygen saturation in Cheyne-Stokes respiration. J Appl Physiol 1997; 83: 1184-91.

[108]   Trinder J, Merson R, Rosenberg JI, *et al.* Pathophysiological interactions of ventilation, arousals, and blood pressure oscillations during cheyne-stokes respiration in patients with heart failure. Am J Respir Crit Care Med 2000; 162: 808-13.

[109]   Naughton MT, Benard DC, Liu PP, *et al.* Effects of nasal CPAP on sympathetic activity in patients with heart failure and central sleep apnea. Am J Respir Crit Care Med 1995; 152: 473-9.

[110]   Bucca CB, Brussino L, Battisti A, *et al.* Diuretics in obstructive sleep apnea with diastolic heart failure. Chest 2007; 132: 440-6.

[111]   Dark DS, Pingleton SK, Kerby GR, *et al.* Breathing pattern abnormalities and arterial oxygen desaturation during sleep in the congestive heart failure syndrome. Improvement following medical therapy. Chest 1987; 91: 833-6.

[112]   Walsh JT, Andrews R, Starling R, *et al.* Effects of captopril and oxygen on sleep apnoea in patients with mild to moderate congestive cardiac failure. Br Heart J 1995; 73: 237-41.

[113]   Gabor JY, Newman DA, Barnard-Roberts V, *et al.* Improvement in Cheyne-Stokes respiration following cardiac resynchronisation therapy. Eur Respir J 2005; 26: 95-100.

[114]   Sinha AM, Skobel EC, Breithardt OA, *et al.* Cardiac resynchronization therapy improves central sleep apnea and Cheyne-Stokes respiration in patients with chronic heart failure. J Am Coll Cardiol 2004; 44: 68-71.

[115]   Luthje L, Unterberg-Buchwald C, Dajani D, *et al.* Atrial overdrive pacing in patients with sleep apnea with implanted pacemaker. Am J Respir Crit Care Med 2005; 172: 118-22.

[116]   Braver HM, Brandes WC, Kubiet MA, *et al.* Effect of cardiac transplantation on Cheyne-Stokes respiration occurring during sleep. Am J Cardiol 1995; 76: 632-4.

[117]   Abe H, Takahashi M, Yaegashi H, *et al.* Valve repair improves central sleep apnea in heart failure patients with valvular heart diseases. Circ J 2009; 73: 2148-53.

[118]   Bradley TD, Logan AG, Kimoff RJ, *et al.* Continuous positive airway pressure for central sleep apnea and heart failure. N Engl J Med 2005; 353: 2025-33.

[119]   Arzt M, Floras JS, Logan AG, *et al.* Suppression of central sleep apnea by continuous positive airway pressure and transplant-free survival in heart failure: a post hoc analysis of the Canadian Continuous Positive Airway Pressure for Patients with Central Sleep Apnea and Heart Failure Trial (CANPAP). Circulation 2007; 115: 3173-80.

[120]   Fietze I, Blau A, Glos M, *et al.* Bi-level positive pressure ventilation and adaptive servo ventilation in patients with heart failure and Cheyne-Stokes respiration. Sleep Med 2008; 9: 652-9.

[121]   Pepperell JC, Maskell NA, Jones DR, *et al.* A randomized controlled trial of adaptive ventilation for Cheyne-Stokes breathing in heart failure. Am J Respir Crit Care Med 2003; 168: 1109-14.

[122]   Appels A, de Vos Y, van Diest R, *et al.* Are sleep complaints predictive of future myocardial infarction? Act Nerv Super (Praha) 1987; 29: 147-51.

[123]   Eaker ED, Pinsky J, Castelli WP. Myocardial infarction and coronary death among women: psychosocial predictors from a 20-year follow-up of women in the Framingham Study. Am J Epidemiol 1992; 135: 854-64.

[124]   Schwartz SW, Cornoni-Huntley J, Cole SR, *et al.* Are sleep complaints an independent risk factor for myocardial infarction? Ann Epidemiol 1998; 8: 384-92.

[125]   Liu Y, Tanaka H. Overtime work, insufficient sleep, and risk of non-fatal acute myocardial infarction in Japanese men. Occup Environ Med 2002; 59: 447-51.

[126]   King CR, Knutson KL, Rathouz PJ, *et al.* Short sleep duration and incident coronary artery calcification. JAMA 2008; 300: 2859-66.

[127] Knutson KL, Van Cauter E, Rathouz PJ, *et al.* Association between sleep and blood pressure in midlife: the CARDIA sleep study. Arch Intern Med 2009; 169: 1055-61.

[128] Ferrie JE, Shipley MJ, Cappuccio FP, *et al.* A prospective study of change in sleep duration: associations with mortality in the Whitehall II cohort. Sleep 2007; 30: 1659-66.

[129] Gottlieb DJ, Punjabi NM, Newman AB, *et al.* Association of sleep time with diabetes mellitus and impaired glucose tolerance. Arch Intern Med 2005; 165: 863-7.

[130] Gottlieb DJ, Redline S, Nieto FJ, *et al.* Association of usual sleep duration with hypertension: the Sleep Heart Health Study. Sleep 2006; 29: 1009-14.

[131] Grandner MA, Drummond SP. Who are the long sleepers? Towards an understanding of the mortality relationship. Sleep Med Rev 2007; 11: 341-60.

[132] Hublin C, Partinen M, Koskenvuo M, Kaprio J. Sleep and mortality: a population-based 22-year follow-up study. Sleep 2007; 30: 1245-53.

[133] Kojima M, Wakai K, Kawamura, T *et al.* Sleep patterns and total mortality: a 12-year follow-up study in Japan. J Epidemiol 2000; 10: 87-93.

[134] Patel SR, Ayas NT, Malhotra MR, *et al.* A prospective study of sleep duration and mortality risk in women. Sleep 2004; 27: 440-4.

[135] Tamakoshi A, Ohno Y. Self-reported sleep duration as a predictor of all-cause mortality: results from the JACC study, Japan. Sleep 2004; 27: 51-4.

[136] Youngstedt SD, Kripke DF. Long sleep and mortality: rationale for sleep restriction. Sleep Med Rev 2004; 8: 159-74.

[137] Suzuki E, Yorifuji T, Ueshima K, *et al.* Sleep duration, sleep quality and cardiovascular disease mortality among the elderly: a population-based cohort study. Prev Med 2009; 49: 135-41.

[138] Chien KL, Chen PC, Hsu HC, *et al.* Habitual sleep duration and insomnia and the risk of cardiovascular events and all-cause death: report from a community-based cohort. Sleep 2010; 33: 177-84.

[139] Elwood P, Hack M, Pickering J, *et al.* Sleep disturbance, stroke, and heart disease events: evidence from the Caerphilly cohort. J Epidemiol Community Health 2006; 60: 69-73.

[140] Meisinger C, Heier M, Lowel H, *et al.* Sleep duration and sleep complaints and risk of myocardial infarction in middle-aged men and women from the general population: the MONICA/KORA Augsburg cohort study. Sleep 2007; 30: 1121-7.

[141] Qureshi AI, Giles WH, Croft JB, Bliwise DL. Habitual sleep patterns and risk for stroke and coronary heart disease: a 10-year follow-up from NHANES I. Neurology 1997; 48: 904-11.

[142] Phillips B, Mannino DM. Do insomnia complaints cause hypertension or cardiovascular disease? J Clin Sleep Med 2007; 3: 489-94.

[143] Lanfranchi PA, Pennestri MH, Fradette L, *et al.* Nighttime blood pressure in normotensive subjects with chronic insomnia: implications for cardiovascular risk. Sleep 2009; 32: 760-6.

[144] Vgontzas AN, Liao D, Bixler EO, *et al.* Insomnia with objective short sleep duration is associated with a high risk for hypertension. Sleep 2009; 32: 491-7.

[145] Vgontzas AN, Liao D, Pejovic S, *et al.* Insomnia with objective short sleep duration is associated with type 2 diabetes: A population-based study. Diabetes Care 2009; 32: 1980-5.

[146] Knutsson A, Akerstedt T, Jonsson BG, Orth-Gomer K. Increased risk of ischaemic heart disease in shift workers. Lancet 1986; 2: 89-92.

[147] Karlsson B, Knutsson A, Lindahl B. Is there an association between shift work and having a metabolic syndrome? Results from a population based study of 27,485 people. Occup Environ Med 2001; 58: 747-52.

[148] Tuchsen F, Hannerz H, Burr H. A 12 year prospective study of circulatory disease among Danish shift workers. Occup Environ Med 2006; 63: 451-5.

[149] Kroenke CH, Spiegelman D, Manson J, *et al.* Work characteristics and incidence of type 2 diabetes in women. Am J Epidemiol 2007; 165: 175-83.

[150] Morikawa Y, Nakagawa H, Miura K, *et al.* Effect of shift work on body mass index and metabolic parameters. Scand J Work Environ Health 2007; 33: 45-50.

[151] Buijs RM, Scheer FA, Kreier F, *et al.* Organization of circadian functions: interaction with the body. Prog Brain Res 2006; 153: 341-60.

[152] Kohsaka A, Bass J. A sense of time: how molecular clocks organize metabolism. Trends Endocrinol Metab 2007; 18: 4-11.

[153] Scheer FA, Hilton MF, Mantzoros CS, Shea SA. Adverse metabolic and cardiovascular consequences of circadian misalignment. Proc Natl Acad Sci U S A 2009; 106: 4453-8.

[154] Ulfberg J, Nystrom B, Carter N, Edling C. Prevalence of restless legs syndrome among men aged 18 to 64 years: an association with somatic disease and neuropsychiatric symptoms. Mov Disord 2001; 16: 1159-63.

[155] Ohayon MM, Roth T. Prevalence of restless legs syndrome and periodic limb movement disorder in the general population. J Psychosom Res 2002; 53: 547-54.

[156] Phillips B, Hening W, Britz P, Mannino D. Prevalence and correlates of restless legs syndrome: results from the 2005 National Sleep Foundation Poll. Chest 2006; 129: 76-80.

[157] Winkelman JW, Shahar E, Sharief I, Gottlieb DJ. Association of restless legs syndrome and cardiovascular disease in the Sleep Heart Health Study. Neurology 2008; 70: 35-42.

[158] Walters AS, Rye DB. Review of the relationship of restless legs syndrome and periodic limb movements in sleep to hypertension, heart disease, and stroke. Sleep 2009; 32: 589-97.

[159] Arnardottir ES, Mackiewicz M, Gislason T, *et al.* Molecular signatures of obstructive sleep apnea in adults: a review and perspective. Sleep 2009; 32: 447-70.

[160] Narkiewicz K, van de Borne PJ, Cooley RL, *et al.* Sympathetic activity in obese subjects with and without obstructive sleep apnea. Circulation 1998; 98: 772-6.

[161] Grassi G, Facchini A, Trevano FQ, *et al.* Obstructive sleep apnea-dependent and -independent adrenergic activation in obesity. Hypertension 2005; 46: 321-5.

[162] Waradekar NV, Sinoway LI, Zwillich CW, Leuenberger UA. Influence of treatment on muscle sympathetic nerve activity in sleep apnea. Am J Respir Crit Care Med 1996; 153: 1333-8.

[163] Narkiewicz K, Kato M, Phillips BG, *et al.* Nocturnal continuous positive airway pressure decreases daytime sympathetic traffic in obstructive sleep apnea. Circulation 1999; 100: 2332-5.

[164] Donadio V, Liguori R, Vetrugno R, *et al.* Daytime sympathetic hyperactivity in OSAS is related to excessive daytime sleepiness. J Sleep Res 2007; 16: 327-32.

[165] Fletcher EC, Miller J, Schaaf JW, Fletcher JG. Urinary catecholamines before and after tracheostomy in patients with obstructive sleep apnea and hypertension. Sleep 1987; 10: 35-44.

[166] McArdle N, Hillman D, Beilin L, Watts G. Metabolic risk factors for vascular disease in obstructive sleep apnea: a matched controlled study. Am J Respir Crit Care Med 2007; 175: 190-5.

[167] Heitmann J, Ehlenz K, Penzel T, *et al.* Sympathetic activity is reduced by nCPAP in hypertensive obstructive sleep apnoea patients. Eur Respir J 2004; 23: 255-62.

[168] Ziegler MG, Mills PJ, Loredo JS, *et al.* Effect of continuous positive airway pressure and placebo treatment on sympathetic nervous activity in patients with obstructive sleep apnea. Chest 2001; 120: 887-93.

[169] Hedner J, Darpo B, Ejnell H, *et al.* Reduction in sympathetic activity after long-term CPAP treatment in sleep apnoea: cardiovascular implications. Eur Respir J 1995; 8: 222-9.

[170] Minoguchi K, Yokoe T, Tanaka A, *et al.* Association between lipid peroxidation and inflammation in obstructive sleep apnoea. Eur Respir J 2006; 28: 378-85.

[171] Carpagnano GE, Kharitonov SA, Resta O, *et al.* Increased 8-isoprostane and interleukin-6 in breath condensate of obstructive sleep apnea patients. Chest 2002; 122: 1162-7.

[172] Carpagnano GE, Kharitonov SA, Resta O, *et al.* 8-Isoprostane, a marker of oxidative stress, is increased in exhaled breath condensate of patients with obstructive sleep apnea after night and is reduced by continuous positive airway pressure therapy. Chest 2003; 124: 1386-92.

[173] Jordan W, Cohrs S, Degner D, *et al.* Evaluation of oxidative stress measurements in obstructive sleep apnea syndrome. J Neural Transm 2006; 113: 239-54.

[174] Lavie L, Vishnevsky A, Lavie P. Evidence for lipid peroxidation in obstructive sleep apnea. Sleep 2004; 27: 123-8.

[175] Dyugovskaya L, Lavie P, Lavie L. Increased adhesion molecules expression and production of reactive oxygen species in leukocytes of sleep apnea patients. Am J Respir Crit Care Med 2002; 165: 934-9.

[176] Svatikova A, Wolk R, Lerman LO, *et al.* Oxidative stress in obstructive sleep apnoea. Eur Heart J 2005; 26: 2435-9.

[177] Ozturk L, Mansour B, Yuksel M, *et al.* Lipid peroxidation and osmotic fragility of red blood cells in sleep-apnea patients. Clin Chim Acta 2003; 332: 83-8.

[178] Alzoghaibi MA, Bahammam AS. Lipid peroxides, superoxide dismutase and circulating IL-8 and GCP-2 in patients with severe obstructive sleep apnea: a pilot study. Sleep Breath 2005; 9: 119-26.

[179] Ciftci TU, Kokturk O, Bukan N, Bilgihan A. The relationship between serum cytokine levels with obesity and obstructive sleep apnea syndrome. Cytokine 2004; 28: 87-91.

[180] Vgontzas AN, Papanicolaou DA, Bixler EO, *et al.* Elevation of plasma cytokines in disorders of excessive daytime sleepiness: role of sleep disturbance and obesity. J Clin Endocrinol Metab 1997; 82: 1313-6.

[181] Ryan S, Taylor CT, McNicholas WT. Predictors of elevated nuclear factor-kappaB-dependent genes in obstructive sleep apnea syndrome. Am J Respir Crit Care Med 2006; 174: 824-30.

[182] Liu H, Liu J, Xiong S, *et al.* The change of interleukin-6 and tumor necrosis factor in patients with obstructive sleep apnea syndrome. J Tongji Med Univ 2000; 20: 200-2.

[183] Shamsuzzaman AS, Winnicki M, Lanfranchi P, *et al.* Elevated C-reactive protein in patients with obstructive sleep apnea. Circulation 2002; 105: 2462-4.

[184] Yokoe T, Minoguchi K, Matsuo H, *et al.* Elevated levels of C-reactive protein and interleukin-6 in patients with obstructive sleep apnea syndrome are decreased by nasal continuous positive airway pressure. Circulation 2003; 107: 1129-34.

[185] Minoguchi K, Tazaki T, Yokoe T, *et al.* Elevated production of tumor necrosis factor-alpha by monocytes in patients with obstructive sleep apnea syndrome. Chest 2004; 126: 1473-9.

[186] Guilleminault C, Kirisoglu C, Ohayon MM. C-reactive protein and sleep-disordered breathing. Sleep 2004; 27: 1507-11.

[187] Sharma SK, Mishra HK, Sharma H, *et al.* Obesity, and not obstructive sleep apnea, is responsible for increased serum hs-CRP levels in patients with sleep-disordered breathing in Delhi. Sleep Med 2008; 9: 149-56.

[188] Roytblat L, Rachinsky M, Fisher A, *et al.* Raised interleukin-6 levels in obese patients. Obes Res 2000; 8: 673-5.

[189] Vgontzas AN, Papanicolaou DA, Bixler EO, *et al.* Sleep apnea and daytime sleepiness and fatigue: relation to visceral obesity, insulin resistance, and hypercytokinemia. J Clin Endocrinol Metab 2000; 85: 1151-8.

[190] Imagawa S, Yamaguchi Y, Ogawa K, *et al.* Interleukin-6 and tumor necrosis factor-alpha in patients with obstructive sleep apnea-hypopnea syndrome. Respiration 2004; 71: 24-9.

[191] Barcelo A, Barbe F, Llompart E, *et al.* Effects of obesity on C-reactive protein level and metabolic disturbances in male patients with obstructive sleep apnea. Am J Med 2004; 117: 118-21.

[192] Clement K, Langin D. Regulation of inflammation-related genes in human adipose tissue. J Intern Med 2007; 262: 422-30.

[193] Wisse BE. The inflammatory syndrome: the role of adipose tissue cytokines in metabolic disorders linked to obesity. J Am Soc Nephrol 2004; 15: 2792-800.

[194] Kohler M, Craig S, Nicoll D, *et al.* Endothelial function and arterial stiffness in minimally symptomatic obstructive sleep apnea. Am J Respir Crit Care Med 2008; 178: 984-8.

[195] Jelic S, Lederer DJ, Adams T, *et al.* Vascular inflammation in obesity and sleep apnea. Circulation 2010; 121: 1014-21.

CHAPTER 18

Sleep and Metabolic Syndrome

Alexander Babayeuski, M.D.[1,*] and Octavian C. Ioachimescu, M.D., Ph.D.[2]

[1]*Atlanta Medical Center 303 Parkway Dr NE, Atlanta, GA 30312, USA and* [2]*Assistant Professor of Medicine - Emory University, Adjunct Clinical Assistant Professor of Medicine – Morehouse School of Medicine, Medical Director, Atlanta Veterans' Affairs Sleep Disorders Center, Division of Pulmonary, Critical Care and Sleep Medicine, Emory University School of Medicine, Atlanta Veterans Affairs Medical Center, Atlanta, GA 30033, USA*

Abstract: On average, human beings spend approximately one third of their life sleeping. Many individuals are chronically sleep deprived, while many individuals with primary sleep illnesses, such as obstructive sleep apnea (OSA) are unaware of their condition; as a result, without treatment, they suffer from serious negative physical, neurobehavioral and metabolic consequences. Obstructive sleep apnea is now a well recognized chronic disorder that leads to multiple cardiovascular and metabolic complications.

During the last decades there has been a mounting body of data that established a better characterized link between OSA and insulin resistance, diabetes mellitus and/or metabolic syndrome. Likely mechanistic mediators of this connection are intermittent hypoxia and sleep fragmentation. Through sympathetic system activation, oxidative stress, hypoxia/re-oxigenation, systemic inflammation, production of harmful adipokines from metabolically active visceral fat and complex endocrine changes, sleep apnea and obesity lead to a vicious cycle of abnormal glucose metabolism, which likely contributes to an increase in cardiovascular morbidity and mortality. When appropriate, physicians should have a low threshold to assess sleep apnea, as effective therapy is readily available (CPAP, mandibular advancement devices, etc). In this chapter we will summarize and analyze the most current data in this rapidly growing field of sleep medicine.

TOPIC DISCUSSION (CLINICAL OUTLOOK)

During the last century, life of the human beings has changed dramatically, with major individual, socio-economic and societal consequences. These transformations have been driven by several major changes: (1) increased food availability, the emergence of processed foods (*e.g.*, high-fructose corn syrup, etc), with progressively increased caloric intake, frequent snacking and feeding in the immediate period before sleep; (2) improved economic status/power of the standard family, due to a 2-salary earning family model, work during night shifts, better social infrastructure for children education and after-school programs, etc; (3) curtailment in overall physical activity; (4) progressive shortening of the total sleep time in parallel with the introduction of electricity; (5) increased exposure to light and circadian misalignments driven by work and cultural habits (*e.g.*, night shifts, watching TV, work on computer, etc).

In our very competitive, success-driven, 24/7 model of society and compared to only half a century ago, individuals tend to sleep less and weigh significantly more. The lack of sleep and the increase in body weight has a profound effect on hormonal and metabolic health [1,2]. In addition, parallel epidemics of obesity and diabetes are exploding [3,4], making the pathogenic link between them very likely. How sleep misaligned with the light-dark cycle, insufficient sleep or sleep affected by various primary sleep disorders lead to metabolic consequences which constitute the metabolic syndrome, will be reviewed in the next pages of this chapter.

Background

Obstructive Sleep Apnea

Obstructive sleep apnea (OSA) is a common chronic sleep disorder that often needs lifelong therapy [5]. OSA causes intermittent and repetitive closures of the upper airway during sleep, leading to intermittent hypoxia (IH) and sleep fragmentation. OSA is a relatively common condition, but significantly under-diagnosed. About 1 in 5 US

*****Address correspondence to Alexander Babayeuski:** Atlanta Medical Center 303 Parkway Dr NE, Atlanta, GA 30312, USA; Tel: (404) 265-4000; E-mail: babasasha@yahoo.com

adults have at least mild OSA, when defined only by apnea hypopnea index (AHI) between 5 and 14, and 1 in 15 have moderate OSA (AHI 15-29) [6]. In another study, OSA (defined as AHI ≥ 5, and not necessarily associated with any symptoms) was very frequent among both middle-aged women (9%) and men (24%). At the very least, about 4% of men and 2% of women meet minimal diagnostic criteria for OSA (AHI ≥ 5 and common symptoms of excessive daytime sleepiness) [7]. Other studies report even higher prevalence rates, of about 9% [8].

The following demographic and anthropometric parameters are currently known as the main risk factors for OSA:

- Age: OSA prevalence increases from young adulthood and peaks around 50-60s [7].

- Male gender: Men tend to have higher prevalence of OSA compared to women (at least pre-menopausal females).

- Obesity: More than 50-55% of people with BMI ≥ 40 have OSA [9,10].

- Large neck size: Individuals with neck sizes greater than 17 inches (in men) and 16 inches (in women) are at risk for OSA [11].

- Craniofacial abnormalities and chronic nasal congestion

- Socioeconomic status

- Ethnicity: African-Americans and Mexican-Americans [12]

- Smoking, alcohol and the use/abuse of sedatives.

- Family history of sleep apnea

- Snoring: it has been shown that habitual snorers have up to seven times higher risk of developing OSA (risk factor or manifestation of the disease?).

- Diabetes: OSA is much common in people with diabetes and insulin resistance [13,14].

The most common clinical symptoms of OSA are loud snoring and excessive daytime sleepiness (EDS). Nevertheless, many patients become aware of the problem only because their sleeping partner alerts them about the issue due to loud snoring and/or witnessed apneas. Other symptoms include restless legs, morning headaches, poor concentration and deteriorating memory, nocturnal angina and frequent urination, dry mouth and sore throat, nocturnal gasping and choking, and/or persistent daytime fatigue or tiredness.

OSA pathophysiology is complex and still not completely understood. Overall, it does seem to be related to a combination of reduced upper airway size [15], altered shape [16,17], and/or highly compliant airway. Pharyngeal muscle weakness may be the main factor leading to airway collapse during sleep, as muscle tone decreases with diminished neural output at night, resulting in snoring and partial or complete airway collapse. Arousal from sleep (partial or complete) is then needed to overcome collapsed airway. Another reason may be the variability of the respiratory drive in patients with OSA. This may also be explained by what is called "loop gain" in sleep apnea. Campana et al., found a very good analogy with room temperature variation, i.e., an extremely sensitive thermostat and very fast and powerful heater [18]. During apnea, ventilatory drive is increased until inspiration occurs again. At times this can result in ventilation "overshot" that can drive carbon dioxide too low, lower than inspiration threshold resulting in next apnea.

OSA is usually diagnosed based on history and clinical examination, corroborated with an overnight polysomnography (gold standard for diagnosis). OSA is characterized by recurrent apneas and hypopneas [19]. In adults, apnea is an airflow reduction to less than 10% from baseline for 10 seconds or more. Hypopnea, or partial apnea, is an airflow reduction by 30% to 90% from the baseline for 10 seconds or more, accompanied by at least a 4% oxyhemoglobin desaturation; alternatively, hypopnea is defined as a drop between 50% and 90% from baseline for 10 seconds or more and associated with at least a 3% desaturation or an arousal [19,20]. Apnea-hypopnea index (AHI) is the total number of apneas and hypopneas per hour of sleep. The AHI is a well-known OSA severity metric; another one is oxygen desaturation index score (ODI), which is the number oxygen desaturations (drops in SpO_2 of at least 3% or 4% in other publications) per hour of sleep. According to AHI, OSA is classified as mild, when the AHI is between 5 and 14; moderate, when AHI is between 15 to 29; and severe, when AHI is 30 or higher.

OSA is strongly associated with increased cardiovascular risk and morbidity [21-23]. In an 18-year follow-up of the Wisconsin Sleep Cohort (n=1,522), all cause mortality risk, adjusted for BMI and gender, was significantly increased [24]. It has also been noted over the last decades that OSA is strongly linked to development of diabetes [25], cardiovascular diseases [26,27], hypertension [28], obesity [29,30], depression [31], etc. A subgroup of OSA patients may not have any symptoms; nevertheless, these patients still carry the risk of developing hypertension and have an increased risk of all-cause mortality. Treatment with CPAP, which acts as pneumatic splint for the upper airway, seems to reduce the above risks.

Obesity

Obesity has become a global epidemic of historic proportions [32], with very high medical, social and healthcare costs [33-35]. The prevalence of obesity in the US is very high, exceeding 30% in most gender and age groups. Results from the National Health and Nutrition Examination Survey (NHANES), indicate that an estimated 34.2% of U.S. adults aged 20 years and over are overweight, 33.8% are obese, and 5.7% are extremely obese (see Fig. 1). In 2007-2008, the prevalence of obesity among adult Americans was 32.2% in men and 35.5% in women [36]. Comparisons between Canada and USA show that obesity prevalence is higher in the US, with the difference largely due to higher obesity rates in women [35]. A review of prevalence estimates in European countries found that the prevalence of obesity is overall lower than in the US and that it varies widely from country to country, with higher rates in Southern, Central and South-Eastern European countries [36,37].

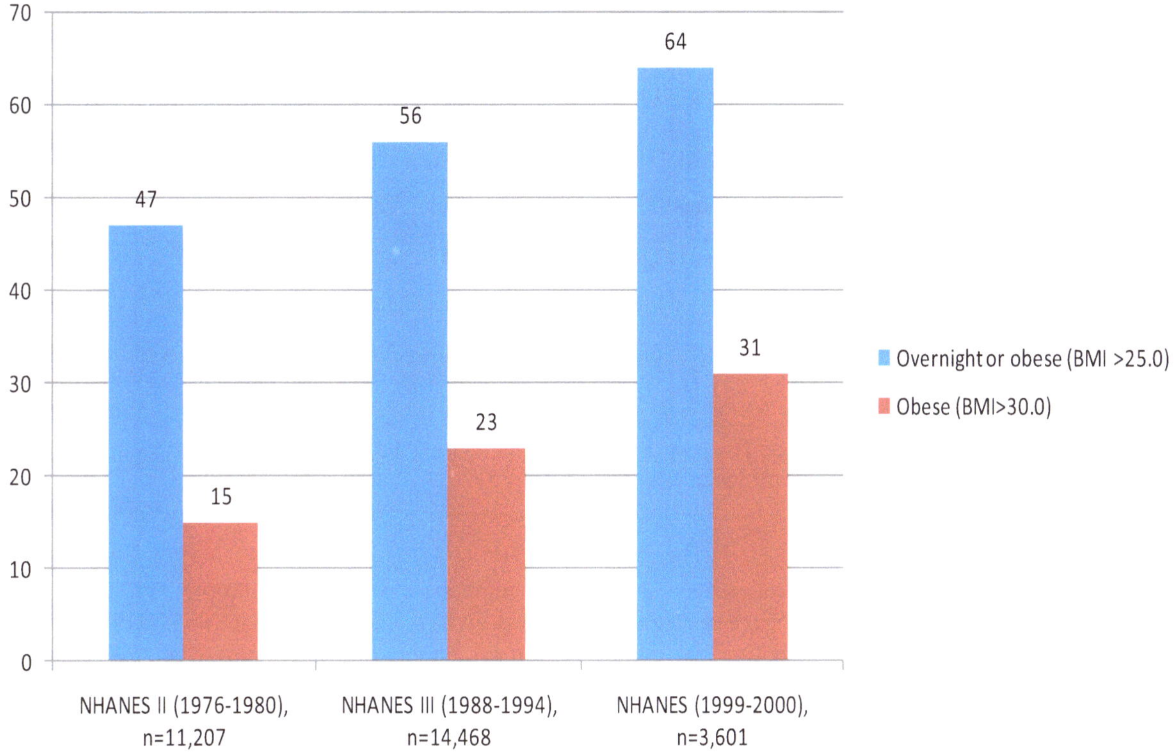

Figure 1: Rates of overweight and obesity in the USA according to National Health and Nutrition Examination Survey (NHANES); available online at:http://www.cdc.gov/nchs/data/hestat/obesity_adult_07_08/obesity_adult_07_08.htm

Obesity is a leading cause of mortality, morbidity, disability, healthcare utilization and costs in the US [33,38,39]. Obesity is associated with more than 30 medical conditions, of which coronary artery disease, hypertension, stroke, type 2 diabetes, cancer, depression, and sleep apnea are the most important. Each year at least 300,000 deaths in the US are considered to be the result of obesity, and The Center for Disease Control and Prevention (CDC) currently estimates that approximately 23.6 million people in the US (7.8% of population) suffer from diabetes. Consequently, in 2006 diabetes represented the 7th leading cause of death in the US.

Diabetes Mellitus

According to National Diabetes Fact Sheet 2007 [38,40], issued by the American Diabetes Association (ADA), *diabetes mellitus* is a group of disorders defined by high levels of blood glucose resulting from defects in insulin production, action or both. ADA recognizes four different sub-types of diabetes:

- Type 1 diabetes (T1DM), previously called insulin-dependent diabetes mellitus (IDDM) or juvenile-onset diabetes. T1DM constitutes 5-10% of all cases and is thought to be secondary to an autoimmune destruction of the pancreatic beta cells, which secrete insulin. Risk factors for T1DM may be autoimmune, genetic, and/or environmental. Currently, there is no known way to prevent T1DM. Several clinical trials for primary prevention of T1DM are currently in progress or in the planning phase.

- Type 2 diabetes (T2DM), previously called non–insulin-dependent diabetes mellitus (NIDDM) or adult-onset diabetes. In adults, T2DM accounts for about 90% to 95% of all diagnosed cases. It usually begins as insulin resistance (IR), a disorder in which the cells do not use insulin properly despite hyperinsulinemia. In time, the pancreas gradually loses its ability to produce insulin and then T2DM may become ketosis-prone and insulin-requiring. T2DM is associated with older age, obesity, family history of diabetes, history of gestational diabetes, impaired glucose metabolism, physical inactivity, and race/ethnicity. African Americans, Hispanic Americans, American Indians, some Asian Americans and Native Hawaiians or Other Pacific Islanders are at particularly high risk for developing T2DM and its complications. T2DM in children and adolescents, although still rare, is being diagnosed more frequently among American Indians, African Americans, Hispanic Americans, and Asians/Pacific Islanders.

- Gestational diabetes (GD) is a form of glucose intolerance diagnosed during pregnancy. GD occurs more frequently among African Americans, Hispanic Americans, and American Indians. It is also more common among obese women and women with a family history of diabetes. Post-pregnancy, 5% to 10% of women with GD remain diabetic, usually T2DM. Furthermore, women who have had GD have a 40% to 60% chance of developing diabetes in the next 5–10 years.

- Other types of diabetes result from specific genetic conditions (such as maturity-onset diabetes of youth), surgery, medications, infections, pancreatic disease, and other illnesses. Such types of diabetes account for 1% to 5% of all diagnosed cases.

Pre-Diabetes Includes Two Different Entities:

- impaired fasting glucose (IFG), which is characterized by fasting serum glucose between 100 and 126 mg/dL, and

- impaired glucose tolerance (IGT), when the glycemic levels are between 140 and 200 mg/dL two hours after a 75-g oral glucose tolerance test (OGTT).

Metabolic Syndrome:

Worldwide and in the last decades, metabolic syndrome has become a major public health problem. Currently, it seems that 25% to 40% of individuals between 25 and 65 years of age have metabolic syndrome [41-45]. Metabolic syndrome (MetS), or syndrome X, is defined by a constellation of abnormalities, including central or abdominal obesity, dyslipidemia, hyperglycemia, and hypertension [41-50]. Metabolic syndrome is further defined by the presence of other components, including elevated circulating levels of triglycerides, reduced levels of high-density lipoprotein cholesterol, and impaired fasting glucose. Elevated circulating levels of pro-inflammatory and/or thrombotic markers (C-reactive protein, tumor necrosis factor-alpha, interleukin-6, and plasminogen activator inhibitor type 1) and/or reduced levels of anti-inflammatory molecules (*e.g.*, adiponectin, interleukin-10, *etc.*) are sometimes used as additional biomarkers of MetS [41,42]. Together, the metabolic abnormalities comprising MetS seem to confer additive risk in terms of cardiovascular mortality and morbidity, *i.e.*, higher than the risk attributable to any individual component. Understandably, MetS shares many common risks factors with atherosclerosis and cardiovascular diseases, but it still adds variable contributions to the variance of the mortality indices.

Excessive food intake and lack of physical activity, which led to the growing epidemic of obesity and MetS, happened not only in western, industrialized nations, but also in developing countries. Furthermore, several clinical epidemiological studies have raised the hypothesis that one of the major changes that contributes to the pathogenesis of the MetS in the industrialized world stems from the introduction of artificial light and work during the night, in addition to the progressive sleep duration shortening [46]. Indeed, these common disorders of circadian behavior and sleep are associated with increased hunger, decreased glucose and lipid metabolism, and broad changes in the hormonal signals involved in satiety [29]. Remarkably, obesity and high-fat feeding also reciprocally affect the circadian system in mice, indicating that metabolism, circadian rhythms, and possibly sleep are interconnected through complex behavioral and molecular pathways [51]. Thus, alterations in energy homeostasis associated with obesity may set in motion a "vicious cycle" of circadian disruption, in turn leading to exacerbation of the original metabolic disturbances.

The MetS can be explained as the end-result of the abdominal visceral adiposity, which acts as a vast endocrine gland, releasing into circulation several hormonal and metabolically active biologic mediators, such as free fatty acids (FFAs), adipokines, angioitensin II

Of note, according to the American Diabetes Association [52], normal fasting plasma glucose is defined as < 100 mg/dL (5.6 mmol/L), impaired fasting glucose (IFG): glycemic levels between 100 and 125 mg/dL (5.6-6.9 mmol/L), and provisional diagnosis of diabetes when fasting plasma levels are ≥ 126 mg/dL (7 mmol/L). When interpreting the 75-g oral glucose tolerance test (OGTT) [52], at 2-hour time mark, normal glucose tolerance is defined as plasma levels < 140 mg/dL (7.8 mmol/L), impaired glucose tolerance (IGT) when the plasma glucose level is between 140 and 199 mg/dL (7.8-11.1 mmol/L), and provisional diagnosis of diabetes when plasma glucose level is 200 mg/dL (11.1 mmmol/L) or above.

Although there are many different definitions for MetS, they all have in common insulin resistance (IR) or its surrogates. These are several available defitions of MetS:

- **World Health Organization definition, 1999** [53]: Diabetes, impaired fasting glucose or impaired glucose tolerance or Insulin Resistance (IR, assessed by clamp studies) *plus* at least two of the following:

    1. BMI>30 and/or waist hip ratio >0.90 in men and >0.85 in women

    2. Triglycerides ≥ 150 mg/dL (1.7 mmol/L)

    3. HDL cholesterol< 35 mg/dL (0.9 mmol/L) in men and < 39 mg/dL (1.0 mmol/L) in women

    4. Blood pressure ≥ 140/90 mm Hg or therapy

    5. Urine albumin excretion rate >20 µg/min or albumin/creatinine ratio ≥ 30mg/g

- **2001 National Cholesterol Education Program/Adult Treatment Panel III, 2005 update** [54]. Presence of any three:

    1. Abdominal obesity- waist circumference > 102 cm (40 inches) in men and > 88 cm (35 inches) in women

    2. Serum Triglycerides ≥ 150 mg/dL (1.7 mmol/L) or therapy

    3. Fasting plasma glucose ≥ 100 mg/dL (5.6 mmol/L) (impaired fasting glucose) or therapy

    4. Serum HDL cholesterol < 39 mg/dL (1.0 mmol/L) in men and < 50 mg/dL (1.3 mmol/L) in women or therapy

    5. Blood pressure ≥ 130/85 mm Hg or therapy

- **International Diabetes Federation (IDF), 2005** [41]: Increased waist circumference (ethnicity specific) plus 2 of the following:

    1. Serum Triglycerides > 150 mg/dL (1.7 mmol/L) or specific therapy for lipid abnormality

    2. HDL cholesterol < 40 mg/dl in men (1.03 mmol/L) or < 50 mg/dL (1.29 mmol/L) in women or therapy

    3. Blood pressure ≥ 130/85 mm Hg or therapy

    4. Fasting plasma glucose ≥ 100 mg/dL (5.6 mmol/L) or diabetes

Others are now advocating for inclusion in the definition of the MetS of a pro-thrombotic state and/or a pro-inflammatory state [54]. Despite many available definitions for MetS, insulin resistance (IR) is thought to be the most important metabolic abnormality and which has a strong positive correlation with the amount of visceral fat [55-57].

Steady-state measurements of IR are flawed with the inherent errors introduced by the static nature of the assessments; an alternative to this is a methodology that uses the tissues' response to insulin, as modeled by infusions of glucose and/or insulin. This way, the pancreatic output of insulin and the tissue response are assessed in conjunction; hence a more realistic model of what constitutes IR.

As described by DeFronzo [58], two methods have been designed to evaluate dynamic glucose metabolism by assessing beta-cell sensitivity to glucose (hyperglycemic clamp technique) and of tissue sensitivity to insulin (euglycemic insulin clamp technique):

1. Hyperglycemic clamp technique: the plasma glucose level is acutely raised to 125 mg/dL above baseline by a priming infusion of glucose. The desired hyperglycemic plateau is subsequently maintained by adjustment of a variable glucose infusion. Because the plasma glucose concentration is held constant, the glucose infusion rate can be used as an index of glucose metabolism. Under these conditions of constant hyperglycemia, the plasma insulin response is biphasic with an early discharge of insulin release during the first 6 minutes, followed by a gradually progressive increase in plasma insulin concentration.

2. Euglycemic insulin clamp technique: the plasma insulin concentration is acutely raised and maintained at approximately 100 μU/mL by a priming continuous infusion of insulin. The plasma glucose concentration is then held constant at basal levels by a variable glucose infusion using the negative feedback principle. Under these steady-state conditions of euglycemia, the glucose infusion rate equals glucose uptake by all the tissues in the body and is therefore a measure of tissue sensitivity to exogenous insulin. The euglycemic-hyperinsulinemic clamp [58] is the gold standard technique for characterization of global IR.

Against the euglycemic-hyperinsulinemic clamp, which is laborious and complex, other tests have been devised to assess IR, with variable performance; for example: insulin levels [59], homeostasis model assessment of insulin resistance (HOMA-IR) [60], fasting plasma glucose-to-insulin ratio [61], quantitative insulin sensitivity check index (QUICKI) [62,63], *etc.*

If it is poor sleep quality and/or short sleep duration, that is/are associated with obesity and metabolic syndrome, it is still unclear. Poor sleep quality can be described in various ways, from qualitative assessments to more refined quantitative methodologies, but, in the end, it is a specific change or deviation from the "normal" sleep architecture seen in healthy individuals. This may be illustrated by a change in the amount or proportion of various sleep stages, increase in the arousal index, time spent in wake after sleep onset, *etc.* The common sleep conditions that lead ultimately to poor sleep quality and/or quantity and are known to be associated (if not pathogenically linked) to obesity and metabolic syndrome are sleep disordered breathing, sleep movement disorders, *etc.*

We will briefly discuss here the 3 main mechanisms of sleep alteration, as exemplified by the disruption of the circadian system (chronodisruption), sleep deprivation and primary sleep conditions such as sleep disordered breathing.

A. CHRONODISRUPTION

Life is almost equivalent to rhythm(s). The majority of the biologic functions in the body follow certain oscillations in time. Circadian rhythms (from Latin *circa diem*, about a day) are part of the complex biology of life and are dictated by multiple factors. In humans, these oscillations are the final output of a "machinery" that inputs circadian rhythms (as dictated by central and peripheral biologic clocks), internal (hormones, cytokines, etc) and external cues (light, temperature, food intake, etc). The endogenous master pacemaker is located in the suprachiasmatic nucleus (SCN) of the hypothalamus, while other circadian oscillators have been identified in the peripheral tissues (*e.g.*, heart, liver, lungs, skeletal muscles, adrenal glands, etc) [64]. The SCN seemed to have evolved to synchronize physical activity, food consumption and sleep within circadian and circannual cycles through hormones and autonomic nervous system.

It has also long been recognized that serious adverse cardiovascular events, including myocardial infarction (MI), sudden death, major arrhythmias, venous thromboembolic disease, peripheral vascular disease, and aortic aneurysmal ruptures have all pronounced circadian rhythmicity, reaching a peak during the early morning [65]. More recent evidence has shown that chronic circadian disruption may also increase susceptibility to develop these disorders. For example, in individuals between 45 and 55 years of age, shift work was found to be associated with a 1.6-fold increased risk of cardiovascular disease for men and a 3.0-fold increased risk for women [66]. Cardiovascular disease and hypertension are also associated with sleep loss [67]; it seems that the risk of a fatal MI increases by 45% in individuals who sleep habitually 5 hours per night or less [68]. Interestingly, the incidence of MI was also significantly increased for the first 3 week days after the transition from standard time (ST) to daylight saving time (DST) in the spring [69]. This may be related to the chrono-disruptive effect of transitions involved in DST. Another reported adverse aspect of sleep chrono-impairment is represented by various alterations of the immune system [70-72]. For instance, sleep deprivation increases monocytes' production of several proinflammatory cytokines, including interleukin-6 and tumor necrosis factor-alpha [73,74]. This seems to add further in support of the theory that obesity, a frequent comorbid condition, is an inflammatory condition [75]. On the other hand, the inflammatory process itself can induce sleep disturbance [70]. Other metabolic disorders may be induced by a phase shift, such as altered postprandial lipid excursions, thereby providing a partial explanation for the increased occurrence of cardiovascular disease reported in shift workers [76].

More recently, Sheer and collaborators [77] investigated the mechanistic links between circadian misalignment and metabolic homeostasis using a controlled simulation of "shift-work" in the clinical laboratory. In this study, 10 subjects underwent a progressive misalignment of the behavioral and the circadian cycles. Their behavioral cycle was extended to a dim-light 28-hour day, with 14 hours of rest and fasting alternating with 14 hours of wake, and with 4 evenly spaced, isocaloric meals. When subjects were approximately 12 hours out of phase from their habitual times, decreased leptin levels, hyperglycemia and hyperinsulinemia (some of them to the degree of prediabetes) were noted. In addition, their daily cortisol rhythm was also reversed, arterial pressure was elevated, and sleep efficiency was decreased [77]. Thus, this study suggested that synchrony between behavioral and physiological rhythms is advantageous to maintain normal glucose metabolism in otherwise healthy persons [78].

Furthermore, primary sleep disorders impacting circadian timing, quality and/or duration of sleep are also associated with metabolic disorders. For example, sleep apnea, a condition that is highly prevalent in individuals with metabolic disorders [79], was thought to lead to clock gene dysfunctions [80], while effective treatments of sleep apnea with CPAP has been found to improve glucose metabolism and energy balance [81].

RESEARCH OUTLOOK

What do we know:

In addition to circadian rhythm disorders (*e.g.*, shift work disorder), genetic polymorphisms in several clock genes have also been linked to sleep disorders [82,83]. As such, polymorphisms in genes *Clock* and *Bmal1*, which are involved in complex circadian regulations, have been linked to some features of the metabolic syndrome. In small sample populations, polymorphisms in the *Clock* gene have been correlated with predisposition to obesity [84,85] and two *Bmal1* haplotypes have been associated with type 2 diabetes mellitus and with hypertension [86]. Polymorphisms in clock genes *Per2* and *Npas2* have also been associated with hypertension and high fasting blood glucose in studies of similar sample size [87]. On the flip side, a rare variant of *Nampt*, clock gene which is involved in a negative feedback loop [88,89], seems to be protective for obesity development [90].

Several recent genome-wide association (GWA) studies pointed out to an interesting finding of the fact that melatonin, an essential pineal hormone implicated in circadian alignment, may be important in the regulation of serum glucose levels [91,92]. These studies have also shown that the presence of a variant of melatonin receptor 1B (*mtnr1b*) is associated with insulin and glucose concentrations. The gene for the common variant *mtnr1b* is in fact expressed in the pancreatic islet (beta) cells, where melatonin seems to modulate the glucose-stimulated insulin secretion [93]. Lyssenko *et al* [93] have shown that the genotype of this single nucleotide polymorphism (SNP) predicts future type 2 diabetes in two large prospective studies. Specifically, this genotype was associated with impairment of early insulin response to both oral and intravenous glucose administration and with faster decrement of insulin secretion over time. Non-diabetic individuals carrying the risk allele and individuals with type 2 diabetes mellitus showed increased expression of the receptor in islets (quantitatively). On the other hand, insulin release from beta cells in response to glucose administration was inhibited in the presence of melatonin. These data suggest that the circulating hormone melatonin, which is predominantly released from the pineal gland (with a certain circadian pattern), is involved in the pathogenesis of diabetes. Given the increased expression of *mtnr1b* in individuals at risk of developing diabetes, the pathogenic effects are likely exerted *via* a direct inhibitory effect on beta cells. Consequently, modulating the melatonin/*mtnr1b* biologic pathway may become a future therapeutic avenue in diabetes. Furthermore, melatonin secretion seems to be impaired in diabetics [94], and the melatonin profile relative to the feeding/fasting cycle is reversed when individuals are subjected to forced dys-synchrony [77].

Taken together, these recent papers raise the hypothesis that chronodisruption, either directly at the level of the circadian clock "machinery", or indirectly through effects of melatonin, may contribute to the development of metabolic syndrome and/or cardiovascular complications.

What we don't know:

- We are still in need to differentiate between the metabolic effects of pure chronodisruption, short sleep duration and fragmented sleep

- So far, there has been a number of publications pointing towards particular core clock gene polymorphisms and different metabolic phenotypes; their importance in the general population and their contribution to development of cardiovascular pathology are still to be clarified

- Is is currently unclear to what extent the melatoninergic pathways are involved in physiology and/or pathology, specifically in the generation of IR

B. SLEEP DEPRIVATION

In the western society, sleep deprivation is by far the most common chronic sleep condition [95-98]. At the turn of the 20th century, young adults slept about 9 hours per night [99], while about 50 years later, in the 1960s, sleep duration was curtailed to around 7.7 hours [100]. This may all be the result of the introduction of electricity and the accelerated industrialization, although the exact cause of this major behavioral change is still unclear. More recently, National Sleep Foundation reported that, in 1998 only 35% of American adults were sleeping 8 hours per night during week days and that number had fallen to 26% by 2005 [101]. On the other hand, the percentage of adult Americans sleeping less than 6 hours each night has increased from 12% in 1998, to 16% in 2005 [101]. Interestingly, the decrease in habitual sleep duration in the United States has occurred over the same time period as the increase in the prevalence of metabolic disease [101]. Furthermore, accumulating epidemiological evidence connects chronic sleep loss with obesity and diabetes [102-104].

At least three common causes of short sleep duration exist and the biological effects of chronic sleep restriction may be very different in these situations:

(1) Voluntary curtailment of sleep in order to spend more time in professional and family-related activities, despite perceived adverse neurocognitive effects of the sleep deprivation;

(2) Insomnia, restless legs, etc, characterized by an inability to sleep longer despite a desire to do so; and

(3) Not perceiving the need to sleep longer because of feeling fully rested with less than 7 hours of sleep (adaptation?, preconditioning?).

Sleep Deprivation and Obesity

Besides neurocognitive and behavioral changes, recent research suggests that chronic sleep restriction may have important metabolic effects, including an increased risk of obesity. Over the past decade, a number of cross-sectional and longitudinal epidemiological studies have identified an association between self-reported sleep habits and obesity (or increased body weight) [1,2,105-115]. Unfortunately, it is difficult to establish causality because obesity is a risk factor for diseases such as OSA (not always carefully assessed in these studies), osteoarthritis, asthma and depression, known factors that can adversely impact one's ability to sleep. Furthermore, self-reported sleep duration may also be highly inaccurate [115-117]. Patel *et al*[105] addressed some of these limitations by analyzing cross-sectionally the data from Osteoporotic Fractures in Men Study (MrOS) [118,119] and the Study of Osteoporotic Fractures (SOF) study [105]. In both cohorts, objective assessment of sleep was performed using actigraphy. Sleep duration was inferred from recordings over a mean of 5 nights in MrOS and 4 nights in SOF. Using this methodology for sleep duration assessment, short sleep remained associated with an elevated BMI in both cohorts, even after adjustment for covariates [105]. Besides anthropometric data such as height and weight (with resultant BMI), waist and hip circumferences were also used in both cohorts to provide information about fat distribution patterns. In analyses adjusted for covariates, men sleeping less than 5 hours had 6.7 and 4.7 cm greater waist and hip circumferences, respectively, versus those sleeping 7 to 8 hours. In women, the corresponding differences were 5.4 and 5.0 cm, respectively. In the MrOS study, dual energy X-ray absorptiometry (DEXA) scans were also performed to assess lean/fat body mass composition. The results showed that, overall, shorter sleep durations were associated with an increased amount of fat mass. In addition, the increase in fat was attributed to an increase in abdominal fat, implying a possible increased risk for diabetes and heart disease. Indeed, two separate studies have confirmed that short sleep duration is as a risk factor for both of these complications, at least in women [68,120].

Sleep Deprivation and Diabetes

Numerous cross-sectional and longitudinal clinical studies have demonstrated so far that short duration and poor-quality sleep predict development of T2DM, even after correcting for age, body mass index (BMI) and other potential confounding parameters [1,2,111-113]. The relationship between chronic sleep deprivation, weight gain and diabetes may involve, at least in part, alterations in glucose metabolism, increase in appetite and hunger, and/or decreased energy expenditures.

Sleep Deprivation and Metabolic Syndrome

For example, healthy individuals submitted to partial (4-hour) sleep deprivation for 6 nights exhibited impaired insulin sensitivity (or IR) following a glucose challenge [114,115]. Sleep deprivation-induced sensation of hunger may be, at least in part, related to reduced serum levels of leptin (an adipose tissue–specific hormone or adipokine which promotes satiety) and increased levels of the hormone ghrelin (a peptide released primarily from the stomach). Both hormones may also impact energy expenditures [116,117].

RESEARCH OUTLOOK:

What do we know:

A significant body of literature has shown consistent correlations between sleep onset and a reduced activity of the hypothalamo-pituitary-adrenal (HPA) axis and that sleep loss may increase serum cortisol levels. Both acute total sleep deprivation (forced wakefulness up to 72 hours) and subacute partial sleep deprivation (consistent reduction of the nocturnal total sleep time for a variable number of days) have been employed to test these associations [121].

Acute (Total) Sleep Deprivation

Several studies have reported an elevation of serum cortisol levels during the nights of total sleep deprivation [237,238,122] and during the following afternoons or evenings if wake state was further maintained [240,241]. Hypercortisolemia after acute sleep loss has been postulated to reflect the stress of prolonged wakefulness and has been found to be associated with high frequency EEG activity during wake [241]. Nevertheless, these findings have not been found by all groups which investigated the relationship between several nights of total sleep deprivation and hormonal changes described above [242-247]. These differences may have multiple explanations: (1) inappropriate hormonal level circadian characterization through insufficient sampling; (2) lack of control group; (3) confounders such as physical activity level, light exposure and even dietary factors, such as alcohol intake; (4) inappropriate sleep characterization [total sleep time attained through undetected or undocumented (micro)naps?]; (5) possible biphasic HPA responses to sleep deprivation [241] (with an acute response, followed by an early subacute response from HPA, and possible severe blunting of the HPA axis activity later on).

Several studies have examined serum cortisol profiles during the recovery sleep after a night of total sleep deprivation, with similar discrepancies: in some studies the cortisol profiles were normal during recovery nights after prolonged wakefulness [248-250], while others (*e.g.*, Vgontzas *et al* [251]) found a significant decrease of cortisol levels, which appeared to be negatively correlated with the slow wave sleep (SWS) rebound. Some have hypothesized that the different circadian timing of the recovery sleep may have played a role in these conflicting findings [121].

Subacute (Partial) Sleep Deprivation

Chronic sleep deprivation has become a widespread problem in modern, western society and its hormonal and metabolic consequences have only begun to be appreciated. The first systematic study of HPA axis activity in a state of sleep debt assessed the effect of 6 consecutive nights of 4 hours in bed in eleven young men [48]. The sleep debt condition was compared with controls undergoing testing after 6 nights of 12 hours in bed. Plasma and salivary cortisol were measured under both conditions. The state of sleep deprivation, as compared to controls of fully rested individuals, was associated with elevated cortisol concentrations in the afternoon and in the early evening and with a slower rate of decline of salivary free cortisol concentrations between 4 PM and 9 PM. Nine of the eleven subjects of the previous study participated later on in a separate protocol, with 8-hour time in bed testing conditions; interestingly, evening cortisol levels observed under 8-hour in bed conditions were intermediate between those measured under 4-hour and 12-hour bedtime conditions [123]. Consistent findings indicative of an elevation of evening cortisol levels following partial sleep loss had been previously reported even after one night of sleep restriction to 4 hours in bed [124]. In this study, plasma cortisol levels between 6 PM and 11 PM were 37% higher on the day following the night with restricted sleep than on the day before. Thus, sleep deprivation appears to be associated with an elevation in evening cortisol levels that may reflect decreased efficacy of the negative feedback loop regulation of the HPA axis. Even if modest, this elevation may result, under conditions of chronic sleep loss, in a significant corticosteroid overload and consequently expose the body to the central and peripheral deleterious effects of these stress hormones.

Similar to the situations described in these experiments, it is notable that chronic short sleepers have been found to have higher nocturnal cortisol levels compared with chronic long sleepers [125], suggesting that mechanisms of long-term adaptation and/or down-regulation of the HPA axis do not seem to occur. In a cross-sectional analysis of the Whitehall II study, the relationship between self-reported sleep duration, sleep disturbances, and salivary cortisol levels has been assessed in a cohort of more than 2,700 middle-aged men and women [126]. Short sleep duration was associated with an elevated cortisol level upon awakening (in AM) and both short sleep duration and disturbances were independently associated with a slower rate of decline of cortisol levels throughout the day, with subsequent increased evening levels.

Altered Sleep Architecture

Slow Wave Sleep (SWS) Restriction

The two recent studies that examined the impact of SWS suppression on the cortisol secretion profiles had negative findings:

An earlier study [127], conducted in young individuals, compared the effects of delayed sleep onset and temporary slow wave sleep (SWS) deprivation on nocturnal growth hormone (GH) and cortisol release in humans. Polysomnographic recordings and blood samples were obtained from 10 men, each participating on three experimental nights. On all nights the subjects went to bed at 11 PM and were wakened at 7 AM. On the baseline night, the lights were turned off at 11 PM, enabling the subjects to fall asleep. To delay sleep onset, on the second night, the subjects were kept awake until 2 AM. On the third night, the subjects were deprived of SWS between 11 PM and 2 AM. SWS deprivation was accomplished by sounding a tone as soon as it appeared the subject was going into stage N3 of sleep. The order of experimental conditions was random. During the unrestricted nights, the occurrence of SWS coincided with the surge in GH secretion, and low plasma cortisol levels. Delaying sleep onset after 2 AM lead to a delayed GH secretion, which coincided also with the initial period of SWS. Selective SWS deprivation between 11 PM and 2 AM did not significantly reduce the overall time spent in SWS, because it recovered after unrestricted sleep was restored (SWS rebound). On these nights, the GH secretory peaks were not significantly changed in amplitude, but they were dissociated from SWS, because they occurred mostly subsequent to sleep onset rather than during the main epochs of SWS occurring after 2 AM. Nocturnal cortisol release was distinctly delayed with delayed sleep onset, whereas SWS suppression had no significant effect. Thus, the timing of both nocturnal GH and cortisol secretion seemed more dependent on sleep onset than on SWS [127].

A more recent study [128] investigated 24-hour cortisol profiles in a group of young individuals (men and women) after two nights of normal sleep and after three nights of selective suppression of SWS sustained throughout the night (using the same methodology, which managed to replace SWS with non-N3 sleep, without increase in wake after sleep onset). No significant changes in cortisol profiles were found in this study.

Rapid Eye Movement Sleep (REM, R) Restriction

Decreased cortisol levels have been reported in a study of selective REM suppression [129], but, unfortunately, REM sleep suppression was achieved through brief awakenings, resulting in a significant increase in wake after sleep onset (WASO) time.

Sleep Fragmentation

A recent experiment of sleep fragmentation on 11 healthy volunteers led to interesting findings [130]. Not surprisingly, following two nights of experimental sleep fragmentation across all stages, an increase in morning cortisol levels was observed and a shift in sympathovagal balance toward an increase in sympathetic nervous system activity. Markers of systemic inflammation and serum adipokines were unchanged with sleep fragmentation. More interestingly, insulin sensitivity decreased significantly, as the ability of glucose to mobilize itself independent of an insulin response, also decreased [130].

What we don't know:

- Understanding the molecular pathophysiology of metabolic abnormalities in states of disrupted sleep remains a major challenge.

- There is a mounting body of literature that shows that sleep loss can impair significantly various metabolic pathways [46,48]. For example, several studies [47,48] have shown that normal individuals placed in controlled experimental sleep deprivation develop IR, hypercortisolism or activation of the hypothalamic-pituitary-adrenal axis (HPA), significant sympathetic autonomic activation, as well as increased appetite and hunger, probably associated with decreased leptin and elevated ghrelin levels. A more recent publication has also shown that even selective slow wave sleep restriction can alter glucose sensitivity in normal individuals [128]. Several other studies have confirmed these observations and pointed out that, in the general population, short sleep duration is associated with abnormal leptin and ghrelin levels and higher body mass indices (BMI) [1,49,131]. While this has spurred the speculation that the increase in the prevalence of obesity may be related to a progressive, culturally-driven sleep shortening in the same populations, there are still significant controversies [132-135] and unknowns [136-138] about the possible mechanistic relationships and the exact link between obesity and habitual sleep duration [132-134,139-141]. Furthermore, besides the overall sleep duration, several population cohorts have suggested that difficulty falling asleep and/or staying asleep can be associated with an increase in diabetes, at least in men [50,142]. These mechanistic connections are overall difficult to prove or disprove, especially based on observational studies' data.

- A recent and intriguing theory suggested that a voracious intestinal absorbtion of nutrients may contribute to obesity and, possibly, metabolic syndrome [143]. According to this animal study, mice genetically deficient in Toll-like receptor 5 (TLR5, a component of the innate immune system that is expressed in the gut mucosa and which serves to defend against infections), exhibit hyperphagia and develop hallmark features of metabolic syndrome, including hyperlipidemia, hypertension, insulin resistance (IR), and increased adiposity. These metabolic changes correlated with changes in the composition of the gut microflora, and transfer of the gut microflora from TLR5-deficient mice to wild-type, germ-free mice conferred many features of metabolic syndrome to the recipients. Food restriction prevented obesity, but not IR, in the TLR5-deficient mice. These results support the emerging view that the gut microflora contributes to metabolic disease and suggest that malfunction of the innate immune system may lead, at least in a subgroup of patients, to metabolic syndrome [143].

- Because the prevalence of chronic sleep deprivation is increasing in modern society, with negative health consequences and because the observed association between short sleep and obesity, a clinical study was designed and is under way to assess the feasibility of increasing sleep duration to a "healthy" duration (approximately 7.5 hours) and to determine the effect of sleep extension on body weight (Sleep Extension Group). This proof-of-concept study on a randomized sample will assess 'whether sleep extension is feasible and whether it influences BMI [144]. While many groups are interested in conducting intervention studies in which short sleepers are randomized to either a treatment that prolongs their sleep or a control condition, given the long timeframe needed to observe measurable differences in weight, it may be difficult to conduct such trials among individuals who do not perceive a need to increase their sleep.

C. OBSTRUCTIVE SLEEP APNEA (OSA)

OSA is independently associated with the main components of the MetS, such as insulin resistance (IR) and obesity, augmenting further the morbid risk attributable to MetS on cardiovascular mortality. Generally, it is thought that OSA affects the metabolism indirectly, through IH and sleep fragmentation.

Because of the described definition discrepancies, there are patients who have MetS according to one definition, and not according to other definitions. This affects significantly the reported prevalence of MetS. Using the ATP III definition, the overall prevalence of MetS in the National Health and Nutritional Examination Survey 1999-2002 database was 34.5% [145]. Furthermore, given the obesity epidemic, the prevalence of MetS is, undoubtedly, on the rise.

OSA has very high prevalence among patients with MetS, hinting to a causal relationship [146]. As early as 2004, Coughlin *et al* [147] found that MetS is 9.1 times more common in individuals with OSA versus healthy individuals. Since then, many others confirmed a strong association between these conditions [148-159]; the main references which reported the incidence of MetS in OSA are listed in Table **1**.

Table 1: Main studies reporting the prevalence of MetS in OSA patients [BMI: body mass index; CI: confidence interval; Contr: Controls; Def: definition; HOMA: homeostasis model assessment; IDF: International Diabetes Federation; IGF-1: insulin growth factor-1; IR: insulin resistance; MetS: metabolic syndrome, NCEP-ATP III: National Cholesterol Education Program, Expert Panel on Detection, Evaluation and Treatment of High Blood Cholesterol in Adults (Adult Treatment Panel III); NS: non-significant; OR: odds ratio; OSA: obstructive sleep apnea; Ref: reference; S_pO_2: arterial oxygen saturation; WHO: World Health Organization; Yr: year]

Yr/Ref	Author	Def/Methods	OSA	MetS (%)	Results (OR for MetS)
2004[147]	Coughlin, SR (UK)	NCEP-ATP III HOMA	43 Obese non-OSA (Contr) 61 Obese OSA	35% 87%	OR MetS 9.1 (95%CI: 2.6-31.2)
2006[150]	Gruber, A (UK)	IDF HOMA	38 Non-OSA (Contr) 41 OSA	24% 74%	OR MetS 5.9 (95%CI: 2.0-17.6); IR not assoc with OSA independent of obesity
2006[293]	Lam, JCM (Hong Kong)	NCEP-ATP III, modified	160 Non-OSA (Contr) 95 OSA	21% 58%	OR MetS 5.3 (95%CI: 3.0-9.2)
2006[157]	Sasanabe, R (Japan)	Japanese definition	89 Non-OSA (Contr) 819 OSA	22% 49%	OR MetS: 6.6 (95% CI: 1.5-29.3)
2006[158]	Shiina, K (Japan)	Japanese definition	90 Non-OSA (Contr) 94 OSA	16% 43%	OSA associated with high risk for MetS
2007[151]	Kono, M (Japan)	Japanese definition	52 Non-OSA (Contr) 42 OSA	4% 19%	AHI correlated with # of MetS components, BMI and SpO2 (NS)
2007[153]	McArdle, N (Australia)	WHO HOMA	21 Non-OSA Males (Contr) 21 OSA Males	5% 24% (p=0.19)	Confirmed an independent association between MetS and OSA after controlling for central obesity, age, and alcohol consumption, with a trend for IGF-1
2007[156]	Peled, N (Israel)	NCEP-ATP III HOMA	98 males for PSG: 9 Snorers (Contr)	0% 11%	OSA severity correlates with the MetS AHI correlates with IR better than SpO2

			9 mild OSA	21%	
			27 moderate OSA	30%	
			53 severe OSA		
2007[155]	Parish, JM (USA)	NCEP-ATP III	54 no OSA (Contr)	43%	Prevalence of MetS and hypertension correlated with the severity of OSA
			57 mild OSA	49%	
			57 moderate OSA	49%	
			60 severe OSA	70%	
2008[159]	Tkacova, R (Slovakia)	IDF HOMA	28 no OSA (Contr)	46%	OR for NCEP ATP-III risk>10%:
			38 mild-moderate OSA	51%	1.0
			31 severe OSA	77%	1.4 (95% CI: 0.4-4.8)
					4.0 (95% CI: 1.02-16.2)
2008[149]	Chin, K (Japan)	NCEP-ATP III/ Japanese def.	275 males:	7%/14%	OR adjusted for age and BMI:
			114 no OSA (Contr)	23%/18%	1
			103 mild OSA	33%/31%	1.0 (95% CI: 0.4-2.1)
			42 moderate OSA	69%/62%	0.7 (95% CI: 0.3-1.9)
			16 severe OSA		2.5 (95% CI: 0.6-9.6)
2009[154]	Nieto, FJ (USA)	NCEP-ATP III HOMA	313 no OSA (Contr)	32% overall	OR adjusted for age, sex and BMI:
			150 mild OSA	38% females	2.5 (95% CI: 1.5-4.2)
			103 moderate/severe OSA	27% males	2.2(95%CI: 1.2-3.9)
2010[148]	Angelico, F (USA)	NCEP-ATP III HOMA	48 snorers (Contr)	43%	MetS increased in frequency with severity of SDB; IR was the only independent predictor of oxygen desaturation index (ODI)
			54 mild OSA	44%	
			51 moderate OSA	55%	
			73 severe OSA	60%	

Since OSA patients have MetS even in the absence of diabetes, hypertension or dyslipidemia, the immediate therapeutic implication is that initiating CPAP at lower AHI may prevent cardiovascular disease [160]. OSA patients generally carry long lists of metabolic problems, and OSA is well known to be an independent risk factor for cardiovascular disease [161-163], hence some advocate screening for OSA [164,165]. OSA has been linked to hypertension [28], heart failure [166] and ischemic heart disease [27], arrhythmias, and stroke. CPAP therapy may improve the above conditions and decrease cardiovascular risk [167,168].

The CIRCS study published recently (2010) demonstrated that nocturnal IH (as OSA marker) is associated with metabolic risk factor accumulation, increased CRP, and increased risk of T2DM and MetS overall [169-171]. Also, the presence of MetS is well correlated to AHI as an OSA severity marker, confirming the role of IH and sleep fragmentation in metabolic disturbances caused by OSA.

We will review below briefly the connection (as we know it) between different components of MetS and OSA.

OSA and Abnormal Glucose Metabolism, Insulin Resistance and Diabetes

While hypertension does not seem be the only mechanism by which OSA can lead to cardiovascular and overall morbidity and mortality [24,172-174], it has been proposed that an additional possible pathogenic pathway is *via* abnormal glucose metabolism [128,175,176]. Insulin resistance (IR) is by far the most important component of MetS. Recently, there has been a lot of attention on the relationship between OSA and abnormal glucose metabolism, since sleep apnea can induce IR, a known major cardiovascular risk factor [177,178], even in the absence of obesity [176,179]. This pathogenic connection is perfectly plausible, given that:

(1)   OSA and diabetes are morbid conditions frequently associated [175,176,180,181];

(2)   Up to 23% of patients with T2DM have OSA by overnight oximetry [182];

(3)   Sleep fragmentation secondary to OSA can lead to activation of HPA, autonomic sympathetic system and counter-regulatory hormones [130,183]. Sleep fragmentation is likely a function of arousals and/or hypoxia, but other factors such as painful diabetic peripheral neuropathy can disrupt sleep cycle as well. Previous studies have found that insulin sensitivity decreases after 2 nights of fragmented sleep in healthy volunteers [130]; furthermore, durations of sleep less than 6 hours and more than 9 hours increase the prevalence of diabetes [183].

(4)   Shorter sleep duration induced by OSA may be a risk factor for IR [184,185] and for developing diabetes in select populations [128].

(5)   Multiple studies have shown a role of intermittent hypoxia (IH) in the development of IR [184,186,187], MetS [171,188], and T2DM [170,189]. IH has been shown to even cause the death of beta-cells through oxidative stress [190]. Interestingly, IH affected insulin levels in leptin deficient, obese mice, but not in lean mice [187], suggesting that obesity or obesity related adipokines might have been involved, at least in that particular model.

(6)   Punjabi *et al* [191] have shown in a study on 118 non-diabetic subjects that those with mild, moderate and severe OSA have a reduction in insulin sensitivity of 26.7%, 36.5% and 43.7%, respectively, independent of age, gender, race, and body fat composition. Interestingly, the reduction in insulin sensitivity and the observed reduced disposition index, which is an integrated measurement of pancreatic insulin output, were correlated with the average degree of oxihemoglobin desaturation.

(7)   Australian Busselton Health Study showed that moderate-severe OSA presents both at baseline (prevalence data) and at 4-year follow-up (incident data) increased likelihood to have diabetes as a comorbidity [192]. The longitudinal model remained significant after adjustment for age, gender, BMI, waist circumference and mean arterial pressure [192]. By contrast, the longitudinal analyses of the Wisconsin Sleep Cohort study [181], with similar duration of follow-up (4 years) and similar age at baseline, did not find moderate-severe OSA to be a risk factor for incident diabetes after adjusting for age, gender and waist circumference. On the other hand, in both cohorts, mild OSA had an odds ratio of developing diabetes higher than 1, but did not remain significant after adjustment for age, gender and body habitus. However, the increased risk of incident diabetes in mild OSA compared to no OSA group pointed out that the risk of diabetes increases with OSA severity and that the exact risk assessment may need larger studies, with greater statistical power.

(8)   So far, very few studies were able to show or to support the hypothesis of reverse causation (*i.e.*, that diabetes leads to OSA).

For a comprehensive review of the complex relationships between OSA, IR and MetS, we recommend consulting the review written by N. Punjabi and published in 2009 [193].

OSA as a part of Metabolic Syndrome

OSA and MetS have such a high prevalence and strong correlation to IR, that some experts propose that sleep apnea is included in the MetS (or syndrome Z) [154,194,195]. While OSA is a systemic, rather than a local disease, it is heralded by a number of inflammatory markers that are elevated independent from obesity. It is the visceral fat amount and metrics of IR that have the strongest correlation with OSA severity markers such as AHI and EDS [196-198]. To date, evidence exists for all three scenarios: OSA being a manifestation of MetS, OSA and MetS related to IH as a common denominator [199] or MetS as a risk factor for OSA development [200,201].

Dyslipidemia as a part of MetS and OSA

Evidence shows that IH can cause dyslipidemia in lean mice. Several cross-sectional studies suggest that OSA is independently associated with increased levels of total cholesterol, low-density lipoprotein and triglycerides, whereas others report no such relationship. Some nonrandomized and randomized studies show that OSA treatment with continuous positive airway pressure (CPAP) may have a beneficial effect on lipid profile [202,203], while others do not [204]. In summary, there is increasing evidence that IH is independently associated with dyslipidemia. However, the role of OSA in causality of dyslipidemia remains to be established. More research is needed in this field to provide better evidence of the role of OSA in dyslipidemia [203].

OSA and Hypertension

Another important component of MetS is hypertension. While OSA is known to be strongly associated with increased cardiovascular risk and morbidity [21-23], OSA is known to cause hypertension independent of obesity [170] and up to 30% of hypertensive patients have OSA. Potential mechanism may be the carotid body response to hypoxia and subsequent sympathetic activation [205,206]. The severity of hypertension also seems to correlate with the OSA severity [207].

A recent study from Brazil found that MetS posed an odds ratio for developing OSA of 19.04 (95% confidence interval 5.25 to 69.03) in OSA patients with hypertension, much higher than the ones conferred by the typical clinical features that characterize OSA, including snoring and excessive daytime sleepiness [203]. OSA may also cause concentric LV geometry without hypertension, thus increasing cardiovascular risk [208,209].

Short sleep duration itself can be a factor for developing hypertension. Sleep duration of 5 hours or less has been associated with hypertension in otherwise healthy subjects, even after controlling for obesity and diabetes [67]. Interestingly, prolonged sleep can also cause hypertension, and it is important to keep in mind that if sleep can affect through different metabolic pathways the weight gains, IR and blood pressure, then improving sleep quality should translate into improved cardiovascular mortality.

The pathogenic connection between OSA and hypertension is also supported by the fact that effective CPAP therapy leads to improved systemic arterial pressures [208,210,211]. Nevertheless, this effect is not always clinically relevant, has not been reproduced consistently and depends on baseline blood pressure and patient compliance with treatment.

OSA and Atherosclerosis

Atherosclerosis is another part of MetS that is closely linked to OSA. Recent studies have shown evidence of endothelial dysfunction and apoptosis in patients with OSA [212,213], resulting in vasoconstriction and acceleration of atherosclerosis. The overall effect of OSA on vascular function may be as deleterious as diabetes; vascular function seems to be improved when assessed by flow mediated dilatation [214,215] after CPAP therapy [214]. Treatment of OSA with CPAP may improve early atherosclerosis, as there have been improvements in carotid medial thickness, pulse wave velocity, CRP, and catecholamines levels [216].

One of the deadliest events related to atherosclerosis is myocardial infarction (MI). In a recent study, OSA was suggested to be a trigger for MI because of the very high likelihood of nocturnal and early morning MIs in OSA patients, a result of shifted sympthathetic activity and circadian rhythms in these patients. Several authors have suggested more targeted assessments of the nocturnal MI patients for OSA [217].

OSA and Obesity

Obesity is a worldwide growing epidemic that has increased rapidly in the last 20 years. According to estimates, by 2030 86.3% of US adult population will be overweight or obese [218]. OSA and sleep duration have a profound effect on body weight [2]. As the obesity epidemic grows new data is becoming available. Obesity is considered one of the main risk factors for OSA. According to one study, more than 50-55% of obese patients (BMI >40) had OSA – an enormous number of patients [9,10]. Obesity can cause OSA by fat deposition in the upper airway region; and as a result predispose individuals to upper airway collapse while sleeping. However, not all adipose tissue is equal and obese people differ in their fat distribution and their metabolic risks. Subcutaneous fat is most abundant adipose tissue. Most important, however, is the distribution. Prospective studies have shown that visceral intraabdominal fat rather than neck or parapharyngeal fat correlated positively with OSA severity markers like AHI [219] and metabolic parameters [220]. Even in people without diabetes the amount of visceral fat is considered the most important predictor of insulin resistance [57]. Visceral fat surround the inner organs, mainly the omentum and mesentery. It is more cellular and more metabolically active than subcutaneous fat as it secretes different proinflammatory cytokines. It also carries with it a greater mortality rate than subcutaneous fat [221].

Sleep duration affects appetite through the complex interaction of leptin and sleep cycle [102]. In a Wisconsin sleep cohort study, the subgroup (n=1,024) showed that sleeping less than 8 hours increases BMI proportionally to the decrease in sleep. Also, leptin and ghrelin levels were low (the main appetite regulating hormones with opposite action) resulting in increased appetite and increased BMI [131]. In a recent pilot study the severity of OSA was positively correlated with visceral fat (r=0.73, p<0.001) [222] and OSA markers such as AHI correlated with visceral fat. Another study provided evidence that sleep duration ≤5 hours and ≥8 hours are associated with increased amounts (CT defined) of visceral fat [223]. Supporting evidence is also the fact that CPAP therapy has been shown to reduce the amount of visceral adipose tissue [224,225]. In short, individuals overall decreasing sleep duration can contribute to the increasing obesity prevalence, and weight loss (medical intervention like diet and exercise or bariatric surgery) remains a very effective treatment of OSA [226,227] in obese OSA patients.

Adversely, there are number of studies that do not support the link between obesity and sleep duration [228,229]. Larger studies are needed to either confirm or disprove the relationship between obesity and sleep duration.

Even a correlation between OSA and obesity (especially morbid obesity) should make health care providers vigilant to screen and diagnose OSA. Inexpensive screening tools (like clinical symptoms and physical signs) are readily available to identify patients at risk [10].

RESEARCH OUTLOOK

What do we know:

The question is how exactly IH and sleep fragmentation affect metabolism and cause IR? The most studied pathogenic theories are represented by: sympathetic activity [230], neuroendocrine dysfunction [121,231], systemic inflammation [194,232], oxidative stress [233], endothelial dysfunction [212,213] and adipokine dysregulation [175].

- Increased sympathetic activity in patients with OSA [234-239] has insulin antagonizing effect [240-243], resulting in hyperglycemia from decreased muscle uptake and increased glycogenolysis. It also antagonizes the antilipolytic action of insulin [243], resulting in increased lipolysis and non-esterified fatty acid production, which alone can cause IR [244]. Furthermore, sympathetic overactivity exerts direct effect on blood vessels, causing vasoconstriction, and thus further worsening glucose metabolism.

- It is well known that hypothalamic-pituitary-adrenal axis (HPA) can affect human metabolism, and cortisol is well known for its hyperglycemic effects. There is sufficient evidence that OSA can influence HPA axis, which in turn influences glucose metabolism. A study by D. Henley demonstrated improvement of ACTH and cortisol levels after 3 months of CPAP therapy, suggesting that untreated OSA is associated with elevated ACTH and cortisol [245]. Beneficial effects of CPAP were also confirmed in other studies [246-248].

- Oxidative stress has been suggested as one of the pathogenic pathways by which OSA can lead to glucose abnormalities and IR [249,250]. Oxidative stress (or redox stress) is thought to be caused by an imbalance between the production of reactive oxygen species (ROS) and other free radicals and antioxidant defenses. Constant exposure to hypoxemia-reoxygenation cycles generates plenty of ROS. Moreover, CPAP can work as an antioxidant therapy in OSA patients, reducing lipid peroxidation and restoring reduced glutathione levels, which are the main measures of oxidative stress [251]. This study also provided evidence that there was improvement in daytime symptoms, as assessed by Epworth Sleepiness Scale (ESS) after oral intake of antioxidants vitamin C and E. Multiple other studies confirmed this hypothesis as well [252-255].

- There is sufficient evidence to support the hypothesis that sleep disturbances cause pro-inflammatory state. Systemic inflammation has been linked to cardiovascular and thrombophilic disorders, as well as diabetes. Inflammatory markers like CRP are currently being used to assess cardiovascular risk. Systemic inflammation plays an important role in OSA pathogenesis, as evident by increased in inflammatory markers in OSA patients and their response to CPAP therapy [74,256,257]. Underlying systemic inflammation also explains greater atherosclerosis progression in OSA patients. Markers of systemic inflammation in OSA patients include interleukin-6 (IL-6), tumor necrosis factor- alpha (TNF-α), CRP, and different adhesion molecules. Again, the main underlying causes are IH and sleep fragmentation, but obesity and especially visceral obesity, which is very prevalent among OSA patients, can also contribute to systemic inflammation [258]. A special study, however, showed that CRP, independent of obesity, is associated with nocturnal hypoxia [143]. All three mechanisms (IH, sleep fragmentation and obesity) seem to contribute to systemic inflammation.

- The view of adipose tissue as a "fat depot" has changed over the last decade, especially after the discovery of leptin in 1994. Adipose tissue, especially visceral fat, is a metabolically active and secretes different metabolic and proinflammatory cytokines (adipokines). In obesity, adipose tissue becomes dysfunctional [259] and adipose tissue hypoxia and hypoperfusion occur [260]. Increased production of inflammatory markers by adipose tissue may be the result of slow angiogenesis, compared with the growth of adipose tissue itself [261]. Also, adipose tissue, in individuals who are obese, show higher infiltration of macrophages, which often are the main sources of inflammatory molecules. This is important because it opens a window for specifically targeting macrophages with PPAR (peroxisome proliferator-activated receptor) agonists [262].

- The most important adipokines are leptin, adiponectin, and resistin. Leptin regulates body weight, energy expenditure, and sympathetic activity and is associated with insulin resistance [202]. Leptin is elevated in OSA patients, and CPAP therapy has been found decrease leptin levels [202,263-265]. In the study of IH in OSA patients (obese controls), higher levels of leptin made endothelial inflammation more severe, meaning that obesity and intermittent hypoxia may act synergistically by leptin being a synergistic factor [266]. Adiponectin, however, appears to have anti-inflammatory and insulin-sensitizing actions and is decreased in OSA [267-269] due to IH. It improves with CPAP therapy [255,267] likely due to hypoxia reduction. Other adipokines of recent interest are chemerin and resistin, which appear to correlate with insulin resistance; however, their role in OSA is not clear [270], and studies have shown an association of insulin resistance and diabetes between OSA independently of obesity [186,203,222,271,272].

- Snoring is another common symptom of OSA; in the general population, approximately 9% of men snore occasionally [273]. Still, there are very few studies relating snoring with metabolic abnormalities. One study, however, demonstrated that habitual snoring was associated with impaired glucose tolerance (IGT) even in non-obese, normoglycemic men with elevated HbA1c levels [274]. Snoring has also been independently associated with hypertension, even in non-obese adults [275,276], and it seems to increase the risk of vascular disease [277]. Overall, snoring is not a benign symptom, and it may be associated with CVD and metabolic risk. Further research is needed in this area in order to establish a direct relationship between snoring in OSA pathophysiology.

- The main therapy of OSA is CPAP, which improves daytime sleepiness, the quality of life of patients with OSA [278] and their bed partners [279], cardiovascular mortality [280] and ejection fraction [281], hypertension [204,282], driving performance [283,284], and mental function [285]. It also reduces oxidative stress [253] and enhances sexual performance [286,287]. There is sufficient evidence demonstrating that CPAP therapy improves insulin sensitivity and other metabolic parameters [288-293]. In patients with moderate to severe OSA consistent use of CPAP improves insulin secretion, reduces leptin and cholesterol levels. The effect remains after 8 weeks of therapy [202]. However, some smaller studies that have tried to show that CPAP does not affect significantly IR and glucose control [204,294] and there is no improvement in systemic inflammatory markers with CPAP therapy [295].

- Given the global expansion of epidemic of diabetes and the undeniably strong correlation between diabetes and OSA, the International Diabetes Federation (IDF) Task Force on Epidemiology and Prevention recommended assessing patients with diabetes for clinical signs and symptoms of OSA (like snoring and witnessed apneas) and vice versa [296]. Therefore, OSA patients should be screened for diabetes, hypertension, dyslipidemia, and MetS, and even asymptomatic patients with diabetes should be screened for OSA (Berlin and/or ESS questionnaires) [297].

What we don't know:

- There is overwhelming evidence that OSA may cause IR and diabetes. Interestingly, the opposite relationship, *i.e.*, diabetes or IR causing sleep disturbances—may be true as well, as painful diabetic peripheral neuropathy may cause sleep impairment [13]. In one case-control study, diabetes was an independent risk factor for severe nocturnal hypoxemia in obese patients [14]. Another small study suggested that diabetic neuropathy may affect respiration during sleep [298].

- An interesting suggestion was raised by A. Vgontzas *et al*, who questioned that excessive daytime sleepiness (EDS) and fatigue are the result of sleep apnea and sleep disruption *per se* [199]. The alternative explanation posits that obesity alone can cause EDS and fatigue [9], even in the absence of sleep apnea. In the general population, the average prevalence of EDS is between 5 and 20%. A study in 1998 revealed that obese patients who do not suffer from sleep apnea are sleepier than non-obese controls, despite the fact that the percentage of total sleep time was higher among the obese patients [299]. Another recent study found that sleepy OSA patients tend to be more obese than non-sleepy patients, and to have higher AHIs [198]. Even snoring can contribute to EDS independent of AHI and BMI [300]. The importance of EDS against other OSA symptoms was demonstrated in a study which showed EDS as the only sleep symptom associated with increased cardiovascular morbidity and mortality [301]. EDS can be a marker of IR independent of obesity and can help identify OSA patients who are at risk for MetS [197]. Furthermore, compliance with CPAP therapy is better in OSA patients with EDS, as these patients are likely to benefit more from therapy. Further research is needed in this area, but current data suggests that factors other than number of apneas may play a role in EDS pathogenesis [302].

- Another interesting theory states that hyperinsulinemia and IR may precede the development of apnea in obesity [200,303]. An illustrative example is that of the women suffering from polycystic ovarian syndrome (PCOS), who seem to have a 30-fold increased risk of developing sleep disordered breathing [223], have higher rates of EDS [196] and in whom IR seem to be the main initial metabolic abnormality. One possible mechanism of this pathogenic connection may be related to the observation that the pharyngeal dilator muscle activity may be diminished in the presence of hyperinsulinemia or IR, as is the case with the vascular muscle tone in obesity [201].

REFERENCES

[1] Hasler G, Buysse DJ, Klaghofer R, *et al.* The association between short sleep duration and obesity in young adults: a 13-year prospective study. Sleep 2004; 27(4): 661-6.

[2] Gangwisch JE, Malaspina D, Boden-Albala B, Heymsfield SB. Inadequate sleep as a risk factor for obesity: analyses of the NHANES I. Sleep 2005; 28(10): 1289-96.

[3] Ginter E, Simko V. Adult obesity at the beginning of the 21st century: epidemiology, pathophysiology and health risk. Bratisl Lek Listy 2008; 109(5): 224-30.

[4] Ginter E, Simko V. Diabetes type 2 pandemic in 21st century. Bratisl Lek Listy 2010; 111(3): 134-7.

[5] Epstein LJ, Kristo D, Strollo PJ Jr., *et al.* Clinical guideline for the evaluation, management and long-term care of obstructive sleep apnea in adults. J Clin Sleep Med 2009; 5(3): 263-76.

[6] Shamsuzzaman AS, Gersh BJ, Somers VK. Obstructive sleep apnea: implications for cardiac and vascular disease. JAMA 2003; 290(14): 1906-14.

[7] Young T, Palta M, Dempsey J, Skatrud J, Weber S, Badr S. The occurrence of sleep-disordered breathing among middle-aged adults. N Engl J Med 1993; 328(17): 1230-5.

[8] Jennum P, Riha RL. Epidemiology of sleep apnoea/hypopnoea syndrome and sleep-disordered breathing. Eur Respir J 2009; 33(4): 907-14.

[9] Resta O, Foschino-Barbaro MP, Legari G, *et al.* Sleep-related breathing disorders, loud snoring and excessive daytime sleepiness in obese subjects. Int J Obes Relat Metab Disord 2001; 25(5): 669-75.

[10] Sergi M, Rizzi M, Comi AL, *et al.* Sleep Apnea in Moderate-Severe Obese Patients. Sleep Breath 1999; 3(2): 47-52.

[11] Plywaczewski R, Bielen P, Bednarek M, Jonczak L, Gorecka D, Sliwinski P. [Influence of neck circumference and body mass index on obstructive sleep apnoea severity in males]. Pneumonol Alergol Pol 2008; 76(5): 313-20.

[12] Mezick EJ, Matthews KA, Hall M, *et al.* Influence of race and socioeconomic status on sleep: Pittsburgh SleepSCORE project. Psychosom Med 2008; 70(4): 410-6.

[13] Zelman DC, Brandenburg NA, Gore M. Sleep impairment in patients with painful diabetic peripheral neuropathy. Clin J Pain 2006; 22(8): 681-5.

[14] Lecube A, Sampol G, Lloberes P, *et al.* Diabetes is an independent risk factor for severe nocturnal hypoxemia in obese patients. A case-control study. PLoS One 2009; 4(3): e4692.

[15] Enciso R, Nguyen M, Shigeta Y, Ogawa T, Clark GT. Comparison of cone-beam CT parameters and sleep questionnaires in sleep apnea patients and control subjects. Oral Surg Oral Med Oral Pathol Oral Radiol Endod 2010; 109(2): 285-93.

[16] Abramson Z, Susarla S, Troulis M, Kaban L. Age-related changes of the upper airway assessed by 3-dimensional computed tomography. J Craniofac Surg 2009; 20 Suppl 1: 657-63.

[17] Abramson Z, Susarla S, August M, Troulis M, Kaban L. Three-dimensional computed tomographic analysis of airway anatomy in patients with obstructive sleep apnea. J Oral Maxillofac Surg 2010; 68(2): 354-62.

[18] Campana L, Eckert DJ, Patel SR, Malhotra A. Pathophysiology & genetics of obstructive sleep apnoea. Indian J Med Res 2010; 131: 176-87.

[19]   Iber C, Ancoli-Israel S, Chesson A, Quan SF. The AASM Manual for the Scoring of Sleep and Associated Events (Rules, Terminology and Technical Specifications). 1. 2007. Westchester, IL, American Academy of Sleep Medicine.

[20]   Meoli AL, Casey KR, Clark RW, *et al.* Hypopnea in sleep-disordered breathing in adults. Sleep 2001; 24(4): 469-70.

[21]   Somers VK, White DP, Amin R, *et al.* Sleep apnea and cardiovascular disease: an American Heart Association/american College Of Cardiology Foundation Scientific Statement from the American Heart Association Council for High Blood Pressure Research Professional Education Committee, Council on Clinical Cardiology, Stroke Council, and Council On Cardiovascular Nursing. In collaboration with the National Heart, Lung, and Blood Institute National Center on Sleep Disorders Research (National Institutes of Health). Circulation 2008; 118(10): 1080-111.

[22]   Newman AB, Nieto FJ, Guidry U, *et al.* Relation of sleep-disordered breathing to cardiovascular disease risk factors: the Sleep Heart Health Study. Am J Epidemiol 2001; 154(1): 50-9.

[23]   Marin JM, Carrizo SJ, Vicente E, Agusti AG. Long-term cardiovascular outcomes in men with obstructive sleep apnoea-hypopnoea with or without treatment with continuous positive airway pressure: an observational study. Lancet 2005; 365(9464): 1046-53.

[24]   Young T, Finn L, Peppard PE, *et al.* Sleep disordered breathing and mortality: eighteen-year follow-up of the Wisconsin sleep cohort. Sleep 2008; 31(8): 1071-8.

[25]   Knutson KL, Ryden AM, Mander BA, Van CE. Role of sleep duration and quality in the risk and severity of type 2 diabetes mellitus. Arch Intern Med 2006; 166(16): 1768-74.

[26]   Kasasbeh E, Chi DS, Krishnaswamy G. Inflammatory aspects of sleep apnea and their cardiovascular consequences. South Med J 2006; 99(1): 58-67.

[27]   King CR, Knutson KL, Rathouz PJ, Sidney S, Liu K, Lauderdale DS. Short sleep duration and incident coronary artery calcification. JAMA 2008; 300(24): 2859-66.

[28]   Peppard PE, Young T, Palta M, Skatrud J. Prospective study of the association between sleep-disordered breathing and hypertension. N Engl J Med 2000; 342(19): 1378-84.

[29]   Knutson KL, Van CE. Associations between sleep loss and increased risk of obesity and diabetes. Ann N Y Acad Sci 2008; 1129: 287-304.

[30]   Van CE, Knutson KL. Sleep and the epidemic of obesity in children and adults. Eur J Endocrinol 2008; 159 Suppl 1: S59-S66.

[31]   Schwartz DJ, Kohler WC, Karatinos G. Symptoms of depression in individuals with obstructive sleep apnea may be amenable to treatment with continuous positive airway pressure. Chest 2005; 128(3): 1304-9.

[32]   World Health Organization. Obesity and overweight. 2006. Available at: www.who.int/mediacentre/factsheets/fs311/en/index.html

[33]   Finkelstein EA, Trogdon JG, Cohen JW, Dietz W. Annual medical spending attributable to obesity: payer-and service-specific estimates. Health Aff (Millwood) 2009; 28(5): w822-w831.

[34]   Trogdon JG, Finkelstein EA, Hylands T, Dellea PS, Kamal-Bahl SJ. Indirect costs of obesity: a review of the current literature. Obes Rev 2008; 9(5): 489-500.

[35]   Tjepkema M. Adult obesity. Health Rep 2006; 17(3): 9-25.

[36]   Flegal KM, Carroll MD, Ogden CL, Curtin LR. Prevalence and trends in obesity among US adults, 1999-2008. JAMA 2010; 303(3): 235-41.

[37]   Berghofer A, Pischon T, Reinhold T, Apovian CM, Sharma AM, Willich SN. Obesity prevalence from a European perspective: a systematic review. BMC Public Health 2008; 8: 200.

[38]   American Obesity Association. Obesity in US Adults: 2007. Available at: http://www.obesity.org/statistics/.

[39]   Ogden CL, Carroll MD, McDowell MA, Flegal KM. Obesity among adults in the United States- no change since 2003-2004. NCHS data brief no 1. http://www.cdc.gov/obesity/data/index.html. 2007. Hyattsville, MD, National Center for Health Statistics.

[40]   American Diabetes Association National Diabetes Fact Sheet. American Diabetes Association, 1-14. 2007. Available at: www.who.int/mediacentre/factsheets/fs311/en/index.html

[41]   Alberti KG, Zimmet P, Shaw J. The metabolic syndrome--a new worldwide definition. Lancet 2005; 366(9491): 1059-62.

[42]   Zimmet P, Magliano D, Matsuzawa Y, Alberti G, Shaw J. The metabolic syndrome: a global public health problem and a new definition. J Atheroscler Thromb 2005; 12(6): 295-300.

[43]   Lorenzo C, Williams K, Hunt KJ, Haffner SM. The National Cholesterol Education Program - Adult Treatment Panel III, International Diabetes Federation, and World Health Organization definitions of the metabolic syndrome as predictors of incident cardiovascular disease and diabetes. Diabetes Care 2007; 30(1): 8-13.

[44]   Klein S, Allison DB, Heymsfield SB, *et al.* Waist circumference and cardiometabolic risk: a consensus statement from shaping America's health: Association for Weight Management and Obesity Prevention; NAASO, the Obesity Society; the American Society for Nutrition; and the American Diabetes Association. Diabetes Care 2007; 30(6): 1647-52.

[45]   Buijs RM, Kreier F. The metabolic syndrome: a brain disease? J Neuroendocrinol 2006; 18(9): 715-6.

[46]   Knutson KL, Spiegel K, Penev P, Van Cauter E. The metabolic consequences of sleep deprivation. Sleep Med Rev 2007; 11(3): 163-78.

[47]   Spiegel K, Tasali E, Penev P, Van Cauter E. Brief communication: Sleep curtailment in healthy young men is associated with decreased leptin levels, elevated ghrelin levels, and increased hunger and appetite. Ann Intern Med 2004; 141(11): 846-50.

[48]   Spiegel K, Leproult R, Van Cauter E. Impact of sleep debt on metabolic and endocrine function. Lancet 1999; 354(9188): 1435-9.

[49]   Chaput JP, Despres JP, Bouchard C, Tremblay A. Short sleep duration is associated with reduced leptin levels and increased adiposity: Results from the Quebec family study. Obesity (Silver Spring) 2007; 15(1): 253-61.

[50]   Nilsson PM, Roost M, Engstrom G, Hedblad B, Berglund G. Incidence of diabetes in middle-aged men is related to sleep disturbances. Diabetes Care 2004; 27(10): 2464-9.

[51]   Kohsaka A, Laposky AD, Ramsey KM, *et al.* High-fat diet disrupts behavioral and molecular circadian rhythms in mice. Cell Metab 2007; 6(5): 414-21.

[52]   Diagnosis and classification of diabetes mellitus. Diabetes Care 2008; 31 Suppl 1: S55-S60.

[53]   World Health Organization. Definition, diagnosis and classification of diabetes mellitus and its complications: report of a WHO Consultation. 1999. Available at: http://whqlibdoc.who.int/hq/1999/WHO_NCD_NCS_99.2.pdf

[54]   Third Report of the National Cholesterol Education Program (NCEP) Expert Panel on Detection, Evaluation, and Treatment of High Blood Cholesterol in Adults (Adult Treatment Panel III) final report.http://circ.ahajournals.org/cgi/reprint/106/25/3143. Circulation 2002; 3188.

[55]   Despres JP. Abdominal obesity as important component of insulin-resistance syndrome. Nutrition 1993; 9(5): 452-9.

[56]   Hayashi T, Boyko EJ, McNeely MJ, Leonetti DL, Kahn SE, Fujimoto WY. Visceral adiposity, not abdominal subcutaneous fat area, is associated with an increase in future insulin resistance in Japanese Americans. Diabetes 2008; 1269-75.

[57]   Usui C, Asaka M, Kawano H, Aoyama T, Ishijima T, Sakamoto S, Higuchi M. Visceral fat is a strong predictor of insulin resistance regardless of cardiorespiratory fitness in non-diabetic people. J Nutr Sci Vitaminol (Tokyo) 2010; 56(2): 109-16.

[58]   DeFronzo RA, Tobin JD, Andres R. Glucose clamp technique: a method for quantifying insulin secretion and resistance. Am J Physiol 1979; 237(3): E214-E223.

[59]   Laakso M. How good a marker is insulin level for insulin resistance? Am J Epidemiol 1993; 137(9): 959-65.

[60]   Matthews DR, Hosker JP, Rudenski AS, Naylor BA, Treacher DF, Turner RC. Homeostasis model assessment: insulin resistance and beta-cell function from fasting plasma glucose and insulin concentrations in man. Diabetologia 1985; 28(7): 412-9.

[61]   Legro RS, Finegood D, Dunaif A. A fasting glucose to insulin ratio is a useful measure of insulin sensitivity in women with polycystic ovary syndrome. J Clin Endocrinol Metab 1998; 83(8): 2694-8.

[62]   Katz A, Nambi SS, Mather K, Baron AD, Follmann DA, Sullivan G, Quon MJ. Quantitative insulin sensitivity check index: a simple, accurate method for assessing insulin sensitivity in humans. J Clin Endocrinol Metab 2000; 85(7): 2402-10.

[63]   Mather KJ, Hunt AE, Steinberg HO, Paradisi G, Hook G, Katz A *et al.* Repeatability characteristics of simple indices of insulin resistance: implications for research applications. J Clin Endocrinol Metab 2001; 86(11): 5457-64.

[64]   Hastings M, O'Neill JS, Maywood ES. Circadian clocks: regulators of endocrine and metabolic rhythms. J Endocrinol 2007; 195(2): 187-98.

[65]   Oishi K. Plasminogen activator inhibitor-1 and the circadian clock in metabolic disorders. Clin Exp Hypertens 2009; 31(3): 208-19.

[66]   Knutsson A. Health disorders of shift workers. Occup Med (Lond) 2003; 53(2): 103-8.

[67]   Gangwisch JE, Heymsfield SB, Boden-Albala B, Buijs RM, Kreier F, Pickering TG *et al.* Short sleep duration as a risk factor for hypertension: analyses of the first National Health and Nutrition Examination Survey. Hypertension 2006; 47(5): 833-9.

[68]   Ayas NT, White DP, Manson JE, Stampfer MJ, Speizer FE, Malhotra A, Hu FB. A prospective study of sleep duration and coronary heart disease in women. Arch Intern Med 2003; 163(2): 205-9.

[69]   Janszky I, Ljung R. Shifts to and from daylight saving time and incidence of myocardial infarction. N Engl J Med 2008; 359(18): 1966-8.

[70]   Imeri L, Opp MR. How (and why) the immune system makes us sleep. Nat Rev Neurosci 2009; 10(3): 199-210.

[71]   Vgontzas AN, Papanicolaou DA, Bixler EO, *et al.* Circadian interleukin-6 secretion and quantity and depth of sleep. J Clin Endocrinol Metab 1999; 84(8): 2603-7.

[72]   Vgontzas AN, Zoumakis M, Papanicolaou DA, *et al.* Chronic insomnia is associated with a shift of interleukin-6 and tumor necrosis factor secretion from nighttime to daytime. Metabolism 2002; 51(7): 887-92.

[73]   Krueger JM. The role of cytokines in sleep regulation. Curr Pharm Des 2008; 14(32): 3408-16.

[74]   Ryan S, Taylor CT, McNicholas WT. Systemic inflammation: a key factor in the pathogenesis of cardiovascular complications in obstructive sleep apnoea syndrome? Thorax 2009; 64(7): 631-6.

[75]   Hotamisligil GS, Erbay E. Nutrient sensing and inflammation in metabolic diseases. Nat Rev Immunol 2008; 8(12): 923-34.

[76]   Ribeiro DC, Hampton SM, Morgan L, Deacon S, Arendt J. Altered postprandial hormone and metabolic responses in a simulated shift work environment. J Endocrinol 1998; 158(3): 305-10.

[77]   Scheer FA, Hilton MF, Mantzoros CS, Shea SA. Adverse metabolic and cardiovascular consequences of circadian misalignment. Proc Natl Acad Sci U S A 2009; 106(11): 4453-8.

[78]   Ramsey KM, Bass J. Obeying the clock yields benefits for metabolism. Proc Natl Acad Sci U S A 2009; 106(11): 4069-70.

[79]   de Sousa AG, Cercato C, Mancini MC, Halpern A. Obesity and obstructive sleep apnea-hypopnea syndrome. Obes Rev 2008; 9(4): 340-54.

[80]   Burioka N, Koyanagi S, Endo M, *et al.* Clock gene dysfunction in patients with obstructive sleep apnoea syndrome. Eur Respir J 2008; 32(1): 105-12.

[81]   Kawakami N, Takatsuka N, Shimizu H. Sleep disturbance and onset of type 2 diabetes. Diabetes Care 2004; 27(1): 282-3.

[82]   Ptacek LJ, Jones CR, Fu YH. Novel insights from genetic and molecular characterization of the human clock. Cold Spring Harb Symp Quant Biol 2007; 72: 273-7.

[83]   Cuninkova L, Brown SA. Peripheral circadian oscillators: interesting mechanisms and powerful tools. Ann N Y Acad Sci 2008; 1129: 358-70.

[84]   Scott EM, Carter AM, Grant PJ. Association between polymorphisms in the Clock gene, obesity and the metabolic syndrome in man. Int J Obes (Lond) 2008; 32(4): 658-62.

[85]   Sookoian S, Gemma C, Gianotti TF, Burgueno A, Castano G, Pirola CJ. Genetic variants of Clock transcription factor are associated with individual susceptibility to obesity. Am J Clin Nutr 2008; 87(6): 1606-15.

[86]   Woon PY, Kaisaki PJ, Braganca J, *et al.* Aryl hydrocarbon receptor nuclear translocator-like (BMAL1) is associated with susceptibility to hypertension and type 2 diabetes. Proc Natl Acad Sci U S A 2007; 104(36): 14412-7.

[87]   Englund A, Kovanen L, Saarikoski ST, *et al.* NPAS2 and PER2 are linked to risk factors of the metabolic syndrome. J Circadian Rhythms 2009; 7: 5.

[88]   Ramsey KM, Yoshino J, Brace CS, *et al.* Circadian clock feedback cycle through NAMPT-mediated NAD+ biosynthesis. Science 2009; 324(5927): 651-4.

[89]   Nakahata Y, Sahar S, Astarita G, Kaluzova M, Sassone-Corsi P. Circadian control of the NAD+ salvage pathway by CLOCK-SIRT1. Science 2009; 324(5927): 654-7.

[90]   Blakemore AI, Meyre D, Delplanque J, *et al.* A rare variant in the visfatin gene (NAMPT/PBEF1) is associated with protection from obesity. Obesity (Silver Spring) 2009; 17(8): 1549-53.

[91]   Bouatia-Naji N, Bonnefond A, Cavalcanti-Proenca C, *et al.* A variant near MTNR1B is associated with increased fasting plasma glucose levels and type 2 diabetes risk. Nat Genet 2009; 41(1): 89-94.

[92]   Prokopenko I, Langenberg C, Florez JC, *et al.* Variants in MTNR1B influence fasting glucose levels. Nat Genet 2009; 41(1): 77-81.

[93]   Lyssenko V, Nagorny CL, Erdos MR, *et al.* Common variant in MTNR1B associated with increased risk of type 2 diabetes and impaired early insulin secretion. Nat Genet 2009; 41(1): 82-8.

[94]   Radziuk J, Pye S. Diurnal rhythm in endogenous glucose production is a major contributor to fasting hyperglycaemia in type 2 diabetes. Suprachiasmatic deficit or limit cycle behaviour? Diabetologia 2006; 49(7): 1619-28.

[95]   Bonnet MH, Arand DL. We are chronically sleep deprived. Sleep 1995; 18(10): 908-11.

[96]   Quick-stats: percentage of adults who reported an average of < 6 hours of sleep per 24-hour period, by sex and age group - United States 1985-2004. Morbidity and Mortality Weekly Report 54[Article 533]. 2005.

[97]   Mindell JA, Meltzer LJ, Carskadon MA, Chervin RD. Developmental aspects of sleep hygiene: findings from the 2004 National Sleep Foundation Sleep in America Poll. Sleep Med 2009; 10(7): 771-9.

[98]   Foley D, Ancoli-Israel S, Britz P, Walsh J. Sleep disturbances and chronic disease in older adults: results of the 2003 National Sleep Foundation Sleep in America Survey. J Psychosom Res 2004; 56(5): 497-502.

[99]   Terman L, Hocking A. The sleep of school children, its distribution according to age, and its relationship to physical and mental efficiency. J Educ Psychol 4, 269-282. 1913.

[100] Tune GS. Sleep and wakefulness in normal human adults. Br Med J 1968; 2(5600): 269-71.

[101] National Sleep Foundation. 2005 Sleep in America Poll. 2005. Washington, National Sleep Foundation. Available at: http://www.sleepfoundation.org/

[102] Leproult R, Van CE. Role of Sleep and Sleep Loss in Hormonal Release and Metabolism. Endocr Dev 2010; 17: 11-21.

[103] Copinschi G. Metabolic and endocrine effects of sleep deprivation. Essent Psychopharmacol 2005; 6(6): 341-7.

[104] Gangwisch JE. Epidemiological evidence for the links between sleep, circadian rhythms and metabolism. Obes Rev 2009; 10 Suppl 2: 37-45.

[105] Patel SR. Reduced sleep as an obesity risk factor. Obes Rev 2009; 10 Suppl 2: 61-8.

[106] Vioque J, Torres A, Quiles J. Time spent watching television, sleep duration and obesity in adults living in Valencia, Spain. Int J Obes Relat Metab Disord 2000; 24(12): 1683-8.

[107] Sekine M, Yamagami T, Handa K, *et al.* A dose-response relationship between short sleeping hours and childhood obesity: results of the Toyama Birth Cohort Study. Child Care Health Dev 2002; 28(2): 163-70.

[108] von KR, Toschke AM, Wurmser H, Sauerwald T, Koletzko B. Reduced risk for overweight and obesity in 5- and 6-y-old children by duration of sleep--a cross-sectional study. Int J Obes Relat Metab Disord 2002; 26(5): 710-6.

[109] Cournot M, Ruidavets JB, Marquie JC, Esquirol Y, Baracat B, Ferrieres J. Environmental factors associated with body mass index in a population of Southern France. Eur J Cardiovasc Prev Rehabil 2004; 11(4): 291-7.

[110] Patel SR, Malhotra A, White DP, Gottlieb DJ, Hu FB. Association between reduced sleep and weight gain in women. Am J Epidemiol 2006; 164(10): 947-54.

[111] Willett W, Stampfer MJ, Bain C, *et al.* Cigarette smoking, relative weight, and menopause. Am J Epidemiol 1983; 117(6): 651-8.

[112] Patel SR, Ayas NT, Malhotra MR, *et al.* A prospective study of sleep duration and mortality risk in women. Sleep 2004; 27(3): 440-4.

[113] Reilly JJ, Armstrong J, Dorosty AR, *et al.* Early life risk factors for obesity in childhood: cohort study. BMJ 2005; 330(7504): 1357.

[114] Agras WS, Hammer LD, McNicholas F, Kraemer HC. Risk factors for childhood overweight: a prospective study from birth to 9.5 years. J Pediatr 2004; 145(1): 20-5.

[115] Lauderdale DS, Knutson KL, Yan LL, *et al.* Objectively measured sleep characteristics among early-middle-aged adults: the CARDIA study. Am J Epidemiol 2006; 164(1): 5-16.

[116] Lauderdale DS, Knutson KL, Yan LL, Liu K, Rathouz PJ. Self-reported and measured sleep duration: how similar are they? Epidemiology 2008; 19(6): 838-45.

[117] Walsleben JA, Kapur VK, Newman AB, *et al.* Sleep and reported daytime sleepiness in normal subjects: the Sleep Heart Health Study. Sleep 2004; 27(2): 293-8.

[118] Blank JB, Cawthon PM, Carrion-Petersen ML, *et al.* Overview of recruitment for the osteoporotic fractures in men study (MrOS). Contemp Clin Trials 2005; 26(5): 557-68.

[119] Orwoll E, Blank JB, Barrett-Connor E, *et al.* Design and baseline characteristics of the osteoporotic fractures in men (MrOS) study--a large observational study of the determinants of fracture in older men. Contemp Clin Trials 2005; 26(5): 569-85.

[120] Ayas NT, White DP, Al-Delaimy WK, *et al.* A prospective study of self-reported sleep duration and incident diabetes in women. Diabetes Care 2003; 26(2): 380-4.

[121] Balbo M, Leproult R, Van Cauter E. Impact of sleep and its disturbances on hypothalamo-pituitary-adrenal axis activity. Int J Endocrinol 2010; 2010: 759234.

[122] von Treuer K, Norman TR, Armstrong SM. Overnight human plasma melatonin, cortisol, prolactin, TSH, under conditions of normal sleep, sleep deprivation, and sleep recovery. J Pineal Res 1996; 20(1): 7-14.

[123] Spiegel K, Leproult R, L'hermite-Baleriaux M, Copinschi G, Penev PD, Van CE. Leptin levels are dependent on sleep duration: relationships with sympathovagal balance, carbohydrate regulation, cortisol, and thyrotropin. J Clin Endocrinol Metab 2004; 89(11): 5762-71.

[124] Leproult R, Copinschi G, Buxton O, Van Cauter E. Sleep loss results in an elevation of cortisol levels the next evening. Sleep 1997; 20(10): 865-70.

[125] Spath-Schwalbe E, Scholler T, Kern W, Fehm HL, Born J. Nocturnal adrenocorticotropin and cortisol secretion depends on sleep duration and decreases in association with spontaneous awakening in the morning. J Clin Endocrinol Metab 1992; 75(6): 1431-5.

[126] Kumari M, Badrick E, Ferrie J, Perski A, Marmot M, Chandola T. Self-reported sleep duration and sleep disturbance are independently associated with cortisol secretion in the Whitehall II study. J Clin Endocrinol Metab 2009; 94(12): 4801-9.

[127] Born J, Muth S, Fehm HL. The significance of sleep onset and slow wave sleep for nocturnal release of growth hormone (GH) and cortisol. Psychoneuroendocrinology 1988; 13(3): 233-43.

[128] Tasali E, Leproul R, Ehrmann DA, Van Cauter E. Slow-wave sleep and the risk of type 2 diabetes in humans. Proc Natl Acad Sci U S A 2008; 105(3): 1044-9.

[129] Born J, Schenk U, Spath-Schwalbe E, Fehm HL. Influences of partial REM sleep deprivation and awakenings on nocturnal cortisol release. Biol Psychiatry 1988; 24(7): 801-11.

[130] Stamatakis KA, Punjabi NM. Effects of sleep fragmentation on glucose metabolism in normal subjects. Chest 2010; 137(1): 95-101.

[131] Taheri S, Lin L, Austin D, Young T, Mignot E. Short sleep duration is associated with reduced leptin, elevated ghrelin, and increased body mass index. PLoS Med 2004; 1(3): e62.

[132] Bliwise DL, Young TB. The parable of parabola: what the U-shaped curve can and cannot tell us about sleep. Sleep 2007; 30(12): 1614-5.

[133] Marshall NS, Glozier N, Grunstein RR. Reply to Taheri and Thomas: is sleep duration associated with obesity-U cannot be serious. Sleep Med Rev 2008; 12(4): 303-5.

[134] Cappuccio FP, Taggart FM, Kandala NB, et al. Meta-analysis of short sleep duration and obesity in children and adults. Sleep 2008; 31(5): 619-26.

[135] Stranges S, Cappuccio FP, Kandala NB, et al. Cross-sectional versus prospective associations of sleep duration with changes in relative weight and body fat distribution: the Whitehall II Study. Am J Epidemiol 2008; 167(3): 321-9.

[136] Horne J. Short sleep is a questionable risk factor for obesity and related disorders: statistical versus clinical significance. Biol Psychol 2008; 77(3): 266-76.

[137] Horne J. Too weighty a link between short sleep and obesity? Sleep 2008; 31(5): 595-6.

[138] Young T. Increasing sleep duration for a healthier (and less obese?) population tomorrow. Sleep 2008; 31(5): 593-4.

[139] Marshall NS, Glozier N, Grunstein RR. Is sleep duration related to obesity? A critical review of the epidemiological evidence. Sleep Med Rev 2008; 12(4): 289-98.

[140] Patel SR, Hu FB. Short sleep duration and weight gain: a systematic review. Obesity (Silver Spring) 2008; 16(3): 643-53.

[141] Taheri S, Thomas GN. Is sleep duration associated with obesity-where do U stand? Sleep Med Rev 2008; 12(4): 299-302.

[142] Mallon L, Broman JE, Hetta J. High incidence of diabetes in men with sleep complaints or short sleep duration: a 12-year follow-up study of a middle-aged population. Diabetes Care 2005; 28(11): 2762-7.

[143] Vijay-Kumar M, Aitken JD, Carvalho FA, et al. Metabolic syndrome and altered gut microbiota in mice lacking Toll-like receptor 5. Science 2010; 328(5975): 228-31.

[144] Cizza G, Marincola P, Mattingly M, et al. Treatment of obesity with extension of sleep duration: a randomized, prospective, controlled trial. Clin Trials 2010; 7(3): 274-85.

[145] Ford ES, Giles WH, Dietz WH. Prevalence of the metabolic syndrome among US adults: findings from the third National Health and Nutrition Examination Survey. JAMA 2002; 287(3): 356-9.

[146] Angelico F, del BM, Augelletti T, et al. Obstructive sleep apnoea syndrome and the metabolic syndrome in an internal medicine setting. Eur J Intern Med 2010; 21(3): 191-5.

[147] Coughlin SR, Mawdsley L, Mugarza JA, Calverley PM, Wilding JP. Obstructive sleep apnoea is independently associated with an increased prevalence of metabolic syndrome. Eur Heart J 2004; 25(9): 735-41.

[148] Angelico F, del BM, Augelletti T, et al. Obstructive sleep apnoea syndrome and the metabolic syndrome in an internal medicine setting. Eur J Intern Med 2010; 21(3): 191-5.

[149] Chin K, Oga T, Takahashi K, et al. Associations between obstructive sleep apnea, metabolic syndrome, and sleep duration, as measured with an actigraph, in an urban male working population in Japan. Sleep 2010; 33(1): 89-95.

[150] Gruber A, Horwood F, Sithole J, Ali NJ, Idris I. Obstructive sleep apnoea is independently associated with the metabolic syndrome but not insulin resistance state. Cardiovasc Diabetol 2006; 5: 22.

[151] Kono M, Tatsumi K, Saibara T, et al. Obstructive sleep apnea syndrome is associated with some components of metabolic syndrome. Chest 2007; 131(5): 1387-92.

[152] Lam JC, Lam B, Lam CL, et al. Obstructive sleep apnea and the metabolic syndrome in community-based Chinese adults in Hong Kong. Respir Med 2006; 100(6): 980-7.

[153] McArdle N, Hillman D, Beilin L, Watts G. Metabolic risk factors for vascular disease in obstructive sleep apnea: a matched controlled study. Am J Respir Crit Care Med 2007; 175(2): 190-5.

[154] Nieto FJ, Peppard PE, Young TB. Sleep disordered breathing and metabolic syndrome. WMJ 2009; 108(5): 263-5.

[155] Parish JM, Adam T, Facchiano L. Relationship of metabolic syndrome and obstructive sleep apnea. J Clin Sleep Med 2007; 3(5): 467-72.

[156] Peled N, Kassirer M, Shitrit D, et al. The association of OSA with insulin resistance, inflammation and metabolic syndrome. Respir Med 2007; 101(8): 1696-701.

[157] Sasanabe R, Banno K, Otake K, *et al.* Metabolic syndrome in Japanese patients with obstructive sleep apnea syndrome. Hypertens Res 2006; 29(5): 315-22.

[158] Shiina K, Tomiyama H, Takata Y, *et al.* Concurrent presence of metabolic syndrome in obstructive sleep apnea syndrome exacerbates the cardiovascular risk: a sleep clinic cohort study. Hypertens Res 2006; 29(6): 433-41.

[159] Tkacova R, Dorkova Z, Molcanyiova A, Radikova Z, Klimes I, Tkac I. Cardiovascular risk and insulin resistance in patients with obstructive sleep apnea. Med Sci Monit 2008; 14(9): CR438-CR444.

[160] Oktay B, Akbal E, Firat H, Ardic S, Kizilgun M. CPAP treatment in the coexistence of obstructive sleep apnea syndrome and metabolic syndrome, results of one year follow up. Acta Clin Belg 2009; 64(4): 329-34.

[161] McNicholas WT, Bonsigore MR. Sleep apnoea as an independent risk factor for cardiovascular disease: current evidence, basic mechanisms and research priorities. Eur Respir J 2007; 29(1): 156-78.

[162] Wolk R, Somers VK. Sleep and the metabolic syndrome. Exp Physiol 2007; 92(1): 67-78.

[163] Selim B, Won C, Yaggi HK. Cardiovascular consequences of sleep apnea. Clin Chest Med 2010; 31(2): 203-20.

[164] Butt M, Dwivedi G, Khair O, Lip GY. Obstructive sleep apnea and cardiovascular disease. Int J Cardiol 2010; 139(1): 7-16.

[165] Cherniack EP, Cherniack NS. Obstructive sleep apnea, metabolic syndrome, and age: will geriatricians be caught asleep on the job? Aging Clin Exp Res 2010; 22(1): 1-7.

[166] Ferreira S, Marinho A, Patacho M, *et al.* Prevalence and characteristics of sleep apnoea in patients with stable heart failure: Results from a heart failure clinic. BMC Pulm Med 2010; 10: 9.

[167] Bradley TD, Floras JS. Obstructive sleep apnoea and its cardiovascular consequences. Lancet 2009; 373(9657): 82-93.

[168] Abe H, Takahashi M, Yaegashi H, *et al.* Efficacy of continuous positive airway pressure on arrhythmias in obstructive sleep apnea patients. Heart Vessels 2010; 25(1): 63-9.

[169] Muraki I, Tanigawa T, Yamagishi K, *et al.* Nocturnal intermittent hypoxia and C reactive protein among middle-aged community residents: a cross-sectional survey. Thorax 2010; 65(6): 523-7.

[170] Muraki I, Tanigawa T, Yamagishi K, *et al.* Nocturnal intermittent hypoxia and the development of type 2 diabetes: the Circulatory Risk in Communities Study (CIRCS). Diabetologia 2010; 53(3): 481-8.

[171] Muraki I, Tanigawa T, Yamagishi K, *et al.* Nocturnal intermittent hypoxia and metabolic syndrome; the effect of being overweight: the CIRCS study. J Atheroscler Thromb 2010; 17(4): 369-77.

[172] Shahar E, Whitney CW, Redline S, *et al.* Sleep-disordered breathing and cardiovascular disease: cross-sectional results of the Sleep Heart Health Study. Am J Respir Crit Care Med 2001; 163(1): 19-25.

[173] Marin JM, Carrizo S. Mortality in obstructive sleep apnea. Sleep Med Clin 2007; 2: 593-601.

[174] Marshall NS, Wong KK, Liu PY, Cullen SR, Knuiman MW, Grunstein RR. Sleep apnea as an independent risk factor for all-cause mortality: the Busselton Health Study. Sleep 2008; 31(8): 1079-85.

[175] Tasali E, Mokhlesi B, Van CE. Obstructive sleep apnea and type 2 diabetes: interacting epidemics. Chest 2008; 133(2): 496-506.

[176] Punjabi NM, Polotsky VY. Disorders of glucose metabolism in sleep apnea. J Appl Physiol 2005; 99(5): 1998-2007.

[177] Balkau B, Eschwege E. Insulin resistance: an independent risk factor for cardiovascular disease? Diabetes Obes Metab 1999; 1 Suppl 1: S23-S31.

[178] Stoney RM, O'Dea K, Herbert KE, *et al.* Insulin resistance as a major determinant of increased coronary heart disease risk in postmenopausal women with Type 2 diabetes mellitus. Diabet Med 2001; 18(6): 476-82.

[179] Tasali E, Ip MS. Obstructive sleep apnea and metabolic syndrome: alterations in glucose metabolism and inflammation. Proc Am Thorac Soc 2008; 5(2): 207-17.

[180] Resnick HE, Redline S, Shahar E, *et al.* Diabetes and sleep disturbances: findings from the Sleep Heart Health Study. Diabetes Care 2003; 26(3): 702-9.

[181] Reichmuth KJ, Austin D, Skatrud JB, Young T. Association of sleep apnea and type II diabetes: a population-based study. Am J Respir Crit Care Med 2005; 172(12): 1590-5.

[182] West SD, Nicoll DJ, Stradling JR. Prevalence of obstructive sleep apnoea in men with type 2 diabetes. Thorax 2006; 61(11): 945-50.

[183] Gottlieb DJ, Punjabi NM, Newman AB, *et al.* Association of sleep time with diabetes mellitus and impaired glucose tolerance. Arch Intern Med 2005; 165(8): 863-7.

[184] Donga E, van DM, van Dijk JG, *et al.* A single night of partial sleep deprivation induces insulin resistance in multiple metabolic pathways in healthy subjects. J Clin Endocrinol Metab 2010; 95(6): 2963-8.

[185] Donga E, van DM, van Dijk JG, *et al.* Partial sleep restriction decreases insulin sensitivity in type 1 diabetes. Diabetes Care 2010.

[186] Chen L, Cao ZL, Han F, Gao ZC, He QY. Chronic intermittent hypoxia from pedo-stage decreases glucose transporter 4 expression in adipose tissue and causes insulin resistance. Chin Med J (England) 2010; 123(4): 463-70.

[187] Polotsky VY, Li J, Punjabi NM, *et al.* Intermittent hypoxia increases insulin resistance in genetically obese mice. J Physiol 2003; 552(Pt 1): 253-64.

[188] Punjabi NM, Ahmed MM, Polotsky VY, Beamer BA, O'Donnell CP. Sleep-disordered breathing, glucose intolerance, and insulin resistance. Respir Physiol Neurobiol 2003; 136(2-3): 167-78.

[189] Tuomilehto H, Peltonen M, Partinen M, *et al.* Sleep duration is associated with an increased risk for the prevalence of type 2 diabetes in middle-aged women - The FIN-D2D survey. Sleep Med 2008; 9(3): 221-7.

[190] Xu J, Long YS, Gozal D, Epstein PN. Beta-cell death and proliferation after intermittent hypoxia: role of oxidative stress. Free Radic Biol Med 2009; 46(6): 783-90.

[191] Punjabi NM, Beamer BA. Alterations in Glucose Disposal in Sleep-disordered Breathing. Am J Respir Crit Care Med 2009; 179(3): 235-40.

[192] Marshall NS, Wong KK, Phillips CL, Liu PY, Knuiman MW, Grunstein RR. Is sleep apnea an independent risk factor for prevalent and incident diabetes in the Busselton Health Study? J Clin Sleep Med 2009; 5(1): 15-20.

[193] Punjabi NM. Do sleep disorders and associated treatments impact glucose metabolism? Drugs 2009; 69 Suppl 2: 13-27.

[194] Aurora RN, Punjabi NM. Sleep Apnea and Metabolic Dysfunction: Cause or Co-Relation? Sleep Med Clin 2007; 2(2): 237-50.

[195] Vgontzas AN, Bixler EO, Chrousos GP. Sleep apnea is a manifestation of the metabolic syndrome. Sleep Med Rev 2005; 9(3): 211-24.

[196] Vgontzas AN, Legro RS, Bixler EO, Grayev A, Kales A, Chrousos GP. Polycystic ovary syndrome is associated with obstructive sleep apnea and daytime sleepiness: role of insulin resistance. J Clin Endocrinol Metab 2001; 86(2): 517-20.

[197] Barcelo A, Barbe F, de la *et al.* Insulin resistance and daytime sleepiness in patients with sleep apnoea. Thorax 2008; 63(11): 946-50.

[198] Oksenberg A, Arons E, Nasser K, Shneor O, Radwan H, Silverberg DS. Severe obstructive sleep apnea: sleepy versus nonsleepy patients. Laryngoscope 2010; 120(3): 643-8.

[199] Bonsignore MR, Eckel J. Metabolic aspects of obstructive sleep apnoea syndrome. http://err.ersjournals.com/cgi/content/full/18/112/113. European Respiratory Review 2009; 18(112): 113-24.

[200] Balkau B, Vol S, Loko S, *et al.* High baseline insulin levels associated with 6-year incident observed sleep apnea. Diabetes Care 2010; 33(5): 1044-9.

[201] Yki-Jarvinen H, Westerbacka J. Vascular actions of insulin in obesity. Int J Obes Relat Metab Disord 2000; 24 Suppl 2: S25-S28.

[202] Cuhadaroglu C, Utkusavas A, Ozturk L, Salman S, Ece T. Effects of nasal CPAP treatment on insulin resistance, lipid profile, and plasma leptin in sleep apnea. Lung 2009; 187(2): 75-81.

[203] Drager LF, Genta PR, Pedrosa RP, *et al.* Characteristics and predictors of obstructive sleep apnea in patients with systemic hypertension. Am J Cardiol 2010; 105(8): 1135-9.

[204] Coughlin SR, Mawdsley L, Mugarza JA, Wilding JP, Calverley PM. Cardiovascular and metabolic effects of CPAP in obese males with OSA. Eur Respir J 2007; 29(4): 720-7.

[205] Rey S, Valdes G, Iturriaga R. [Pathophysiology of obstructive sleep apnea-associated hypertension]. Rev Med Chil 2007; 135(10): 1333-42.

[206] Iturriaga R, Moya EA, Del RR. Cardiorespiratory alterations induced by intermittent hypoxia in a rat model of sleep apnea. Adv Exp Med Biol 2010; 669: 271-4.

[207] He QY, Feng J, Zhang XL, *et al.* Relationship of daytime blood pressure and severity of obstructive sleep apnea among Chinese: a multi-center investigation in China. Chin Med J (Engl) 2010; 123(1): 18-22.

[208] Baguet JP, Nadra M, Barone-Rochette G, Ormezzano O, Pierre H, Pepin JL. Early cardiovascular abnormalities in newly diagnosed obstructive sleep apnea. Vasc Health Risk Manag 2009; 5: 1063-73.

[209] Cioffi G, Russo TE, Stefenelli C, *al.* Severe obstructive sleep apnea elicits concentric left ventricular geometry. J Hypertens 2010; 28(5): 1074-82.

[210] Rao M, Rajda G, Uppuluri S, Beck GR, Liu L, Bisognano JD. The role of continuous positive airway pressure in the treatment of hypertension in patients with obstructive sleep apnea-hypoapnea syndrome: a review of randomized trials. Rev Recent Clin Trials 2010; 5(1): 35-42.

[211] Barbe F, Duran-Cantolla J, Capote F, *et al.* Long-term effect of continuous positive airway pressure in hypertensive patients with sleep apnea. Am J Respir Crit Care Med 2010; 181(7): 718-26.

[212] Jelic S, Lederer DJ, Adams T, *et al.* Endothelial repair capacity and apoptosis are inversely related in obstructive sleep apnea. Vasc Health Risk Manag 2009; 5: 909-20.

[213] Jelic S, Lederer DJ, Adams T, *et al.* Vascular inflammation in obesity and sleep apnea. Circulation 2010; 121(8): 1014-21.

[214] Bayram NA, Ciftci B, Keles T, *et al.* Endothelial function in normotensive men with obstructive sleep apnea before and 6 months after CPAP treatment. Sleep 2009; 32(10): 1257-63.

[215] Yim-Yeh S, Rahangdale S, Nguyen AT, *et al.* Vascular Dysfunction in Obstructive Sleep Apnea and Type 2 Diabetes Mellitus. Obesity (Silver Spring) 2010.

[216] Drager LF, Bortolotto LA, Figueiredo AC, Krieger EM, Lorenzi GF. Effects of continuous positive airway pressure on early signs of atherosclerosis in obstructive sleep apnea. Am J Respir Crit Care Med 2007; 176(7): 706-12.

[217] Kuniyoshi FH, Garcia-Touchard A, Gami AS, *et al.* Day-night variation of acute myocardial infarction in obstructive sleep apnea. J Am Coll Cardiol 2008; 52(5): 343-6.

[218] Wang Y BMLLCBKS. Will all Americans become overweight or obese? estimating the progression and cost of the US obesity epidemic. Obesity (Silver Spring) 2008;16:2323-2330. Obesity (Silver Spring) 2008.

[219] Schafer H, Pauleit D, Sudhop T, Gouni-Berthold I, Ewig S, Berthold HK. Body fat distribution, serum leptin, and cardiovascular risk factors in men with obstructive sleep apnea. Chest 2002; 122(3): 829-39.

[220] Casazza K, Dulin-Keita A, Gower BA, Fernandez JR. Intrabdominal fat is related to metabolic risk factors in Hispanic Americans, African Americans and in girls. Acta Paediatr 2009; 98(12): 1965-71.

[221] Ibrahim MM. Subcutaneous and visceral adipose tissue: structural and functional differences. Obes Rev 2009.

[222] Hannon TS, Lee S, Chakravorty S, Lin Y, Arslanian SA. Sleep-disordered breathing in obese adolescents is associated with visceral adiposity and markers of insulin resistance. Int J Pediatr Obes 2010.

[223] Vgontzas AN, Bixler EO, Chrousos GP. Metabolic disturbances in obesity versus sleep apnoea: the importance of visceral obesity and insulin resistance. J Intern Med 2003; 254(1): 32-44.

[224] Chin K, Shimizu K, Nakamura T, *et al.* Changes in intra-abdominal visceral fat and serum leptin levels in patients with obstructive sleep apnea syndrome following nasal continuous positive airway pressure therapy. Circulation 1999; 100(7): 706-12.

[225] Trenell MI, Ward JA, Yee BJ, Phillips CL, Kemp GJ, Grunstein RR, Thompson CH. Influence of constant positive airway pressure therapy on lipid storage, muscle metabolism and insulin action in obese patients with severe obstructive sleep apnoea syndrome. Diabetes Obes Metab 2007; 9(5): 679-87.

[226] Dixon JB, Schachter LM, O'brien PE. Polysomnography before and after weight loss in obese patients with severe sleep apnea. Int J Obes (Lond) 2005; 29(9): 1048-54.

[227] Rao A, Tey BH, Ramalingam G, Poh AG. Obstructive sleep apnoea (OSA) patterns in bariatric surgical practice and response of OSA to weight loss after laparoscopic adjustable gastric banding (LAGB). Ann Acad Med Singapore 2009; 38(7): 587.

[228] Patel SR, Malhotra A, Gottlieb DJ, White DP, Hu FB. Correlates of long sleep duration. Sleep 2006; 29(7): 881-9.

[229] Patel SR, Hu FB. Short sleep duration and weight gain: a systematic review. Obesity (Silver Spring) 2008; 16(3): 643-53.

[230] Peled N, Greenberg A, Pillar G, Zinder O, Levi N, Lavie P. Contributions of hypoxia and respiratory disturbance index to sympathetic activation and blood pressure in obstructive sleep apnea syndrome. Am J Hypertens 1998; 11(11 Pt 1): 1284-9.

[231] Bratel T, Wennlund A, Carlstrom K. Pituitary reactivity, androgens and catecholamines in obstructive sleep apnoea. Effects of continuous positive airway pressure treatment (CPAP). Respir Med 1999; 93(1): 1-7.

[232] Larkin EK, Rosen CL, Kirchner HL, *et al.* Variation of C-reactive protein levels in adolescents: association with sleep-disordered breathing and sleep duration. Circulation 2005; 111(15): 1978-84.

[233] Lavie L. Oxidative stress--a unifying paradigm in obstructive sleep apnea and comorbidities. Prog Cardiovasc Dis 2009; 51(4): 303-12.

[234] Somers VK, Dyken ME, Clary MP, Abboud FM. Sympathetic neural mechanisms in obstructive sleep apnea. J Clin Invest 1995; 96(4): 1897-904.

[235] Leuenberger UA, Brubaker D, Quraishi S, Hogeman CS, Imadojemu VA, Gray KS. Effects of intermittent hypoxia on sympathetic activity and blood pressure in humans. Auton Neurosci 2005; 121(1-2): 87-93.

[236] Ziegler MG, Nelesen R, Mills P, Ancoli-Israel S, Kennedy B, Dimsdale JE. Sleep apnea, norepinephrine-release rate, and daytime hypertension. Sleep 1997; 20(3): 224-31.

[237] Bao X, Nelesen RA, Loredo JS, Dimsdale JE, Ziegler MG. Blood pressure variability in obstructive sleep apnea: role of sympathetic nervous activity and effect of continuous positive airway pressure. Blood Press Monit 2002; 7(6): 301-7.

[238] Narkiewicz K, van de Borne PJ, Montano N, Dyken ME, Phillips BG, Somers VK. Contribution of tonic chemoreflex activation to sympathetic activity and blood pressure in patients with obstructive sleep apnea. Circulation 1998; 97(10): 943-5.

[239] Narkiewicz K, van de Borne PJ, Cooley RL, Dyken ME, Somers VK. Sympathetic activity in obese subjects with and without obstructive sleep apnea. Circulation 1998; 98(8): 772-6.

[240] Peles E, Akselrod S, Goldstein DS, Nitzan H, Azaria M, Almog S *et al.* Insulin resistance and autonomic function in traumatic lower limb amputees. Clin Auton Res 1995; 5(5): 279-88.

[241] Barth E, Albuszies G, Baumgart K, *et al.* Glucose metabolism and catecholamines. Crit Care Med 35, S508-S518. 2007.

[242] Egan BM. Insulin resistance and the sympathetic nervous system. Curr Hypertens Rep 2003; 5(3): 247-54.

[243] Navegantes LC, Sjostrand M, Gudbjornsdottir S, Strindberg L, Elam M, Lonnroth P. Regulation and counterregulation of lipolysis *in vivo*: different roles of sympathetic activation and insulin. J Clin Endocrinol Metab 2003; 88(5515): 5520.

[244] Roden M, Price TB, Perseghin G, *et al.* Mechanism of free fatty acid-induced insulin resistance in humans. J Clin Invest 1996; 97(12): 2859-65.

[245] Henley DE, Russell GM, Douthwaite JA, *et al.* Hypothalamic-pituitary-adrenal axis activation in obstructive sleep apnea: the effect of continuous positive airway pressure therapy. J Clin Endocrinol Metab 2009; 94(11): 4234-42.

[246] Vgontzas AN, Pejovic S, Zoumakis E, *et al.* Hypothalamic-pituitary-adrenal axis activity in obese men with and without sleep apnea: effects of continuous positive airway pressure therapy. J Clin Endocrinol Metab 2007; 92(11): 4199-207.

[247] Carneiro G, Togeiro SM, Hayashi LF, *et al.* Effect of continuous positive airway pressure therapy on hypothalamic-pituitary-adrenal axis function and 24-h blood pressure profile in obese men with obstructive sleep apnea syndrome. Am J Physiol Endocrinol Metab 2008; 295(2): E380-E384.

[248] Schmoller A, Eberhardt F, Jauch-Chara K, *et al.* Continuous positive airway pressure therapy decreases evening cortisol concentrations in patients with severe obstructive sleep apnea. Metabolism 2009; 58(6): 848-53.

[249] Eriksson J.W. Metabolic stress in insulin's target cells leads to ROS accumulation - a hypothetical common pathway causing insulin resistance. FEBS Lett 2007; 581(3734): 3742.

[250] Lee K.U. Oxidative stress markers in Korean subjects with insulin resistance syndrome. Diabetes Res Clin Pract 2001;(54): 29-33.

[251] Singh TD, Patial K, Vijayan VK, Ravi K. Oxidative stress and obstructive sleep apnoea syndrome. Indian J Chest Dis Allied Sci 2009; 51(4): 217-24.

[252] Murri M, Alcazar-Ramirez J, Garrido-Sanchez L, *et al.* Oxidative stress and metabolic changes after continuous positive airway pressure treatment according to previous metabolic disorders in sleep apnea-hypopnea syndrome patients. Transl Res 2009; 154(3): 111-21.

[253] Hernandez C, Abreu J, Abreu P, Colino R, Jimenez A. [Effects of nasal positive airway pressure treatment on oxidative stress in patients with sleep apnea-hypopnea syndrome]. Arch Bronconeumol 2006; 42(3): 125-9.

[254] Lima AM, Franco CM, Castro CM, Bezerra AA, Ataide L Jr., Halpern A. [Obstructive sleep apnea contribution to oxidative stress in obesity]. Arq Bras Endocrinol Metabol 2008; 52(4): 668-76.

[255] de Lima AM, Franco CM, de Castro CM, Bezerra AA, Ataide L Jr., Halpern A. Effects of nasal continuous positive airway pressure treatment on oxidative stress and adiponectin levels in obese patients with obstructive sleep apnea. Respiration 2010; 79(5): 370-6.

[256] Ryan S, McNicholas WT. Intermittent hypoxia and activation of inflammatory molecular pathways in OSAS. Arch Physiol Biochem 2008; 114(4): 261-6.

[257] Ryan S, McNicholas WT. Inflammatory cardiovascular risk markers in obstructive sleep apnoea syndrome. Cardiovasc Hematol Agents Med Chem 2009; 7(1): 76-81.

[258] Faber DR, van der Graaf Y, Westerink J, Visseren FL. Increased visceral adipose tissue mass is associated with increased C-reactive protein in patients with manifest vascular diseases. Atherosclerosis 2010; 212(1): 274-80.

[259] Bluher M. Adipose tissue dysfunction in obesity. Exp Clin Endocrinol Diabetes 2009; 117(6): 241-50.

[260] Hosogai N, Fukuhara A, Oshima K, Miyata Y, Tanaka S, Segawa K. Adipose tissue hypoxia in obesity and its impact on adipocytokine dysregulation. Diabetes 2007; 56: 901-11.

[261] Trayhurn P Wood IS. Adipokines: inflammation and the pleiotropic role of white adipose tissue. Br J Nutr 2004; 92: 347-55.

[262] Heilbronn LK, Campbell LV. Adipose tissue macrophages, low grade inflammation and insulin resistance in human obesity. Curr Pharm Des 2008; 14(12): 1225-30.

[263] Ip MS, Lam KS, Ho C, Tsang KW, Lam W. Serum leptin and vascular risk factors in obstructive sleep apnea. Chest 2000; 118(3): 580-6.

[264] Ozturk L, Unal M, Tamer L, Celikoglu F. The association of the severity of obstructive sleep apnea with plasma leptin levels. Arch Otolaryngol Head Neck Surg 2003; 129(5): 538-40.

[265] Shimura R, Tatsumi K, Nakamura A, *et al* Fat accumulation, leptin, and hypercapnia in obstructive sleep apnea-hypopnea syndrome. Chest 2005; 127(2): 543-9.

[266] Feng J, Chen BY, Cui LY, *et al.* Inflammation status of rabbit carotid artery model endothelium during intermittent hypoxia exposure and its relationship with leptin. Sleep Breath 2009; 13(3): 277-83.

[267] Carneiro G, Togeiro SM, Ribeiro-Filho FF, *et al.* Continuous positive airway pressure therapy improves hypoadiponectinemia in severe obese men with obstructive sleep apnea without changes in insulin resistance. Metab Syndr Relat Disord 2009; 7(6): 537-42.

[268] Magalang UJ, Cruff JP, Rajappan R, *et al.* Intermittent hypoxia suppresses adiponectin secretion by adipocytes. Exp Clin Endocrinol Diabetes 2009; 117(3): 129-34.

[269] Kanbay A, Kokturk O, Ciftci TU, Tavil Y, Bukan N. Comparison of serum adiponectin and tumor necrosis factor-alpha levels between patients with and without obstructive sleep apnea syndrome. Respiration 2008; 76(3): 324-30.

[270] Pfau D, Stepan H, Kratzsch J, *et al.* Circulating Levels of the Adipokine Chemerin in Gestational Diabetes Mellitus. Horm Res Paediatr 2010.

[271] Ip MS, Lam B, Ng MM, Lam WK, Tsang KW, Lam KS. Obstructive sleep apnea is independently associated with insulin resistance. Am J Respir Crit Care Med 2002; 165(5): 670-6.

[272] Caminiti C, Evangelista P, Leske V, Loto Y, Mazza C. [Obstructive sleep apneas in symptomatic obese children: polisomnographic confirmation and its association with disturbances in carbohydrate metabolism]. Arch Argent Pediatr 2010; 108(3): 226-33.

[273] Teculescu D, Hannhart B, Aubry C, *et al.* Who are the "occasional" snorers? Chest 2002; 122(2): 562-8.

[274] Joo S, Lee S, Choi HA, Kim J, Kim E, Kimm K, *et al.* Habitual snoring is associated with elevated hemoglobin A1c levels in non-obese middle-aged adults. J Sleep Res 2006; 15(4): 437-44.

[275] Kim J, Yi H, Shin KR, Kim JH, Jung KH, Shin C. Snoring as an independent risk factor for hypertension in the nonobese population: the Korean Health and Genome Study. Am J Hypertens 2007; 20(8): 819-24.

[276] Park CG, Shin C. Prevalence and association of snoring, anthropometry and hypertension in Korea. Blood Press 2005; 14(4): 210-6.

[277] Thomas GN, Jiang CQ, Lao XQ, McGhee SM, Zhang WS, Schooling CM, *et al.* Snoring and vascular risk factors and disease in a low-risk Chinese population: the Guangzhou Biobank Cohort Study. Sleep 2006; 29(7): 896-900.

[278] Siccoli MM, Pepperell JC, Kohler M, Craig SE, Davies RJ, Stradling JR. Effects of continuous positive airway pressure on quality of life in patients with moderate to severe obstructive sleep apnea: data from a randomized controlled trial. Sleep 2008; 31(11): 1551-8.

[279] Doherty LS, Kiely JL, Lawless G, McNicholas WT. Impact of nasal continuous positive airway pressure therapy on the quality of life of bed partners of patients with obstructive sleep apnea syndrome. Chest 2003; 124(6): 2209-14.

[280] Doherty LS, Kiely JL, Swan V, McNicholas WT. Long-term effects of nasal continuous positive airway pressure therapy on cardiovascular outcomes in sleep apnea syndrome. Chest 2005; 127(6): 2076-84.

[281] Burgess KR. Central sleep apnoea and heart failure (part II). Respirology 1998; 3(1): 1-11.

[282] Pepperell JC, Ramdassingh-Dow S, Crosthwaite N, *et al.* Ambulatory blood pressure after therapeutic and subtherapeutic nasal continuous positive airway pressure for obstructive sleep apnoea: a randomised parallel trial. Lancet 2002; 359(9302): 204-10.

[283] Hoekema A, Stegenga B, Bakker M, *et al.* Simulated driving in obstructive sleep apnoea-hypopnoea; effects of oral appliances and continuous positive airway pressure. Sleep Breath 2007; 11(3): 129-38.

[284] George CF. Reduction in motor vehicle collisions following treatment of sleep apnoea with nasal CPAP. Thorax 2001; 56(7): 508-12.

[285] Carratu P, Karageorgiou G, Bonfitto P, *et al.* Long-term evaluation of mental fatigue by Maastricht Questionnaire in patients with OSAS treated with CPAP. Monaldi Arch Chest Dis 2007; 67(1): 6-9.

[286] Karkoulias K, Perimenis P, Charokopos N, Efremidis G, Sampsonas F, Kaparianos A, *et al.* Does CPAP therapy improve erectile dysfunction in patients with obstructive sleep apnea syndrome? Clin Ter 2007; 158(6): 515-8.

[287] Taskin U, Yigit O, Acioglu E, Aricigil M, Toktas G, Guzelhan Y. Erectile dysfunction in severe sleep apnea patients and response to CPAP. Int J Impot Res 2010; 22(2): 134-9.

[288] Harsch IA, Schahin SP, Radespiel-Troger M, *et al.* Continuous positive airway pressure treatment rapidly improves insulin sensitivity in patients with obstructive sleep apnea syndrome. Am J Respir Crit Care Med 2004; 169(2): 156-62.

[289] Dawson A, Abel SL, Loving RT, *et al.* CPAP therapy of obstructive sleep apnea in type 2 diabetics improves glycemic control during sleep. J Clin Sleep Med 2008; 4(6): 538-42.

[290] Dorkova Z, Petrasova D, Molcanyiova A, Popovnakova M, Tkacova R. Effects of continuous positive airway pressure on cardiovascular risk profile in patients with severe obstructive sleep apnea and metabolic syndrome. Chest 2008; 134(4): 686-92.

[291] Wang H, Wang L, Liu J. [The effect of short-time continuous positive airway pressure treatment on insulin sensitivity in patients with obstructive sleep apnea-hypopnea syndrome and type 2 diabetes]. Lin Chung Er Bi Yan Hou Tou Jing Wai Ke Za Zhi 2008; 22(13): 597-9.

[292] Schahin SP, Nechanitzky T, Dittel C, *et al.* Long-term improvement of insulin sensitivity during CPAP therapy in the obstructive sleep apnoea syndrome. Med Sci Monit 2008; 14(3): CR117-CR121.

[293] Lam JC, Lam B, Yao TJ, *et al.* A randomised controlled trial of nasal continuous positive airway pressure on insulin sensitivity in obstructive sleep apnoea. Eur Respir J 2010; 35(1): 138-45.

[294] West SD, Nicoll DJ, Wallace TM, Matthews DR, Stradling JR. Effect of CPAP on insulin resistance and HbA1c in men with obstructive sleep apnoea and type 2 diabetes. Thorax 2007; 62(11): 969-74.

[295] Kohler M, Ayers L, Pepperell JC, *et al.* Effects of continuous positive airway pressure on systemic inflammation in patients with moderate to severe obstructive sleep apnoea: a randomised controlled trial. Thorax 2009; 64(1): 67-73.

[296] Shaw JE, Punjabi NM, Wilding JP, Alberti KG, Zimmet PZ. Sleep-disordered breathing and type 2 diabetes: a report from the International Diabetes Federation Taskforce on Epidemiology and Prevention. Diabetes Res Clin Pract 2008; 81(1): 2-12.

[297] Idris I, Hall AP, O'Reilly J, *et al.* Obstructive sleep apnoea in patients with type 2 diabetes: aetiology and implications for clinical care. Diabetes Obes Metab 2009; 11(8): 733-41.

[298] Neumann C, Martinez D, Schmid H. Nocturnal oxygen desaturation in diabetic patients with severe autonomic neuropathy. Diabetes Res Clin Pract 1995; 28(2): 97-102.

[299] Vgontzas AN, Bixler EO, Tan TL, Kantner D, Martin LF, Kales A. Obesity without sleep apnea is associated with daytime sleepiness. Arch Intern Med 1998; 158(12): 1333-7.

[300] Svensson M, Franklin KA, Theorell-Haglow J, Lindberg E. Daytime sleepiness relates to snoring independent of the apnea-hypopnea index in women from the general population. Chest 2008; 134(5): 919-24.

[301] Newman AB, Spiekerman CF, Enright P, *et al.* Daytime sleepiness predicts mortality and cardiovascular disease in older adults. The Cardiovascular Health Study Research Group. J Am Geriatr Soc 2000; 48(2): 115-23.

[302] Alexandros N, Vgontzas A. Excessive Daytime Sleepiness in Sleep Apnea: It's Not Just Apnea Hypopnea Index. Sleep Med. 2008; 9(7), 712-714.

[303] Pillar G, Shehadeh N. Abdominal fat and sleep apnea: the chicken or the egg? Diabetes Care 2008; 31 Suppl 2: S303-S309

CHAPTER 19

Sleep Apnea and Cerebrovascular Disorders

Henry Klar Yaggi, M.D. M.P.H.[*]

Associate Professor of Medicine, Yale University School of Medicine, Section of Pulmonary and Critical Care Medicine, Medical Director, VA CT Center for Sleep Medicine, Clinical Epidemiology Research Center, 950 Campbell Ave, Building 35 annex, West Haven, CT 06516, USA

Abstract: When considered separately from cardiovascular disease, stroke is the third leading cause of death and ranks as the leading cause of long-term disability [1]. Strategies for stroke treatment and prevention have helped to reduce the burden of disease, but it remains an important public health challenge. Therefore, understanding underlying pathophysiology and developing novel therapeutic approaches for cerbrovascular disease is of crucial importance.

Understanding the link between sleep and cerebrovascular disease may represent one such novel approach. A recent Institute of Medicine report, entitled *Sleep Disorders and Sleep Deprivation: an Unmet Public Health Challenge*, estimated that 50-70 million Americans suffer from a chronic sleep disorder. A major aspect of this "unmet public health challenge" is the cerebrovascular health consequences of sleep-disordered breathing. Obstructive sleep apnea (OSA), a common form of sleep-disordered breathing, has a high and rising prevalence in the general adult population, attributable in part to the emerging epidemic of obesity and enhanced awareness. OSA has also been independently linked to important health outcomes, including hypertension [2], fatal and nonfatal cardiovascular events [3-5], stroke [6-8], sudden cardiac death [5] and all cause mortality [9, 10], while therapy for sleep apnea may help to reduce cerebrovascular risk.

TOPIC DISCUSSION (CLINICAL OUTLOOK)

Autonomic Changes in Cardiovascular System during Sleep, and the Circadian Occurrence of Sudden Death Events

Studies in normal humans using microneurography (which allows for direct recording of peripheral sympathetic nerve traffic) suggest that the cardiovascular influence of sleep is more complex than a generalized inhibition of the sympathetic nervous system [11]. The most striking example is REM sleep which replaces non-REM sleep for several minutes at regular intervals and is accompanied by skeletal muscle atonia and bursts of rapid eye movements and muscles twitches. During REM sleep, sympathetic-nerve activity increases significantly and blood pressure and heart rate return to levels similar to those during wakefulness. Conversely, there are marked reductions in blood pressure ("nocturnal dipping"), heart rate, and sympathetic activity during non-REM sleep (which accounts for most of sleep time), that are progressive with deeper stages of non-REM (*i.e.*, slow wave sleep). These observations might explain why myocardial ischemia, infarction, and stroke are less common during the night than during daytime periods of similar duration, particularly the morning hours [12]. In contrast, this observed morning circadian pattern of adverse cardiovascular events appears to be inverted among patients with obstructive sleep apnea, where the peak circadian time for sudden death occurs during the sleeping hours between midnight and 6:00 am [5]. These sudden death events likely consist, in part, of acute strokes.

Obstructive Sleep Apnea and Cerebrovascular Outcomes

Overnight polysomnography is considered the gold standard diagnostic test to evaluate the presence of sleep apnea. A number of cross-sectional and case-control studies [3, 13-19] have used overnight polysomnography in order to evaluate the association between sleep apnea and cerebrovascular disease. One cross-sectional study demonstrating the association between sleep-disordered breathing and cerebrovascular disease comes from the results of Sleep Heart Health Study [3]. This community-based study explored the association between sleep-disordered breathing and prevalent self-reported cardiovascular disease (myocardial infarction, angina, coronary revascularization

*Address correspondence to Henry Klar Yaggi: Associate Professor of Medicine, Yale University School of Medicine, Section of Pulmonary and Critical Care Medicine, Medical Director, VA CT Center for Sleep Medicine, Clinical Epidemiology Research Center, 950 Campbell Ave, Building 35 annex, West Haven, CT 06516, USA; E-mail: henry.yaggi@yale.edu

Octavian C. Ioachimescu (Ed)

procedures, heart failure, or stroke) in a large cohort of 6,424 individuals who underwent unattended overnight polysomnography at home. This study revealed indepepdnent associations between sleep apnea and cardiovascular risk after adjusting for 'traditional' cardiovascular risk factors

An inarguable criterion for causal inference is that exposure must precede the onset of the disease. Although in general, case-control and cross-sectional studies are efficient study designs for evaluating strength of association, they have a significant limitation in their ability to establish the temporal course in a cause-and-effect relationship. Such study designs might reflect reverse causal pathways whereby sleep-disordered breathing has been the consequence rather than the cause of vascular disease. This is particualrly true for stroke, where several case reports of sleep apnea after bulbar stroke have been reported in the literature [20-22]. Therefore, it is difficult to be certain whether sleep apnea is a cause or consequence of the cardiovascular outcome. The direction of this arrow of causation can ultimately only be definitively determined by analysis of incident cerebrovascular disease events.

Recently, prospective observational cohort studies have clarified this temporal reltionship and have demonstrated that sleep apnea increases the risk for stroke [6, 8], stroke and all-cause-mortality [9, 10], and fatal and nonfatal cardiovascular events (including stroke) [4]. In one study, after excluding prevalent stroke and adjusting for traditional cerbrovascular risk factors (including hypertension which itself may be on the causal pathway between sleep apnea stroke), sleep apnea was associated with a 2-fold increased risk for transient ischemic attack (TIA), stroke, or all-cause-mortality [7]. In a trend analysis, increasing severity of sleep apnea at baseline was associated with an increased risk for the development of the composite endpoint (p = 0.005) [7]. Those patients in the highest severity quartile of the cohort (AHI > 36) had a greater than three-fold increased risk for the devlopment of stroke or death. A similar magnitude of risk has recently been described in other population population-based cohort studies, including the Sleep Heart Health Study [6, 8].

Therefore, there is a strong association between sleep apnea and cerebrovascular outcomes, which has been consistently observed using different study designs and in different populations This risk appears to increase with increasing severity of sleep apnea, and persists even after adjustment for 'traditional' vascular risk factors. This independent association implies that there are mechanisms specific to sleep apnea that confer cerebrovascular risk and which are discussed in more detail below.

RESEARCH OUTLOOK

What do we know:

Pathophysiologic Mechanisms of Cardiovascular Disease in Sleep Apnea

Patients with sleep apnea have recurrent "cycles" of sleep, airway obstruction, arousal, and resumption of ventilation. Several physiologic stresses arise from this intermittent airway occlusion during sleep including: cyclical hypoxemia of varying duration and severity, strenuous respiratory efforts against an occluded airway resulting in the generation of severely negative intra-thoracic pressures, sympathetic activation, reduced total sleep time, and snoring with potential vibratory injury. These stresses, unique to sleep apnea, serve as potential mechanisms for the increased risk of adverse cerebrovascular events and are discussed in further detail below.

Inflammation and Intermittent Hypoxia

Systemic inflammation plays an important role in the development of atherosclerosis. The pathogenesis of inflammation and atherosclerosis in sleep apnea has not been entirely elucidated, however, intermittent hypoxia followed by re-oxygenation (common to sleep apnea) appears to play a key role. Repetitive episodes of hypoxia may selectively activate vascular inflammatory pathways [23, 24]. A higher frequency of repetitive oxygen desaturations has been correlated with increasing severity of atherosclerosis [25]. It is suggested that intermittent hypoxia promotes the formation of reactive oxygen species (ROS), particularly during the re-oxygenation period, which can be deleterious to cell endothelial cells, leukocytes, and platelets. These cells, in turn, express adhesion molecules and pro-inflammatory cytokines that may lead to endothelial injury and dysfunction and consequently to atherosclerosis [26-31].

Nocturnal Sympathetic Activation

Sympathetic over-activity of obstructive sleep apnea has been suggested for several years and evidence continues to accumulate for a role in the pathogenesis of cerebrovascular complications. Early reports found increased plasma and urinary catecholamine levels in patients with sleep apnea and a fall in these levels after treatment with tracheostomy [32]. Others employed more direct measures of sympathetic nerve activity through the use of a tungsten microelectrode in the peroneal nerve. This methodology demonstrated increased muscle sympathetic nerve activity following acute apneic events [33]. Superimposed on these bursts of sympathetic activation are 'surges' of blood pressure of up to 240 mm Hg at apnea termination. These acute blood pressure elevations during apnea appear to be driven by changes in baroreceptor sensitivity during sleep and chemoreceptor responses to progressive hypoxia [34]. Considering that humans typically spend one-third of their lives sleeping, these nocturnal increases in blood pressure might in themselves contribute to hypertensive cardiovascular and cerebrovascular consequences. Indeed, patients with sleep apnea commonly do not have the normal nocturnal fall or 'dipping' in blood pressure [35]. Among patients with hypertension, those who exhibit a diminished nocturnal decline in blood pressure, or 'non-dippers' [36] have been reported to have more cardiovascular target-organ damage than dippers [37, 38], including silent cerebrovascular damage [39]. Three longitudinal studies conducted in patients with hypertension have confirmed that a diminished nocturnal decline in blood pressure predicted cardiovascular events [40, 41], including worse stroke prognosis [42]. Moreover, diminished nocturnal decline of blood pressure is a risk factor for cardiovascular mortality, independent of overall blood pressure load during a 24-hour period, with 5% decrease in nocturnal dipping being associated with a 20% increase in cardiovascular mortality [43].

Sleep Apnea and Daytime Hypertension

In addition to acute blood pressure swings at night, evidence supports that sustained *diurnal* hypertension can arise from obstructive apnea. This appears to be in part related to a "carryover" phenomenon of heightened sympathetic activity [33]. In the Sleep Heart Health Study [44], sleep apnea was associated with prevalent hypertension, even after controlling for potential confounders such as age, gender, body mass index (BMI) and other measures of adiposity, alcohol, and smoking. Overall, the odds of hypertension appeared to increase with increases in respiratory distress index in a dose-response fashion. From the prospective results of the Wisconsin Sleep Cohort, the presence of sleep apnea at baseline was accompanied by a substantially increased risk for future hypertension at 4-year follow-up [2]. Even after adjusting for baseline hypertension status, age, gender, BMI, waist and neck circumference, weekly alcohol and cigarette use, the risk for hypertension remained elevated (2-3 fold). The Seventh Report of the Joint Committee on Prevention, Detection, Evaluation, and Treatment of High Blood Pressure (JCN 7) recognizes the etiologic role of sleep apnea as an identifiable cause of hypertension [45].

Cardiac Arrhythmia

Sleep apnea is associated with cardiac arrhythmias, conduction abnormalities such as second-degree atrioventricular block [46], and potentially life threatening arrhythmias such as ventricular tachycardia [47]. Sleep apnea has also been specifically associated with atrial fibrillation [48-50]. This risk of atrial fibrillation among OSA patients is predicted best by the severity of nocturnal hypoxemia [50]. In a recent analysis of participants from the Sleep Heart Health Study, individuals with severe sleep-disordered breathing had a two to four-fold odds of complex arrhythmia (atrial fibrillation, non-sustained ventricular tachycardia, complex ventricular ectopy), compared to patients without sleep-disordered breathing, even after adjustment for potential confounders. The association between sleep apnea and atrial fibrillation provides and indirect mechanism for stroke *via* embolic phenomenon.

Mechanical Load

Large negative intra-pleural pressures are generated as a result of attempting to inspire against an obstructed upper airway. This large negative intrapleural pressure results in an elevated transmural pressure or afterload (difference between intraventricular pressure and intrapleural pressure) [51]. Thus, increases in afterload and associated decreases in cardiac output are also associated with individual obstructive apneas and may predispose to ischemia and vascular events.

Short Sleep Duration and Metabolic Dysregulation

There is significant overlap between sleep apnea and the cluster of cardiovascular risk factors that constitutes the "metabolic syndrome." In fact there is accumulating evidence to suggest that sleep restriction may worsen these metabolic abnormalities. Sleep curtailment has been linked to impaired carbohydrate tolerance and insulin resistance [52], and even the development of type 2 diabetes [53]. Recently, short sleep duration has also been linked to the development of incident coronary artery calcification. Several studies have also demonstrated sleep-disordered breathing increases the risk for glucose intolerance [54], insulin resistance [55, 56] and even overt clinical diabetes [57]. Hypoxia may explain some of this risk [54].

Snoring and Carotid Atherosclerosis

A novel mechanism has recently emerged linking sleep apnea to stroke *via* a direct pathogenetic relationship between snoring and carotid atherosclerosis. Snores originate from the upper airway during sleep and are a result of vibrations of the pharyngeal wall and associated structures. It has been hypothesized that oscillatory pressure waves/vibrations originating in the upper airway during snoring may be transmitted through the surrounding tissue to the carotid artery wall. The proximity of the carotid artery bifurcation to the lateral pharyngeal wall is such that it is likely exposed to these vibrations and may cause pathologic damage to the arterial wall endothelium, triggering an inflammatory cascade leading to early atherosclerosis or worse embolic phenomenon. In this context, a recent cross-sectional study [58] was conducted on 110 patients who underwent overnight polysomnography with quantification of snoring, carotid artery ultrasound, and also simultaneous quantification of femoral artery atherosclerosis as a distant (from the upper airway) control artery. A significant association was observed (in a dose-response fashion) between percent of time snoring and the prevalence of carotid artery atherosclerosis (but not femoral atherosclerosis), even after adjustment for confounding variables. Of note, early epidemiologic studies linking sleep-disordered breathing to stroke used snoring as a "proxy measure" for sleep disordered breathing, however this data suggest a more direct pathogenetic relationship.

Therapy for Sleep Apnea and Impact on Cardiovascular Risk

Compared with control, CPAP (the main medical therapy for sleep apnea) shows significant improvements in objective and subjective measures of sleepiness, quality of life, cognitive function [58]. CPAP has also been demonstrated to improve left ventricular function in patients with congestive heart failure and sleep apnea [59-62], and decrease automobile accidents [63]. To date no published *long-term* prospective randomized controlled trials have demonstrated that the treatment of sleep apnea decreases the risk of cerebrovascular events in terms of either primary or secondary prevention. However, *long-term* longitudinal observational cohort studies have evaluated the impact of CPAP therapy on cardiovascular outcomes, and *short-term* randomized controlled trials have evaluated the impact of CPAP on hypertension and intermediate cerebrovascular endpoints in patients with sleep apnea.

Long- term Observational Studies

An early study that gives some insight into the impact of treatment of sleep apnea on the risk of stroke (and myocardial infarction) was a retrospective cohort study of patients who were diagnosed with sleep apnea with polysomnography in the 1970s, *i.e.*, prior to the availability of CPAP, when the only known definitive therapy for sleep apnea consisted of tracheostomy [64]. In this study, seven years of follow-up was provided on 198 patients, of which 71 patients received tracheostomy (considered 'effective treatment') and 127 received 'conservative treatment' consisting of recommended weight loss (the only alternative). Any new hypertension, myocardial infarction or stroke occurring since the original polysomnography was considered the main vascular morbidity outcome. Despite the fact that at study entry the tracheostomy group included more patients with a history of hypertension, myocardial infarction or stroke, it was the conservatively treated group who developed considerably more vascular outcomes [64].

More recently, prospective observational cohorts designed to examine the impact of treatment on long-term cardiovascular outcomes in patients with sleep apnea have demonstrated that CPAP therapy may reduce mortality in severe sleep apnea [65] and protect against death from cardiovascular disease [66]. In a study conducted by Marin *et al* [4] the incidence of fatal and nonfatal cardiovascular events (including stroke) was highest in patients with severe untreated sleep apnea. Patients who received and complied with CPAP (who largely had severe sleep apnea) had a significantly reduced cardiovascular risk, suggesting that long-term therapy with CPAP may reduce risk of fatal and nonfatal cardiovascular events. CPAP compliance has been similarly associated with reduced stroke mortality [68].

Short-term Randomized Controlled Trials with CPAP and the Endpoint of Blood Pressure

Short-term (up to 3 months) randomized controlled trials have been published looking at arterial blood pressure as the outcome. Although the studies vary with respect to the magnitude of blood pressure reduction, overall there appears to be a clinically important blood pressure reduction in both 24-hour systolic and diastolic pressures. The characteristics of the patients selected for these trials give clues to those most likely to gain any blood pressure lowering benefits. In general, those more likely to experience benefit have more severe and symptomatic sleep apnea, are hypertensive or on hypertensive therapy at baseline, receive more effective therapy for sleep apnea (longer use), and have more frequent oxygen desaturations [60-62]. Those less likely to experience benefit are normotensive at baseline, asymptomatic, and more likely have mild sleep apnea [67, 68]. A systematic literature review conducted by the Cochrane Collaboration [58] found that mean 24-hour systolic and diastolic pressures were significantly lower on CPAP (-7.24 mm Hg systolic, -3.07 mm Hg diastolic). Other meta-analyses have indicated that magnitude of the blood pressure reduction increases significantly with more severe sleep apnea and longer effective nighttime use of CPAP [69]. When extrapolated to antihypertensive epidemiologic data, such BP lowering effects would be predicted to significantly reduce stroke and coronary heart disease event risk [62, 70].

CPAP treatment and Intermediate Cerebrovascular Endpoints

In addition to reduction of blood pressure, CPAP therapy has been demonstrated to improve a number of "intermediate" cerebrovascular endpoints. Effective CPAP therapy eliminates cyclic hypoxia, decreases inflammatory markers of atherosclerosis [29], reduces sympathetic activity and catecholamines [61], reduces recurrent atrial fibrillation [71], and improves left ventricular function [59]. Recently, a short-term randomized controlled trial demonstrated that CPAP also significantly decreases early signs of atherosclerosis as measured by carotid intima-media thickness and arterial stiffness [72]. Therefore, the potential cerebrovascular event risk reduction of CPAP therapy may be more than that conferred just by its blood pressure lowering effects; however, this question awaits the results of future longer-term randomized controlled trials.

What we don't know:

- A major area of uncertainty exists regarding whether the treatment of sleep apnea with CPAP helps to reduce risk of cerebrovascular events both in terms of primary prevention as well as secondary prevention among patients with existing TIA and stroke, both in acute and chronic setting.

- Primary Prevention: previous observational cohort studies have demonstrated a risk reduction in fatal and nonfatal cardiovascular events (including stroke) associated with the regular use of CPAP therapy. A criticism of these types of observational studies is that, in these studies, patients who are complying with CPAP therapy are also complying with other medical co-therapies (e.g., other medication adherence, leading healthier lifestyle), resulting in an overestimation of the beneficial effects of CPAP therapy. However, methodological work comparing the results of observational studies with the results of randomized controlled trials on a variety of different clinical topics (where both types of studies existed), showed that the results of observational studies tend not to overestimate the impact of treatment [75]. But whether longer-term randomized controlled trials will confirm the results of observational studies regarding the primary prevention benefit of CPAP treatment awaits further investigation. Challenges exist in designing longer term randomized controlled trials including strategies to increase CPAP compliance, determining appropriate control groups, and safety considerations of patients with sleep apnea in long-term control groups; but ongoing trials are using a variety of strategies to examine the impact of this therapy.

- Secondary Prevention (TIA): Patients with TIA are ideal candidates for the prevention of recurrent vascular events. There are over 300,000 TIAs annually in the United States and, importantly, patients with TIA are at high risk for poor outcomes, despite current prevention strategies (25% will have stroke, cardiovascular event, or death 90 days post-TIA, with half of these events occurring within the first 72 hours). New approaches to reduce recurrent vascular event rate are needed, particularly in acute post-TIA period. Sleep apnea occurs in 60-80% of patients post TIA/stroke and is associated with poor outcomes post-stroke. A variety of physiologic sequelae of sleep apnea (intermittent hypoxia, sympathetic activation, platelet aggregation, and alterations in cerebral blood flow) may account for this risk. CPAP safely and effectively treats sleep apnea and attenuates these physiologic sequelae. Whether CPAP may decrease the high risk of recurrent vascular events among patients with sleep apnea is an important unanswered question.

- Secondary prevention (stroke): Stroke is the third leading cause of death in the United States and, importantly, it is the leading cause of long-term disability. Strategies for stroke prevention including controlling hypertension, smoking cessation, treating diabetes and atrial fibrillation have helped to reduce the burden of stroke, but still remains an important public health challenge. Therefore, there is a need for developing novel therapeutic approaches. Treating obstructive sleep apnea with CPAP may represent one such approach. Currently, few therapeutic strategies are available for patients in the acute stroke setting, with only 5% of patients being candidates for thrombolytic therapy. The treatment of sleep apnea may represent a novel therapeutic strategy for patients with acute stroke that can be applied in the acute setting, to the majority of post-stroke patients, and is well tolerated with a good safety profile. Whether CPAP therapy improves outcomes among post-stroke patients using a randomized controlled trial design is an important unanswered question.

Summary/Public Health Implications

Multiple prospective observational cohort studies have demonstrated that obstructive sleep apnea significantly increases the risk of stroke independent of potential confounding risk factors. This implies that there are mechanisms mediated by sleep apnea that confer vascular risk. The current literature suggests that such mechanisms include: intermittent hypoxia, systemic inflammation, and athersclerosis; nocturnal sympathetic activation; diurnal hypertension; cardiac arrythmia (including atrial fibrillation); mechanical load, metabolic dysregulation, and snoring-induced vibratory injury.

The increasing prevalence of sleep-disordered breathing in the population suggests that the population attributable risk percent is high (the percentage of the total risk of cerebrovascular disease and stroke due to sleep apnea), making this an important public health issue. This is particularly true, given that sleep apnea is a potentially modifiable risk factor. Indeed, guidelines from the American Heart Association/American Stroke Association Stroke Council regarding the primary prevention of ischemic stroke recommend "questioning bed partners and patients, particularly those with abdominal obesity and hypertension, about symptoms of sleep-disordered breathing and referring to a sleep specialist as appropriate" [76].

Short-term randomized controlled trials of CPAP in hypertension/intermediate cardiovascular endpoints and long-term observational cohort studies with follow-up of cerebrovascular and cardiovascular outcomes suggest a clinically significant risk reduction associated with the use of CPAP. However, there are currently no published long term randomized studies demonstrating the efficacy of treating sleep apnea in reducing cerebrovascular outcome events. Such studies are critical prior to instituting large-scale sleep-apnea screening guidelines. In the meantime, clinicians should have a low threshold for evaluating symptoms in their patients consistent with sleep-disordered breathing.

REFERENCES

[1]   AHA. 2005 Heart and Stroke Statistical Update. In: Dallas, Texas.: American Heart Association; 2005.

[2]   Peppard P, Young T, Palta M, Skatrud J. Prospective study of the association between sleep-disordered breathing and hypertension. N Engl J Med 2000; 342: 1378-84.

[3]   Shahar E, Whitney C, Redline S, *et al.* Sleep-disordered breathing and cardiovascular disease: cross-sectional results of the Sleep Heart Health Study. Am J Respir Crit Care Med 2001; 163: 19-25.

[4]   Marin JM, Carrizo SJ, Vicente E, Agusti AG. Long-term cardiovascular outcomes in men with obstructive sleep apnoea-hypopnoea with or without treatment with continuous positive airway pressure: an observational study. Lancet 2005; 365: 1046-53.

[5]   Gami AS, Howard DE, Olson EJ, Somers VK. Day-night pattern of sudden death in obstructive sleep apnea. N Engl J Med 2005; 352: 1206-14.

[6]   Arzt M, Young T, Finn L, *et al.* Association of Sleep-Disordered Breathing and the Occurrence of Stroke. Am J Respir Crit Care Med 2005.

[7]   Yaggi H, Concato J, Kernan W, *et al.* Obstructive Sleep Apnea as a Risk Factor for Stroke and Death. NEJM 2005; 353: 2034-2041.

[8]   Munoz R, Duran-Cantolla J, Martinez-Vila E, *et al.* Severe Sleep Apnea and Risk of Ischemic Stroke in the Elderly. Stroke 2006.

[9]   Marshall NS, Wong KK, Liu PY, *et al.* Sleep apnea as an independent risk factor for all-cause mortality: the Busselton Health Study. Sleep 2008; 31: 1079-85.

[10]   Young T, Finn L, Peppard PE, *et al.* Sleep disordered breathing and mortality: eighteen-year follow-up of the Wisconsin sleep cohort. Sleep 2008; 31: 1071-8.

[11]   Somers VK, Dyken ME, Mark AL, Abboud FM. Sympathetic-nerve activity during sleep in normal subjects. N Engl J Med 1993; 328: 303-7.

[12]   Marler JR, Price TR, Clark GL, *et al.* Morning increase in onset of ischemic stroke. Stroke 1989; 20: 473-6.

[13]   Mohsenin V, Valor R. Sleep apnea in patients with hemispheric stroke. Arch Phys Med Rehabil 1995; 76: 71-6.

[14]   Dyken M, Somers V, Yamada T, *et al.* Investigating the relationship between stroke and obstructive sleep apnea. Stroke. 1996; 27:401-7.

[15]   Bassetti C, Aldrich M. Sleep apnea in acute cerebrovascular diseases: final report on 128 patients. Sleep 1999; 22: 217-23.

[16]   Bassetti C, Aldrich M, Chervin R, Quint D. Sleep apnea in patients with transient ischemic attack and stroke: a prospective study of 59 patients. Neurology. 1996; 47: 1167-73.

[17]   Parra O, Arboix A, Bechich S, *et al.* Time course of sleep-related breathing disorders in first-ever stroke or transient ischemic attack. Am J Respir Crit Care Med 2000; 161: 375-80.

[18]   Mooe T, Rabben T, Wiklund U, *et al.* Sleep-disordered breathing in women: occurrence and association with coronary artery disease. Am J Med 1996; 101: 251-6.

[19]   Peker Y, Kraiczi H, Hedner J, *et al.* An independent association between obstructive sleep apnoea and coronary artery disease. Eur Respir J 1999; 14: 179-84.

[20]   Chaudhary B, Elguindi A, King D. Obstructive sleep apnea after lateral medullary syndrome. South Med J 1982; 75: 65-7.

[21]   Askenasy J, Goldhammer I. Sleep apnea as a feature of bulbar stroke. Stroke 1988; 19: 637-9.

[22]   Waller P, Bhopal R. Is snoring a cause of vascular disease? An epidemiological review. Lancet 1989; 1: 143-6.

[23]   Ryan S, Taylor CT, McNicholas WT. Selective activation of inflammatory pathways by intermittent hypoxia in obstructive sleep apnea syndrome. Circulation 2005; 112: 2660-7.

[24]   Savransky V, Nanayakkara A, Li J, *et al.* Chronic intermittent hypoxia induces atherosclerosis. Am J Respir Crit Care Med 2007; 175: 1290-7.

[25]   Hayashi M, Fujimoto K, Urushibata K, *et al.* Nocturnal oxygen desaturation correlates with the severity of coronary atherosclerosis in coronary artery disease. Chest 2003; 124: 936-941.

[26]   Dyugovskaya L, Lavie P, Lavie L. Increased adhesion molecule expression and production of reactive oxygen species in leukocytes of sleep apnea patients. Am J Respir Crit Care Med 2002; 165: 934-939.

[27]   El-Solh A, Mador M, Sikka P, *et al.* Adhesion molecules in patients with coronary artery disease and moderate-to-severe obstructive sleep apnea. Chest 2002; 121: 1541-1547.

[28]   Ohga E NT, Tomita T, *et al.* Increased levels of circulating I-CAM-1, VCAM-1, and L-selectin in obstructive sleep apnea syndrome. J Appl Physiol 1999; 87: 10-14.

[29]   Lavie L. Obstructive sleep apnoea syndrome--an oxidative stress disorder. Sleep Med Rev 2003; 7: 35-51.

[30]   Lavie L, Dyugovskaya L, Lavie P. Sleep-apnea-related intermittent hypoxia and atherogenesis: adhesion molecules and monocytes/endothelial cells interactions. Atherosclerosis 2005; 183: 183-4.

[31]   Lavie L. Sleep-disordered breathing and cerebrovascular disease: a mechanistic approach. Neurol Clin 2005; 23:1059-75.

[32]   Fletcher E, Miller J, Schaaf J. Urinary catecholamines before and after tracheostomy in patients with obstructive sleep apnea and hypertension. Sleep 1987; 10: 35-44.

[33]   Somers V, Dyken M, Clary M, Abboud F. Sympathetic neural mechanisms in obstructive sleep apnea. J Clin Invest 1995; 96: 1897-904.

[34]   O'Donnell C, King E, Schwartz A, *et al.* Relationship between blood pressure and airway obstruction during sleep in the dog. J. Appl. Physiol. 1994; 77: 1819-1828.

[35]   Hla KM, Young T, Finn L, *et al.* Longitudinal association of sleep-disordered breathing and nondipping of nocturnal blood pressure in the Wisconsin Sleep Cohort Study. Sleep 2008; 31: 795-800.

[36]   O'Brien E, Sheridan J, O'Malley K. Dippers and non-dippers. Lancet 1988; 2: 397.

[37]   Bianchi S, Bigazzi R, Baldari G, *et al.* Diurnal variations of blood pressure and microalbuminuria in essential hypertension. Am J Hypertens 1994; 7: 23-9.

[38]   Verdecchia P, Schillaci G, Guerrieri M. Circadian blood pressure changes and left ventricular hypertrophy. Circulation 1990; 81: 528-536.

[39]   Shimada K, Kawamoto A, Matsubayashi K, Ozawa T. Silent cerebrovascular disease in the elderly. Correlation with ambulatory pressure. Hypertension 1990; 16: 692-9.

[40]   Verdecchia P, Porcellati C, Schillaci G, *et al.* Ambulatory blood pressure. An independent predictor of prognosis in essential hypertension. Hypertension 1994; 24: 793-801.

[41]   Staessen JA, Thijs L, Fagard R, *et al.* Predicting cardiovascular risk using conventional vs ambulatory blood pressure in older patients with systolic hypertension. Systolic Hypertension in Europe Trial Investigators. JAMA 1999; 282: 539-46.

[42]   Kario K, Pickering TG, Matsuo T, *et al.* Stroke prognosis and abnormal nocturnal blood pressure falls in older hypertensives. Hypertension 2001; 38: 852-7.

[43]   Ohkubo T, Hozawa A, Yamaguchi J, *et al.* Prognostic significance of the nocturnal decline in blood pressure in individuals with and without high 24-h blood pressure: the Ohasama study. J Hypertens 2002; 20: 2183-9.

[44]   Neito F, Young T, Lind B, *et al.* Association of sleep-disordered breathing, sleep anea, and hypertension in a large community based study. JAMA 2000; 283: 1829-36.

[45]   Chobanian AV, Bakris GL, Black HR, *et al.* The Seventh Report of the Joint National Committee on Prevention, Detection, Evaluation, and Treatment of High Blood Pressure: the JNC 7 report. JAMA 2003; 289: 2560-72.

[46]   Zwillich C, Devlin T, White D, *et al.* Bradycardia during sleep apnea. Characteristics and mechanism. J Clin Invest 1982; 69: 1286-92.

[47]   Fichter J, Bauer D, Arampatzis S, *et al.* Sleep-related breathing disordes are associated with ventricular arrhythmias in patients with an implantable cardioverter defibrillator. Chest 2002; 122: 558-561.

[48]   Javaheri S, Parker T, Liming J, *et al.* Sleep apnea in 81 ambulatory male patients with stable heart failure: types and their prevalences, consequences, and presentations. Circulation 1998; 97: 2154-59.

[49]   Kanagala R, Murali N, Friedman P, *et al.* Obstructive sleep apnea and the recurrence of atrial fibrillation. Circulation 2003; 107: 2589-94.

[50]   Gami AS, Pressman G, Caples SM, *et al.* Association of atrial fibrillation and obstructive sleep apnea. Circulation 2004; 110: 364-7.

[51]   Bradley T. Right and left ventricular functional impairment and sleep apnea. Clin Chest Med 1992; 13: 459-479.

[52]   Spiegel K, Leproult R, Van Cauter E. Impact of sleep debt on metabolic and endocrine function. Lancet 1999; 354: 1435-9.

[53]   Yaggi HK, Araujo AB, McKinlay JB. Sleep duration as a risk factor for the development of type 2 diabetes. Diabetes Care 2006; 29: 657-61.

[54]   Sulit L, Storfer-Isser A, Kirchner HL, Redline S. Differences in polysomnography predictors for hypertension and impaired glucose tolerance. Sleep 2006; 29: 777-83.

[55]   Ip MS, Lam B, Ng MM, *et al.* Obstructive sleep apnea is independently associated with insulin resistance. Am J Respir Crit Care Med 2002; 165: 670-6.

[56]   Punjabi N, Sorkin J, Katzel L, *et al.* Sleep-disordered breathing and insulin resistance in middle-aged and overweight men. Am J Respir Crit Care Med 2002; 165: 677–682.

[57]   Reichmuth KJ, Austin D, Skatrud JB, Young T. Association of sleep apnea and type II diabetes: a population-based study. Am J Respir Crit Care Med 2005; 172:1590-5.

[58]   Giles T, Lasserson T, Smith B, *et al.* Continuous positive airways pressure for obstructive sleep apnoea in adults. Cochrane Database Syst Rev 2006; 3: CD001106.

[59]   Kaneko Y, Floras J, Usui K, *et al.* Cardiovascular effects of continuous positive airway pressure in patients with heart failure and obstructive sleep apnea. N Engl J Med 2003; 348: 1233-41.

[60]   Becker H, Jerrentrup A, Ploch T, *et al.* Effect of nasal continuous positive airway pressure treatment on blood pressure in patients with obstructive sleep apnea. Circulation 2003; 107: 68-73.

[61]   Faccenda J, Mackay T, Boon N, Douglas N. Randomized placebo-controlled trial of continuous positive airway pressure on blood pressure in the sleep apnea-hypopnea syndrome. Am J Respir Crit Care Med 2001; 163: 344-348.

[62]   Pepperell J, Ramdassingh-Dow S, Crosthwaite N, *et al.* Ambulatory blood pressure after therapeutic and subtherapeutic nasal continuous positive airway pressure for obstructive sleep apnoea: a randomised parallel trial. Lancet 2002; 359: 204-10.

[63]   Findley L, Smith C, Hooper J, *et al.* Treatment with nasal CPAP decreases automobile accidents in patients with sleep apnea. Am J Respir Crit Care Med 2000; 161: 857-9.

[64]   Partinen M, Guilleminault C. Daytime sleepiness and vascular morbidity at seven-year follow-up in obstructive sleep apnea patients. Chest 1990; 97: 27-32.

[65]   Marti S, Sampol G, Munoz X, *et al.* Mortality in severe sleep apnoea/hypopnoea syndrome patients: impact of treatment. Eur Respir J 2002; 20: 1511-8.

[66]   Doherty LS, Kiely JL, Swan V, McNicholas WT. Long-term effects of nasal continuous positive airway pressure therapy on cardiovascular outcomes in sleep apnea syndrome. Chest 2005; 127: 2076-84.

[67]   Barbe F, Mayoralas LR, Duran J, *et al.* Treatment with continuous positive airway pressure is not effective in patients with sleep apnea but no daytime sleepiness. a randomized, controlled trial. Ann Intern Med 2001; 134: 1015-23.

[68]   Monasterio C, Vidal S, Duran J, *et al.* Effectiveness of continuous positive airway pressure in mild sleep apnea-hypopnea syndrome. Am J Respir Crit Care Med 2001; 164: 939-43.

[69]   Haentjens P, Van Meerhaeghe A, Moscariello A, *et al.* The impact of continuous positive airway pressure on blood pressure in patients with obstructive sleep apnea syndrome: evidence from a meta-analysis of placebo-controlled randomized trials. Arch Intern Med 2007; 167: 757-64.

[70] MacMahon S, Peto R, Cutler J, *et al.* Blood pressure, stroke, and coronary heart disease. Part 1, Prolonged differences in blood pressure: prospective observational studies corrected for the regression dilution bias. Lancet 1990; 335: 765-74.

[71] Kanagala R, Murali N, Friedman P, *et al.* Obstructive Sleep Apnea and the Recurrence of Atrial Fibrillaiton. Circulation 2003; 107: 2589-2594.

[72] Drager LF, Bortolotto LA, Figueiredo AC, *et al.* Effects of continuous positive airway pressure on early signs of atherosclerosis in obstructive sleep apnea. Am J Respir Crit Care Med 2007; 176: 706-12.

CHAPTER 20

Sleep and Epilepsy

Silvia Neme-Mercante, M.D.[1] and Nancy Foldvary-Schaefer, D.O., M.S.[2,*]

[1]*Associate Staff, Cleveland Clinic Sleep Disorders Center, 9500 Euclid Avenue, FA20, Cleveland, Ohio 44195, USA and* [2]*Associate Professor of Medicine, Cleveland Clinic Lerner College of Medicine of Case Western Reserve University, Director, Cleveland Clinic Sleep Disorders Center, Cleveland Clinic Neurological Institute, 9500 Euclid Avenue, FA20, Cleveland, Ohio 44195, USA*

Abstract: Over a century of work has confirmed critical links between sleep and epilepsy. Seizures can have profound effects on sleep, typically causing awakenings, arousals and shifts to lighter stages. However, sleep continuity is disrupted in people with epilepsy even in the absence of seizures, suggesting that sleep instability may be an inherent component of certain forms of epilepsy. Antiepileptic drugs (AEDs) can adversely affect sleep and wakefulness. At least some of the newer AEDs appear to have more favorable sleep-wake profiles than the older agents. In turn, sleep is an important modulator of seizures and epileptic discharges on the electroencephalogram (EEG). Sleep instability can promote seizures and sleep deprivation provokes seizures and EEG abnormalities. Synchronized Non-REM (NREM) sleep facilitates seizures, whereas the clinical and EEG manifestations of epilepsy are suppressed in REM sleep. The sleep EEG is useful in the diagnosis and localization of epilepsy. New epileptic foci can appear in sleep and REM sleep demonstrates the most precise localization of the epileptic discharge. Polysomnography combined with video and EEG (VEEG-PSG) aids in the differentiation of seizures and parasomnias. Daytime sleepiness and sleep disorders such as sleep apnea are common in people with epilepsy. Treating sleep apnea has been shown to reduce EEG abnormalities and seizures in some cases. These observations underscore the importance of a routine sleep assessment in case of all the people with epilepsy.

TOPIC DISCUSSION (CLINICAL OUTLOOK)

Summary

The relationship between sleep and epilepsy has been recognized since ancient times. Attention to the effects of sleep on seizures and the EEG and the effects of seizures and AEDs on sleep and wakefulness has important implications on the diagnosis and treatment of epilepsy. Whether sleep disruption is caused by seizures, AED therapy, or a co-existing sleep disorder, an adverse impact on daily functioning is likely. The sleep history should be considered when choosing an AED, as some agents are likely to stabilize sleep, while others destabilize or have no effect. Polysomnography should be considered in people with epilepsy and sleep disorder symptoms, most importantly daytime sleepiness and fatigue.

Epilepsy Basics

Epilepsy, derived from the Greek '*epilepsia*', is characterized by a spontaneous tendency for recurrent seizures [1]. The second most common chronic neurological disorder, epilepsy affects 8.0 per 1000 people in the U.S and over 50 million people worldwide, with 2 million new cases developing annually [2]. Although the majority of patients can be treated successfully with medical therapy, an estimated 30% to 40% of people with epilepsy are drug resistant [3]. Intractable seizures substantially impair quality of life, limiting academic, social and employment opportunities and posing a risk for seizure-related injury and death. Some of the more common epilepsy risk factors include head injury, stroke, central nervous system infection, congenital lesions, febrile seizures and a positive family history of epilepsy.

Seizures are classified as focal or generalized; some types of seizures have characteristic electrographic manifestations, natural history, risk factors, neuroimaging and/or genetic features, facilitating thus the diagnosis of

*Address correspondence to Nancy Foldvary-Schaefer: Associate Professor of Medicine, Cleveland Clinic Lerner College of Medicine of Case Western Reserve University, Director, Cleveland Clinic Sleep Disorders Center, Cleveland Clinic Neurological Institute, 9500 Euclid Avenue, FA20, Cleveland, Ohio 44195; Tel: 216/445-2990; Fax: 216/636-0090, USA; E-mail: foldvan@ccf.org

epilepsy syndromes [4]. Focal seizures originate primarily within networks limited to one cerebral hemisphere.The symptoms and signs in focal seizures are variable, depending on the location of the epileptic focus and the nature of ictal propagation. In contrast, generalized seizures originate within bilaterally distributed networks.

Early Observations on the Relationship Between Sleep and Epilepsy

Before the discovery of the EEG, observations regarding sleep and epilepsy focused on the relation of seizures to clock time and sleep. In 1885, Gowers studied seizure timing in 850 institutionalized people with epilepsy [5]. He noted that 21% patients had seizures exclusively at night (nocturnal epilepsy), 42% had seizures exclusively during the day (diurnal epilepsy), and the remaining 37% had seizures either during the day or at night. Nocturnal seizures seemed to peak 1 to 2 hours after sleep onset and at 5 to 6 AM, near the end of the sleep period, whereas diurnal seizures clustered in the early morning and late afternoon.

Decades later, Janz described a form of idiopathic epilepsy characterized by generalized tonic-clonic seizures (GTCs) on awakening, and coined the term 'awakening epilepsy [6]. He felt that the pattern of seizure occurrence in relation to sleep and wake had etiological significance, as awakening epilepsies were unlikely to have a known organic cause (10%), whereas sleep and random (seizures occurring during sleep and wakefulness) epilepsy more often did (23% and 54%, respectively). Since these early observations, several epilepsy syndromes have been described, in which seizures occur predominately or exclusively from sleep or upon awakening (Table 1).

Table 1: Sleep and Wake Epilepsies

Sleep Epilepsies	Wake Epilepsies
Benign rolandic epilepsy of childhood	Juvenile myoclonic epilepsy
Autosomal dominant nocturnal frontal lobe epilepsy	Absence epilepsy
Symptomatic frontal lobe epilepsy	Epilepsy with grand mal seizures on awakening
Supplementary sensorimotor area epilepsy	
Lennox Gastaut Syndrome (tonic seizures)	
Epilepsy with continuous spike wave during sleep	

Effect of Sleep on Seizures and EEG

Published in 1947, the first systematic study analyzing the diagnostic yield and localizing value of sleep recordings involved 500 patients with various types of epilepsy [7]. Interictal epileptic discharges were observed in 36% of waking EEGs, increasing to 82% during sleep. Sleep recordings revealed additional epileptic foci in some patients who had only one focus during wakefulness. The increased yield of sleep recordings was greatest for patients with focal seizures and least for those with non-convulsive generalized seizures. Countless publications on the effects of sleep on the EEG in epilepsy have since been published.

Many studies have demonstrated that NREM sleep activates epileptic discharges and seizures in focal epilepsy. A recent prospective study analyzed the distribution of more than 600 seizures across the sleep-wake cycle of 133 temporal lobe epilepsy (TLE) patients undergoing video-EEG monitoring [8]. Forty-three percent of seizures arose from sleep and secondary generalized motor seizures arose more often from sleep (55%) than complex partial (42%) and simple partial (35%) seizures. Sleep appears to activate frontal seizures more often than temporal seizures [9]. Furthermore, secondary generalization of focal seizures tends to occur more often during sleep compared to wake and frontal lobe seizures tend not to secondarily generalize during sleep.

Many studies have described the influence of sleep stage on interictal epileptic discharge expression in focal epilepsy. Interictal spike rate increases at sleep onset, gradually peaks in stage non-REM 3 (N3), and then falls in REM (R) sleep to levels lower than seen in wakefulness [10]. In addition, the field of an interictal discharge typically expands during NREM sleep, occasionally accompanied by the appearance of new foci, becoming more diffuse in stage N3 compared to N1 and N2, and more constricted in REM sleep.

Patients with generalized epilepsy also show variation in the occurrence of seizures and epileptic activity on the EEG with sleep and wakefulness [11]. However, sleep may be a less important activator in generalized epilepsy than in the focal epilepsy since epileptic discharges are often present on routine awake EEG recordings. Generalized epileptic discharges usually increase with sleep onset, continue to increase through stage N3, diminish sharply in REM sleep, and increase sharply in the morning after awakening. During NREM sleep, generalized spike-wave discharges often become more disorganized, increasing in amplitude and slowing in frequency; whereas the morphology of discharges in REM sleep is similar to wakefulness. The EEG is most abnormal after awakening in patients with awakening epilepsy (*e.g.* juvenile myoclonic epilepsy). In contrast, the EEG in the sleep epilepsies tends to be normal during wakefulness but shows a marked increase in epileptic discharges during sleep.

Effects of Sleep Deprivation on Seizures and the EEG

Sleep deprivation is one of the most critical public health issues of our time and of major importance for people with epilepsy. The effect of sleep deprivation on epilepsy has been the subject of extensive investigation. Sleep deprivation is recognized as a seizure precipitant, reported by up to one-third of adults with epilepsy, more often in those with awakening epilepsy [6, 12]. In a recent diary study involving 71 adults with focal epilepsy, the odds of a seizure the next day decreased for each hour of sleep the prior night, suggesting that modest amounts of sleep loss can precipitate seizures [12].

In addition to recording sleep, sleep deprivation activates epileptic discharges on the EEG. In a series of studies from the 1980s, the effects of total sleep deprivation (at least 24 hours) was compared in subjects with different seizure types and epilepsy syndromes [13]. For most types of seizures, spontaneous sleep and sleep-deprived recordings produced similar activation rates. However, seizures were more likely to be activated by sleep or sleep deprivation in patients with generalized epilepsy than focal epilepsy.

Whether EEG activation produced by sleep deprivation is due to the recording of sleep itself or an independent activating effect has been the subject of debate. One of the few studies addressing this question found a significantly greater yield of epileptic abnormalities following sleep deprivation compared to routine wake and drug-induced sleep EEGs [14]. Epileptic discharges were seen only on sleep deprived recordings in 28% of subjects and sleep deprivation activated a new epileptic focus in 7% of cases. Comparative studies confirm that sleep deprivation activates epileptic abnormalities on EEG in 23-93% of patients with definite or suspected seizures [15].

Sleep Organization in Epilepsy and the Effects of Seizures, Antiepileptic Drugs and Vagus Nerve Stimulation on Sleep

Numerous studies have described abnormal sleep patterns in people with epilepsy. In general, these include prolonged sleep and REM latency, reduced percentage of REM sleep, increased wake after sleep onset, total sleep time and sleep efficiency, and increased arousals, awakenings and stage shifts [16]. These findings hold true even the absence of seizures and are observed in patients with idiopathic generalized and TLE, although more so in the latter.

Both focal and generalized seizures affect sleep continuity. Nocturnal generalized motor seizures decrease total sleep time and REM sleep, prolong REM latency, and increase stages N1 and N2, time wake after sleep onset and arousals [16]. In a TLE series, a significant decrease in REM sleep was found on nights following daytime seizures, an even greater decrease in REM sleep on nights of seizures, and the greatest amount of REM suppression on nights in which seizures occurred before the first REM period [17]. Both diurnal and nocturnal seizures prolonged REM sleep latency. Nocturnal, but not diurnal, seizures increased stage N1 and decreased N3 sleep. These findings suggest that sleep is inherently unstable in people with epilepsy. Sleep instability promotes seizures and in turn, seizures fragment sleep, thus facilitating the epileptic process.

Antiepileptic drugs (AEDs) have variable effects on sleep and wakefulness, as summarized in Table **2**. The antiepileptic effect of some of these agents may in part be due to a consolatory effect on sleep. In general, the second-generation AEDs are believed to have fewer side effects than older agents. However, no adequately-designed trials have compared the effects of AEDs on sleep or wakefulness. Gabapentin, pregabalin and tiagabine have been used off-label for the treatment of insomnia and restless legs syndrome.

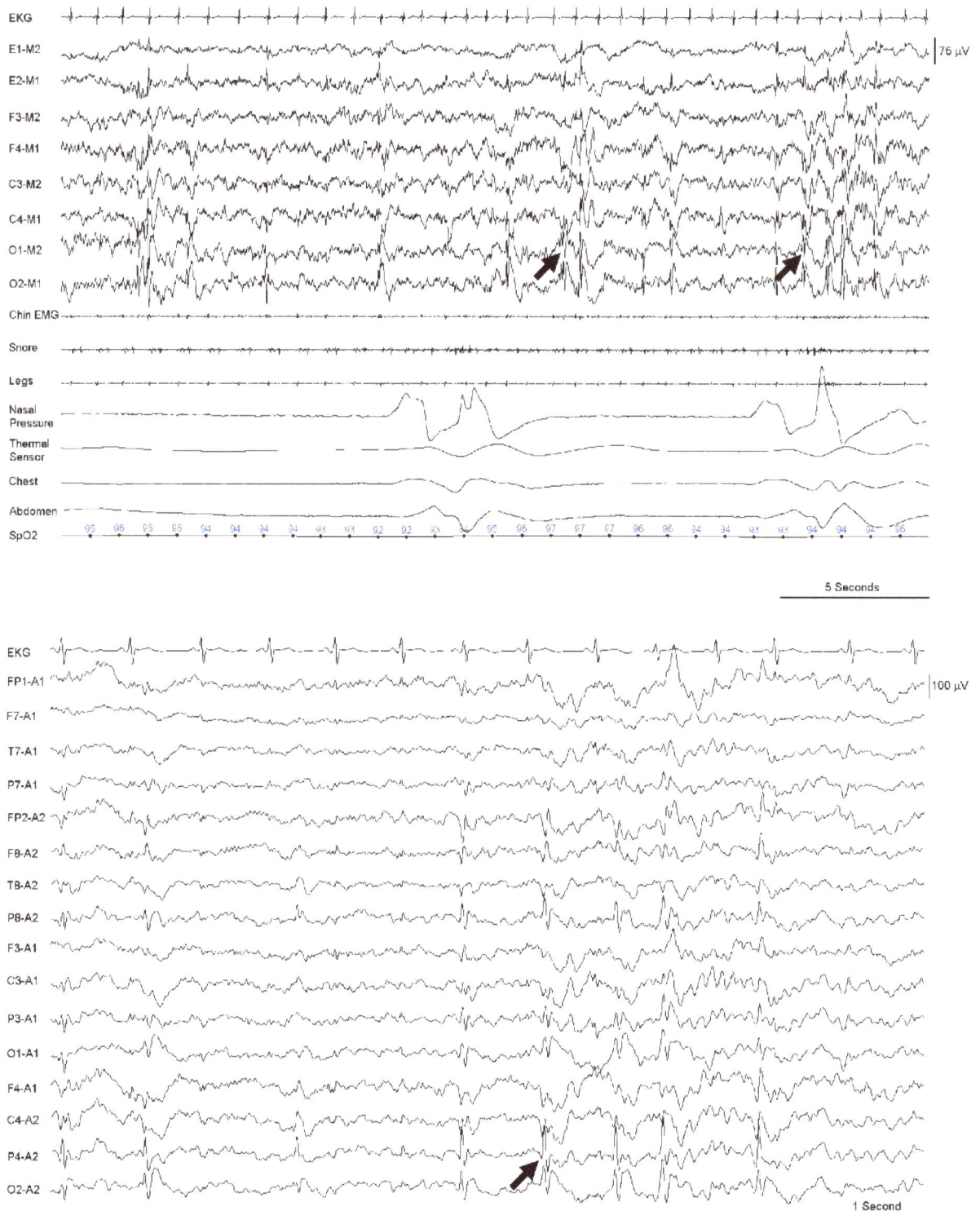

Figure 1: Interictal epileptic discharges in a 9 year old boy with benign rolandic epilepsy of childhood displayed on a routine PSG montage (A) and an expanded EEG in a 10-second epoch (B). Note the poorly localized sharp waves on the PSG recording (arrows) compared to the expanded EEG where sharp waves are observed in the right centro-temporo-parietal region (arrow). The discharges have a stereotypical morphology and dipole when viewed on a referential recording with a positivity (downward deflection) anteriorly (FP2) and a negativity (upward deflection) posteriorly (P8, P4).

Table 2: Effects of Antiepileptic Drugs on Sleep Architecture NA not available; --no change; ↓ decrease; ↑increase

Drug	Sleep latency	Sleep efficiency	Arousals	N1	N2	N3	REM
1st Generation							
Phenobarbital	↓	↑	↓	NA	↑	--	↓
Primidone	↓	NA	NA	NA	NA	↑	↓
Benzodiazepines		NA	NA	↓	↑	↓	NA
Ethoxusamide	NA	NA	NA	↑	NA	↓	NA
Phenytoin	↓	--	↑	↓	↑	↑	↓
Carbamazepine	--	--	↓	--	--	↑	↓
Valproic acid	--	--	--	↑	↑	--	--
2nd Generation							
Felbamate		NA	NA	NA	NA	NA	NA
Gabapentin	NA	--	↓	↓	--	↑	↑
Lamotrigine	NA	--	↓	--	↑	↓	↑
Topiramate	↓	↓	NA	--	--	--	--
Tiagabine		NA	NA	NA	↓	↑	NA
Levetiracetam	--	NA	↑	NA	↑	↓	NA
Oxcarbazepine	NA	NA	NA	NA	NA	↑	↑
Zonisamide	NA	NA	NA	NA	NA	NA	NA
Pregabalin	NA	NA	NA	NA	NA	↑	NA
Lacosamide	NA	NA	NA	NA	NA	NA	NA

Approved by the FDA in 1997 as adjunctive therapy for focal epilepsy in patients over 12 years of age, vagus nerve stimulation (VNS) also produces changes in sleep patterns and daytime wakefulness. The VNS device consists of a pulse generator (implanted subcutaneously in the left infraclavicular region), a spiral bipolar lead (attached around the left vagus nerve), a handheld magnet, and a programming wand with a handheld computer. Although the precise mechanism is unknown, VNS reduces the frequency and severity of seizures by delivering small pulses of electrical stimulation at preset regular intervals, interrupted by periods of no stimulation. In clinical trials, approximately a third of subjects experienced a 50% or greater reduction in seizures. VNS has a variety of effects on sleep and wakefulness in people with epilepsy. Sleep architectural changes including decreased REM sleep and increased awakenings, wake after sleep onset, and stage N1 sleep were observed with stimulation currents over 1.5 mA [18]. Improved daytime alertness and sleep-related decreases in airflow and effort coinciding with VNS activation in patients with epilepsy have also been reported [18-20]. In a study involving 16 patients with intractable epilepsy, sleep apnea emerged after VNS therapy in 4 cases [20]. VNS may produce apneas by altering upper airway muscle tone and/or interfering with central respiratory mechanisms. Lowering the VNS stimulus frequency from 30 Hz to 20 Hz was found to ameliorate VNS-induced respiratory events [21]. A sleep assessment including sleep history followed by diagnostic PSG in cases of suspected obstructive sleep apnea (OSA) should be performed prior to implantation.

Sleep and Wake Disorder Symptoms in Epilepsy

The causes of sleep disturbance and sleep symptoms in patients with epilepsy are many, including factors that are relevant to the general population, such as insufficient sleep, inadequate sleep hygiene and co-existing sleep disorders. Seizures can disrupt sleep, even those occurring during waking hours. Antiepileptic drugs can cause or exacerbate daytime sleepiness, fatigue, insomnia and disturbed nocturnal sleep.

Excessive daytime sleepiness (EDS) is the most common sleep-wake complaint in people with epilepsy. Several studies have found that one-third to one-half of epilepsy patients report EDS [22, 23]. Epworth Sleepiness Scale scores of 10 or greater are seen in as many as 25% of cases [24]. Among 30 consecutive patients with epilepsy who underwent multiple sleep latency testing, the mean sleep latency (MSL) was found to be 8.4 minutes, borderline by standard criteria, and 10% of subjects had a MSL less than 5 minutes [25]. Using the Awake Maintenance Task, treated epilepsy patients were found to be significantly drowsier than untreated patients with epilepsy, patients with multiple sclerosis and normal controls [26].

Results of several studies illustrate the spectrum of sleep and wake complaints in people with epilepsy. In a series of 100 adults with epilepsy, sleep complaints were reported by 30% of patients versus only 10% of controls, with sleep maintenance insomnia, EDS and sleep apnea and restless legs syndrome symptoms predominating [27].

A recent study found that only 39% of 148 patients rated their sleep as always good compared with 79% of 100 healthy control subjects [28]. Patients with epilepsy were significantly more likely to report nocturnal and early morning awakenings, even though their total hours slept was comparable to control subjects. In an earlier study, poor sleep was reported by 37% of epilepsy patients [29]. These individuals exercised less, had more irregular sleep patterns, more naps, and consumed more caffeine, alcohol, and tobacco within 6 hours of bedtime than those without sleep complaints. Epilepsy patients with poor sleep were less likely to be seizure free and more likely to have daytime sleepiness than those without sleep complaints.

Sleep Disorders in Epilepsy

Primary sleep disorders are an important, underappreciated cause of sleepiness and sleep disruption in people with epilepsy. Recent reports suggest that OSA is more common in patients with epilepsy than suspected. Using PSG, 33% of 39 unselected patients with medically resistant focal epilepsy, including 50% of males and 19% of females, had OSA defined by an apnea-hypopnea index (AHI) >10 [30]. Patients with OSA were more likely to be male, have a higher body mass index, and a history of snoring, witnessed apnea or nocturnal seizures. In a study involving older people with epilepsy, the presence of sleep apnea was associated with worsening seizure control or the development of epilepsy later in life [31]. Proposed mechanisms for the increased prevalence of OSA in epilepsy patients include AEDs' effects on central nervous system depression (barbiturates, benzodiazepines) upper airway tone (possibly phenytoin), and weight gain (carbamazepine, valproic acid, gabapentin, pregabalin, among others), reduced physical activity of people with epilepsy leading them to be generally heavier than age-matched controls, and co-morbid endocrinopathies, such as hypothyroidism and polycystic ovarian syndrome.

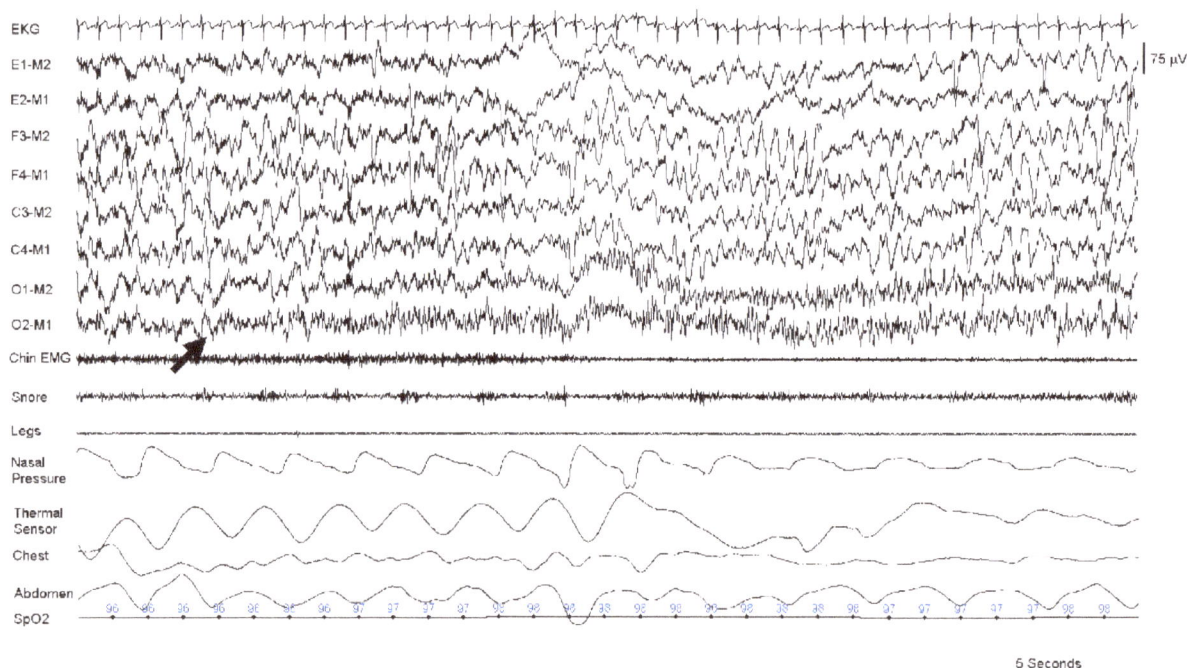

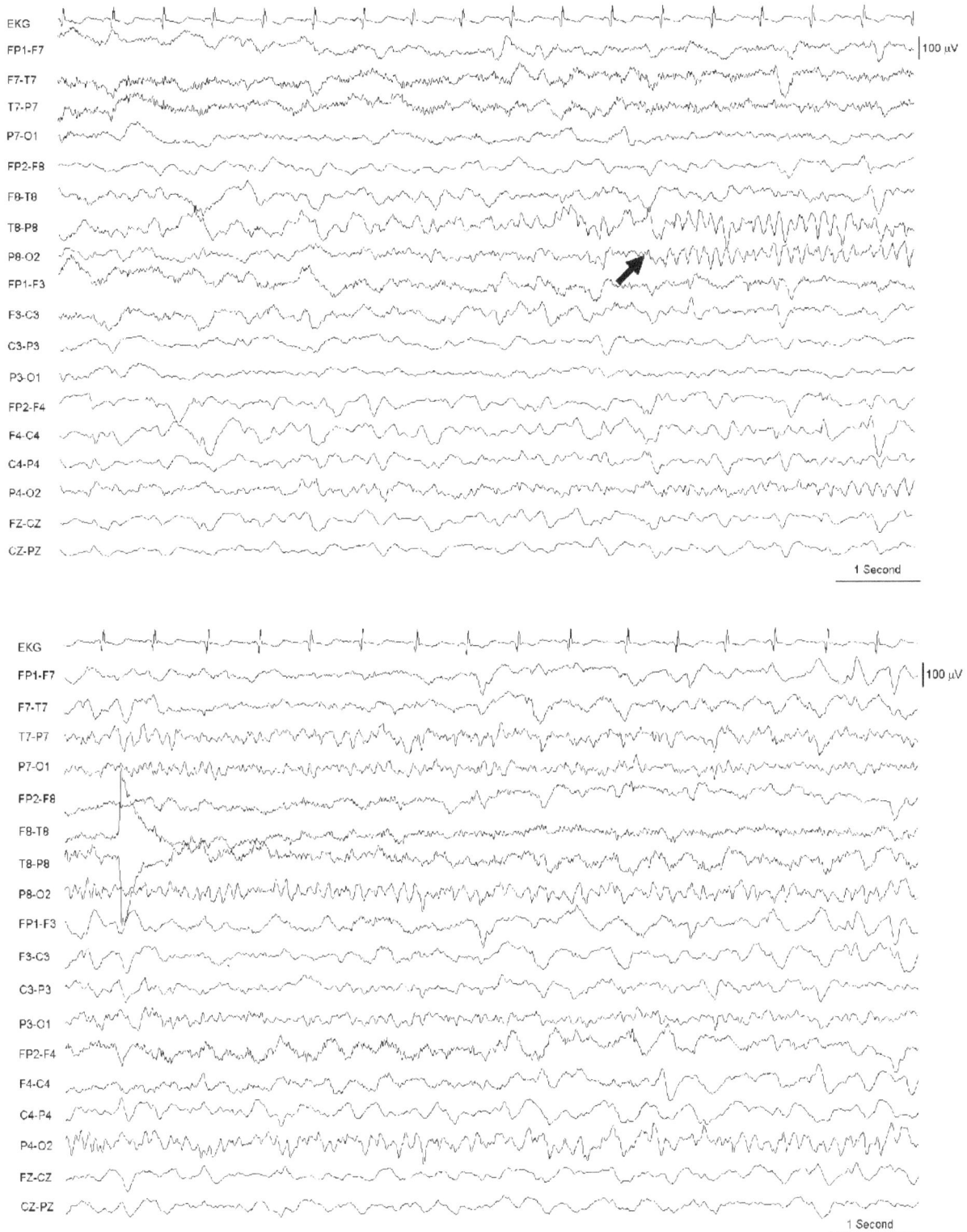

Figure 2: The figures illustrate a right parietal lobe seizure in a 3 year old boy with intractable epilepsy who presented with recurrent awakenings from sleep displayed on a routine PSG montage (A) and an 18-channel EEG (B,C). No clearly recognizable change other than arousal is seen on the PSG recording (A; arrow denotes EEG seizure onset). On the expanded EEG, the EEG onset (B; arrow) consists of rhythmic alpha activity in the right temporo-parietal region that evolves to faster frequencies and superimposed diffuse slow waves in both cerebral hemispheres (C) in the next 10 seconds of the seizure.

The treatment of OSA has since been shown to reduce seizures in 40- 86% of adults with epilepsy [32,33]. A recent randomized pilot trial was published investigating the impact of OSA treatment in epilepsy [34]. Adults with intractable epilepsy and OSA were randomized to therapeutic or sham continuous positive airway pressure (CPAP) for 10 weeks. Subjects maintained seizure calendars and AED therapy were held constant. Thirty- five subjects were randomized to therapeutic (22) or sham (13) CPAP. The baseline AHI and CPAP adherence were comparable between groups. While the study was not powered to detect differences in seizure frequency between groups, a seizure reduction of 50% or greater occurred in 28% of therapeutic CPAP subjects and only 15% of controls.

Possible explanations for improved seizure control with OSA therapy include improvement or resolution of sleep fragmentation, sleep deprivation, cerebral hypoxemia, cardiac output and cardiac arrhythmias. A study involving 8 subjects with focal epilepsy and OSA or hypoxia in sleep found that CPAP not only normalized the AHI, but markedly reduced spike rate (number of interictal discharges per unit time in sleep) [35]. These findings support the concept that sleep related breathing increase excitability in the epileptic brain.

Differentiating Seizures and Parasomnias – The Use of Video Electroencephalography-Polysomnography (VEEG-PSG)

The differential diagnosis of unusual behaviors and movements in sleep includes epilepsy (most often nocturnal frontal lobe epilepsy [NFLE]), NREM arousal disorders (confusional arousals, sleep terrors and sleepwalking), REM sleep behavior disorder, nocturnal panic attacks, psychogenic disorders and movement disorders (Table 3). The diagnosis of nocturnal spells is challenging because of the overlapping features of epileptic seizures, parasomnias and other nonepileptic events in sleep. Seizure recognition during PSG is particularly difficult due to the limited number of channels dedicated to EEG. In contrast to parasomnias, nocturnal frontal lobe seizures typically have an abrupt onset, are accompanied by sustained asymmetric dystonic, tonic posturing and hypermotor behaviors including thrashing, pedaling and kicking, tend to be stereotyped for the individual, are brief, typically lasting 20-30 seconds, are associated with preserved awareness, and have no postictal confusion or amnesia [36]. In contrast, panic attacks, nonepileptic psychogenic seizures, and arousal disorders tend to be less stereotyped and more variable in duration and clinical manifestations. Movement disorders typically present during wakefulness and are associated with abnormalities on neurological examination.

Table 3: Differential Diagnosis of Abnormal Behaviors in Sleep

Disorder	Time of onset	Event recollection	Stereotypy	PSG/EEG findings
Disorders of Arousal	First 1/3 of sleep period	No	No	N3 sleep arousal
REM sleep behavior disorder	Last 1/3 of sleep period	Dream recall	No	REM sleep without atonia
Nocturnal frontal lobe seizures	Any	Usually	Yes	Epileptic activity, slow waves or no EEG change
Nonepileptic psychogenic seizures	During wake time	Variable	No	Normal awake EEG despite behavioral sleep
Nocturnal panic disorder	Any	Yes	No	Arousal from light NREM with normal awake EEG

Over recent decades, the use video- electroencephalography combined with PSG (VEEG-PSG) has begun to elucidate the spectrum of abnormal behaviors in sleep. VEEG-PSG has several advantages over standard PSG including the ability to analyze motor behavior, correlate behavior with EEG, and more accurately detect seizure activity due to the additional scalp electrodes. VEEG-PSG is particularly valuable in patients with frequent sleep-related spells that fail to respond to conventional treatments, normal awake EEGs and suspected sleep disorders.

Among 122 patients with suspected parasomnias that underwent video PSG with 12 to 16 channels of EEG, 35% were given a definite diagnosis of epilepsy or a sleep disorder and 30% had supportive evidence of one or the other diagnosis [37]. We performed two investigations to compare the yield of abbreviated EEG montages to the 18-

channel EEG in patients with abnormal sleep-related behaviors [38, 39]. In both studies, electroencephalographers were better able to differentiate seizures from non-epileptic events using 18-channel recordings. Seizures arising from the temporal or parietal-occipital regions were more likely to be correctly identified and localized than those arising from the frontal lobe. This is particularly important since seizures localized to the frontal region are most often confused with parasomnias and nonepileptic, psychogenic events.

The challenge of identifying epileptic discharges and seizures during PSG is compounded by a variety of factors including the number of available EEG electrodes, location of the epileptic generator, display speed, video quality and experience of the polysomnographer. Differentiating frontal lobe seizures and parasomnias by EEG alone is difficult, since only about one-third of frontal lobe seizures are accompanied by clear ictal rhythms on scalp EEG; another one-third are characterized by diffuse, nonlateralized EEG changes not unlike that of the arousal disorders; and the remainder by no recognizable EEG changes other than those attributed to muscle artifact.

The frontal lobe epilepsies are perhaps the most studied of all sleep-related epilepsies. In 1981, Lugaresi reported a series of patients with stereotyped movements in sleep consisting of asymmetric tonic or dystonic posturing and bizarre behaviors having choreoathetoid or ballistic features lasting 20 to 30 seconds without associated EEG abnormalities [40]. He questioned whether this disorder, initially called hypnogenic paroxysmal dystonia, and later nocturnal paroxysmal dystonia (NPD), represented a previously unrecognized form of epilepsy. Subsequently, detailed analyses of seizures arising from the orbitofrontal and mesial frontal regions confirmed that the semiology of Lugaresi's cases overlapped with that of frontal lobe epilepsy. The epileptic nature of NPD was confirmed by intracranial EEG recordings and the term nocturnal frontal lobe epilepsy (NFLE) was coined.

NFLE is a heterogeneous disease [41]. Familial, sporadic, idiopathic, cryptogenic and symptomatic forms have been observed. The familial form, known as autosomal dominant nocturnal frontal lobe epilepsy (ADNFLE), constitutes as many as 25% of cases. Linkage studies have localized genes for ADNFLE to chromosomes 20q13 and 15q24 with mutations in the transmembrane region of the neuronal nicotinic acetylcholine receptor (nAChR) alpha4-subunit (CHRNA4), beta2-subunit (CHRNB2), and alpha2-subunit (CHRNA2). The nAChRs are ion channels distributed widely on neuronal and glial membranes in cortical and subcortical regions of the brain. These channels regulate the release of acetylcholine, gamma-hydroxybutyric acid and glutamate and have a modulatory effect on arousals at the cortical and thalamic levels. It is hypothesized that these receptor mutations cause changes in neuronal excitability preferentially affecting the mesial prefrontal area and regulate microarousals thereby destabilizing sleep [42].

Seizures in patients with NFLE occur exclusively or predominately during sleep and can be of virtually any type. In a series of 100 consecutive patients with NFLE, three subgroups of clinical presentation were identified [41]. Paroxysmal arousals, consisting of brief episodes of sudden eye opening, head raising or sitting up in bed, often with a frightened expression and sometimes vocalization; nocturnal paroxysmal dystonia described as episodes of intermediate duration characterized by wide, often ballistic movements, dystonic posturing or choreoathetoid movements of head, trunk, limbs and vocalization; and episodic nocturnal wandering characterized by longer duration paroxysmal ambulation, accompanied by screaming and bizarre, dystonic movements. Most attacks were brief and repetitive with sudden onset and offset and accompanied by marked autonomic activation. Consciousness was usually preserved, and motor features were stereotyped. The age at onset ranged from infancy to adolescence, and there was a slight male predominance. A personal or family history of parasomnia was present in more than one-third of cases. Epileptic activity was not observed in the EEGs of nearly half the affected individuals.

The Frontal Lobe Epilepsy and Parasomnias (FLEP) scale has been proposed as an adjunct in the diagnosis of NFLE [43]. This is an 11-item tool completed by the clinician addressing clinical features of sleep-related behaviors. A total score of zero or less is very unlikely to be seen in epilepsy, whereas, patients scoring 3 or greater generally have epilepsy. Video EEG monitoring or PSG is recommended for those with intermediate FLEP scores of +1 to +3. The sensitivity and specificity of the FLEP in the identification of NFLE was 71.4% and 100%, respectively [44].

RESEARCH OUTLOOK

Summary:

Seizures preferentially occur during sleep and in some types of epilepsy. The most extensively investigated of these disorders is ADNFLE. Patients with ADNFLE have seizures with clinical manifestations that can be indistinguishable from disorders of arousal. A better understanding the pathophysiology of ADNFLE and similar sleep-related seizure disorders will help to elucidate the mechanisms by which sleep regulates the expression of seizures and EEG abnormalities in people with epilepsy. It remains uncertain as to whether there is a common substrate for nocturnal seizures and parasomnias.

Few well-designed studies have explored the effects of AEDs on sleep and wakefulness. Equally important are studies examining the prevalence and predictors of primary sleep disorders, such as insomnia, restless legs syndrome and sleep apnea in adults and children with epilepsy. A better understanding of these effects and relationships might influence the choice of therapy in people with epilepsy, ultimately having a positive impact on seizure control and quality of life.

What do we know:

Synchronized NREM sleep facilitates and desynchronized REM sleep discourages seizure occurrence. Sleep deprivation provokes seizures and epileptic activity in some patients with epilepsy.

Seizures, interictal epileptic discharges and some AEDs adversely affect sleep quality and quantity in patients with epilepsy.

Excessive daytime sleepiness is the most common complaint of patients with epilepsy likely due to seizures, epilepsy treatments and co-morbid sleep disorders.

Obstructive sleep apnea is more common in epilepsy patients than the general population. Treatment of OSA has been shown to improve seizure control in some patients.

VEEG-PSG is a valuable tool for the evaluation of patients with abnormal sleep-related movements and behaviors and should be considered in patients who fail to respond to conventional therapy and when routine and sleep-deprived EEG fails to establish a diagnosis.

What we don't know:

Systematic trials to determine the incidence of primary sleep disorders in epilepsy are needed.

A better understanding of the effects of the newer AEDs on sleep and wakefulness is required. This would permit clinicians to choose agents by taking into account a patient's sleep history.

Given the prevalence of daytime sleepiness in the epilepsy population, further studies are needed to determine the effect of sleepiness on quality of life in epilepsy and develop appropriate management strategies for sleepy people with epilepsy.

The effect of melatonin on epilepsy is still unclear; future studies need to assess the intrinsic circadian derangements attributable to melatonin secretory cycle disruption, AEDs and seizures.

The complex regulation of circadian clock genes can be disrupted by seizures, although no studies so far have evaluated these regulatory patterns in epilepsy.

Virtually no studies have focused on the relationships between sleep and epilepsy in pediatric patients.

REFERENCES

[1]	World Health Organization: Neurological disorders: Public health challenges: Global burden of neurological disorders. http://www.who.int/mental_health/neurology/neurodiso/en/index.html, accessed on 2/17/2010.
[2]	Hirtz D, Thurman DJ, Gwinn-Hardy K, *et al.* How common are the "common" neurologic disorders? Neurology 2007; 68: 326-37.
[3]	Mohanraj R, Brodie MJ. Diagnosing refractory epilepsy: Response to sequential treatment schedules. Eur J Neurol 2006; 13: 277-82.

[4]   Berg AT, Berkovic SF, Brodie MJ, *et al.* Revised terminology and concepts for organization of seizures and epilepsies: Report of the ILAE Commission on Classification and Terminology, 2005–2009. *Epilepsia* 2010; 51: 676–85.

[5]   Gowers W. Course of epilepsy. In: Gowers, W, Ed. Epilepsy and other chronic convulsive diseases: their causes, symptoms and treatment. New York: William Wood 1885; 157-64.

[6]   Janz D. The grand mal epilepsies and the sleep waking cycle. Epilepsia 1962; 3: 69–109.

[7]   Gibbs EL, Gibbs FA. Diagnostic and localizing value of electroencephalographic studies in sleep. Nerv Ment Dis 1947; 26: 366-76.

[8]   Herman ST, Walczak TS, Bazil CW. Distribution of partial seizures during the sleep-wake cycle: differences by seizure onset site. Neurology 2001; 56: 1453-9.

[9]   Crespel A, Coubes P, Baldy-Moulinier M. Sleep influence on seizures and epilepsy effects on sleep in partial frontal and temporal lobe epilepsies. Clin Neurophysiol 2000; 111(Suppl 2): S54-9.

[10]   Sammaritano M, Gigli GL, Gotman J. Interictal spiking during wakefulness and sleep and the localization of foci in temporal lobe epilepsy. Neurology 1991; 41: 290-7.

[11]   Ross JJ, Johnson L, Walter RD. Spike and wave discharges during stages of sleep. Arch Neurol 1966; 14: 399-407.

[12]   Haut SR, Hall CB, Masur J, Lipton RB. Seizure occurrence: precipitants and prediction. Neurology 2007; 69: 1905-10.

[13]   Degen R, Degen HE. Sleep and sleep deprivation in epileptology. Epilepsy Res Suppl 1991; 2: 235–60.

[14]   Rowan AJ, Veldhuisen RJ, Nagelkerke NJD. Comparative evaluation of sleep deprivation and sedated sleep EEGs as diagnostic aids in epilepsy. Electroencephalogr Clin Neurophysiol 1982; 54: 357–64.

[15]   Foldvary-Schaefer N, Grigg-Damberger M. Sleep and Epilepsy: What We Know, Don't Know, and Need to Know. J Clin Neurophysiol 2006; 23: 4-20.

[16]   Touchon J, Baldy-Moulinier M, Billiard M, Besset A, Cadilhac J. Sleep organization and epilepsy. In: Degen R and Rodin EA, eds. Epilepsy, sleep and sleep deprivation, 2nd ed. Amsterdam: Elsevier Science Publishers 1991; 73-81.

[17]   Bazil, CW, Castro, LHM, Walczak, TS. Reduction of rapid eye movement sleep by diurnal and nocturnal seizures in temporal lobe epilepsy. Arch Neurol 2000; 57: 363-8.

[18]   Rizzo P, Beelke M, De Carli F, *et al.* Chronic vagal nerve stimulation improves alertness and reduces rapid eye movement sleep in patients affected by refractory epilepsy. Sleep 2003; 26: 607-11.

[19]   Galli R, Bonanni E, Pizzanelli C, *et al.* Daytime vigilance and quality of life in epileptic patients treated with vagal nerve stimulation. Epilepsy Beh 2003; 4: 185-91.

[20]   Marzec M, Edwards J, Sagher O, Fromes G, Malow BA. Effects of vagal nerve stimulation on sleep related breathing in epilepsy patients. Epilepsia 2003; 44: 930-5.

[21]   Malow BA, Edwards J, Marzec M, *et al.* Effects of vagus nerve stimulation on respiration during sleep: a pilot study. Neurology 2000; 55: 1450–4.

[22]   Collaborative Group for the Study of Epilepsy. Adverse reactions to antiepileptic drugs: a multicenter survey of clinical practice. Epilepsia 1986; 27: 323-30.

[23]   Weintraub DB, Resor SR, Bazil CW, Hirsch LJ. Head to head comparison of the sedating effect of antiepileptic durgs in adults with epilepsy. Neurology 2005; 64: A22-3.

[24]   Malow BA, Bowes RJ, Lin X. Predictors of sleepiness in epilepsy patients. Sleep 1997; 20: 1105-10.

[25]   Drake ME, Weate SJ, Newell SA, Padamadan H, Pakalnis A. Multiple sleep latency tests in epilepsy. Clin Electroencephalogr 1994; 25: 59-62.

[26]   Salinsky MC, Oken BS, Binder LM. Assessment of drowsiness in epilepsy patients receiving chronic antiepileptic drug therapy. Epilepsia 1996; 37: 181-7.

[27]   Khatami R, Zutter D, Siegel A, *et al.* Sleep-wake habits and disorders in a series of 100 adult epilepsy patients: A prospective study. Seizure 2006; 15: 299-306.

[28]   Abad-Alegria F, Lopez-Mallen ME, de Francisco-Maqueda P. Insomnio y somnolencia en epilepsia. Rev Neurol 1997; 25: 1171–2.

[29]   Lannon SL, Vaughn BV. Sleep hygiene in people with epilepsy. Epilepsia 1997; 38: 227.

[30]   Malow BA, Levy K, Maturen K, Bowes R. Obstructive sleep apnea is common in medically refractory epilepsy patients. Neurology 2000; 55: 1002-7.

[31]   Chihorek AM, Abou-Khalil B, Malow BA. Obstructive sleep apnea is associated with seizure occurrence in older adults with epilepsy. Neurology 2007; 69: 1823-7.

[32]   Devinsky O, Ehrenberg B, Barthlen GM, Abramson HS, Luciano D. Epilepsy and sleep apnea syndrome. Neurology 1994; 44: 2060-4.

[33]   Vaughn BV, D'Cruz OF, Beach R, Messenheimer JA. Improvement of epileptic seizure control with treatment of obstructive sleep apnea. Seizure 1996; 5: 73-8.

[34]   Malow BA, Foldvary-Schaefer N, Vaughn BV, *et al.* Treating Obstructive Sleep Apnea in Adults with Epilepsy: A Randomized Pilot Trial. Neurology 2008; 71: 572-7.

[35]   Oliveira AJ, Zamagni M, Dolso P, Bassetti MA, Gigli GL. Respiratory disorders during sleep in patients with epilepsy: Effect of ventilatory therapy on EEG nterictal epileptiform discharges. Clin Neurophysiol 2000; 111: S141-5.

[36]   Zucconi M, Oldani A, Ferini-Strambi L, Bizzozero D, Smirne S. Nocturnal paroxysmal arousals with motor behaviors during sleep: frontal lobe epilepsy or parasomnia? J Clin Neurophysiol 1997; 14: 513-522.

[37]   Aldrich MS, Jahnke B. Diagnostic value of video-EEG polysomnography. Neurology 1991; 41: 1060-6.

[38]   Foldvary-Schaefer N, De Ocampo J, Mascha E, Burgess R, Dinner D, Morris H. Accuracy of seizure detection using abbreviated EEG during polysomnography. J Clin Neurophysiol 2006; 23: 68-71.

[39]   Foldvary N Sleep Caruso AC; Mascha E; Perry M; Klem G; McCarthy V; Qureshi F; Dinner D. Identifying montages that best detect electrographic seizure activity during polysomnography. Sleep 2000; 23: 221-9.

[40]   Lugaresi E, Cirignotta F.Hypnogenic paroxysmal dystonia: epileptic seizure or a new syndrome? Sleep 1981; 4: 129-38.

[41]   Provini F, Plazzi G, Tinuper P, Vandi S, Elio Lugaresi E, Montagna P. Nocturnal frontal lobe epilepsy: A clinical and polygraphic overview of 100 consecutive cases. Brain 1999; 122: 1017–31.

[42]   Romcy-Pereira RN, Leite JP, Garcia-Cairasco N. Synaptic plasticity along the sleep–wake cycle: Implications for epilepsy. Epilepsy Behav 2009; 14: 47–53.

[43]   Derry CP, Davey M, Johns M *et al.* Distinguishing sleep disorders from seizures: diagnosing bumps in the night. Arch Neurol 2006; 63: 705-9.

[44]   Manni R, Terzaghi M, and Repetto A. The FLEP scale in diagnosing nocturnal frontal lobe epilepsy, NREM and REM parasomnias: Data from a tertiary sleep and epilepsy unit. Epilepsia 2008; 49: 1581–5.

CHAPTER 21

Pediatric Sleep Issues

Paul R. Carney, M.D.[1,*], Sachin S. Talathi, Ph.D.[2] and James D. Geyer, M.D.[3]

[1]Wilder Professor and Chief, Division of Pediatric Neurology, Departments of Pediatrics, Neurology and Neuroscience, J Crayton Pruitt Department of Biomedical Engineering, University of Florida Mc Knight Brain Institute, Gainesville, Florida, USA; [2]Assistant Professor, Division of Pediatric Neurology, Department of Pediatrics, University of Florida, Gainesville, Florida, USA and [3]Director, Sleep Program, Associate Professor of Neurology and Sleep Medicine, Alabama Neurology and Sleep Medicine, Tuscaloosa, Alabama, USA

Abstract: Pediatric sleep disorders are quite common and often disturbing to either the patient or the child's family. As the patient matures into adult, sleep disorders continue to be common and an important factor in development, both social and cognitive. Sleep disorders can adversely impact physical and mental health. Non-restorative sleep can hamper a child's ability to concentrate and control emotions and behavior. Sleep disorders vary among age groups, but most can occur with varying frequency at any age.

Several disorders are typically seen only during the first few years of life, including colic, excessive nighttime feedings, and sleep onset association disorder. A number of conditions are common during childhood but begin to improve as the child ages. The non-REM sleep parasomnias, including sleepwalking, confusional arousals, and night terrors, are the most common in the pediatric category. Nightmares are also common in childhood but can occur at any age.

Sleep-related breathing disorders including obstructive sleep apnea, central sleep apnea, central alveolar hypoventilation syndrome, and Cheyne-Stokes respirations are not found only in adults but are, in fact, quite common in the pediatric population. While these disorders can occur at any age, treatment options vary substantially by age.

TOPIC DISCUSSION (CLINICAL OUTLOOK)

Disorders During the First 3 Years of Life

The most common sleep-related problems for children between ages 6 months and 3 years arise because of difficulty initiating or maintaining sleep [1]. Numerous factors have been implicated in the occurrence of repetitive nocturnal waking and inability to fall asleep: infant temperament, nutrition, physical discomfort, mild allergy, and parental marital conflict [2, 3].

Sleep-Onset Association Disorder

Clinical Features

Sleep complaints in the infant and young child usually come from the parents, not the child. Nighttime awakenings often become worrisome to parents. However, as might be expected, the problems often reflect certain established patterns of interaction between the parent and the child at the time of sleep transition. Nighttime arousals are very common in all ages; however, older children and adults are usually unaware of these disruptions.

Causes/Pathogenesis

Parents may incorrectly conclude that nocturnal awakenings are abnormal, and become involved in the sleep transition process. The child may then become accustomed to parental intervention and become unable to make the transition back to sleep alone. This is known as sleep-onset association disorder. The child is then reliant on the parent to help complete the sleep transition regardless of the time of night.

*****Address correspondence to Paul R. Carney:** Wilder Professor and Chief, Division of Pediatric Neurology, Departments of Pediatrics, Neurology and Neuroscience, J Crayton Pruitt Department of Biomedical Engineering, University of Florida Mc Knight Brain Institute, Gainesville, Florida, USA; E-mail: carnepr@peds.ufl.edu

Diagnosis and Treatment

Diagnosis is made with a careful history. Children with this disorder usually respond rapidly to simple gradual behavioral interventions, which helps the child learn a new set of sleep- associated habits [4].

Difficulties Learning to Sleep Alone

Clinical Features

The ability to sleep alone throughout the night without parental intervention is a learned process. Children typically awaken 5 to 8 times per night, at the end of each sleep cycle, but some children are able to put themselves back to sleep without parental awareness or intervention. Most infants are capable of learning this process by about 5 to 7 months of age [1].

Diagnosis and Treatment

The key to this process is to gradually withdraw the amount of parental involvement at sleep onset. This same parental behavior response is required for middle-of-the-night awakenings. Consistency is of critical importance if the treatment plan is going to work, especially in conditioning the child to sleep throughout the night. When fear is affecting the progression of this process, it is important to address the child's and/or parent's anxiety effectively. Fear on the part of the child can prevent sleep. In such cases, it is important for the parents to problem-solve about their child's fear and how to best accommodate the behavioral treatment plan. Fear regarding the safety of one's child can alter a planned behavioral intervention. Parents must be aware of their own fears and anxieties so that these do not cause the sleep disturbance in the child.

Excessive Nighttime Feedings

Clinical Features

An increase in nighttime awakenings among infants and toddlers may be related to nighttime feedings. Infants fed large quantities at night (8-32 oz) tend to have frequent awakenings, ranging up to eight per night [4-7]. Repeated awakenings for feeding disrupt the functioning of circadian-modulated systems, which may cause further deleterious effects on sleep-wake stabilization [4, 8, 9].

Diagnosis and Treatment

Diagnosis relies on a characteristic history: multiple nocturnal awakenings, return to sleep only with feeding, significant fluid intake during the night, and extremely wet diapers. Treatment consists of a gradual decrease in the frequency of feedings during the night [4]. Frequent awakenings, three or more per night in a child over 6 months of age, may cause sleep fragmentation that has a deleterious effect on a child. As feedings decrease and associated habits are eliminated over several weeks, sleep consolidation usually promptly occurs [7].

Limit Setting

Clinical Features

Inability to set limits at bedtime can also cause sleep deterioration. Typical bedtime struggles may consist of requests for water, stories, use of the bathroom, and adjustment of lights [4, 7]. A diagnosis of this sort can be made from the history alone. The parents are typically unable to enforce nighttime rules with enough consistency to keep the child in bed and quiet so that he or she can initiate asleep.

Diagnosis and Treatment

Parents have to learn to be firm in their limit setting, enforcing a regular bedtime ritual with sleep onset as the goal. The child should also be kept in his or her bedroom with the use of a gate or closure of the door if necessary. Positive behavior modification using techniques such as a sticker or star chart, as well as other prizes for staying in bed, may elicit a positive response [4].

Fear

Clinical Features

Fear and nightmares are also common in early childhood, and represent an element of normal development. A truly anxious child at night should be handled in the same manner whether the child's fears were initially expressed during waking or sleep.

Diagnosis and Treatment

Mild fears often respond to supportive firmness and a stable social setting. Positive reinforcement, with rewards for staying in bed, may help motivate the child. Treatment may also consist of sleep schedule correction, progressive relaxation [10], and progressive desensitization [11]. Only in rare instances are medications indicated.

Colic

Clinical Features

Colic is the most common medical condition affecting the sleep of young infants. It causes an inconsolable fussiness and crying, typically in the late afternoon and evening. Although symptoms usually resolve spontaneously by 3 to 4 months of age, the sleep disturbances often persist, secondary to altered sleep schedules and habitual patterns of the parental responsiveness [7].

Diagnosis and Treatment

Colic is diagnosed when there are unexplained spells of crying in healthy infants. Treatment mainly focuses on education and management strategies for helping the parents cope with the stresses of caring for the infant [12].

PARASOMNIAS—NOCTURNAL EVENTS

In the course of clinical practice many unusual nocturnal phenomena may be described by the child or parents. The correct diagnosis can usually be ascertained from the clinical history alone but in some cases video polysomnography may be necessary. Additional EEG leads should be used if a seizure disorder is suspected and additional EMG leads can be useful in patients with movement disorders.

Nocturnal movement disorders are extremely common in the pediatric population. In some cases, these events are so common that they may be considered a normal component of childhood and are usually "outgrown".

Restless Legs Syndrome

Clinical Features

Restless legs syndrome is a disorder composed of four principal diagnostic criteria; 1) Intense, irresistible desire to move limbs, usually with uncomfortable feeling in the limbs, 2) Symptoms worsen with decreased activity, 3) Symptoms improve with activity, and 4) Symptoms are typically worse at night [13]. Restless legs syndrome may cause significant sleep onset insomnia.

Adult patients often have difficulty describing the symptoms. Children have even greater difficulty describing the symptoms and are frequently ignored by adults (including physicians). Patients may described the subjective symptoms of RLS in a number of ways including creepy, painful, burning, aching, electrical, crawly, tingly, like worms or bugs crawling under the skin, *etc.* In children, these symptoms can easily be mistaken for "growing pains". Children may get into trouble at school or at home because they can have difficulty sitting still. Restless legs syndrome is significantly underdiagnosed or mis-diagnosed because of these factors.

Epidemiology

Restless legs syndrome has an age-adjusted prevalence of up to 10% of adults. While it is less common in children and increases with increasing age, the syndrome is underdiagnosed in children. The symptom severity also typically worsens with increasing age. Primary restless legs syndrome is a genetic disorder with an autosomal dominant pattern. Secondary restless legs syndrome, associated with a precipitating factor, is less common in younger patients. Renal failure, iron deficiency, and diabetes may contribute to the restlessness. In children, growing pains may mimic or cause restless legs.

Evaluation

The laboratory evaluation of RLS includes serum ferritin, screening for uremia and screening for diabetes. Low normal ferritin levels (20-60 ng/mL) may be associated with RLS and frequently respond to treatment with iron

[14]. Other vitamin, hormone and mineral derangements can also contribute to the symptoms. Polysomnography is not indicated in the evaluation of RLS, unless there is suspicion of a comorbid sleep disorder.

Treatment

Dopamine agonist therapy is the mainstay of RLS treatment in adults. No agents have been FDA approved for treatment of RLS in children. Fortunately, the use of simple non-pharmacological therapies may be of significant benefit including teaching the child to visualize an activity or simply allowing the child to move/swing the legs. Teachers should be informed of the condition. The fact that it is not a form of attention deficit disorder should be reinforced. Symptoms may be caused by an underlying iron or vitamin deficiency and supplementing with iron, vitamin B_{12}, or folate (as indicated) may be sufficient to relieve symptoms in these specific cases.

Periodic Limb Movement Disorder

Clinical Features

Periodic limb movement disorder (PLMD) is "characterized by periodic episodes of repetitive and highly stereotyped limb movements that occur during sleep" ([15], [16]). While these movements usually occur in the legs they can also occur in the arms. There is typically extension of the toe and flexion of the ankle, and possibly the knee and hip as well. Most patients are unaware of the movements. The sleep disruption associated with the movements can lead to insomnia or daytime somnolence. There is a repetitive increase in EMG activity (most often measured over the anterior tibialis muscle) lasting 0.5 to 5 seconds. The periodic limb movement index is the total number of periodic limb movements divided by the total hours of sleep. A PLM index over 5 is considered abnormal. Periodic limb movements may be associated with arousals. While many assume that the higher the PLM-arousal index the more like one is to suffer from daytime sleepiness this has not been proven ([15], [16]).

Epidemiology

Periodic leg movements often accompany restless leg syndrome (RLS), narcolepsy and obstructive sleep apnea. While all patients with PLMD and most patients with RLS have periodic limb movements on a sleep study only the RLS patients have the daytime annoying sensations in their limbs that improve with movement. Use of caffeine, neuroleptics, alcohol, monoamine oxidase inhibitors or tricyclic antidepressants can cause periodic limb movements. Withdrawal of benzodiazepines, barbiturates and certain hypnotics can also cause or aggravate periodic limb movements. Periodic limb movements are reportedly rare in children but increases in prevalence with age.

There are several conditions that mimic periodic limb movements. Sleep starts or hypnic jerks are frequently mentioned by patients. These occur in drowsiness, may be associated with a feeling of falling and do not recur repetitively during sleep. Seizures can cause nighttime kicking movements but may also cause nocturnal enuresis, morning musculoskeletal soreness, or bleeding from oral laceration. An expanded additional 16 lead EEG on the polysomnogram is invaluable in identifying these patients.

Treatment

There are no FDA approved treatments for PLMD in children. Limiting the consumption of caffeine can improve or completely control periodic limb movements. Limiting the use of other aggravating substances and medications is also important. Adequate treatment of underlying sleep disorders including obstructive sleep apnea and RLS can improve the limb movements.

Rhythmic Movement Disorder

Clinical Features

Rhythmic movement disorder (RMD) "comprises a group of stereotyped, repetitive movements involving large muscles, usually of the head and neck; the movements typically occur immediately prior to sleep onset and are sustained into light sleep" (ICSD [16]). This can be manifest as repetitive head banging, leg banging or body rolling. The movements typically begin during drowsiness. Movements typically occur with a frequency of 0.5 to 2 times per second.

While this is very common in normal infants, it is sometimes associated with a static encephalopathy, autism or psychopathology in older children and adults. It appears to be more common in males. The movements are thought to have a self-soothing effect for some individuals. The noise from the movements can be disturbing to family members. While injuries, even serious injury such as subdural hematoma, are possible, they are not common. It is very important to have the technologist accurately document what was seen at the time this occurs in the sleep laboratory. Continuous video monitoring usually easily confirms the diagnosis.

The differential includes nocturnal seizures, masturbation, bruxism, and periodic limb movement disorder. Bruxism and PLMD are usually easily distinguished on the sleep study. Gasping respirations from sleep apnea can cause rhythmic movements.

Treatment

The primary treatment is to ensure the safety of the patient. The family should be counseled about the diagnosis.

Nocturnal Bruxism

Clinical Features

Nocturnal bruxism is "a stereotypical movement disorder characterized by grinding or clenching of the teeth during sleep" (ICSD [16]). This often leads to abnormal destruction of the surface of teeth which may first be noticed by a dentist. It often causes headaches or jaw and facial pain. Its prevalence has been estimated at 5-20 percent or even higher [17]. It is relatively common in patients with a static encephalopathy [18]. It occurs equally in males and females. Most people with bruxism are of normal intelligence. While a link has been questioned with anxiety and psychosocial stress, psychological problems are not more common in patients with bruxism. There is a familial tendency toward bruxism. Temporal-mandibular joint dysfunction and malocclusion are sometimes accredited as being an underlying cause or result of bruxism. There is no guarantee that correction of these abnormalities will cure bruxism in a particular individual. It can occur in all stages of sleep and is often disturbing to family members. Rhythmic muscle artifact is usually noted on most electrodes placed on the head during polysomnography.

The only significant differential diagnosis is a seizure disorder. Seizure disorders can cause masticatory movements in some individuals. Usually, there is additional history to lead to this diagnosis.

Treatment

The primary treatment is to protect the teeth with a bite block if necessary.

REM Sleep Behavior Disorder

Clinical Features

REM sleep behavior disorder (RBD) is characterized "by the intermittent loss of REM sleep electromyographic atonia and by the appearance of elaborate motor activity associated with dream mentation" (ICSD [16]). The patient physically acts out a dream, leading to a variety of movements and actions and some episodes can be violent. It is more common in males. Although it can be seen at any age it is most prevalent in the sixth and seventh decade, occurring more frequently in patients with Parkinson's disease. REM sleep behavior disorder is uncommon in childhood but may be seen in patients with narcolepsy.

The polysomnogram shows episodes of sustained increased muscle tone in REM sleep instead of the decreased tone normally seen at this time. The polysomnogram should be preformed with continuous time-locked video. The video may show movements including punching and guttural utterances. If carefully awakened during an episode, the patient may, in some cases, recall the content of the dream and a reason for the movements can sometimes be ascertained. There is often an increase in NREM periodic limb movement index and in the REM density.

A careful general medical and neurological history is necessary. Tricyclic antidepressants and other anti-cholinergic medications may lead to RBD symptoms. There are also reports of transient RBD symptoms following hypnotic or alcohol withdrawal. The differential includes nocturnal seizures. Concomitant 16-channel EEG can be useful in this situation. Another REM related parasomnia, the nightmare, is sometimes confused with RBD. A nightmare is a frightening dream that often awakens the sleeper. Rarely, striking out can be part of a nightmare. RBD patients tend to be more explosive and usually do not awaken with the frightening aspect so common in a true nightmare. The differential also includes other NREM parasomnias including sleep walking, confusional arousals, and sleep terrors.

Sleep Terrors

Clinical Features

Sleep terrors are "characterized by a sudden arousal from slow-wave sleep with a piercing scream or cry, accompanied by autonomic and behavioral manifestations of intense fear" (ICSD [16]). Various autonomic phenomena may occur, including tachycardia, mydriasis, diaphoresis, and flushing. Patients often sit up in bed and scream inconsolably. The patient typically appears fearful and is difficult to awaken. Once awakened, the child often seems confused. While some type of dream may be recalled, it is often simple, fragmented, has no plot and usually makes no sense. The patient is amnestic for the event.

It is usually seen between ages 4 and 12 years of age, occurring in approximately 3% of children. In rare cases, sleep terrors may persist into adulthood. Like most NREM parasomnias, it usually disappears in adolescence. It is more common in males than in females. Other family members often have a history of a NREM parasomnia [19]. Sleep terrors begin in slow wave sleep, and are therefore more common in the first third of the night, but can happen anytime during the night.

The differential diagnosis is broad and includes nightmares, confusional arousals, and epileptic seizures. When people awaken from nightmares, they are usually clear of mind and often can remember a dream with some detail. While some children may remember a simple image when awakened from a sleep terror, there is no frightening story such as with a nightmare. Nightmares are more common in the last third of the night where REM sleep is more prevalent. Nightmares typically have less associated autonomic phenomena than do sleep terrors. If there is a partial arousal during slow wave sleep the person often seems stuck in a confused state without the fear seen in sleep terrors. This is called a confusional arousal. These people also do not have the autonomic phenomena represented in sleep terrors. Epileptic seizures can present with a cry and the patient can be confused afterward. Ictal fear can be seen in certain epileptic syndromes. Most epileptics do not have seizures solely in sleep. Focal dystonic posturing or tonic-clonic activity points to a seizure as the likely diagnosis. In some cases, continuous video-EEG monitoring is needed to distinguish a night terror from a nocturnal seizure.

Treatment

The primary treatment is to ensure the safety of the patient. The family should be counseled about the diagnosis.

Confusional Arousals

Clinical Features

Confusional arousals "consist of confusion during and following arousals from sleep, usually from deep sleep in the first part of the night" (ICSD [16]). Patients may not respond at all or when they do, the response is inappropriate and they are usually amnestic for the event. Confusional arousals usually arise in the first third of the night from slow wave sleep (Fig. **1**). They are sometimes associated with incontinence. Typical of most NREM parasomnias, confusional arousals are common in young children and usually disappear with adolescence. While usually seen in children, it can be seen in adults when there is interference with awakening. Examples include sleep deprivation, metabolic encephalopathies, and use of medications that suppress the central nervous system. It is seen equally in both sexes. There is a familial predisposition to NREM parasomnias in general.

The differential includes sleep terrors, sleepwalking and nocturnal seizures. Sleep terrors are associated with a frightful scream and more autonomic phenomena as described above. Sleepwalking is very similar to confusional arousals except that patients get up and walk with sleep walking. Most epileptics with nocturnal seizures also have diurnal seizures. Video-EEG monitoring may be necessary to distinguish nocturnal seizures from parasomnias.

Treatment

Reassurance for the patient and the patient's family is the most important component of care. In rare cases pharmacotherapy may be necessary. It was recommended that children with confusional arousals and sleeping walking may be safer not using a bunk bed.

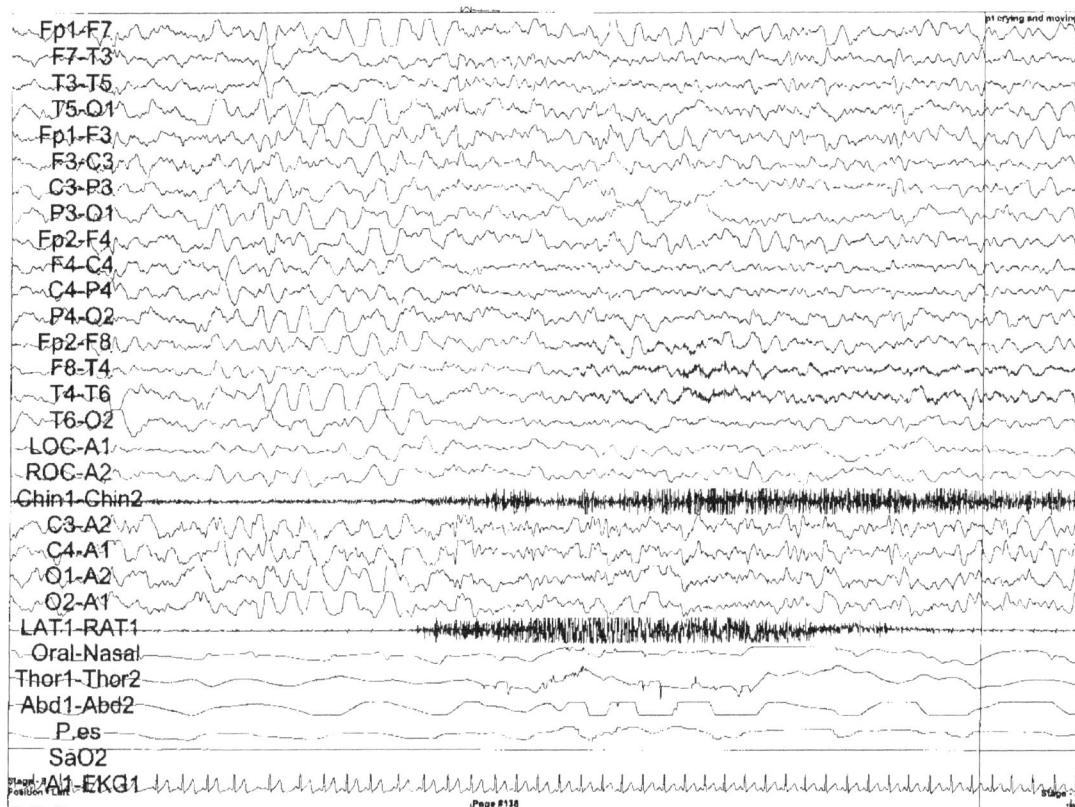

Figure 1: Polysomnogram: Expanded EEG montage with esophageal manometry pressure monitoring; 30-second page. Eight year old boy with confusional arousals. Staging: Stage 3 to stage 4 sleep. Following the arousal, the EEG shows continued delta activity intermixed with faster frequencies, associated with moving and crying. The observed behavior was typical of a confusional arousal. In the 5 to 6 seconds preceding the arousal, the EEG shows delta activity that is more rhythmic and synchronous than the delta activity with usually occurs in slow-wave sleep. Rhythmic, synchronous delta activity sometimes precedes or accompanies arousals from slow-wave sleep in patients with arousal disorders. (Used by permission, "Atlas of Polysomnography", 2nd Edition Eds. J. Geyer MD, T. Payne MD, P. Carney MD Lippincott Williams & Wilkins, 2010) [39].

Nocturnal Epilepsy

Clinical Features

Epilepsy is "a disorder characterized by an intermittent, sudden discharge of cerebral neuronal activity" (ICSD [16]). Almost any seizure type can occur during sleep [20]. In some epileptic syndromes, the seizures occur primarily during sleep (e.g. benign epilepsy with central-temporal spikes or Rolandic epilepsy and nocturnal frontal lobe epilepsy). The manifestation of the seizure depends on its neuroanatomic origin. Generalized tonic-clonic seizures are associated with loss of awareness, tonic flexion and then extension, a forced expiratory "cry", and then clonic rhythmic jerking of the extremities. Focal (partial) seizures may or may not be associated with alteration of consciousness but are associated with unilateral sensory or motor phenomena. Automatisms consisting of repetitive picking movements or lip smacking may be seen. Some partial seizures can secondarily generalize. Sleep deprivation, noncompliance with anti-epileptic medication, fever and alcohol can contribute to breakthrough seizures. Epilepsy can be idiopathic or symptomatic of an underlying discernable brain lesion. The lesions could be a tumor, stroke, brain dysgenesis, hippocampal sclerosis or due to post-traumatic changes. The EEG may show generalized, bilateral synchronous spike and wave activity or generalized polyspike activity in patients with generalized seizures. The EEG often shows focal, regional epileptiform activity including spikes or sharp waves and focal slowing of background activity in patients with focal (partial) seizures. Focal epileptiform activity is more common in NREM sleep and suppressed in REM sleep. Epileptiform activity is much more common in sleep than wakefulness in children with Rolandic epilepsy. A diurnal EEG may be all

330 *Contemporary Sleep Medicine for Physicians*

that is needed to confirm the diagnosis. An EEG after sleep deprivation or overnight continuous video-EEG may be needed in more complicated cases. Sleep deprivation from other sleep disorders such as sleep apnea has been shown to worsen seizures in some patients.

The differential includes nocturnal paroxysmal dystonia, sleepwalking, rhythmic movement disorder and REM behavior disorder. Nocturnal paroxysmal dystonia occurs in a short form (15-60 seconds) and a longer form (up to 60 minutes). It is characterized by repeated stereotypical dyskinetic episodes of ballismus or choreoathetosis often associated with vocalizations in NREM sleep [21]. Sleepwalking, rhythmic movement disorder and REM behavior disorder are not associated with epileptiform activity.

Table 1: Main parasomnias (sleep terror vs. nightmares) and differentiating characteristics

	Sleep Terror	**Nightmare**
Prevalence	Uncommon	Common
Sleep stage	SWS	REM
Onset	First 90 minutes of sleep	Second half of night
Features	Intense; vocalization, fear, motor activity	Less intense; vocalization, fear, motor activity
Mental content	Sparse	Elaborate
Violent behavior	Common	None
Injury	More likely	Unlikely
Amnesia	Often	Rare
Ability to arouse	Difficult	Easy
On awakening	Confused	Oriented

Table 2: Other parasomnias (confusional arousals vs. sleep walking vs. REM Sleep Behavior Disorder) and main differentiating characteristics

	Confusional Arousals	**Sleep Walking**	**REM Sleep Behavior Disorder**
Prevalence	Uncommon	Common	0.5%. More common in Parkinson's, MSA
Sleep stage	SWS	SWS	REM
Onset, typically	First 1/3 of the night	First 1/3 of the night	Last 1/3 of the night
Features	Complex behavior. Slow confused speech.	Complex behaviors not limited to walking.	Acting out dreams. May be violent. Increased EMG tone.
Violent behavior	Occasional	Rare	Frequent
Injury	Rare	Rare	Occasional
Treatment	Benzodiazepines	Benzodiazepines. TCA's.	Clonazepam. Carbamazepine.

Tables adapted from "Neurology for the Boards", 3rd Edition Eds. JD Geyer, J Keating, PR Carney, Lippincott Williams & Wilkins, (2006).

DISORDERS OF EXCESSIVE DAYTIME SLEEPINESS

Narcolepsy

Clinical Features

Narcolepsy is a disorder of excessive sleepiness with a loss of control of the boundaries between sleep and wakefulness. The classic tetrad of symptoms defining narcolepsy includes 1) excessive daytime sleepiness, 2) cataplexy, 3) sleep paralysis, and 4) hypnapompic or hypnagogic hallucinations [16]. Most patients will display only some of these symptoms, while a minority of patients, between 10% and 15%, will actually have the entire tetrad of symptoms. Excessive sleepiness is the most common symptom (present in almost 100% of cases). Sleep attacks, sudden and unpredictable episodes of severe sleepiness or sleep, are less common but can result in serious accidents and injury.

Diagnostic Criteria:

- excessive daytime sleepiness
- cataplexy
- sleep paralysis
- hypnapompic or hypnagogic hallucinations
- fragmented sleep

Epidemiology

Narcolepsy occurs in approximately 1 in 2000 persons and peaks in the second decade of life. Subtle symptoms may be present much earlier. Parents often refer the child with narcolepsy as having been a "sleepy head" as a young child. There is no significant gender difference for narcolepsy but there is a significant ethnic difference with the disorder occurring much more frequently in Japan. Monozygotic twins are discordant for narcolepsy. Eighty-six percent of narcoleptics with definite cataplexy have HLA DQB1-0602 on chromosome 6, but greater than 99% of patients with these haplotypes do not have narcolepsy. Orexin or hypocretin may also be involved in narcolepsy [22].

Treatment

Several treatment options are available but are not FDA approved for use in the child. Treatment of the excessive sleepiness is vital to improve daytime function and school performance. Modafinil (Provigil[+] or Nuvigil[+]) is a pro-alerting drug that can dramatically improve daytime sleepiness. If modafinil proves ineffective, traditional stimulants such as methylphenidate, and dextroamphetamine may also be of benefit. Sodium oxybate (Xyrem[+]) may also be an option for the sleepiness, especially when there is concomitant cataplexy. In an off label use, tricyclic antidepressants (and by extension, serotonin and/or norepinephrine reuptake inhibitors) may also be quite effective for cataplexy.

Circadian Rhythm Sleep Disorders

For optimal sleep and alertness, desired sleep time and wake times should be synchronized with the timing of the endogenous alertness promoting circadian rhythm. Misalignment between the circadian rhythm and the 24 hour physical environment can result in symptoms of insomnia and/or excessive daytime sleepiness. Circadian rhythm sleep disorders arise when the physical environment is altered relative to the internal circadian timing system, such as in jet lag and shift work, or when the timing of endogenous circadian rhythms are altered, such as in circadian rhythm sleep phase disorders. The latter, is thought to occur predominantly because of chronic alterations in the circadian clock or its entrainment mechanisms. This section focuses on this second group of disorders, which is the most common in childhood.

The essential feature of a Circadian Rhythm Sleep Disorder (CRSD) is that the sleep disturbance is due primarily to alterations of the circadian time-keeping system or a misalignment between the endogenous circadian rhythm and exogenous factors that affect the timing or duration of sleep. The circadian related sleep disruption leads to insomnia or excessive daytime sleepiness that causes functional impairment or distress. Furthermore, maladaptive behaviors often influence the presentation and clinical course of circadian rhythm sleep disorders.

Delayed Sleep Phase Syndrome

Clinical Features

Delayed Sleep Phase Syndrome (DSPS) is characterized by bedtimes and wake times that are usually delayed 3-6 hours relative to desired or socially acceptable sleep/wake times. The patient typically cannot fall asleep before 2-6am and has difficulty waking up earlier than 10 am - 1 pm [23, 24]. In most cases, attempts to advance the patient's sleep times are unsuccessful. When allowed to follow their preferred schedule, circadian phase of sleep is delayed, but relatively stable and sleep quality is reported to be normal. Patients with DSPS often report feeling most alert in the evening and most sleepy in the early morning. They score as definite "evening" types on the Horne and Ostberg questionnaire of diurnal preference and often are described as "night" people, or "night owls" [25]. Most patients seeking treatment do so because of enforced socially acceptable bed times and wake up times result in insomnia, excessive sleepiness and functional impairments, particularly during the morning hours [23].

Clinical Epidemiology

DSPS is probably the most common of the primary circadian rhythm sleep disorders in children [26]. Although the actual prevalence of DSPS in the general population is unknown, it has been reported that among adolescents and young adults, the prevalence is 7-16% [23, 27].

Differential Diagnosis

Delayed Sleep Phase Syndrome must be distinguished from "normal" sleep patterns, particularly in adolescents and young adults who exhibit delayed schedules without impaired functioning. Social and behavioral factors play an important role in the development and maintenance of the delayed sleep patterns. Attempts to fall asleep earlier result in prolonged sleep latency and may promote as well as perpetuate features of conditioned insomnia. Exposure to bright light in the evening may promote the inability to sleep and exacerbate the delayed circadian phase. Furthermore, the role of school avoidance, social maladjustment and family dysfunction must be considered as precipitating and contributing factors, especially in adolescents. Individuals may use alcohol and excessive caffeine to cope with symptoms of insomnia and excessive sleepiness, which in turn, may exacerbate the underlying circadian rhythm sleep disorder.

A family history may be present in approximately 40% of individuals with DSPS, and the DSPS phenotype has been an autosomal dominant trait [28].

Diagnostic Evaluation

The diagnosis of DSPS depends primarily on the clinical history. However, diagnostic studies such as actigraphy and sleep diaries can be very useful to confirm the delayed sleep phase pattern. Recordings of sleep diaries and actigraphy over a period of at least 2 weeks demonstrate delayed sleep onset and sleep offset, with sleep onsets typically delayed until 2-6 AM and wake up times in the late morning or early afternoon. Daily work or school schedules may result in earlier than desired wake time during weekdays, but a delay in bedtime and wake up time is almost always seen during weekends and while on vacation. Polysomnographic (PSG) parameters of sleep architecture, when performed at the natural delayed sleep times, are essentially normal for age. However, if a conventional bedtime and wake up time is scheduled, PSG recording will show prolonged sleep latency and decreased total sleep time.

Clinical Management

Approaches aimed at resetting circadian rhythms, such as chronotherapy, timed bright light and melatonin have been employed for the treatment of DSPS. Chronotherapy is a treatment in which sleep times are progressively delayed by approximately 3 hours per day until the desired earlier bedtime schedule is achieved [29]. Although effective, the length and repeated nature of treatment and need for adherence to restrictive social and professional schedules limit practicality in the clinical setting. However, in adolescents, in which behavioral factors often contribute to the delayed sleep phase, chronotherapy in conjunction with enforcement of regular sleep and wake times are important components of the clinical management.

Exposure to bright light for 1-2 hours in the morning results in an advance of the phase of circadian rhythms, whereas evening light exposure causes phase delays. Therefore, bright light exposure during the early morning hours and avoidance of bright light in the evening have been shown to be effective treatments for DSPS [30]. Following 2 weeks of exposure to 2 hours of bright light of 2500 lux each morning and restricted evening light, individuals with DSPS showed earlier sleep times and reported improved morning alertness level. However, many patients, particularly those who are severely delayed, find it difficult to awaken earlier for the 1-2 hour of bright light therapy. Despite potential utility of bright light therapy, the timing, intensity and duration of treatment remain to be defined.

Exposure to broad spectrum light of 2,000 to 10,000 lux for approximately 1-2 hours is generally recommended for use in clinical practice.

Due to the practical limitations of chronotherapy and phototherapy, melatonin, taken orally in the evening, has been increasingly investigated as a treatment for DSPS. Several studies have demonstrated the potential benefits of melatonin administered in the evening [31]. However, because the timing of administration and dose varied between studies, and the relative lack of large scale controlled clinical trials, clinical guideline for the use of melatonin in the treatment of DSPS is not available. The treatment of DSPS with melatonin is an unapproved use and remains empirical. Treatment success depends on many variables including severity of the delayed sleep phase, co-morbid psychopathology, ability and willingness of the patient to comply with the treatment, school schedule, work obligations, and social pressures.

Advanced Sleep Phase Syndrome

Advanced Sleep Phase Syndrome (ASPS) is characterized by habitual sleep-onset and wake-up times that are several hours earlier relative to conventional and desired times (ICSD [16], [32-34]). It is rarer in children versus older adults (reason for not treating it *in extenso* in this chapter) and can be treated by phase advance chronotherapy ([32-34]).

Pediatric Obstructive Sleep Apnea

Epidemiology

Pediatric OSA occurs with a prevalence of 2-4% for children between the ages of 2 and 18 [35, 36]. Obstructive apnea is relatively uncommon in normal children. In the past obstructive sleep apnea was primarily seen in patients with significant adenotonsillar hypertrophy or neurological dysfunction [37]. More recently, obstructive sleep apnea has been associated with obesity in children.

The symptoms of obstructive sleep apnea are different in children compared to adults. Although daytime sleepiness and fatigue are reported in children, behavioral problems, hyperactivity and neurocognitive deficits are much more common in children with sleep apnea compared to normal controls or adults with obstructive sleep apnea [38].

Diagnosis

Pediatric OSA can be confirmed with overnight polysomnography. The severity of OSA has been defined by use of AHI criteria alone. This approach is, however, flawed. This problem becomes more pronounced in the pediatric population. The criteria are different than adults, with an apnea index of > 1/hr considered abnormal.

In children a cessation of airflow for two or more respiratory cycles is considered an apnea when the event is obstructive [35-39]. Of note, the respiratory rate in children (20-30/min) is greater than adults (12-15/min). The obstructive apnea hypopnea index (AHI) > 1 is considered abnormal in children as opposed to 5 in adults. There is usually only a mild decrease in the arterial oxygen saturation.

The importance of central apnea in older children is less certain than in infants. Most pediatric sleep specialists do not consider central apneas following sighs (big breaths) to be abnormal. Some central apnea is most likely normal in children especially during REM sleep. In one study, up to 30% of normal children had at least occasional central apneas. Central apneas longer than 20 seconds or those of any length associated with arterial oxygen desaturation below 90% are often considered abnormal although a few such events have been noted in normal children [38]. Therefore, in most cases, observation is recommended unless the events are frequent or the arterial oxygen desaturations severe.

There is a shortage of sleep laboratories that can accommodate children appropriately. Other potential screening techniques have not proved successful thus far. Therefore, in a child with behavioral problems, hyperactivity or daytime sleepiness, a polysomnogram should be considered especially if obesity, adenotonsillar hypertrophy or other upper airway anatomic anomalies are present.

Treatment

The treatment of choice for the majority of pediatric OSA cases is adenotonsillectomy. There are some specific groups who are at increased risk for postoperative morbidity: children < 3 years of age; severe OSA; and those with underlying medical disorders. Weight loss and nasal CPAP are also used in pediatric OSA for those cases who do not improve after adenotonsillectomy or are not surgical candidates. CPAP is used as the primary treatment modality much less frequently in children than in adults. Craniofacial surgeries are also an option in selected children with anatomic abnormalities.

RESEARCH OUTLOOK

What we don't know:

Many disorders that have been well characterized in the adult population have yet to be fully described in the pediatric population. For example, restless legs syndrome is known to occur in children but is poorly recognized. When it is identified, no FDA approved treatments are available.

The relationship between nocturnal epilepsy and the circadian cycle has been preliminarily studied but remains insufficiently studied. Carney *et al* continue to delve into this complex relationship.

For many years, surgical intervention has been the mainstay of pediatric obstructive sleep apnea treatment. With the obesity epidemic among children, these surgical options are no longer adequate for large numbers of patients. Better and more tolerable treatments must be developed.

REFERENCES

[1]   Anders TF, Halpern LF, Hua J. Sleeping through the night: a developmental perspective. Pediatrics 1992; 90: 554-60.
[2]   Beltramini AU, Hertzig ME. Sleep and bedtime behavior in preschool-aged children. Pediatrics 1983; 71: 153-8.
[3]   Dahl RE. The development and disorders of sleep. Adv Pediatr 1998; 45: 73-90.
[4]   Anders TF, Eiben LA. Pediatric sleep disorders: a review of the past 10 years. J Am Acad Child Adolesc Psychiatry 1997; 36: 9-20.
[5]   Carskadon MA. Patterns of sleep and sleepiness in adolescents. Pediatrician 1990; 17: 5-12.
[6]   Feber R. Introduction: pediatric sleep disorders medicine. In: Feber R, Kryger M, Eds. Principles and Practice of Sleep Medicine in the Child. Philedelphia 1995.
[7]   Feber R. Assessment of sleep disorders in the child. In: Feber R, Kryger M, Eds. Principles and Practice of Sleep Medicine in the Child. Philadelphia. Philadelphia 1995.
[8]   Beal VA. Termination of night feeding in infancy. J Pediatr 1969; 75: 690-2.
[9]   Zuckerman B, Stevenson J, Bailey V. Sleep problems in early childhood: continuities, predictive factors, and behavioral correlates. Pediatrics 1987; 80: 664-71.
[10] Feber R. Sleeplessness in children. In: Feber R, Kryger M, Eds. Principles and Practice of Sleep Medicine in the Child. Philadelphia: Saunders 1995.
[11] Van Tassel EB. The relative influence of child and environmental characteristics on sleep disturbances in the first and second years of life. J Dev Behav Pediatr 1985; 6: 81-6.
[12] Richman N. A community survey of characteristics of one- to two- year-olds with sleep disruptions. J Am Acad Child Psychiatry 1981; 20: 281-91.
[13] Feber R. Solve your childs sleep problem. New York: Simon & Schuster 1985.
[14] Feber R. Sleeplessness, night awakening, and night crying in the infant and toddler. Pediatr Rev 1987; 9: 69-82.
[15] Mendelson WB. Are periodic leg movements associated with clinical sleep disturbance? Sleep 1996; 19: 219-23.
[16] The International Classification of Sleep Disorders In: Rochester: 1997.
[17] Glaros AG. Incidence of diurnal and nocturnal bruxism. J Prosthet Dent 1981; 45: 545-9.
[18] Richmond G, Rugh JD, Dolfi R, Wasilewsky JW. Survey of bruxism in an institutionalized mentally retarded population. Am J Ment Defic 1984; 88: 418-21.
[19] Kales A, Soldatos CR, Bixler EO, *et al.* Hereditary factors in sleepwalking and night terrors. Br J Psychiatry 1980; 137: 111-8.
[20] Bazil CW. Sleep and epilepsy. Semin Neurol 2002; 22: 321-7.
[21] Provini F, Plazzi G, Lugaresi E. From nocturnal paroxysmal dystonia to nocturnal frontal lobe epilepsy. Clin Neurophysiol 2000; 111 (Suppl 2): S2-8.

[22]   Oka Y, Inoue Y, Kanbayashi T, *et al.* Narcolepsy without cataplexy: 2 subtypes based on CSF hypocretin-1/orexin-A findings. Sleep 2006; 29: 1439-43.

[23]   Regestein QR, Monk TH. Delayed sleep phase syndrome: a review of its clinical aspects. Am J Psychiatry 1995; 152: 602-8.

[24]   Czeisler CA, Richardson GS, Zimmerman JC, *et al.* Entrainment of human circadian rhythms by light-dark cycles: a reassessment. Photochem Photobiol 1981; 34: 239-47.

[25]   Horne JA, Ostberg O. A self-assessment questionnaire to determine morningness-eveningness in human circadian rhythms. Int J Chronobiol 1976; 4: 97-110.

[26]   Yamadera H, Takahashi K, Okawa M. A multicenter study of sleep-wake rhythm disorders: therapeutic effects of vitamin B12, bright light therapy, chronotherapy and hypnotics. Psychiatry Clin Neurosci 1996; 50: 203-9.

[27]   Pelayo R, Thorpy M, Govinski P. Prevalence of delayed sleep phase syndrome among adolescents. Sleep Res 1988; 17: 372.

[28]   Ancoli-Israel S, Schnierow B, Kelsoe J, *et al.* A pedigree of one family with delayed sleep phase syndrome. 2001; 18: 831.

[29]   Weitzman ED, Czeisler CA, Coleman RM, *et al.* Delayed sleep phase syndrome. A chronobiological disorder with sleep-onset insomnia. Arch Gen Psychiatry 1981; 38: 737-46.

[30]   Chesson AL, Jr., Anderson WM, Littner M, *et al.* Practice parameters for the nonpharmacologic treatment of chronic insomnia. An American Academy of Sleep Medicine report. Standards of Practice Committee of the American Academy of Sleep Medicine. Sleep 1999; 22: 1128-33.

[31]   James SP, Sack DA, Rosenthal NE, Mendelson WB. Melatonin administration in insomnia. Neuropsychopharmacology 1990; 3: 19-23.

[32]   Moldofsky H, Musisi S, Phillipson EA. Treatment of a case of advanced sleep phase syndrome by phase advance chronotherapy. Sleep 1986; 9: 61-5.

[33]   Schrader H, Bovim G, Sand T. The prevalence of delayed and advanced sleep phase syndromes. J Sleep Res 1993; 2: 51-55.

[34]   Reid KJ, Chang AM, Dubocovich ML, *et al.* Familial advanced sleep phase syndrome. Arch Neurol 2001; 58: 1089-94.

[35]   Redline S, Tishler PV, Schluchter M *et al.* Risk factors for sleep-disordered breathing in children. Associations with obesity, race, and respiratory problems. Am J Respir Crit Care Med 1999; 159: 1527-32.

[36]   Guilleminault C, Korobkin R, Winkle R. A review of 50 children with obstructive sleep apnea syndrome. Lung 1981; 159: 275-87.

[37]   Ali NJ, Pitson D, Stradling JR. Sleep disordered breathing: effects of adenotonsillectomy on behaviour and psychological functioning. Eur J Pediatr 1996; 155: 56-62.

[38]   Rosen CL. Clinical features of obstructive sleep apnea hypoventilation syndrome in otherwise healthy children. Pediatr Pulmonol 1999; 27: 403-9.

[39]   Geyer J, Payne T, Carney P. Atlas of Digital Polysomnography. Philadelphia: Lippincott Williams &Wilkins 2000.

Index